Introduction to

HEALTH OCCUPATIONS

TODAY'S HEALTH CARE WORKER

FIFTH EDITION

Introduction to HEALTH OCCUPATIONS

TODAY'S HEALTH CARE WORKER

Shirley A. Badasch, M. Ed, RN

Doreen S. Chesebro, B. Ed, LVN

PRENTICE HALL HEALTH
Upper Saddle River, New Jersey 07458

Library of Congress Cataloging–in–Publication Data
Badasch, Shirley A., 1934–
    Introduction to health occupations : today's health care worker /
Shirley A. Badasch, Doreen S. Cheseboro.—5th ed.
        p. cm.
    Includes bibliographical references and index.
    ISBN 0-13-013147-4
    1. Allied health personnel–Vocational guidance.
        I. Chesebro, Doreen S., 1944– . II. Title.
R697.A4B33 1999   99-38341
610.69—dc21   CIP

Publisher: *Julie Alexander*
Editor-in-Chief: *Cheryl Mehalik*
Acquisitions Editor: *Barbara Krawiec*
Managing Development Editor: *Marilyn Meserve*
Editorial Assistant: *Stephanie Camangian*
Director of Marketing: *Leslie Cavaliere*
Marketing Manager: *Tiffany Price*
Marketing Coordinator: *Cindy Frederick*
Director of Production and Manufacturing: *Bruce Johnson*
Managing Production Editor: *Pat Walsh*
Production Liaison: *Cathy O'Connell*
Production Editor: *Susan Geraghty*
Production Manager: *Ilene Sanford*
Cover Design: *Marianne Frasco*
Cover Illustration: *Timothy Cook*
Interior Design: *Amy Rosen*
Photographers: *Craig Sotres, George Dodson, Michal Heron*
Compositor: *The Clarinda Company*
Printer/Binder: *RR Donnelley and Sons, Roanoke*

Previously titled *HEALTHCARE WORKER: An Introduction to Health Occupations.*

For co-writing Chapter 19, "Medical Clerical Worker," acknowledgments go to Monica Maldonado-Puertas, Education Coordinator, Business Bristol Park Medical Group, Inc., Costa Mesa, California.
For co-writing Chapter 21, "Dental Assistant," acknowledgments go to Vivian Muensterman, Baldy View ROP.

Printed in the United States of America
10 9 8 7 6 5 4 3 2 1

ISBN 0-13-013147-4

Prentice-Hall International (UK) Limited, *London*
Prentice-Hall of Australia Pty. Limited, *Sydney*
Prentice-Hall Canada Inc., *Toronto*
Prentice-Hall Hispanoamericana, S.A., *Mexico*
Prentice-Hall of India Private Limited, *New Delhi*
Prentice-Hall of Japan, Inc., *Tokyo*
Prentice-Hall (Singapore) Pte. Ltd.
Editora Prentice-Hall do Brasil, Ltda., *Rio de Janeiro*

This revision is dedicated:
In Loving Memory of Jerry Badasch
and
To Our Children
DeeAnn, Todd Chesebro, and Candice Verhoeven
Mark Badasch, Jerry, Tim, Kevin, Shaun, Erin Gallagher, and Kelly White
Who have taught us, throughout the years, the value of education.

NOTICE

The procedures described in this textbook are based on consultation with nursing authorities. The author and publisher have taken care to make certain that these procedures reflect currently accepted clinical practice; however, they cannot be considered absolute recommendations.

The material in this textbook contains the most current information available at the time of publication. However, federal, state, and local guidelines concerning clinical practices, including without limitation, those governing infection control and standard precautions, change rapidly. The reader should note, therefore, that new regulations may require changes in some procedures.

It is the responsibility of the reader to familiarize himself or herself with the policies and procedures set by federal, state, and local agencies as well as the institution or agency where the reader is employed. The authors and the publishers of this textbook, and the supplements written to accompany it, disclaim any liability, loss, or risk resulting directly or indirectly from the suggested procedures and theory, from any undetected errors, or from the reader's misunderstanding of the text. It is the reader's responsibility to stay informed of any new changes or recommendations made by any federal, state, and local agency as well as by his or her employing health care institution or agency.

CONTENTS

Part One
Basic Knowledge and Skills

CHAPTER 1
INTRODUCTION TO BEING A HEALTH CARE
WORKER   1

CHAPTER 8
YOUR BODY AND HOW IT FUNCTIONS 146

CHAPTER 9
HUMAN GROWTH AND DEVELOPMENT 196

CHAPTER 10
NUTRITION 215

CHAPTER 11
MEASURING VITAL SIGNS 225

CHAPTER 12
CONTROLLING INFECTION 245

CHAPTER 13
PATIENT AND EMPLOYEE SAFETY   262

CHAPTER 14
EMPLOYABILITY AND LEADERSHIP   299

Part two
Multidisciplinary Skills

CHAPTER 15
NURSE ASSISTANT/PATIENT CAREGIVER   316

UNIT 2   Advanced Roles/Sub-Acute Care   410

Procedures List for Chapter 15 *(see pages xx–xxii)*.

CHAPTER 16
HOME HEALTH AIDE   417

CHAPTER 17
ELECTROCARDIOGRAM TECHNICIAN   431

CHAPTER 18
LABORATORY ASSISTANT/MEDICAL ASSISTANT LABORATORY SKILLS; PHLEBOTOMIST   446

UNIT 1   Laboratory Skills   446

UNIT 2   Phlebotomist   492

CHAPTER 22
HEALTH INFORMATION TECHNICIAN   548

CHAPTER 23
CLINICAL MEDICAL ASSISTANT   582

CHAPTER 24
DENTAL ASSISTANT   654

Procedures

Measuring Vital Signs—Chapter 11

Controlling Infection—Chapter 12

Patient and Employee Safety—Chapter 13

Nurse Assistant/Patient Caregiver—Chapter 15

Home Health Aide—Chapter 16

Electrocardiogram Technician—Chapter 17

Laboratory Assistant/Medical Assistant Laboratory Skills; Phlebotomist—Chapter 18

Physical Therapy Aide—Chapter 19

Central Supply/Central Processing Worker—Chapter 20

Environmental Services Technician/ Housekeeper—Chapter 21

Health Information Technician—Chapter 22

Clinical Medical Assistant—Chapter 23

Dental Assistant—Chapter 24

PREFACE

The increase in longevity and changes in the health care system create an increased need for educated and skilled health care workers. This need for health care workers is expected to continue its growth well into the twenty-first century. Gerontology, rehabilitation, ambulatory care, outpatient services, and managed care are expected to show the greatest growth. The occupations that service these high growth areas include: dental assistants, long-term care nursing assistants, nursing assistants with advanced skills, assistive personnel, home health care aides, medical assistants, laboratory assistants/phlebotomists, physical therapy aides, food service workers, environmental service workers, electrocardiogram technicians, and central supply/central processing workers. Demand for multidisciplinary health care workers is high due to the increasing need to provide appropriate care and customer service that meet patient/client needs and new budgetary restraints. These multiskilled workers may work under a variety of job titles ranging from Unlicensed Assistive Personnel, Assistive Caregivers to Patient Care Partners.

Because preventive health is a key component in twenty-first century health care, preventive health care and patient teaching are emphasized throughout the text. The qualities and values required to become an outstanding health care worker are also interwoven throughout the text and learning system materials. All of the information in this textbook has been carefully reviewed and updated. New areas of emphasis address the continuing changes in healthcare, such as subacute care and assistive caregiving for acute care.

A unique **learning system** divides the text into two parts. The first part, chapters one through fourteen, includes the basic information all health care workers must have to work in any department within the health care environment. The second part, Multidisciplinary Skills, chapters fifteen through twenty-four, span a variety of entry-level occupations. Students can select one occupational area or several occupational areas in Part Two, allowing them an opportunity to become a multiskilled health worker. This **learning system** also provides all areas of training required by the 1987 Omnibus Budget Reconciliation Act (OBRA), it addresses the National Standards, and allows for state differences in curriculum and JACHO Standards such as age-specific communication.

The changing requirements for health care presents educators and students alike with ever-changing challenges. *Introduction to Health Occupations, Fifth Edition*, helps meet the needs of not only the health care system, but all levels of students, from secondary and postsecondary to English as a second language (ESL) students with the following:

■ *Easy readability* meets the learning needs of all students.

■ *Margin Glossary* provides immediate feedback and understanding of vocabulary.

■ *Student Workbook* provides additional reinforcement to help in the retention of content and works in tandem with *Steps to Success* activities at the beginning of each unit to help guide students through new material.

■ *Skills Check-off Sheets* are designed for both practice and competency assessment. These check-off sheets provide step-by-step instructions to help students perform procedures correctly and competently.

■ *Portfolio Connection* helps students develop a vocational portfolio to demonstrate job or higher education readiness.

- ■ *Your Link to Success* encourages students to think critically and apply unit concepts to real life situations.
- ■ *Age-Specific Communication Skills* are addressed throughout.
- ■ *Medical Math Chapter* reviews the basic math concepts which students will need to succeed, such as multiplication, division, percentages, and fractions.
- ■ *Medical Terminology* is addressed throughout the text and workbook.
- ■ *Standard Precautions* are highlighted throughout to safeguard the health of both students and patients.

Instructors and students alike will benefit from our complete learning package that includes:

■ Instructor's Guide

Our instructor's guide is loaded with content, teaching hints, and resources to help make your job as instructor easier. It contains presentation content, suggested activities, points of interest, advance preparation hints, examples, additional discussion topics, and guidelines, as well as resources for program enhancement. These resources include transparency masters to add interest and facilitate learning, worksheet keys, evaluations with keys, and detailed activities and instructions that promote critical thinking. Additional chapters and skills are included for Radiology Aide/Darkroom Attendant, Nursing Assistant–Acute Care Specialists, Assistive Caregiver, and Food Service Worker. In addition, a Test Item File (printed test questions) is also available as part of our complete learning package.

■ Student Workbook

Our student workbook provides students with a variety of practice activities that include worksheets, scenarios, activities, and selected check-off sheets designed for both practice and competency assessment. These check-off sheets provide step-by-step instructions to help students perform procedures correctly and competently. A complete set of check-off sheets can be obtained through the Companion Website described below. All of these Workbook activities will help students successfully learn the skills required for their respective career choices.

■ Companion Website www.prenhall.com/badasch

The Companion Website, tied chapter-by-chapter to the text, gives students an on-line study guide that provides immediate feedback, guides them step-by-step through procedures with skill check-off sheets, and provides links to interesting and relevant sites on the World Wide Web. The Companion Website shell also enables instructors to create a customized syllabus and download Powerpoint slides and transparency masters.

Health care workers provide a valuable service to society. They are responsible for people of all ages and cultures who require a wide array of services. Today's health care worker must fill a variety of roles from caregiver to patient educator and beyond. *Introduction to Health Occupations, Fifth Edition,* prepares students for all these roles by providing the skills information they need to be effective health care workers.

■ 1987 OMNIBUS BUDGET RECONCILIATION ACT (OBRA)

To ensure quality care in long-term care (Skilled Nursing) facilities new guidelines were adopted by the Federal Government. These guidelines are known as OBRA. The OBRA Act of 1987 requires that individuals employed in skilled nursing facilities receive training and be evaluated on their skills. OBRA requires a minimum of 16 hours of instruction before resident contact. These are classroom hours and are identified on the following table with an asterisk.

Omnibus Budget Reconciliation Act of 1987 Requirements Health Care Worker Subject Areas That Satisfy All OBRA Requirements

1. Communication and Interpersonal Communications	Chapter 4:	Meeting Your Needs and the Needs of Others
	Unit 2:	Understanding Human Needs
	Topic:	Meeting the Needs of Co-workers and Other Staff
	Unit 3:	Cultural Competency
	Topics:	Culture and Behavior
		Gestures and Body Language
		Communicating Effectively with Other Cultures
		Folk Medicine
	Chapter 5:	Effective Communications
	Unit 1:	Interpersonal Communication for All Ages
	Topics:	Elements That Influence Your Relationships with Others
		Barriers to Communication
		Elements of Communication
		Good Listening Skills
		Verbal Communication
		Nonverbal Communication
2. Infection Control*	Chapter 12:	Controlling Infection
	Unit 1:	The Nature of Microorganisms
	Topics:	Introduction to Microorganisms
		How Microorganisms Affect the Body
		How Microorganisms Spread
		Signs and Symptoms of Infection
	Unit 2:	Asepsis
	Topics:	Standard Precautions
		Controlling the Spread of Infection
	Unit 3	Standard Precautions
	Topics:	Introduction to Standard Precautions
		Transmission-Based Precaution Rooms
3. Safety and Emergency Procedures*	Chapter 13	Patient and Employee Safety
	Unit 1:	General Safety and Injury and Illness Prevention
	Topics:	OSHA Standards
		General Safety
	Unit 2:	Patient Safety
	Topics:	Identifying the Patient
		Ambulation Devices
		Transporting Devices
		Postural Supports
		Side Rails
	Unit 3:	Disaster Preparedness
	Topics:	Disaster Plan
		Fire Causes and Prevention
	Unit 4:	Principles of Body Mechanics
	Topic:	Body Mechanics
	Unit 5:	First Aid
	Topics:	General Principles of First Aid
		Life-Threatening Situations

Omnibus Budget Reconciliation Act of 1987 Requirements Health Care Worker Subject Areas That Satisfy All OBRA Requirements (continued)

4. Promoting Residents' Independence*	Chapter 9: Unit 3: Topics:	Human Growth and Development Disabilities and Role Changes Importance of Independence Physical Disabilities Roles Changes in the Disabled
5. Respecting Resident Rights*	Chapter 3: Unit 2: Topics:	Medical Ethics and Law Legal Roles and Responsibilities of a Health Care Worker Legal Responsibilities Confidentiality
6. Basic Nursing Skills	Chapter 11: Unit 1: Unit 2: Chapter 15: Unit 1: Topics:	Measuring Vital Signs Temperature, Pulse, and Respiration Blood Pressure Abnormal signs (integrated into chapter when indicated) Nurse Assistant/Patient Caregiver Basic Care Skills/OBRA Standards/Long-Term Care Height and Weight Measuring Intake and Output Abnormal signs (integrated into chapter where appropriate)
7. Personal Care Skills	Chapter 15: Unit 1: Topics:	Nurse Assistant/Patient Caregiver Basic Care Skills/OBRA Standards/Long-Term Care Morning and Evening Care (AM and PM Care) Skin Management Oral Hygiene Offering the Urinal and/or Bedpan Movement and Ambulation of the Resident Positioning and Body Alignment Range of Motion Bathing the Resident Care of Hair and Nails Shaving the Resident Dressing and Undressing the Resident Bedmaking Feeding the Resident Incontinent Resident
8. Mental Health and Social Service Needs	Chapter 3: Unit 2: Topic: Chapter 4: Unit 2: Topics: Chapter 9: Unit 1: Topic: Unit 2: Topic: Unit 3: Topic:	Medical Ethics and Law Legal Roles and Responsibilities of a Health Care Worker Legal Responsibilities Meeting Your Needs and the Needs of Others Understanding Human Needs Meeting the Needs of Patients/Clients Defense Mechanisms Human Growth and Development Development and Behavior Development and Behavior Aging and Role Change Role Changes in the Aging Disabilities and Role Changes Importance of Independence
9. Basic Restorative Services:	Chapter 15: Topics: Chapter 19: Topics:	Nurse Assistant/Patient Caregiver Positioning and Body Alignment Range of Motion Incontinent Resident Prosthetic Devices Special Care Devices Physical Therapy Aide Guarding Techniques Rehabilitation Equipment

Health Care Core and Occupational Cluster

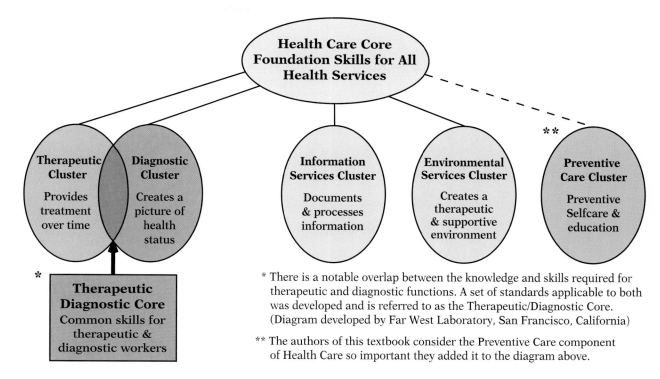

* There is a notable overlap between the knowledge and skills required for therapeutic and diagnostic functions. A set of standards applicable to both was developed and is referred to as the Therapeutic/Diagnostic Core. (Diagram developed by Far West Laboratory, San Francisco, California)

** The authors of this textbook consider the Preventive Care component of Health Care so important they added it to the diagram above.

We reviewed the National Health Care Skill Standards to guide us in determining what information meets the needs of future health care workers: "Health care skill standards are statements which answer the question, 'What does a worker need to know and be able to do to contribute to the safe and effective delivery of health care?' The standards will inform current and future health care workers, employers, and educators what skills and knowledge workers need to succeed—in a job and in a career. It is envisioned that these standards will help provide the foundation for better worker preparation, both in school and on the job" *(Quality & Excellence Health Care Skill Standards)*. We continued to ask the question: What does a worker need to know and be able to do to contribute to the safe and effective delivery of health care? When the authors ask this question about each topic in the text, it focuses the information on key material needed by an entry-level health care worker and eliminates unnecessary material.

Note: State standards/guidelines may divide the health care services differently than the National Standards. For example, Preventive Health Care may be a state cluster (see figure).

THE PARTS OF THIS BOOK

Part One of this book is the core knowledge that all health care workers must learn before entering a health care occupation. Part Two provides you with the knowledge, tasks, and skills for the health care area of your choice. The step-by-step procedures enhance the text's content and reinforce student learning. The procedures prepare you to perform the skills necessary in your chosen health career area. If you cannot complete the objectives or demonstrate the procedures successfully, you are not adequately prepared for work, internship, or the community classroom. When you successfully complete the objectives in Part One and the Objectives for the health career chosen in Part Two, you are prepared for an entry-level position in a health care setting. You may choose to complete one area and then move into another area. Many of the skills are transferable. The emphasis in the workplace today is on multidisciplinary trained workers. The more areas in which you are proficient, the more marketable you are.

■ LIST OF OCCUPATIONS IN PART TWO

- Nurse Assistant/Patient Caregiver
- Home Health Aide
- Electrocardiogram Technician
- Laboratory Assistant/Medical Assistant Laboratory Skills; Phlebotomist
- Physical Therapy Aide
- Central Supply/Central Processing Worker
- Environmental Services Technician/Housekeeper
- Health Information Technician
- Clinical Medical Assistant
- Dental Assistant

Note: Nurse Assistant—Acute Care Specialties/Assistive Personnel, Food Service Worker, and Radiology Aide/Darkroom Attendant chapters are located in the Instructor's Guide. If you are interested in one of these areas, ask your teacher for the chapter.

Start of Unit and Career Basics

STEPS TO SUCCESS

Designed to ensure your success, these exercises guide you through each unit using activities from the student workbook and end-of-chapter Links to Success. These activities can be completed independently or with instructor supervision.

INTRODUCTION TO BEING A HEALTH CARE WORKER

1

UNIT 1 History of Health Care

Steps to success

1. Complete Vocabulary Worksheet 1 in the Student Workbook.
2. Read this unit.
3. Complete Unit 1 Worksheets 2 through 6 as assigned.
4. When you are confident that you can meet each objective for this unit, ask your instructor for the unit evaluation.

Rationale

Health care has developed and changed throughout history. Knowing the history of health care helps you understand current procedures, practices, and philosophies. The experiences and discoveries of the past led to the advances of today. Today's achievements could not have occurred without the trials and errors of the past. When you understand the primitive beginnings of medicine, you appreciate the advances made during the past 5,000 years.

Objectives

When you have completed this unit, you will be able to do the following:

✓ Match vocabulary words with their correct meanings.
✓ Identify nine scientists and explain what they contributed to medicine.

era Period of time.

✓ Choose one **era** in the history of health care and write a paper to explain how health care technology changed.
✓ Discuss advances in medicine in the twentieth century.

1

UNIT 2 • Overview of Careers   41

CAREER BASICS

NURSING SERVICE WORKERS

	Education and/or Experience Required	Average Income
NURSE ASSISTANT/ GERIATRIC AIDE	✓ High school diploma or equivalent (preferred) ✓ Hospital-conducted on-the-job training ✓ Completion of an OBRA-approved nurse assistant program	✓ Annual: $12,500–20,800
UNLICENSED ASSISTIVE PERSONNEL	✓ Additional training in specialty (e.g., EKG, phlebotomy)	✓ Annual: $13,500–21,200
HOME HEALTH AIDE	✓ High school diploma or equivalent (preferred) ✓ Preservice training (40–120 hours) provided by an employing agency ✓ Completion of a vocational education program as a home health aide ✓ State certification may be required	✓ Annual: $10,900–17,200
LICENSED VOCATIONAL NURSE (LVN)/LICENSED PRACTICAL NURSE (LPN)	✓ High school diploma or equivalent ✓ Graduation from a recognized one-year program ✓ License for the state of employment	✓ Annual: $20,200–35,000
REGISTERED NURSE	✓ High school diploma or equivalent ✓ Graduation from a two-year community college ✓ Graduation from a four-year college or university ✓ Graduation from an accredited school of nursing ✓ Graduation from a diploma school (three-year hospital schools are being phased out) ✓ License for the state of employment	✓ Annual: $24,500–63,000
NURSE PRACTITIONER	✓ All requirements for becoming a registered nurse ✓ Completion of an accredited course in nurse practitioner training ✓ License for the state of employment	✓ Annual: $57,000–76,800

CAREER BASICS

What does it take to become a health care professional? Career Basics helps answer this question with an overview of the education/experience requirements for a variety of health careers from all four National Health Care Skill Standards career clusters. This book also covers skills and procedures of ten representative careers to give you a sense of what health care professionals do in the real world.

Chapter Review and Procedures

YOUR LINK TO SUCCESS

These activities will challenge you to think critically and apply chapter concepts to real life situations in areas such as medical math, computers, law and ethics, patient education, communication, cultural competency, medical terminology, and case studies.

PORTFOLIO CONNECTION

How do you plan and prepare for a career? Portfolio Connection will help you by encouraging you to create a vocational portfolio that shows your job and/or higher education readiness.

CHAPTER REVIEW **Your link to success**

Thinking Critically: Check Your Understanding

1. **Legal and Ethical** The field of medical ethics is affected by new technology every day. Explain how the legal system is involved in medical matters today. Think about recent medical cases that lawyers have tried.
2. **Cultural Competency** There are many caregivers from different cultures working in our country today. They come from all over the world. You have a co-worker who does not understand the chain of command because it is a new concept for her. Your co-worker also has difficulty understanding English. Why is it important for her to understand how the chain of command works? What can you do to help her understand?
3. **Communication** You are asked to give a talk to a class of sixth graders about the history and future of medicine. What will you tell the class about how early medical advances influenced today's medical practice? What do you think will happen in medicine in the future? How will you explain your ideas?
4. **Case Study** A new patient is telling you how upset he is about a change in his insurance. His company changed from private insurance to an HMO. The patient is very agitated and worried because the system is new to him. Why do you think the patient is so agitated? What can you do to reassure him?

Portfolio Connection

The history of medicine shows that experience, and evaluation of that experience, helps people plan and develop future health care. The same is true for you. Planning and preparing for a career is a process that allows you to look back on your experiences and learn from them. You can evaluate the things in your past that worked for you and those that did not.

You now have an opportunity to create a file that reflects what you learn. This file is called a *vocational portfolio*. Your portfolio will contain documents that show what you have learned during your vocational preparation. Your work will show the abilities and skills you gain throughout your training. You will also create a job search packet that helps you identify ways to share your portfolio with schools or potential employers. Developing your portfolio provides a chance to express the positive results of your learning experiences in a professional manner.

Think about a time when you surprised yourself by accomplishing something that you were not sure you could do. What caused you to try it when you were unsure about it? What went well in that experience? What would you do differently? Explain your answers in a short paper. Your explanation must clearly identify your self-evaluation and show how you would approach uncertain experiences in the future.

This assignment helps you review and evaluate your past experience. Some of the future assignments for your portfolio will require a similar process, with a focus on your vocational training. Turn this assignment in to your instructor. When you create your portfolio in Chapter 2 your teacher will return it to you. Put it in your portfolio in Section Four, "Written Samples."

Procedure

Denture Care

1. Wash hands.
2. Assemble equipment.
   a. Tissues
   b. Paper towel or gauze squares
   c. Mouthwash
   d. Disposable denture cup
   e. Toothbrush or denture brush
   f. Denture paste or toothpowder
   g. Towel
   h. Disposable nonsterile gloves
   ALERT: Follow Standard Precautions.
3. Identify resident.
4. Explain what you are going to do.
5. Pull privacy curtain.
6. Lower side rails.
7. Raise head of bed if allowed.
8. Place towel across resident's chest.
9. Prepare emesis basin by placing tissue or paper towel in bottom of basin.
10. Put on gloves.
11. Have resident remove his or her dentures.
12. Remove dentures if resident cannot.

Upper Denture
   a. Explain what you are going to do.
   b. Use a gauze square to grip upper denture.
   c. Place your index finger between top ridge of denture and cheek.
   d. Gently pull on denture to release suction.
   e. Remove upper denture.

Lower Denture
   a. Use a gauze square to grip lower denture.
   b. Place your index finger between lower ridge and cheek.
   c. Gently pull on denture to release suction.
   d. Remove lower denture.
13. Place dentures in lined emesis basin and take to sink or utility room.
14. Hold dentures firmly in palm of hand.
15. Put toothpowder or toothpaste on toothbrush.
16. Hold dentures under cold running water and brush dentures until clean.

17. Rinse dentures under cold running water.

18. Place in denture cup.
19. Place a solution of mouthwash and cool water in cup.
20. Help resident rinse mouth with mouthwash; if food particles are between cheek and gumline, gently swab away with gauze.
21. Have resident replace dentures.
22. Place dentures in labeled denture cup next to bed, if dentures are to be left out.
23. Rinse equipment and put away.
24. Remove gloves; dispose of in hazardous waste.
25. Wash hands.
26. Position resident.
27. Raise side rails if required.
28. Secure call bell within resident's reach.
29. Chart procedure and how it was tolerated.

Note: The resident may want to soak dentures overnight after PM care has been given. Place dentures in a solution in a denture cup and store in a safe place.

PROCEDURES

When performing procedures, it's important to do every step correctly. Brightly colored procedure boxes throughout the text clearly outline each procedure, from beginning to end, step by step. When appropriate, procedures are supported with photos and illustrations.

ACKNOWLEDGMENTS

The authors wish to express their sincere thanks to the many people who helped develop this book from the outline to the finished product.

■ To our families—a warm and loving thanks for their willingness to support us throughout this revision.

■ Richmond Ramsey for advising on the Medical Math.

■ Sister Suzanne Sassus, Vice-President, St. Joseph Health System

■ Phyllis Young-Gallagher, R.N. Neonatal and Maternity Health Specialist for Advising on Neonatal and Obstetrics/Maternal Care.

■ Gloria Bizjak for reviewing the First Aid Unit.

■ To the reviewers whose suggestions gave us fresh viewpoints on content and contributed to the overall quality of this book.

■ FOR THE FIFTH EDITION

Nancy Applewhite
Pender High School
Burgaw, NC

Julia Blair
HO Coordinator
Health Science Department
Clara Barton HS
Brooklyn, NY

Kathleen Bode
Chairman, Department of Health and
    Human Services
Flint Hills Technical College
Emporia, KS

Joanne Brogan
Nursing & Health Education
North Idaho College
Coeur D'alene, ID

Karen Cassidy
Adult Ed. Director
United Technology Center
Bangor, ME

Toni Decklkever
HO Coordinator
Cheyenne East High School
Cheyenne, WY

Dr. Sally Flesch
Professor, Department Chair of
    Allied Health
Black Hawk College
Moline, IL

Darlene Henderson
HST Instructor
Lufkin High School
Lufkin, TX

Regina Lohre
Allied Health Instructor
Washington High School
Milwaukee, WI

Rita Melton
Dean of Computer Technology Public
    Service & Health
Aiken Technical College
Aiken, SC

Julie Slack
Instructor, Health Occupations
Dixie College
St. George, UT

John Smith
Assistant Superintendent
Southeast Regional Occupational
    Program
Cerritos, CA

Tom Ward
Tacoma Baptist Schools
Tacoma, WA

■ REVIEWERS FOR PREVIOUS EDITIONS

Julie Abernathy, Instructor
Lodi Career Center—Health Career
Lodi, CA

Gloria Bizjak, Curriculum Specialist
University of Maryland
Maryland Fire & Rescue Institute
College Park, MD

Mary A. Brennan, RN, MS Ed.
Portland Arts & Technology High School
Portland, ME

Merrill Ferguson, CDA, EDOA
Instructor—Cuillier Career Center
Marreto, LA

Ruth Huff, RN
Health Occupations Teacher
High School—Oxford, NC

Lale J. Saltzgaver, RN, Ph.D., Supervisor
Learey Technical Center
Tampa, FL

Nancy G. Sochat, Health Occupations
  Coordinator
Health Professions Academy
Socorro High School
El Paso, TX

Linda T. Teague, RN
Vocational Certification
  NC State University
Enka High School
Enka, NC

Rosemarie Meyer, BSN, RN
Instructor—Lake County High Schools
Grayslake, IL

ABOUT THE AUTHORS

Shirley A. Badasch, M.Ed, RN, is a graduate of California State University at Long Beach. Her career includes acute care nursing, office nursing, industrial nursing, Director of Nursing for a developmentally disabled nursing facility, and Assistant Administrator in Long Term Care. Ms. Badasch's teaching experience includes co-developing the Medical Occupations Program and teaching for nine years in a Regional Occupation Program, and part-time instructor in the Educational Psychology department, California State University at Long Beach. She also taught in the teacher certification program at Cal Poly Pomona and California State University at Sacramento. During her career she worked as a contract consultant to the California State Department of Education, presenting seminars, writing materials, developing programs, and consulting on program development. Ms. Badasch completed her career as the Director of Education for a large medical group. She continues to research and participate in health occupations as a volunteer in her community and as a member of the California Association of Health Career Educators.

Doreen S. Chesebro, B.Ed, LVN, is a graduate of California State University at Long Beach. Her nursing career includes acute care nursing and office nursing. Ms. Chesebro's teaching experience includes co-developing and teaching the Medical Occupations Program in a Regional Occupation Program and as a part-time instructor for teacher certification at California State University at Sacramento and Cal Poly Pomona. Ms. Chesebro also served as a Program Specialist for Regional Occupation, Long Beach Unified School District. During this time she also participated as a member of several committees developing and presenting seminars for medical occupation instructors. She is currently the Director of Education for a large medical group and is active in developing integrated health education systems. Ms. Chesebro works closely with the medical staff and business staff in developing classes and materials for employees and patients.

Introduction to
HEALTH OCCUPATIONS
TODAY'S HEALTH CARE WORKER

INTRODUCTION TO BEING A HEALTH CARE WORKER

1

History of Health Care

S*teps to success*

1. Complete Vocabulary Worksheet 1 in the Student Workbook.
2. Read this unit.
3. Complete Unit 1 Worksheets 2 through 6 as assigned.
4. When you are confident that you can meet each objective for this unit, ask your instructor for the unit evaluation.

Rationale

Health care has developed and changed throughout history. Knowing the history of health care helps you understand current procedures, practices, and philosophies. The experiences and discoveries of the past led to the advances of today. Today's achievements could not have occurred without the trials and errors of the past. When you understand the primitive beginnings of medicine, you appreciate the advances made during the past 5,000 years.

Objectives

When you have completed this unit, you will be able to do the following:

✓ Match vocabulary words with their correct meanings.
✓ Identify nine scientists and explain what they contributed to medicine.

era Period of time.

✓ Choose one **era** in the history of health care and write a paper to explain how health care technology changed.
✓ Discuss advances in medicine in the twentieth century.

✓ Research and report on possible advances in medicine for the twenty-first century.

✓ Explain medical ethics and how it affects health care workers and patients/clients.*

✓ Compare health care in the past with health care in the twentieth and twenty-first centuries.

■ EARLY BEGINNINGS

predators Organisms or beings that destroy.

superstitious Trusting in magic or chance.

exorcise To force out evil spirits.

intravenously Directly into a vein.

Primitive human beings had no electricity, few tools, and poor shelter. Their time was spent protecting themselves against **predators** and finding food. They were **superstitious** and believed that illness and disease were caused by supernatural spirits. In an attempt to heal, tribal doctors performed ceremonies to **exorcise** evil spirits. They used herbs and plants as medicines. Some of the same medicines are still used today. Here are some examples:

■ Digitalis comes from the foxglove plant. Today it is given in pill form, **intravenously,** or by injection. In early times, people chewed the leaves of the foxglove plant to strengthen and slow the heartbeat.

■ Quinine comes from the bark of the cinchona tree. It controls fever, relieves muscle spasms, and helps prevent malaria.

■ Belladonna and atropine are made from the poisonous nightshade plant. They relieve muscle spasm, especially in gastrointestinal (GI) pain.

■ Morphine is made from the opium poppy. It relieves severe pain. It is addicting and is used only when nothing else will help.

■ MEDICINE IN ANCIENT TIMES

accurate Exact, correct, or precise.

The Egyptians were the earliest people to keep **accurate** health records. They were superstitious and called upon the gods to heal them. They also learned to identify certain diseases. They used medicines to heal disease and learned the art of splinting fractures.

The ancient Greeks were the first to study the causes of disease. They kept records on what they observed and what they thought caused illness. The Greeks understood the importance of searching for new information about disease. This research helped eliminate superstition.

observation Act of watching.

During ancient times, religious custom did not allow bodies to be dissected. The father of medicine, Hippocrates (ca. 469–377 B.C.), based his knowledge of anatomy and physiology on **observation** of the external body. He kept careful notes of the signs and symptoms of many diseases. With these records he found that disease was not caused by supernatural forces. Hippocrates wrote the standard of ethics called the Oath of Hippocrates. This standard is the basis for today's medical ethics. Physicians still take this oath.

The Greeks observed and measured the effects of disease. They found that some disease was caused by lack of sanitation. The Romans learned from the Greeks and developed a sanitation system. They brought clean water into their cities by way of aqueducts (waterways). They built sewers to carry off waste. They also built public baths with filtering systems. This was the beginning of public health and sanitation.

*Client is replacing the term patient in many health care areas. We will use the terms combined or interchangeably until the transition is complete.

The Romans were the first to organize medical care. They sent medical equipment and physicians with their armies to care for wounded soldiers. Roman physicians kept a room in their houses for the ill. This was the beginning of hospitals (Figure 1–1). Public buildings for the care of the sick were established. Physicians were paid by the Roman government. It is interesting to note that the Roman physician wore a death mask. This mask had a spice-filled beak, which the Romans believed protected them from infection and bad odors.

FIGURE 1–1.
Roman physician.

■ THE DARK AGES (A.D. 400–800) AND THE MIDDLE AGES (A.D. 800–1400)

When the Roman Empire was conquered by the Huns (nomads from the north), the study of medical science stopped. For a period of 1,000 years, medicine was practiced only in **convents** and **monasteries.** Because the Church believed that life and death were in God's hands, the monks and priests had no interest in how the body functioned. Medication consisted of herbal mixtures, and care was **custodial.** Monks collected and translated the writings of the Greek and Roman physicians.

convents An establishment of nuns.

monasteries Homes for men following religious standards.

custodial Marked by watching and protecting rather than seeking to cure.

Terrible epidemics caused millions of deaths during this period. Bubonic plague (the black death) alone killed 60 million people. Other uncontrolled diseases included smallpox, diphtheria, syphilis, and tuberculosis. Today, these illnesses are not always life threatening. Scientists have discovered vaccines and medications to control these diseases. It is important to remember that some diseases can become epidemic if people are not vaccinated.

■ THE RENAISSANCE (A.D. 1350–1650)

The Renaissance period saw the rebirth of learning. During this period, new scientific progress began. There were many developments during this period:

■ The building of universities and medical schools for research
■ The search for new ideas about disease rather than the unquestioning acceptance of disease as the will of God
■ The acceptance of **dissection** of the body for study
■ The development of the printing press and the publishing of books, allowing greater access to knowledge from research

dissection Act or process of dividing, taking apart.

These changes influenced the future of medical science.

■ THE SIXTEENTH AND SEVENTEENTH CENTURIES

The desire for learning that began during the Renaissance continued through the next two centuries. During this time, several outstanding scientists added new knowledge. Here are some examples:

■ Leonardo da Vinci studied and recorded the anatomy of the body (Figure 1–2).
■ William Harvey used this knowledge to understand physiology, and he was able to describe the circulation of blood and the pumping of the heart.

FIGURE 1–2.
Human body as depicted by Leonardo da Vinci. (Courtesy of Galleria Dell' Accademia.)

- Gabriele Fallopius discovered the fallopian tubes of the female anatomy.
- Bartolommeo Eustachio discovered the tube leading from the ear to the throat (eustachian tube).
- Antonie van Leeuwenhoek invented the microscope, establishing that there is life smaller than the eye can see. Van Leeuwenhoek scraped his teeth and observed the bacteria that cause tooth decay. Although it was not yet realized, the germs that cause disease were now visible.

quackery Practice of pretending to cure diseases.

Unfortunately **quackery,** mass death from childbed fever, and disease continued. The causes of infection and disease were still not understood.

THE EIGHTEENTH CENTURY

Many discoveries were made in the eighteenth century that required a new way of teaching medicine. Students not only attended lectures in the classroom and laboratory, but also observed patients at the bedside. When a patient died, they dissected the body and were able to observe the disease process. This led to a better understanding of the causes of illness and death. The study of physiology continued, and more new discoveries were made:

stethoscope Instrument used to hear sound in the body (e.g., heartbeat, lung sounds, bowel sounds).

- René Laënnec invented the **stethoscope.** The first stethoscope was made of wood. It increased the ability to hear the heart and lungs, allowing doctors to determine if disease was present.
- Joseph Priestley discovered the element oxygen. He also observed that plants refresh air that has lost its oxygen, making it usable for respiration.
- Benjamin Franklin's discoveries affect us in many ways. His discoveries include bifocals, and he found that colds could be passed from person to person.
- Edward Jenner discovered a method of vaccination for smallpox. Smallpox killed many people in epidemics. His discovery saved millions of lives. His discovery also led to immunization and to preventive medicine in public health.

THE NINETEENTH AND TWENTIETH CENTURIES

Medicine continued to progress rapidly, and the nineteenth century was the beginning of the organized advancement of medical science. Important events during the nineteenth and twentieth centuries include the following:

- Ignaz Semmelweis identified the cause of childbed fever (puerperal fever). Large numbers of women died from this fever after giving birth. Semmelweis noted that the patients of midwives (women who delivered babies but were not physicians) had fewer deaths. One of the differences in the care given by the physicians and the midwives was that the physicians went to the "dead room," where they dissected dead bodies. These physicians did not wash their hands or change their aprons before they delivered babies. Their hands were dirty, and they infected the women. Semmelweis realized what was happening, but other physicians laughed at him. Eventually, his studies were proved correct by others, and handwashing and cleanliness became an accepted practice. Today, handwashing is still one of the most important ways that we control the spread of infection.

■ Louis Pasteur discovered that tiny **microorganisms** were everywhere. Through his experiments and studies, he proved that microorganisms cause disease. Before this discovery, doctors thought that microorganisms were *created by* disease. He also discovered that heating milk prevented the growth of bacteria. Pasteurization kills bacteria in milk. We still use this method to treat milk today.

■ Joseph Lister learned about Pasteur's discovery that microorganisms cause infection. He used carbolic acid on wounds to kill germs that cause infection. He became the first doctor to use an **antiseptic** during surgery. Using an antiseptic during surgery helped prevent infection in the incision.

■ Ernst von Bergmann developed **asepsis.** He knew from Lister's and Pasteur's research that germs caused infections in wounds. He developed a method to keep an area germ-free before and during surgery. This was the beginning of asepsis.

■ Robert Koch discovered many disease-causing organisms. He is considered the father of microbiology. He also introduced the importance of cleanliness and sanitation in preventing the spread of disease.

■ Wilhelm Roentgen discovered x-rays in 1895. This discovery allowed doctors to see inside the body and helped them discover what was wrong with the patient.

■ Paul Ehrlich discovered the effect of medicine on disease-causing microorganisms. His treatment was effective against some microorganisms but was not effective in killing other bacteria. His discoveries brought about the use of chemicals to fight disease. In his search to find a chemical to treat syphilis, he completed 606 experiments. On the 606th experiment, he found a treatment that worked.

Before the nineteenth century, pain was a serious problem. Surgery was performed on patients without **anesthesia.** Early physicians used herbs, hashish, and alcohol to help relieve the pain of surgery. They even choked patients to cause unconsciousness to stop pain. Many patients died from shock and pain. During the nineteenth and twentieth centuries, nitrous oxide (for dental care), ether, and chloroform were discovered. These drugs have the ability to put people into a deep sleep so that they do not experience pain during surgery. The knowledge of asepsis and the ability to prevent pain during surgery are the basis of safe, painless surgery today.

Scientists and physicians learn from the discoveries of the past. They continue to study and research new ways to treat diseases, illness, and injury. Some of the most important discoveries in recent times include the following:

■ Gerhard Domagk discovered sulfonamide compounds. These compounds were the first medications effective in killing bacteria. They changed the practice of medicine by killing deadly diseases.

■ In 1892 in Russia, Dmitri Ivanovski discovered that some diseases are caused by microorganisms that cannot be seen with a microscope. They are called *viruses.* These viruses were not studied until the electron microscope was invented in Germany. These are some of the diseases caused by viruses:

• Poliomyelitis • Rabies • Measles • Influenza • Chicken pox • German measles • Herpes zoster • Mumps

■ Sigmund Freud (Figure 1–3) discovered the conscious and unconscious parts of the mind. He studied the effects of the unconscious mind on the body. He determined that the mind and body work together. This led to an understanding of psychosomatic illness (physical illness caused by emotional conflict). His studies were the basis of psychology and psychiatry.

microorganisms Organisms so small that they can only be seen through a microscope.

antiseptic Substance that slows or stops the growth of microorganisms.

asepsis Sterile condition, free from all germs.

anesthesia Loss of feeling or sensation.

FIGURE 1–3.
Sigmund Freud.

■ Alexander Fleming found that penicillin killed life-threatening bacteria. The discovery of penicillin is considered one of the most important discoveries of the twentieth century. Before penicillin was discovered, people died of illnesses that we consider curable today, including pneumonia, gonorrhea, and blood poisoning.

■ Jonas Salk discovered that a dead polio virus would cause immunity to poliomyelitis. This virus paralyzed thousands of adults and children every year. It seemed to attack the most active and athletic people. It was a feared disease, and the discovery of the vaccine saved many people from death or crippling.

■ In contrast to Salk's virus, Albert Sabin used a live polio virus vaccine, which is more effective. This vaccine is used today to immunize babies against this dreaded disease.

The discovery of methods to control whooping cough, diphtheria, measles, tetanus, and smallpox saved many lives. These diseases kill unprotected children and adults. It is important for everyone to be immunized. Immunizations are available from doctors, clinics, hospitals, and public health services.

Our society is discovering new approaches to medical care every year. Patients/clients are being taught more about wellness, and they are learning more about self-care. Family and friends are learning patient care skills, including how to perform detailed procedures. Nurses and technicians are visiting patients/clients at home or caring for them in an ambulatory care setting. Just a few years ago, patients were admitted to the hospital for surgery and recovered in the hospital over a period of several days. Today, many patients enter the hospital, have surgery, and are sent home the same day.

People are living longer and are usually healthier. New inventions and procedures have changed medicine as we once knew it. Here are some examples:

■ The possibility of eliminating disabling disease through genetic research

recipient One who receives.

■ The ability to transplant organs from a donor to a **recipient**

■ The ability to reattach severed body parts

■ The use of computers to aid in diagnosis, accurate record keeping, and research

noninvasive Not involving penetration of the skin.

■ The ability to use **noninvasive** techniques for diagnosis

■ The advancement in caring for the unborn fetus

■ The rediscovery of acupuncture, acupressure, herbal therapy, and healing touch

geriatric Pertaining to old age.

Every day, science makes new progress. We are living in a time of great advancement and new understanding in medicine. People are living longer, creating a need to better understand **geriatric** medicine. Frontiers in medical science include cancer, AIDS, multiple sclerosis, arthritis, and muscular dystrophy.

■ THE ADVANCEMENT OF NURSING

In the nineteenth century, nursing became an important part of medical care. In 1860, Florence Nightingale (1820–1910) attracted well-educated, dedicated women to the Nightingale School of Nursing. The graduates from this school raised the standards of nursing, and nursing became a respectable profession. Before this time, nursing was considered unsuitable for a respectable lady. The people giving care to patients were among the lowest in society—"too old, too weak, too drunken, too dirty, or too bad to do anything else."

Florence Nightingale came from a cultured, middle-class family who opposed her interest in caring for the ill. However, she convinced her father to give her money to live, and she gained experience by volunteering in hospitals. During the Crimean War, she took a group of 38 women to care for soldiers dying from cholera. More soldiers were dying from cholera than from war injuries. She became a legend while she was there because of her dedication to nursing. After the war she devoted much of her life to preparing reports on the need for better sanitation and construction and management of hospitals. Her primary goal was to gain effective training for nurses. The public established a Nightingale fund to pay for the training, protection, and living costs of nurses. This was established in recognition of her services to the military during the Crimean War. She also designed a hospital ward that improved the environment and care of the patients. Prior to this time, patients were crowded into small areas that were often dirty. The ward that she designed allowed for a limited number of beds, permitted circulation of air, had windows on three sides, and was clean.

During this time, Clara Barton (1821–1912) served as a volunteer nurse in the American Civil War. After the war, she established a bureau of records to help search for missing men. She also assisted in the organization of military hospitals in Europe during the Franco-Prussian War. These experiences led her to establish the American Red Cross.

Another step forward in the field of nursing was contributed by Lillian Wald (1867–1940). She was an American public health nurse and social reformer. She established the Henry Street Settlement in New York to bring nursing care into the homes of the poor. This led to the Visiting Nurse Service of New York. Today, visiting nurse services are found in most communities.

■ PATIENT CARE TODAY

Nursing care has changed many times throughout the years. Patients have been cared for by teams that included a registered nurse as team leader, a licensed vocational nurse or practical nurse (LVN/LPN) as a medication nurse, and a nursing assistant who provided personal care. In primary care nursing, which followed team nursing, all patient care was provided by a registered nurse. Today, unlicensed assistive caregivers are part of the patient caregiver team. There are many titles and new job descriptions for these positions, including clinical partner, service partner, nurse extender, health care assistant, and patient care assistant. These new positions extend the role of entry-level employees. The nurse assistant performs additional tasks, such as phlebotomy and recording an electrocardiogram (EKG). Employees from departments other than nursing learn patient care skills. Environmental service workers and food service workers may help with serving food and providing some routine patient care. The registered nurse delegates patient care tasks according to the training and expertise of the assistive personnel.

■ A LOOK BACK AND AN OVERVIEW OF THE FUTURE

In the twentieth century, medicine is making great strides in improving health care. During this century, we experienced many changes, including these:

■ Antibiotics for bacterial diseases
■ Improved life expectancy
■ Organ transplants

■ Healthier hearts (reduced smoking, better diets)
■ Dentistry without pain
■ Childhood immunizations
■ Noninvasive diagnosis with computers (CAT, MRI)
■ End of smallpox
■ Childhood immunizations
■ New understanding of DNA and genetics
■ Control of diabetes
■ Decline in polio

The future of medicine holds many promises for better health. Current and future research will provide us with many new advances, including these:

■ Cure for AIDS
■ Decrease in the cases of malaria, influenza, leprosy, and African sleeping sickness
■ Cure for genetically transferred diseases (e.g., Tay-Sachs, muscular dystrophy, multiple sclerosis, cerebral palsy, Alzheimer's, lupus)
■ Improved treatment for arthritis and the common cold
■ Isolation of the gene that causes depression
■ Use of electronics to allow the disabled to walk
■ Nutritional therapy to decrease the number of cases of schizophrenia

■ MEDICAL ETHICS

Advancement in medicine creates new problems. How will the recipient of an organ be chosen? Who will be allowed to receive experimental drugs? How will the creation of in vitro embryos be ethically managed? Is it ethical to provide continuing confidentiality about AIDS patients, or should they be required to report their condition? Does a terminally ill patient have the right to assisted death (euthanasia)? There are many questions now, and there will be more questions in the future as health care changes.

■ SUMMARY

You have learned that the science of health care has grown and developed over the last 5,000 years. These changes increased the average life expectancy. Our standards of living improved with the progress of medical science. The dedication of the many scientists discussed in this unit is responsible for the improvements in health care that we enjoy today. Their research is the foundation of the high technology that is developing in medicine.

UNIT 2 Health Care Providers

Steps to success

1. Complete Vocabulary Worksheet 1 before beginning the reading.
2. Read this unit.
3. Complete Unit 2 Worksheets 2 through 5 as assigned.
4. When you are confident that you can meet each objective for this unit, ask your instructor for the unit evaluation.
5. Complete "Your Link to Success" at the end of this chapter.

Rationale

It is the responsibility of every health care worker to help patients/clients solve their health problems. Since the health care industry has many delivery systems, it is important for future health care workers to be aware of health care agencies and **facilities,** their delivery systems, their organization, and some of their major services. When you understand how health care facilities and agencies serve the public, you will become a resource person for members of your community.

facilities Places designed or built to serve a special function (e.g., hospital, clinic, doctor's office).

Objectives

When you have completed this unit, you will be able to do the following:

✓ Match vocabulary words with their correct meanings.
✓ Write a report on a volunteer agency.
✓ Define *managed care.*
✓ Define *ambulatory care.*
✓ Evaluate how managed care and ambulatory care meet the needs of the changing health care system.
✓ List six types of outpatient care and the type of treatment given.
✓ Define *wellness* and *preventive care.*
✓ Contrast the current trends with health care in the twentieth century.
✓ Fill in an organizational chart.
✓ Give two reasons why the organization of health care facilities is important.
✓ Explain a chain of command.
✓ List and define the major services in health care.
✓ Identify two departments in each major service.

■ TYPES OF HEALTH CARE PROVIDERS

There are several facilities and agencies that provide medical care. Some are familiar, and others will be new to you. The following descriptions will help you understand the differences among the many providers of medical care.

diagnostic Pertaining to the determination of the nature of a disease or injury by examining (e.g., using x-ray and laboratory tests).

surgical Repairing or removing a body part by cutting.

chronic Continuing over many years or for a long time (e.g., chronic illness).

tuberculosis Disease caused by Tubercle bacilli; may cause death if untreated.

psychiatric Pertaining to the mind.

specialties Fields of study or professional work (e.g., pediatrics, orthopedics, obstetrics).

hydrotherapy Treatment that uses water therapy for disease or injury.

prosthetics Artificial parts made for the body (e.g., teeth, feet, legs, arms, hands, eyes, breasts).

outpatients Patients/clients who do not require hospitalization but are under a physician's care.

immunizations Substances given to make disease organisms harmless to the patient; may be given orally or by injection (e.g., tetanus, polio).

rehabilitation Process that helps people who have been disabled by sickness or injury to recover as many of their original abilities for activities of daily living as possible.

General hospitals are facilities where patients are hospitalized for a short time, a few days to a few weeks. They provide a wide range of **diagnostic,** medical, **surgical,** and emergency care services.

Specialty hospitals provide care for specific illnesses, such as **chronic** diseases, **tuberculosis,** and **psychiatric** problems. Patients/clients in these hospitals are generally hospitalized for a long time.

Convalescent care (e.g., nursing home, long-term care) facilities generally care for elderly people needing nursing services and personal care. They also care for physically ill or injured people of all ages who require an extended convalescence for recovery.

Ambulatory care/clinics are facilities where several physicians with different **specialties** combine their practices. This allows the patient/client to have immediate care for many different illnesses.

Physician and dental facilities provide care that promotes wellness and diagnosis of illness. Simple surgery, bone setting, counseling, and administration of drugs also take place here. Physicians and dentists may choose to provide care in an ambulatory care setting.

Rehabilitation centers provide care for patients/clients who require physical therapy, **hydrotherapy,** and other therapies for loss of limb or organ function. They may receive **prosthetics** and learn how to use adaptive devices. Patients may stay in the center or be treated as **outpatients.**

Health maintenance organizations stress wellness (preventive health care). This avoids unnecessary hospitalization and other unnecessary major medical expenses. They provide health services that include hospitalization, basic medical services, **immunizations,** and basic checkups.

Home health care agencies provide care in the home for patients/clients who need health services but not hospitalization. Services include nursing, physical therapy, personal care (bathing, dressing, etc.), and homemaking (e.g., housecleaning, food shopping, and cooking). Home health care workers provide care for all ages, from infants to the elderly.

Senior day care provides care for those elderly people who are able to live at home with their families but need care when the family is away. These centers provide a place where the elderly can be cared for during the day. They provide activities, **rehabilitation,** and contact with other people. The elderly are given their medications and are aided in mobility.

The *World Health Organization* is a special agency of the United Nations founded in 1948. It is concerned with world health problems and publishes health information, compiles statistics, and investigates serious health problems worldwide.

Hospices are important in our health care system. They are discussed in this book on page 211.

■ GOVERNMENT AGENCIES

The federal, state, and local governments provide health services. These services are funded by taxes. They are responsible for giving direct health care, safeguarding our food and water supplies, and promoting health education.

Veterans Administration hospitals are federally supported and provide care for veterans who served in the armed forces.

The *U.S. Public Health Department* is a federal agency that has six major responsibilities:

■ Performing research on diseases that kill, handicap, or cripple

■ Preventing and treating alcohol and drug abuse

■ Preventing and controlling diseases that are transmitted by insects, animals, air, water, and people

■ Checking the safety of food and drugs that consumers purchase

■ Planning more effective ways to deliver health services

■ Making quality care available and affordable by encouraging health personnel to work in underserved areas

State psychiatric hospitals serve the mentally ill.

State university medical centers provide training for health workers, give medical care, and conduct medical research.

State public health services provide health education materials. They are responsible for water and food purity, **communicable** disease control, alcohol and drug abuse control, **maternal** health, and **licensing** of various health agencies.

County hospitals provide care for the ill and injured, especially those patients/clients who require financial help in order to receive care.

Local *public health departments* provide services to local communities—focusing on the reporting of communicable diseases, public health nursing, health education, **environmental sanitation,** and maternal and child health services.

Senior centers have clinics that provide special services for geriatric patients (e.g., podiatry clinic, hypertension clinic, general medical care).

■ VOLUNTEER AGENCIES

Volunteer organizations receive support from donations, gifts, membership fees, fund-raisers, and **endowments.** They are not supported by the government, and many of the people who work for them are not paid. They raise funds for medical research and for public education about various health problems. Some well-known agencies include these:

■ American Cancer Society

■ March of Dimes

■ American Red Cross

■ American Heart Association

■ American Diabetes Association

■ National Association of Mental Health

All of these agencies and facilities help bring good health to individuals and communities.

■ MANAGED CARE: QUALITY CARE AND MANAGED COSTS

The managed care provider's goals are to give quality care at reasonable costs. Policies help **assure** quality care at minimal cost. Some of these policies are discussed here.

Preventive care, such as routine physicals, well-baby care, immunizations, and wellness education, helps keep patients healthy. Wellness education stresses the

communicable Capable of passing directly or indirectly from one person or thing to another.

maternal Relating to the mother or from the mother.

licensing Giving an agency or person permission to carry on certain activities and telling what they may not do as well as what they are authorized to do.

environmental sanitation Methods used to keep the environment clean and to promote health.

endowments Gifts of property or money given to a group or organization.

assure To guarantee; to promise positively.

importance of good nutrition, weight control, exercise, and healthy living practices. Health education programs, wellness centers, weight-control programs, fitness centers, health food distributors, and health care organizations all promote wellness and preventive care. Being healthy helps prevent serious illness and lowers medical costs.

Primary care providers may include family and general practice physicians, internists, nurse practitioners, and physician's assistants. Primary providers care for all routine medical problems. The providers also **refer** patients/clients to specialists.

refer To send to.

Specialty care is care given by a provider who is trained in one special area. Specialists usually limit their practice to treating one type of problem. Specializing gives them a broad knowledge of that area. A few specialties are

- Surgery
- Podiatry
- Audiology
- Obstetrics
- Orthopedics
- Chiropractic
- Urology

Emergency care and *urgent care* provide different services. Emergency care is for life-threatening conditions that require hospitalization. Urgent care is for non-emergencies that require prompt treatment. Emergencies requiring hospital care are expensive. Excellent care is available in the urgent care setting, and costs are lower.

The *preadmission authorization requirement for hospitalization* allows necessary hospitalization and prevents unnecessary hospitalization. Good-quality outpatient care is encouraged when possible. Outpatient care is much less expensive, and patients/clients often prefer being in their own homes.

■ AMBULATORY CARE

trend General direction or movement.

The current **trend** is to develop large managed care organizations that provide good-quality, cost-effective health care. Ambulatory care providers are following managed care concepts. One change keeps patients/clients at home for their care whenever possible. Most patients like to be at home because it is comfortable and **familiar.** It also reduces health care costs. Only the very ill and severely injured are hospitalized. All other patients are cared for in facilities like these:

familiar Known.

- Rehabilitation centers
- Outpatient surgery
- Outpatient medical centers/clinics
- Physicians' offices
- Day care

Such facilities provide what is called *ambulatory care*. The patient/client goes to a facility for care and returns home. Some patients also need home health care to help with bathing, range of motion, dressing changes, intravenous therapy, and special treatments.

In ambulatory care there are opportunities for health care workers to use their multidisciplinary skills: For example, a person with an EKG certificate, phlebotomy certificate, or limited radiology certificate is an asset to an ambulatory care organization.

■ QUALITY HEALTH CARE COSTS AND PAYMENTS

Health Plan Employer Data Information Set

Under the direction of the National Committee for Quality Assurance (NCQA), the Health Plan Employer Data and Information Set (HEDIS) sets guidelines and gives a report card that

■ Measures health plan performance
■ Helps identify physicians who give high-quality medical care to their patients/clients
■ Helps identify physicians who do not meet the quality care guidelines

Diagnostic-Related Groupings

The federal government passed legislation in 1983 to regulate the price of medical care. This legislation approved the grouping of medical conditions, the reasonable cost for each condition, and its standard treatment. These groupings are known as *diagnostic-related groupings* (DRGs). DRGs help reduce unnecessary procedures and encourage self-care and home care.

Health Insurance: Third-Party Payers

Health care costs, including dental, are so high that most people have some type of insurance plan. These plans are called *third-party payers*. Insurance companies require the subscriber to pay a fee for insurance coverage and in return agree to pay for specific medical and dental care. Each insurance company determines what it will and will not pay for and how much it will pay. The subscriber must pay any fees that the insurance company does not pay.

Health Maintenance Organizations

Health maintenance organizations (HMOs) require members to pay a co-pay for medical services. The member must get medical care from the physicians, labs, hospitals, and so on, that agree to the fee the HMO is willing to pay. If the member gets medical care outside the HMO, he or she will have to pay for the care.

Preferred Provider Organizations

Physician groups and hospitals work together to give comprehensive health care at a reduced cost to various companies. Employees of these companies contract with a preferred provider organization (PPO) and agree to see providers on the PPO list. If they see other providers, they pay a larger fee.

Medicaid

Health insurance is provided by the state and federal government. Benefits and eligibility are different in each state. People who are blind, disabled, or of low income are generally able to get Medicaid insurance.

Medicare

Health insurance is provided to people over the age of 65. Subscribers pay a monthly payment to the Social Security Administration. Some health care providers accept Medicare payments as payment in full for services; others charge more than Medicare pays. To cover the extra costs, many people buy a third-party payer insurance to cover all of their medical costs. There are many programs for Medicare recipients that provide care for a small co-pay.

■ ORGANIZATION

An efficient health care facility must be well organized. An organizational chart shows how each department fits into the system and identifies the line of authority (Figure 1–4). When you look at an organizational chart, you can see who your immediate supervisor is. It tells you the areas of responsibility for all of the employees. The organizational chart also establishes the chain of command.

Chain of Command

The chain of command tells you to whom you take questions, reports, and problems. This is always your immediate supervisor. It is your immediate supervisor's responsibility to resolve any problem that occurs. If your immediate supervisor is unable to find a solution, he or she takes the problem to his or her immediate supervisor. This provides an efficient problem-solving structure. Bypassing a link in the chain causes misunderstanding and is not professional.

FIGURE 1–4.
Sample organizational chart (relates to the National Health Care Skill Standards, Far West Laboratory).

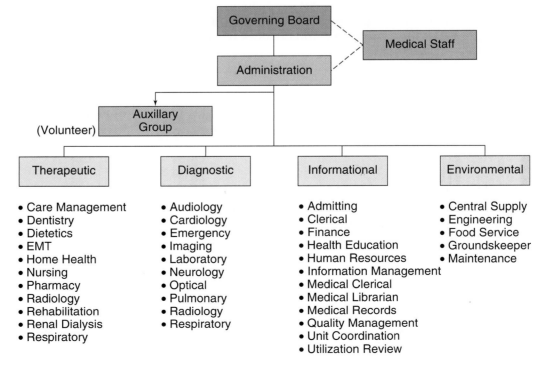

■ MAJOR SERVICES IN HEALTH CARE

As you can see in Figure 1–4, each service has specialized departments. These departments are determined by the type of service they give:

■ *Therapeutic services* provide care over time.
■ *Diagnostic services* create a picture of health status.
■ *Informational services* document and process information.
■ *Environmental services* create a therapeutic and supportive environment.

Services can be organized in several different ways. Your facility's organizational chart is your guideline. To find titles of personnel who are employed in these agencies and facilities, refer to "Overview of Careers" in Chapter 2.

■ SUMMARY

There are many agencies and facilities that help individuals with health problems. They offer many different services and are funded in different ways. There are private agencies as well as those funded by federal, state, and local governments. Each agency meets a special need. The current trend in health care is managed care, outpatient care, and ambulatory care. The emphasis is on wellness and preventive care. All facilities and agencies have an organizational chart to help them be more efficient and to establish a chain of command. In health care facilities, there are four services: **therapeutic,** diagnostic, information, and environmental.

therapeutic Pertaining to the treatment of disease or injury (e.g., physical therapy, radiology, diet, nursing).

Your link to success

Thinking Critically: Check Your Understanding

1. **Legal and Ethical** The field of medical ethics is affected by new technology every day. Explain how the legal system is involved in medical matters today. Think about recent medical cases that lawyers have tried.

2. **Cultural Competency** There are many caregivers from different cultures working in our country today. They come from all over the world. You have a co-worker who does not understand the chain of command because it is a new concept for her. Your co-worker also has difficulty understanding English. Why is it important for her to understand how the chain of command works? What can you do to help her understand?

3. **Communication** You are asked to give a talk to a class of sixth graders about the history and future of medicine. What will you tell the class about how early medical advances influenced today's medical practice? What do you think will happen in medicine in the future? How will you explain your ideas?

4. **Case Study** A new patient is telling you how upset he is about a change in his insurance. His company changed from private insurance to an HMO. The patient is very agitated and worried because the system is new to him. Why do you think the patient is so agitated? What can you do to reassure him?

Portfolio Connection

The history of medicine shows that experience, and evaluation of that experience, helps people plan and develop future health care. The same is true for you. Planning and preparing for a career is a process that allows you to look back on your experiences and learn from them. You can evaluate the things in your past that worked for you and those that did not.

You now have an opportunity to create a file that reflects what you learn. This file is called a *vocational portfolio*. Your portfolio will contain documents that show what you have learned during your vocational preparation. Your work will show the abilities and skills you gain throughout your training. You will also create a job search packet that helps you identify ways to share your portfolio with schools or potential employers. Developing your portfolio provides a chance to express the positive results of your learning experiences in a professional manner.

Think about a time when you surprised yourself by accomplishing something that you were not sure you could do. What caused you to try it when you were unsure about it? What went well in that experience? What would you do differently? Explain your answers in a short paper. Your explanation must clearly identify your self-evaluation and show how you would approach uncertain experiences in the future.

This assignment helps you review and evaluate your past experience. Some of the future assignments for your portfolio will require a similar process, with a focus on your vocational training. Turn this assignment in to your instructor. When you create your portfolio in Chapter 2 your teacher will return it to you. Put it in your portfolio in Section Four, "Written Samples."

FINDING THE RIGHT OCCUPATION FOR YOU

UNIT 1   Career Search

Steps to success

1. Read this unit.
2. Complete Worksheets 1 through 5 as assigned in the Student Workbook.
3. Review the portfolio guidelines and structure in Chapter 2 of your Workbook.
4. Place completed Worksheets 3 through 7 in your Vocational Portfolio.
5. When you are confident that you can meet each objective for this unit, ask your instructor for the unit evaluation.

Rationale

When you consider an occupation in the health care field, it is important to focus on your interests, values, and abilities. When you understand yourself, it is easier to select the right occupation. There are many different career opportunities in the health care field. Researching several careers will help you choose the right career for you. Learning how to use the resources for researching occupations will make it easier for you to choose a career.

Objectives

When you have completed this unit, you will be able to do the following:

✓ Define *interests, values,* and *abilities.*
✓ List five work-related values.
✓ Identify three resources for occupational research.

✓ Research three health careers.
✓ Explain the importance of a vocational portfolio.
✓ Write a paper titled "What I Learned about Selecting a Career."

■ INTERESTS

Your interests tell what you like to do and what you do not like to do. Recognizing your interests helps you make a good career choice. For instance, if you like to work alone, a career in direct patient/client care probably is not right for you. Working in one of the computer areas might be better. When you know your interests early in your career search, you can identify careers that use those interests. If you discover that many of the tasks listed in an occupation are not interesting to you, reconsider your choice, and research careers that require your interests.

■ VALUES

compromising Giving up something important.

prioritize To put in order of importance.

A value is the importance that you place on various elements in your life. Money might be more important to you than leisure time. Working with people might be more important to you than what shift you work. Knowing what values you feel most strongly about helps you avoid **compromising** the things that are most important to you. Recognizing your values also helps you **prioritize** your work-related values, such as job security, leisure time, wages, recognition, creativity, advancement, working environment, home life, responsibility, and management. Ask yourself the following questions.

■ *Job security.* Is it important that you find a job immediately upon the completion of your training program? How important is job availability?

■ *Leisure time.* Is it important for you to have extra time for leisure activities?

■ *Wages.* Is an average wage acceptable if you like your work, or is a very high wage necessary?

■ *Recognition.* Is it important that the job you choose is respected by the people in your community?

■ *Creativity.* Do you like to come up with new ideas to solve problems, or do you prefer a job in which there is exactly one way to do things?

■ *Advancement.* Do you want a career that provides opportunities for promotion?

■ *Working environment.* Do you prefer to work indoors or outdoors?

■ *Home life.* Do you want to work a daytime schedule (9 to 5) with some overtime and with weekends and holidays off, or are you willing to do shift work (all hours, any day of the week)?

■ *Responsibility.* Do you want a job that requires you to make a number of decisions?

■ *Management.* Do you want to be responsible for supervising the work of other people or for organizing many tasks at once?

All of these factors affect your job choice. Make a list of these work values and put them in order of their importance to you. When you research an occupation, refer to your list so you do not choose a job that conflicts with many of your values.

■ ABILITIES

An ability is something you do well. You have many abilities. For example, you may work well with your hands, or you may be very good at mathematics. It is much more pleasant to work in an occupation that uses your abilities. If you choose an occupation that is too far below your ability level, you will be bored. If it is too far above your ability level, you will be frustrated. It is important to evaluate your abilities during your career search. List your abilities, and use the list when researching an occupation. Match your abilities to the job description.

■ RESOURCES FOR OCCUPATIONAL RESEARCH

There are many resources you can use in your research. Two of them are the *Dictionary of Occupational Titles,* which lists job titles, tasks, and duties for 20,000 occupations, and the *Occupational Outlook Handbook,* which discusses the nature of the work, employment outlook, training and qualifications requirements, earnings, and working conditions for a variety of occupations. *Work Briefs* by Science Research Associates, the Career Exploratory Kit, the *Encyclopedia of Careers,* and computer programs are also good resources. In addition, check career-related pamphlets, microfilm, and videos. You can find all of these resources in libraries and career centers. Interview individuals who are already working in health care occupations, as well as looking at written materials.

By conducting occupational research, you learn about the tasks performed, the job outlook, the education required, the working environment, and many other things. It requires time and effort to research the occupations that interest you and to prepare for a specific career. However, your efforts allow you to find a job that gives you satisfaction.

■ HOW TO DO A CAREER SEARCH

1. Choose a health career that interests you. Use the information from the resources listed in this unit and the information in the following unit for your research. Instructions for your research are in the Student Workbook.
2. Interview for information. Interview a worker in the occupation that interests you. Prepare a questionnaire before the interview.
3. Write a paper telling how the occupation you researched matches your interests, abilities, and values.

When you complete your research, you have a guideline to follow that will help you choose an occupation that you enjoy.

■ DEVELOPING A VOCATIONAL PORTFOLIO

A portfolio is a collection of materials that show the knowledge, abilities, skills, and insights you gain in your search for a career. The purpose in developing a portfolio is to show your mastery of vocational requirements to an employer, a college, or a higher-level training program. You also see your own growth and accomplishments over time. Follow the directions in "Vocational Portfolio" at the back of the Student Workbook to assemble your own portfolio.

Completing this project shows your commitment to a set of values and your ability to plan, organize, and create a product. It provides an opportunity to pursue a specific interest and to meet professionals in health care occupations. This project leads you through planning, evidence of progress, final product, and oral presentations.

■ SUMMARY

In this unit you learned that it is important to identify and evaluate your work interests, values, and abilities. You learned how to use this information when you choose a career, how to use many resources to research career possibilities, and the importance of developing a vocational portfolio.

UNIT 2   Overview of Careers

*S*teps to success

1. Complete Vocabulary Worksheet 1 in the Student Workbook.
2. Read this unit.
3. Complete Worksheets 2 and 3 as assigned.
4. When you are confident that you can meet each objective for this unit, ask your instructor for the unit evaluation.
5. Complete "Your Link to Success" at the end of this chapter.

Rationale

There are hundreds of job opportunities in the health care field. The occupations in the four occupational clusters in this unit introduce you to some of the possible health care careers. These occupational clusters follow the National Health Care Skills Standards (see page 14). These standards are a guide to the information you need to be a successful health care worker. Part One of this text provides the health care core foundation skills for all health services that are covered in the national standards. Part Two has entry-level occupations from each cluster in the standards. You can learn the skills from several occupations and become a multidisciplinary/unlicensed assistive personnel health care worker. Finding several areas of interest in the following occupations enhances your education and provides the skills to increase your employability. After carefully researching these careers, you can make an informed decision.

Employment in all of the medical occupations is expected to grow faster than the average for all occupations through the year 2006. Population growth, the increase of middle-aged and elderly people, new medical technology, and the need for more rehabilitation and long-term care make a health care occupation a very good choice for the future.

Objectives

When you have completed this unit, you will be able to do the following:

✓ Define the vocabulary words.
✓ Compare and differentiate the services performed by the therapeutic, diagnostic, information, and environmental services.
✓ Define *therapeutic, diagnostic, information,* and *environmental services.*

You learned in Chapter 1 that there are four major health care service areas, each containing many occupations. On the following pages you will study some of the possible occupations in each service and the duties that you might have as an entry-level employee. Remember that the entry-level jobs are the first step in a career ladder or lattice. The career ladder moves upward in your career. The career lattice allows you to use your transferable skills to move into other career areas. Both allow you many choices. The following information is from the *Dictionary of Occupational Titles*, the *Occupational Outlook Handbook*, and *Descriptions and Organizational Analysis for Hospitals and Related Health Services*.

■ THERAPEUTIC SERVICES

Therapeutic service workers observe the patient/client, instrumentation, and environment. They report results and assist the treatment team by performing procedures accurately. They also assist in reaching treatment goals.

Respiratory Therapy/Respiratory Care Workers

Every breath is the breath of life, and helping patients/clients with their breathing is a very important part of health care. Patients/clients may live without water for a few days. They may live without food for a few weeks. But without air, they will suffer brain damage within a few minutes and may die after nine minutes. Respiratory therapy workers and respiratory care practitioners evaluate, treat, and care for patients/clients of all ages who have breathing problems. Therapists test lung capacity and check blood for oxygen and carbon dioxide content. They give treatments and teach self-care to patients/clients with chronic respiratory problems. They also give emergency care for drowning, stroke, shock, heart failure, and other emergencies. Other duties may include keeping records and making minor repairs to equipment (Figure 2–1).

Respiratory care workers have many career options and work in acute hospitals, cardiopulmonary laboratories, ambulatory care, health maintenance organizations, home health agencies, and nursing homes (Figure 2–2). They work indoors and may be exposed to flammable gases and body fluids. Their jobs may require shift work and weekend work. They stand for long periods of time and carry or push equipment throughout the facility.

FIGURE 2–1. Respiratory assistant/aide cleaning and assembling equipment.

FIGURE 2–2.

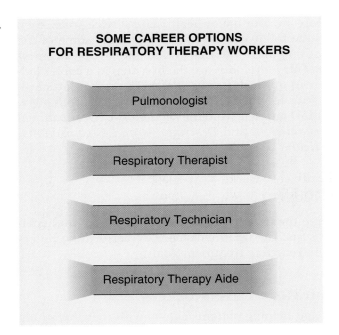

SOME CAREER OPTIONS FOR RESPIRATORY THERAPY WORKERS

Pulmonologist

Respiratory Therapist

Respiratory Technician

Respiratory Therapy Aide

Respiratory Aides/Assistants

Traits

dexterity Skill in using one's hands.

- Possess manual and finger **dexterity** for proper handling of equipment
- Possess some clerical ability for keeping accurate records
- Possess a preference for cleaning and assembling equipment
- Possess the ability to do repetitive procedures
- Possess alertness and accuracy in following set procedures and rules in stressful situations

Tasks

- Spend most time taking care of equipment
- Follow tasks under the direction of a respiratory therapist
- Scrub and wash equipment, such as respirators, intermittent positive-pressure breathing machines, pulmonary function machines, and oxygen administration sets
- Inspect equipment for damage, and report problems to supervisor
- Start and test gauges, and notify supervisor of malfunction
- Deliver oxygen tanks and other equipment where needed
- Assist in administration of gas or aerosol therapy as directed
- Record amount of oxygen used by patient/client, and prepare billing forms
- Assist the respiratory technician and therapist as needed

For more information, write
American Association for Respiratory Care
11030 Ables Lane
Dallas, TX 75229

CAREER BASICS

RESPIRATORY THERAPY WORKERS

	Education and/or Experience Required	Average Income

RESPIRATORY THERAPY AIDE	✓ No educational requirements
	✓ It is desirable to
	  • Have a high school diploma or the equivalent
	  • Have completed a vocational education program in respiratory therapy
		✓ Annual: $18,000–21,000

RESPIRATORY THERAPY TECHNICIAN	✓ High school diploma or equivalent ✓ Completion of respiratory technician training ✓ Certified respiratory therapy technician (CRTT) ✓ Completion of AMA-approved respiratory therapy technician program ✓ One year of work experience ✓ Passing grade on a written examination given by the National Board of Respiratory Therapy	✓ Annual: $22,000–28,000
RESPIRATORY THERAPIST	✓ High school diploma or equivalent ✓ Completion of AMA-approved respiratory therapist training program in a community college or a four-year bachelor's degree program ✓ Registered respiratory therapist (RRT) ✓ Two years of experience in the field following training ✓ Passing grade on a written examination given by the National Board of Respiratory Therapy	✓ Annual: $32,500–48,000

Pharmacy Workers

Pharmacy workers prepare and dispense medications prescribed by physicians, podiatrists, dentists, and other health care professionals (Figure 2–3). They provide information to health care professionals and to the public about medicines. Another important task is to review the medicines that patients/clients are taking. This reduces the chance that the patient/client will have a drug interaction that can cause illness or an allergic reaction. They also help in the strict control of

FIGURE 2–3.
Pharmacy worker
preparing medications.

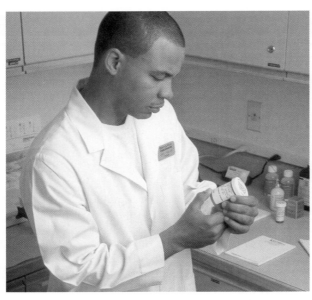

distribution and use of government-controlled products, such as narcotics and barbiturates. Since vaccines and other drugs deteriorate, pharmacy workers are responsible for careful inventory control.

Pharmacy workers have many career options and work in acute hospitals, community pharmacies, health maintenance organizations, home health agencies, and clinics (Figure 2–4). A pharmacist may also work for state and local health departments, as well as for pharmaceutical manufacturers. Pharmacy workers work indoors and may be required to work in a restricted environment, such as areas where sterile solutions are prepared. In large hospitals or community pharmacies, they may work in shifts. Their work requires lifting, carrying, pushing items, and climbing ladders in storage areas. They need good vision for close-up work. They stand for long periods of time and must take proper safety precautions when working with products that can be dangerous.

CAREER BASICS

PHARMACY WORKERS

	Education and/or Experience Required	Average Income
PHARMACY CLERK/PHARMACY HELPER	✓ High school diploma or equivalent ✓ Good typing skills ✓ Two to three months of on-the-job training or completion of a pharmacy vocational program	✓ Annual: $12,000–16,000
PHARMACY TECHNICIAN	✓ Two to 12 months of on-the-job training or completion of a one- to two-year program in a junior college ✓ Some states offer a pharmacy technician certification upon successful completion of an examination	✓ Annual: $13,000–30,000
PHARMACIST	✓ Completion of five years in an accredited pharmacy program ✓ One year of pharmacy internship ✓ License in state of employment	✓ Annual: $59,000–61,317

FIGURE 2-4.

**SOME CAREER OPTIONS
FOR PHARMACY WORKERS**

Pharmacist

Pharmacy Technician/Assistant

Pharmacy Helper

Pharmacy Clerk

Pharmacy Assistants

Traits

■ Possess a working knowledge of basic math, including the metric system

■ Possess the ability to understand important details

■ Possess the desire for routine activities

■ Possess the ability to keep neat, accurate records and to type numbers accurately

■ Possess the capability to perform repetitive activities

■ Possess exactness

■ Possess a willingness to work under direct supervision

Tasks

■ Type labels for medication and records and transactions in the pharmacy log

■ Clip typed labels to medication requests and deliver to the pharmacist

■ Assign prescription numbers

■ List patient's/client's name, physician, and prescription numbers in the log book

■ Copy physician's instructions for use of medication

■ Calculate charges, type billing slips for prescriptions, and enter charges on medication forms

■ Compile periodic reports from log book

■ Mix pharmaceutical preparations using the metric system

■ Label pharmaceutical preparations by using a typewriter, printer, or computer, and maintain records and files

■ Rotate stock to keep dated items current and order supplies

■ Run errands and deliver orders

■ Clean equipment and work areas according to department procedures

■ Destroy damaged drugs according to department standards

■ Use aseptic techniques, follow procedure for working under purification hood, and wear appropriate clothing and disposable caps

FIGURE 2–5.
Occupational therapy worker applying hand support to prevent contractures.

For more information, write
American Association of Colleges
    of Pharmacy
1426 Prince Street
Alexandria, VA 22314

Occupational Therapy Workers

Occupational therapy workers treat people who are mentally, physically, developmentally, or emotionally disabled (Figure 2–5). They evaluate the self-care, work, and leisure skills of their patients/clients. They plan and develop programs that help restore, develop, and maintain patients' ability to manage the activities of daily living. The goal is to improve clients' quality of life by helping them compensate for their limitations.

Occupational therapy workers have many career options and work in general hospitals, schools for handicapped children, nursing homes, outpatient clinics, rehabilitation centers, day care centers, mental health agencies, special workshops, health maintenance organizations, and psychiatric hospitals (Figure 2–6). They work a 40-hour week and may have to work evenings or weekends occasionally. The work environment depends on the type of facility. In a large rehabilitation center, therapists may work in a spacious room equipped with machines, hand

FIGURE 2–6.

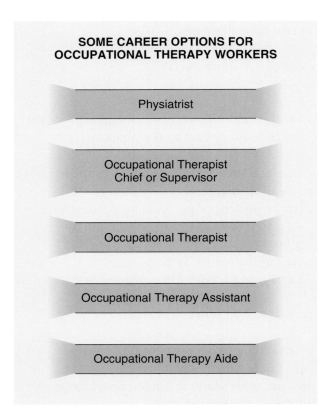

SOME CAREER OPTIONS FOR OCCUPATIONAL THERAPY WORKERS

Physiatrist

Occupational Therapist
Chief or Supervisor

Occupational Therapist

Occupational Therapy Assistant

Occupational Therapy Aide

CAREER BASICS

OCCUPATIONAL THERAPY WORKERS

	Education and/or Experience Required	Average Income
OCCUPATIONAL THERAPY AIDE	✓ High school diploma or equivalent ✓ On-the-job training ✓ Completion of a vocational education program as an occupational therapy aide	✓ Annual: $12,000–16,000
CERTIFIED OCCUPATIONAL THERAPY ASSISTANT (COTA)	✓ High school diploma or equivalent ✓ Completion of a two-year program in a community college ✓ Completion of a certified vocational or technical program ✓ Supervised fieldwork ✓ Completion of a two-year program approved by the American Occupational Therapy Association (COTA)	✓ Annual: $13,000–27,000
OCCUPATIONAL THERAPIST 1	✓ Bachelor's degree in occupational therapy (four-year course in an approved program) ✓ Certification by the Board of Registry of the American Occupational Therapy Association ✓ Up to six months of on-the-job training ✓ Occupational therapist chief or supervisor	✓ Annual: $30,500–45,000
PHYSIATRIST	✓ Graduation from an accredited medical school ✓ License to practice medicine or osteopathy in state of employment ✓ Residency in physical medicine and rehabilitation	✓ Annual: $70,000–120,000

tools, and other devices. In a psychiatric hospital, they may work on the ward. They carry and lift equipment and transfer patients from wheelchairs. Their work requires both standing and sitting.

Occupational Therapy Aides/Assistants

Traits

■ Possess the ability to give written and oral instructions and carry on conversations with patients/clients

■ Possess good coordination and manual dexterity to handle and control tools and materials while instructing patients

■ Prefer working with people, enjoy instructing others in relearning skills, and enjoy creative activities, such as arts and crafts

■ Possess a willingness to do a variety of tasks

■ Possess the ability to follow instructions and to use initiative and judgment in working with clients

■ Possess the ability to communicate the benefits of the project to the patient and to work with a variety of clients

Tasks

Occupational Therapy Aides

■ Transport patients, assemble equipment, and prepare and maintain work areas

■ Perform clerical tasks, restock and order supplies, answer the phone, and schedule appointments

Occupational Therapy Assistants

■ Teach work-related skills (e.g., use of power tools)

■ Help clients with rehabilitative activities and exercises

■ Teach proper method of moving from a wheelchair to bed

■ Observe patient activities for progress and make reports to aid in evaluation of patient progress

■ Assist in adaptation of equipment, splints, and other self-help devices

■ Transport patients

■ Store equipment, clean work areas, and help maintain tools and equipment

■ Perform other clerical duties (e.g., filing)

For more information, write
American Occupational Therapy Association
Division of Credentialing
4720 Montgomery
PO Box 31220
Bethesda, MD 20824-1220
http://www.aota.org

Physical Therapy Workers

Physical therapy workers (Figure 2–7) help people with injuries or diseases of the muscles, nerves, joints, and bones to overcome their disabilities. The client may be disabled from an accident, a stroke, or a disease. Some of the conditions that require treatment are multiple sclerosis, cerebral palsy, nerve injuries, amputations, fractures, arthritis, and heart disease. Patients vary in age from newborn to aged. Physical therapy workers help the patient regain as close to normal activity as possible.

FIGURE 2-7. One of the many duties of a physical therapy aide is assisting patients/ clients with walking.

Physical therapy workers have many career options and work in acute care facilities, long-term care facilities, ambulatory care, health maintenance organizations, rehabilitation centers, schools for the disabled, public health agencies, home health care agencies, and sports medicine centers (Figure 2–8). Some physical therapists are in private practice. They contract to work for health care agencies or may have an office where they provide care. They work in specially equipped

FIGURE 2–8.

SOME CAREER OPTIONS FOR PHYSICAL THERAPY WORKERS

- Physiatrist
- Physical Therapist Chief or Supervisor
- Physical Therapist
- Physical Therapy Assistant
- Physical Therapy Aide

physical therapy departments, in clinics, and in private homes. Their work requires lifting and carrying up to 50 pounds, stooping, pushing, and pulling patients and equipment. They stand and walk during their shifts.

Physical Therapy Aides/Assistants

Traits
- Possess the ability to understand medical terminology
- Possess good verbal and written skills
- Possess manual dexterity and motor coordination for massaging patients and handling therapeutic equipment
- Possess the desire to motivate patients toward recovery
- Possess the ability to perform a variety of tasks following standard procedures

Tasks

Physical Therapy Aides
- Prepare equipment (e.g., hydrotherapy pools, paraffin baths, and hot packs)
- Assist patients/clients to treatment area using a wheelchair or offering a shoulder to lean on
- Inform therapist or assistant if patients/clients are having difficulty with their treatment
- Change linen on beds and tables
- Clean equipment and work area
- Inventory materials and supplies
- Assist with clerical tasks

CAREER BASICS

PHYSICAL THERAPY WORKERS

	Education and/or Experience Required	Average Income
PHYSICAL THERAPY AIDE	✓ High school diploma or equivalent (preferred) ✓ On-the-job training ✓ Completion of a vocational education program as a physical therapy aide	✓ Annual: $13,000–24,000
PHYSICAL THERAPY ASSISTANT	✓ Training requirements are not uniform ✓ 24 states require graduation from an accredited community college ✓ Students may be required to pass a written licensure examination	✓ Annual: $15,600–25,000
PHYSICAL THERAPIST	✓ Four-year degree in physical therapy ✓ Supervised four-month clinical internship ✓ Passing grade on a state licensure examination	✓ Annual: $17,800–53,000

Physical Therapy Assistants
■ Apply heat, cold, and ultrasound
■ Massage and perform therapeutic exercises

For more information, write
American Physical Therapy Association
1111 North Fairfax Street
Alexandria, VA 22314-1488
http://www.apta.org

Emergency Medical Service Workers

First responders are often the first trained people to treat patients/clients. They provide emergency medical care before emergency medical technicians (EMTs) reach the scene. They may be law enforcement officers, members of the fire service, company employees, or private citizens.

Emergency medical technicians are providers of prehospital medical care in an emergency. A heart attack, unscheduled birth, automobile accident, or near drowning all require immediate attention. The EMT administers basic life support and transports sick and injured people to medical facilities (Figure 2–9).

Emergency medical service workers have many career opportunities and may work in rescue, police, and fire departments, ski patrols, hospital emergency departments, and private ambulance services (Figure 2–10). They must usually work shifts and weekends. They work inside and outside in all weather conditions. They may be exposed to body fluids.

Emergency medical service workers must be in good physical condition. For example, they must have good eyesight, hearing, and speech. They must also be able to lift heavy loads, reach, stoop, and climb as the job requires.

FIGURE 2–9. EMTs transporting an injured or sick patient to a medical facility.

First Responders/Emergency Medical Technicians

Traits

■ Possess motor coordination in order to apply bandages and maneuver stretchers in and out of ambulances
■ Possess the ability to determine space in narrow hallways and tight places
■ Possess the ability to perform both routine and nonroutine activities
■ Possess the ability to perform a variety of duties in all kinds of situations
■ Possess the ability to communicate calmly
■ Possess the ability to make judgments about proper basic emergency medical care

FIGURE 2–10.

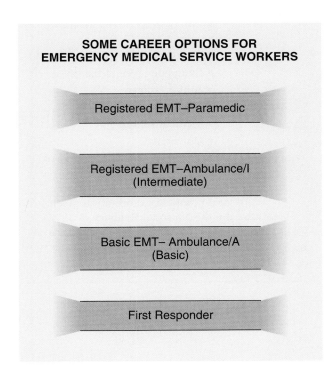

SOME CAREER OPTIONS FOR EMERGENCY MEDICAL SERVICE WORKERS

Registered EMT–Paramedic

Registered EMT–Ambulance/I
(Intermediate)

Basic EMT– Ambulance/A
(Basic)

First Responder

CAREER BASICS

EMERGENCY MEDICAL SERVICE WORKERS

	Education and/or Experience Required	Average Income
BASIC EMT–AMBULANCE/ A (BASIC)	✓ At least 18 years of age ✓ High school diploma or equivalent ✓ Valid driver's license ✓ Completion of a minimum 110-hour program offered in vocational programs ✓ Passing grade on a written and practical exam given by the National Registry of Emergency Medical Technicians or the state emergency medical systems board	✓ Annual: $18,600–23,000
REGISTERED EMT– AMBULANCE/ I (INTERMEDIATE)	✓ Graduation from an approved EMT Basic program and 35–55 hours of additional instruction ✓ Passing grade on a written and practical examination given by the National Registry of Emergency Medical Technicians or the state emergency medical systems board	✓ Annual: $29,000–32,500
REGISTERED EMT–PARAMEDIC	✓ Completion of EMT–paramedic training in an approved program offered by one of the following: • Vocational school • State educational facility • Junior college • Hospital • Medical school • University ✓ Six months of field experience as an EMT–paramedic ✓ Passing grade on a written and practical examination given by the National Registry of Emergency Medical Technicians or the state emergency medical systems board	✓ Annual: $29,000–35,000

Tasks

First Responders

■ Gain access to patient, assess patient, provide appropriate care, and report assessment and care given

■ Lift or move patient to a safe place if necessary

Emergency Medical Technicians/A (Basic)

■ Drive an ambulance

■ Determine the nature of the victim's illness or injury

■ Give appropriate care

   • Open and maintain the airway • Restore breathing • Control bleeding • Treat for shock • Immobilize fractures • Bandage wounds • Assist with childbirth • Give initial care to poison and burn victims • Use automated external defibrillators

■ Use correct equipment and techniques to remove trapped victims safely

■ Transport patients to hospital

   • Place patient on stretcher • Constantly watch patient while in transport • Notify hospital of arrival

■ Report observations of and care given to the victim to the emergency staff

■ Maintain clean, well-equipped ambulance

■ Be certain ambulance is in good running order

   • Check gas, oil, tire pressure, siren, communication equipment

For more information, write
National Association of Emergency Medical Technicians
408 Monroe
Clinton, MS 39056

National Registry of Emergency Medical Technicians
PO Box 29233
Columbus, OH 43229

Medical Assistants

Medical assistants are responsible for the efficient operation of a physician's office. They also work in clinics, health maintenance organizations, and ambulatory care. Medical assistants have varied duties. Some specialize in back office procedures (Figure 2–11), while others choose to work in the front office. They work indoors in a clean environment, 40 hours a week, and some weekends. They have varied job opportunities, and their work requires standing on their feet most of the day

FIGURE 2–11. A back office medical assistant performing one of many duties—taking a client's blood pressure.

(back office), lifting, reaching, and helping patients/clients (Figure 2–12). They may be exposed to body fluids. The front office worker sits at a desk for long periods.

The current trend toward large medical groups has relocated administrative/front office responsibilities. Billing, insurance verification, medical records, appointment scheduling, and payroll have been relocated to departments that specialize in handling work for the increased number of patients/clients. See "Administrative Support Service Workers" later in this unit for more information.

Medical Assistants

Traits

■ Possess the verbal ability to communicate with patients and physicians
■ Possess the ability to follow instructions using good judgment and discretion
■ Possess the manual dexterity for operating equipment
■ Enjoy working with people
■ Possess the desire to give services of help and benefit to others
■ Know the medical terminology
■ Possess the ability to perform a variety of duties
■ Possess the ability to work with people who are ill or anxious

Tasks

Administrative/Front Office Medical Assistants

■ Greet patients/clients
■ Answer phones
■ Handle mail
■ Make appointments
■ Arrange hospital admissions
■ Arrange for laboratory services
■ Prepare insurance forms (e.g., Medicare, medical insurance, workers' compensation)

FIGURE 2–12.

SOME CAREER OPTIONS FOR MEDICAL ASSISTANTS

Office Manager

Clinic—Back Office Medical Assistant

Administrative/Front Office Medical Assistant

CAREER BASICS

MEDICAL ASSISTANTS

	Education and/or Experience Required	Average Income
ADMINISTRATIVE/FRONT OFFICE MEDICAL ASSISTANT	✓ High school diploma or equivalent ✓ On-the-job training in a physician's front office ✓ Completion of an administrative medical assistant program	✓ Annual: $16,500–27,000
CLINICAL/BACK OFFICE MEDICAL ASSISTANT	✓ High school diploma or equivalent ✓ On-the-job training in a physician's back office ✓ Completion of an accredited clinical medical assistant program ✓ Completion of an examination by the American Association of Medical Assistants, which offers a certified medical assistant (CMA) certificate (optional)	✓ Annual: $16,500–27,000

OFFICE MANAGER	✓ Completion of administrative and clinical medical assistant program
	✓ Workshops
	  • Seminars
	  • Home study courses
		✓ Annual: $20,000–34,000

- Type medical reports
- Maintain patient files
- May handle billing and receipts
- Prepare payroll for office staff

Clinical/Back Office Medical Assistants
Tasks vary according to state law.

- Sterilize instruments using an autoclave
- Prepare clients for examination
- Assist physician during examination
- Give injections
- Take and record temperatures, pulse, respiration, and blood pressure
- Measure height and weight
- Perform routine urinalysis
- Collect blood samples
- Perform simple blood tests
- Record electrocardiograms

- Assist with minor surgery
- Direct patients in preparation for x-rays and tests
- Instruct patients about medication and special diets

For more information, write
American Association of Medical Assistants
20 North Wacker Drive, Suite 1575
Chicago, IL 60606-2903

Dental Workers

Dental workers (Figure 2–13) are responsible for maintaining oral health and repairing dental abnormalities. They emphasize treatment and prevention of problems associated with the hard and soft tissues of the mouth.

According to their level of education, dental workers work in private practices, dental schools, hospital dental departments, private clinics, health maintenance organizations, and state and local public health departments (Figure 2–14). Dental laboratory technicians work in a dental laboratory. Dental workers work indoors in a clean environment. They are subject to respiratory infections due to close contact with patients and may be exposed to body fluid. Their work requires standing most of the day, reaching, and handling dental instruments, equipment, and supplies.

Dental Assistants

Traits

- Possess the ability to communicate with the patient/client and the dentist
- Possess good motor coordination
- Possess the manual and finger dexterity to work with small equipment
- Possess good perception of space in order to correctly place x-rays and handle dental prostheses
- Like working with people
- Possess the ability to work with things and objects in order to develop laboratory techniques and dental procedures
- Enjoy scientific and technical activities
- Possess the ability to follow specific directions

FIGURE 2–13. A dental assistant performing one of many tasks—assisting the dentist.

FIGURE 2-14.

SOME CAREER OPTIONS FOR DENTAL WORKERS

Dentist

Dental Hygienist

Dental Laboratory Technician

Dental Assistant

■ Possess the ability to communicate with patients who may be anxious or in pain

Tasks

■ Make the patient comfortable in the dental chair

■ Prepare the client for treatment

■ Hand the dentist proper instruments and materials

■ Suction the patient's mouth

■ Prepare materials for making impressions and restorations

■ Take and process dental x-rays

■ Teach oral health (e.g., flossing, brushing, postoperative care)

■ Prepare instruments for sterilizing

■ Make casts of teeth and mouth from impressions taken by the dentist

■ Apply medications to the teeth and oral tissue, remove cement used in the filling process, and place rubber dams on the teeth (in some states)

■ May manage the office (e.g., make appointments, keep treatment records, send bills, receive payments, and order supplies and materials)

For more information, write
Commission on Dental Accreditation, American Dental Association
211 East Chicago Avenue, Suite 1814
Chicago, IL 60611
http://www.ada.org

National Association of Health Career Schools
750 First Street, NE, Suite 940
Washington, DC 20005
FAX: (202) 842-1565
E-mail: NAHCS@aol.com

American Dental Assistants' Association
203 North Lasalle, Suite 1320
Chicago, IL 60601

CAREER BASICS

DENTAL WORKERS

	Education and/or Experience Required	Average Income
DENTAL ASSISTANT	✓ High school diploma or equivalent ✓ On-the-job training ✓ Completion of a one- or two-year community college or vocational training program ✓ Completion of an examination by the Certifying Board of the Dental Assisting National Board (optional)	✓ Annual: $14,700–24,000
DENTAL HYGIENIST	✓ Graduation from an accredited dental hygienist program in a two-year community college, a four-year bachelor's degree program, or a five-year master's degree program ✓ Passing grade on a written and clinical examination ✓ License in the state of employment (given by the National Board of Dental Examiners)	✓ Annual: $20,000–39,000
DENTAL LABORATORY TECHNICIAN	✓ High school diploma or equivalent ✓ Two-year vocational program ✓ On-the-job training (three to four years) ✓ May become certified by passing a written and practical examination given by the National Board for Certification	✓ Annual: $23,000–50,000
DENTIST	✓ Graduation from a dental school approved by the American Dental Association ✓ Passing grade on written and practical examinations ✓ State licensure by passing written examinations given by the National Board of Examiners	✓ Annual: $109,000–200,000

Nursing Service Workers

Nursing service workers provide many varied and essential services (Figure 2–15). They care for patients who are physically ill or disabled and provide preventive care (e.g., immunizations). They work in industries, community health nursing, general hospitals, long-term care facilities, government agencies, schools, educational institutions, visiting nurse associations, clinics, physicians' offices, ambula-

FIGURE 2–15. Nurse assistants (a and b) and home health aide (c) helping clients.

tory care units, homes, and health maintenance organizations. Nurses work indoors. They may have rotating shifts and work on weekends. Their work requires standing, walking, lifting, and pushing patients, carts, and wheelchairs. They are exposed to unpleasant odors and body fluids.

Nurse Assistants/Home Health Aides

Home health aides care for patients/clients in their homes instead of in a health facility. They care for patients of all ages who need more care than their families can give. Their job requires them to go to different homes. Nurse assistants and home health aides stand, walk, and lift patients and may push wheelchairs. They may be exposed to body fluids. They have many career options ranging from nurse assistant to director of nursing (Figure 2–16).

Traits

- Possess the ability to communicate with patients
- Possess the desire to help others
- Possess the ability to understand instructions given by the nursing staff
- Possess the manual dexterity for operating equipment
- Possess the ability to work with people who are ill

Tasks

Nurse Assistants

- Answer patient/client call lights
- Bathe patients
- Dress and undress clients
- Assist with personal hygiene (e.g., shaving, hair care, oral care, and dental care)
- Serve and collect food trays and feed patients who need help

FIGURE 2–16.

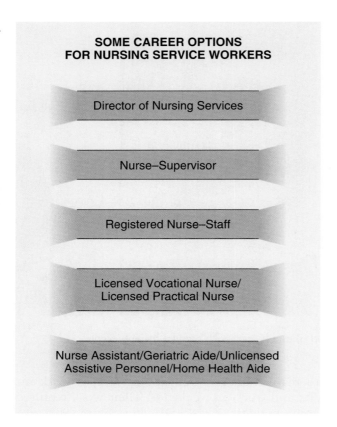

SOME CAREER OPTIONS
FOR NURSING SERVICE WORKERS

Director of Nursing Services

Nurse–Supervisor

Registered Nurse–Staff

Licensed Vocational Nurse/
Licensed Practical Nurse

Nurse Assistant/Geriatric Aide/Unlicensed
Assistive Personnel/Home Health Aide

■ Provide between-meal nourishment and fresh drinking water
■ Transport patients in wheelchair or stretcher or help patients walk
■ Take and record temperature, pulse, and respiration and record blood pressure
■ Record food and liquid intake and output
■ May apply ice bags or heat packs
■ Give back rubs, if appropriate
■ Observe and report any unusual conditions
■ Tidy clients' rooms, change bed linen, and collect soiled linen
■ Write in patients' charts

Home Health Aides
■ Transfer patients from place to place and assist with bathing, walking, and prescribed exercises
■ Assist with medication routines
■ Help with braces or artificial limbs
■ Check and record pulse, respiration, and blood pressure
■ Change nonsterile dressings
■ Provide emotional support and take client outside home as a companion
■ Change bed linen, clean laundry, and clean clients' living quarters
■ Shop for patients' food and prepare meals
■ Report findings and observations to supervisors
■ Act as a companion on shopping trips, doctor visits, and outdoor activities

CAREER BASICS

NURSING SERVICE WORKERS

	Education and/or Experience Required	Average Income
NURSE ASSISTANT/ GERIATRIC AIDE	✓ High school diploma or equivalent (preferred) ✓ Hospital-conducted on-the-job training ✓ Completion of an OBRA-approved nurse assistant program	✓ Annual: $12,500–20,800
UNLICENSED ASSISTIVE PERSONNEL	✓ Additional training in specialty (e.g., EKG, phlebotomy)	✓ Annual: $13,500–21,200
HOME HEALTH AIDE	✓ High school diploma or equivalent (preferred) ✓ Preservice training (40–120 hours) provided by an employing agency ✓ Completion of a vocational education program as a home health aide ✓ State certification may be required	✓ Annual: $10,900–17,200
LICENSED VOCATIONAL NURSE (LVN)/LICENSED PRACTICAL NURSE (LPN)	✓ High school diploma or equivalent ✓ Graduation from a recognized one-year program ✓ License for the state of employment	✓ Annual: $20,200–35,000
REGISTERED NURSE	✓ High school diploma or equivalent ✓ Graduation from a two-year community college ✓ Graduation from a four-year college or university ✓ Graduation from an accredited school of nursing ✓ Graduation from a diploma school (three-year hospital schools are being phased out) ✓ License for the state of employment	✓ Annual: $24,500–63,000
NURSE PRACTITIONER	✓ All requirements for becoming a registered nurse ✓ Completion of an accredited course in nurse practitioner training ✓ License for the state of employment	✓ Annual: $57,000–76,800

For more information, write
National Association of Health Career Schools
750 First Street, NE, Suite 940
Washington, DC 20002
FAX: (202) 842-1565
E-mail: NAHCS@aol.com

National Association for Home Care
228 Seventh Street, SE
Washington, DC 20003

■ DIAGNOSTIC SERVICES

Diagnostic service workers help with the diagnosis of illness and disease. Some diagnostic service workers have direct contact with the patient/client, while others do not. They plan services and prepare and perform tests accurately. They also understand quality control and report results in a timely manner.

Medical Laboratory Workers

Medical laboratory workers (Figure 2–17) perform many varied tests. Some of these tests are highly technical, whereas others are not as technical. In many cases, tests are performed on computerized equipment. Medical laboratory workers determine changes that have occurred in the blood, urine, lymph, and body tissues. They identify increases or decreases in white or red blood cells, cross-match blood for transfusions, identify microscopic changes in cells, and determine the presence of parasites, viruses, or bacteria in the blood, tissue, or urine. These tests help the physician make an accurate diagnosis and correctly treat the patient.

Medical laboratory workers work for acute care hospitals, private laboratories, physicians' offices, clinics, ambulatory care, health maintenance organizations, public health agencies, pharmaceutical firms, and research institutions (Figure 2–18). Their work requires a lot of walking, standing, reaching, stooping, lifting, and carrying of equipment. In addition, they need good eyesight for close work. They work indoors and may be exposed to unpleasant odors and body fluids and

FIGURE 2–17. One of the many duties of a laboratory aide is reading reagent strips.

FIGURE 2–18.

**SOME CAREER OPTIONS FOR
MEDICAL LABORATORY WORKERS**

Pathologist

Laboratory Supervisor

Laboratory Technologist

Laboratory Technician

Laboratory Assistant

Phlebotomist

Laboratory Aide

have frequent contact with water and cleaning solutions. Their jobs often require them to work shifts and weekends.

Laboratory Aides/Phlebotomists

Traits

■ Possess the ability to manipulate small objects, such as glass tubes and slides
■ Possess the ability and willingness to wash and repair glassware and equipment
■ Possess the ability to work under close supervision
■ Possess the ability to be precise and to follow rigid standards while performing job

Tasks

Laboratory Aides

■ Clean laboratory equipment
■ Prepare cleaning solutions
■ Dry glassware and instruments using a cloth, hot-air dryer, or acetone bath
■ Examine clean equipment for cracks or chips and store equipment properly

CAREER BASICS

MEDICAL LABORATORY WORKERS

	Education and/or Experience Required	Average Income
LABORATORY AIDE	✓ High school diploma or equivalent ✓ On-the-job training for at least two months ✓ Completion of a vocational education program as a laboratory aide	✓ Annual: $12,500–15,500
PHLEBOTOMIST	✓ High school graduate or equivalent ✓ 10- to 20-hour certification program in a hospital, physician's office, or laboratory ✓ Completion of a vocational education program as a phlebotomist	✓ Annual: $15,500–23,000
LABORATORY ASSISTANT BLOOD AND PLASMA	✓ High school diploma or equivalent ✓ Completion of an approved 12-month medical laboratory technician certificate program in a community college, vocational school, or private program	✓ Annual: $12,500–24,500
LABORATORY TECHNICIAN	✓ Two years of training in a community college, four-year college or university, or vocational/technical school ✓ Two years of training in a laboratory technician program ✓ Successful completion of requirements for certification (CLT) established by the National Certification Agency for Medical Laboratory Personnel	✓ Annual: $23,500–26,500
LABORATORY TECHNOLOGIST	✓ Graduate of four-year medical technology program in college or university ✓ Graduate of four-year medical technology program and certification (CMT) ✓ Successful completion of a written examination prepared by the Board of Registry of the American Society of Clinical Pathologists, Medical Technologists	✓ Annual: $32,500–45,000

	✓ Registered medical technologist (RMT)	
	✓ Successful completion of a written examination prepared by the International Society of Clinical Laboratory Technology	
LABORATORY SUPERVISOR, ADMINISTRATOR, OR CHIEF PATHOLOGIST, HISTOLOGIST, CYTOLOGIST	✓ Several years of experience as a medical technologist	✓ Annual: $70,000–120,000
	✓ Graduate education in one of the following: • Biological sciences • Chemistry • Management	
PATHOLOGIST	✓ Graduation from a medical school approved by the Council on Medical Education and Hospitals of the American Medical Association	✓ Annual: $70,000–120,000
	✓ State license to practice medicine or osteopathy	
	✓ Certification by the American Board of Pathology	

■ Operate an autoclave to sterilize equipment
■ Prepare stains, solutions, and culture media following appropriate procedures

Phlebotomists/Venipuncture Technicians
■ Draw blood from patients for testing by the technician or technologist

For more information, write
American Society of Blood Banks
8101 Glenbrook Road
Bethesda, MD 20814-2749

International Society for Clinical Laboratory Technology
917 Locust Street, Suite 1100
St. Louis, MO 63101-1413

Board of Certified Laboratory Assistants
9500 South California Avenue
Evergreen Park, IL 60642

Radiology Workers

Radiology workers operate x-ray equipment to take pictures of the internal parts of the body (Figure 2–19). The x-rays provide information for the diagnosis and treatment of patients. For example, x-rays of the chest help detect lung diseases, such as lung cancer and tuberculosis. Some of the diseases or injuries that x-rays help diagnose or treat are ulcers, blood clots, cancer, and fractures. The use of imaging techniques like ultrasound and magnetic resonance imaging (MRI) is

FIGURE 2–19. A radiologic technologist preparing to take an x-ray of a patient.

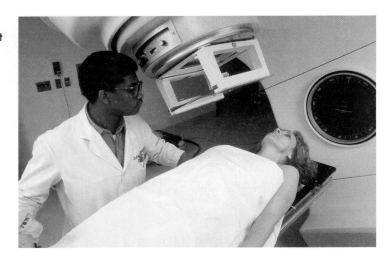

growing. The term *diagnostic imaging* includes these procedures as well as x-ray techniques.

Radiology workers have a variety of job opportunities and may work in general hospitals, physicians' offices, trauma centers, chiropractic offices, private consulting offices, clinics, federal and state agencies, public school systems, health maintenance organizations, and ambulatory care facilities (Figure 2–20). They work indoors and may be in confined areas. They wear protective gloves, aprons, and film badges because the hazards of radiation are present. Shift work and evening work may be part of their schedule. Their work requires the lifting and position-

FIGURE 2–20.

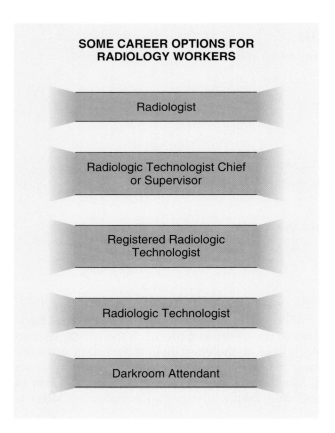

SOME CAREER OPTIONS FOR RADIOLOGY WORKERS

Radiologist

Radiologic Technologist Chief or Supervisor

Registered Radiologic Technologist

Radiologic Technologist

Darkroom Attendant

CAREER BASICS

RADIOLOGY WORKERS

	Education and/or Experience Required	Average Income
DIAGNOSTIC MEDICAL TECHNOLOGIST	✓ High school diploma or equivalent ✓ One-year certificate program ✓ No experience in health occupation	✓ Annual: $24,800–34,900
RADIOLOGIC TECHNOLOGIST/ SONOGRAPHER/ULTRASOUND	✓ Graduation from an accredited program	✓ Annual: $26,600–37,300
RADIOLOGIC TECHNOLOGIST CHIEF	✓ Bachelor's degree in radiologic technology ✓ Experience in two or more radiologic disciplines (e.g., nuclear medicine, radiation therapy) ✓ Should be registered as a radiologic technologist through the American Registry of Radiologic Technologies (ARRT)	✓ Annual: $25,000–50,000
RADIOLOGIST	✓ Graduation from an accredited medical school ✓ License to practice medicine in the state of employment ✓ Three years of special training in radiology recognized and approved by the board and by the Council on Medical Education and Hospitals of the American Medical Association	✓ Annual: $70,000–120,000

ing of patients, standing during most of the shift, and pushing mobile equipment. They may be exposed to body fluids.

The career ladder in the radiology field does not have an aide or assistant position. The following information is included in this book because radiology is an important career for you to consider. Some facilities use transport aides in radiology. Being a transport aide in a radiology department allows you to learn about the radiology department.

Diagnostic Medical Sonographers

Diagnostic medical sonographers use diagnostic ultrasound under the supervision of a physician. They are also called *ultrasound technologists.* They use equipment to transmit sound waves at high frequencies into the patient's body, resulting in an image viewed on a screen and automatically recorded on a printout strip or video. The use of ultrasound is important in prenatal care and for cardiology.

Sonographers work in acute care hospitals, in clinics, and sometimes with a group of obstetrics specialists. They work five-day weeks and generally have weekends and evenings off.

FIGURE 2–21. An EKG technician performing an electrocardiogram.

For more information, write
American Society of Radiologic Technologists
15000 Central Avenue, SE
Albuquerque, NM 87123-3917

American Registry of Radiologic Technologists
1255 Northland Drive
Mendota, MN 55120

Society of Diagnostic Medical Sonographers
12770 Coit Road, Suite 708
Dallas, TX 75251

Electrocardiography Workers
Electrocardiographic Technicians

Electrocardiography workers operate an EKG machine to record the electrical changes that occur during a heartbeat (Figure 2–21). These recordings help physicians diagnose any irregularities or changes in the patient's heartbeat. These tests are done routinely after a certain age, before surgery, and as a diagnostic tool. EKG technicians also apply Holter monitors. EKG technicians have many job opportunities and work in acute care hospitals, clinics, private physicians' offices, health maintenance organizations, and ambulatory care facilities (Figure 2–22). They work indoors and may work shifts, evenings, and weekends. They spend a lot of their time standing and walking.

Electrocardiogram Technicians

Traits

■ Possess the ability to explain procedures to patients/clients
■ Possess the ability to coordinate eye and hand movements when recording electrocardiogram

FIGURE 2–22.

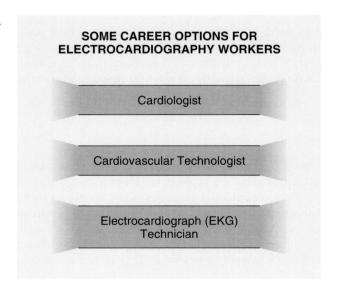

SOME CAREER OPTIONS FOR ELECTROCARDIOGRAPHY WORKERS

Cardiologist

Cardiovascular Technologist

Electrocardiograph (EKG) Technician

CAREER BASICS

ELECTROCARDIOGRAPHY WORKERS

	Education and/or Experience Required	**Average Income**
EKG TECHNICIAN	✓ High school diploma or equivalent ✓ One to six months of on-the-job training ✓ Completion of a vocational education program as an EKG technician ✓ One to two years of study at a community college	✓ Annual: $17,000–23,800
CARDIOVASCULAR TECHNOLOGIST	✓ Completion of a two-year community college program in cardiovascular technology ✓ Completion of a four-year college or university program	✓ Annual: $16,000–28,000
CARDIOLOGIST	✓ Graduation from an accredited school of medicine ✓ One-year internship ✓ One- to two-year residency in internal medicine ✓ One to two years of clinical fellowship in cardiology ✓ Passing grades on examinations for board certification in cardiology	✓ Annual: $70,000–200,000
ELECTROENCEPHALOGRAPHIC TECHNICIAN	✓ High school diploma or equivalent ✓ Twelve months (or more) of specialized training	✓ Annual: $23,200–30,000

■ Possess finger dexterity for attaching electrodes and adjusting equipment

■ Possess the interest in technical and scientific activities to relate testing to the meaning of the heart's activity

■ Prefer routine work

■ Possess the ability to act under pressure in an emergency

■ Possess the ability to deal with people and gain their cooperation

Tasks

■ Escort client to treatment room

■ Take portable equipment to patient's room

■ Explain the test procedure

■ Help client remove necessary clothing

■ Paste or attach electrodes to correct areas on patient's chest, arms, legs; connect leads from EKG machine to electrodes; and operate selector switch on EKG machine

- Reposition chest electrodes to record various positions
- Check recording for accuracy (leads placed incorrectly give an incorrect reading)
- Recognize significant deviations from normal heartbeat and report immediately
- Edit and mount final results
- Send copy of graph to the physician
- Maintain EKG records
- Type physician's diagnosis
- Care for equipment by cleaning electrodes and keeping all equipment well supplied with paper, etc.
- Conduct vectorcardiograms (multidimensional traces), stress testing (exercise tests), and pulse recordings
- Apply Holter monitoring (12- to 24-hour recording of an EKG)

For more information, write
National Society for Cardiovascular Technology
120 Falcon Drive, Suite 3
Fredericksburg, VA 22408

Electroencephalographic Technicians

Electroencephalographic technicians operate an electroencephalograph (EEG) that records the electrical changes that occur in the brain. These recordings help physicians diagnose any irregularities of the electrical impulses in the brain. These changes can occur from disease, injury, brain tumors, stroke, epilepsy, and other neurological changes. They also help with sleep disorders and identifying organic problems like Alzheimer's.

EEG technicians work in acute care hospitals, in neurologists' offices, and in some ambulatory care facilities. EEG technicians usually work in clean environments. They spend about half of their working hours on their feet. They usually work a five-day workweek but may have weekend or after-hours "on-call" time.

Traits

- Possess the ability to explain procedures
- Possess the ability to coordinate eye and hand movement and finger dexterity
- Possess the desire to work with people
- Possess an interest in technical and scientific activities

Tasks

- Record patient's history as relevant to the test
- Apply electrodes properly, operate EEG machine, and record outcome in client's chart

For more information, write
American Society of Electroneurodiagnostic Technologists
204 West Seventh Street
Carroll, IA 51401
http://www.aset.org

■ INFORMATION SERVICES

Information service workers are an important support to all other medical services. These workers analyze, **extract,** and document information using automated systems. They understand the sources, routes, and flow of information within the health care environment.

extract Identify and take out or emphasize.

Administrative Support Service Workers

Administrative support service workers (medical clerical workers) handle complaints, interpret and explain policies or regulations, prepare payrolls, resolve billing disputes, and collect delinquent accounts. They are responsible for the everyday situations that medical organizations must deal with smoothly and efficiently to maintain business operations and good customer service. The following list of occupations are included in administrative support services. See Chapter 19 for more detailed information on these services.

- Claim representative
- Insurance processor or enrollment clerk
- Billing and account collector
- Clerical worker
- Computer or data processor
- Receptionist
- Appointment scheduler
- Material/supply and distribution clerk or purchasing clerk
- Payroll and timekeeping clerk
- Personnel clerk
- Secretary or word processor
- Telephone operator

Admitting Department Workers

Admitting department workers are responsible for the admitting and discharging of patients. They interview patients/clients for information necessary for accurate record keeping (Figure 2–23). The workers in the admitting department are

FIGURE 2–23. One of the many duties of an admitting clerk is interviewing patients/clients.

usually the first hospital employees that the patient sees. Employees in this department help the patient feel confident about the hospital and the care that they will receive.

Admitting workers have a variety of job opportunities and work in an acute care hospital (Figure 2–24). They may assist with lifting patients and carrying their belongings. They may also push wheelchairs or stretchers. Their work is in an office environment and requires sitting and reaching. They may work shifts and evenings.

Admitting Clerks

Traits

■ Possess the ability to understand written admitting procedures
■ Possess the clerical ability to fill out forms and work with business forms and contracts
■ Possess the ability to ask questions in order to compile and evaluate information
■ Enjoy communicating with other professionals and patients/clients
■ Possess the politeness and understanding to deal with clients who may be anxious or in pain

Tasks

■ Interview incoming patients/clients and record information required for admission
■ Assign rooms
■ Prepare identification band
■ Explain hospital rules and policies
■ Store patients' valuables in hospital safe and arrange escort to room
■ Send admitting forms to appropriate departments
■ Prepare daily census and preadmission forms and arrange transfers
■ May act as cashier and receptionist (depending on the size of the facility)
■ Use a computer for records

FIGURE 2–24.

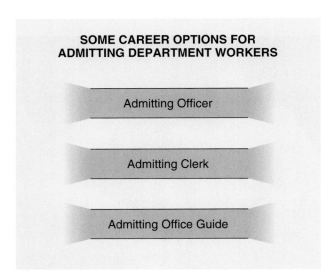

SOME CAREER OPTIONS FOR ADMITTING DEPARTMENT WORKERS

Admitting Officer

Admitting Clerk

Admitting Office Guide

CAREER BASICS

ADMITTING DEPARTMENT WORKERS

	Education and/or Experience Required	Average Income
ADMITTING CLERK	✓ High school diploma or equivalent ✓ Computer skills ✓ One to two months of on-the-job training	✓ Annual: $11,000–21,500
ADMITTING OFFICER	✓ High school diploma or equivalent ✓ Bachelor's degree ✓ Two to three months of on-the-job training ✓ One to two years of experience working in a health care facility (may be required)	✓ Annual: $15,500–27,000

For more information, write
American Hospital Association
840 North Lake Shore Drive
Chicago, IL 60611

Medical Records/Health Information Management Workers

Medical records/health information management workers keep permanent records that describe the patient's condition and the treatment that he or she receives.

Physicians and allied health personnel use medical records to provide care for the patients. Medical records are also legal documents that can be used in a court of law. Insurance companies use the records to determine what they will pay for the patient's care. Records are used in medical research, as well.

Medical records must be accurate and carefully filed (Figure 2–25). Medical records/health information management workers have many job opportunities and are employed by acute care hospitals, long-term care hospitals, public health departments, manufacturers of medical record systems, and insurance companies (Figure 2–26).

Medical records/health information management specialists may have a private practice as a consultant. Their work requires frequent reaching and stretching for files, long periods of time at a desk, and some lifting of records.

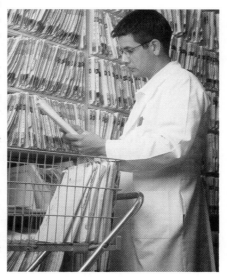

FIGURE 2–25. One of the many duties of a medical records/health information management file clerk is filing and pulling medical records.

FIGURE 2–26.

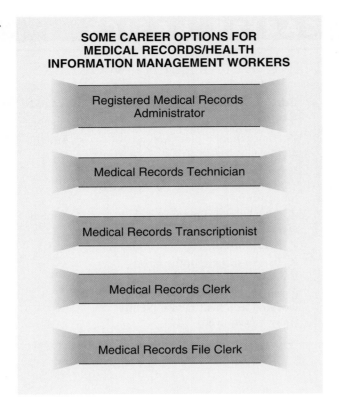

SOME CAREER OPTIONS FOR
MEDICAL RECORDS/HEALTH
INFORMATION MANAGEMENT WORKERS

Registered Medical Records
Administrator

Medical Records Technician

Medical Records Transcriptionist

Medical Records Clerk

Medical Records File Clerk

Medical Records/Health Information Management Clerks

Traits
■ Possess the ability to understand medical terminology, read and understand written medical reports, and separate out information from records
■ Possess the desire to do routine, organized work and follow set procedures and processes
■ Possess the ability to file, sort, and compile statistical reports

Tasks
■ File and pull medical records
■ Maintain a sign-out system for records
■ Update index file of patients and check for prior records of newly admitted clients
■ File cards according to established system and file medical records by numerical system
■ Answer routine staff requests for information about patients
■ Gather statistics for state health department
■ Transcribe reports of operations, x-rays, and laboratory examinations

For more information, write
American Health Information Management Association
919 North Michigan Avenue, Suite 1400
Chicago, IL 60611-1683
http://www.ahima.org

CAREER BASICS

MEDICAL RECORDS/HEALTH INFORMATION MANAGEMENT WORKERS

	Education and/or Experience Required	Average Income
MEDICAL RECORDS/HEALTH INFORMATION MANAGEMENT FILE CLERK	✓ High school diploma or equivalent preferred ✓ On-the-job training ✓ Completion of a vocational education program in the area of admitting file clerk	✓ Annual: $10,000–18,000
MEDICAL RECORDS/HEALTH INFORMATION MANAGEMENT CLERK	✓ High school diploma or equivalent ✓ Typing and filing skills ✓ Knowledge of office methods and medical terminology ✓ Three to six months of on-the-job training ✓ Completion of a vocational education program in the area of medical records clerk	✓ Annual: $10,000–18,000
MEDICAL TRANSCRIPTIONIST	✓ High school diploma or equivalent ✓ On-the-job training ✓ Completion of a vocational education program in the area of medical transcriptionist ✓ Completion of a correspondence course	✓ Annual: $14,000–30,000
MEDICAL RECORDS TECHNICIAN (ART)	✓ Graduation from a program accredited by the American Health Information Management Association (AHIMA) or the AHIMA Independent Study Program and a passing grade on the AHIMA certification exam	✓ Annual: $21,000–31,200
REGISTERED MEDICAL RECORDS ADMINISTRATOR (RRA)	✓ Bachelor's degree from an accredited college program ✓ Passing grade on the certification examination given by the American Health Information Management Association	✓ Annual: $30,200–48,000

Unit Secretaries and Health Unit Coordinators

Unit secretaries and health unit coordinators are responsible for clerical, reception, and communication duties in the nursing unit. One of their main duties is to transcribe physicians' orders. Health unit coordinators are essential to the nursing units, as they relieve the nursing staff of many duties. This gives the nurses more time to devote to patient care.

FIGURE 2–27.

Health unit coordinators have various career options and may be employed in acute care hospitals, long-term care facilities, and clinics (Figure 2–27). Their work is indoors in a clean environment. They may work shifts and weekends. Their work requires sitting at a desk for long periods of time, frequent telephoning, and reaching for and handling charts.

Health Unit Coordinators

Traits

■ Possess the ability to understand routines and instructions
■ Possess the ability to enter numerical and written data correctly on clients' charts
■ Possess the desire to establish a routine in keeping charts
■ Possess the ability to prepare schedules

Tasks

■ Transcribe physicians' orders
■ Prepare and compile records, including patient's name, address, and names of attending physicians
■ Copy information into charts, including patients' temperature, pulse, respiration rate, and blood pressure
■ Prepare requisitions for laboratory tests (e.g., special procedures, diagnostic tests, pharmaceutical orders)
■ Order necessary supplies for the client
■ Answer patients' call lights and send appropriate person for request
■ Provide physicians with clients' charts, check charts for new orders, and keep charts up-to-date
■ Use a computer if applicable

For more information, write
National Association of Health Unit Clerks/Coordinators
709 West Seldon Lane
Phoenix, AZ 85021

CAREER BASICS

HEALTH UNIT COORDINATORS

	Education and/or Experience Required	Average Income
UNIT SECRETARY/HEALTH UNIT COORDINATOR	✓ High school diploma or equivalent ✓ Community college ✓ Hospital training program ✓ Completion of a vocational education program in the area of unit secretary or health unit coordinator	✓ Annual: $10,900–19,000
MANAGER OF HEALTH UNIT COORDINATORS	✓ High school diploma or equivalent ✓ Associate's degree from a community college in unit management as a health unit coordinator	✓ Annual: $14,000–23,000

■ ENVIRONMENTAL SERVICES

Environmental service workers provide a therapeutic environment for the delivery of care. They repair and maintain medical and general equipment, follow aseptic procedures, and ensure high-quality food.

Central Processing/Supply Workers

Central processing/supply workers supply various departments with equipment and materials (Figure 2–28). The equipment must be in working condition. Malfunctioning equipment is life threatening. The workers keep an inventory of supplies and equipment. Supplies and equipment are properly packaged, cleaned, and sterilized. The workers in this department are key members of the health care team (Figure 2–29). Other health care workers cannot give necessary care without proper tools. Central processing/supply workers work in acute care hospitals and large outpatient clinics. The department is often in a basement or at the rear of the building. Lifting and moving articles and equipment are required. The workers stand on their feet for long periods of time and may be exposed to body fluids.

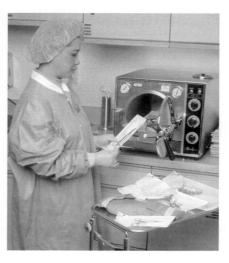

FIGURE 2–28. A central supply worker loading an autoclave.

FIGURE 2–29.

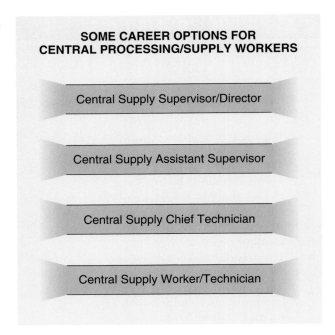

SOME CAREER OPTIONS FOR
CENTRAL PROCESSING/SUPPLY WORKERS

Central Supply Supervisor/Director

Central Supply Assistant Supervisor

Central Supply Chief Technician

Central Supply Worker/Technician

Central Processing/Supply Technicians

Traits

■ Possess the ability to count correctly so that trays and dressings are assembled with the correct number of items

■ Possess some clerical abilities to maintain records and prepare labels correctly

■ Possess manual and finger dexterity for proper handling of equipment and supplies

■ Possess the ability to identify color for recognition of equipment and its location

CAREER BASICS

CENTRAL PROCESSING/SUPPLY WORKERS

	Education and/or Experience Required	Average Income
TECHNICIAN	✓ High school diploma or equivalent ✓ On-the-job training (three to six months) ✓ Completion of a vocational education program as a central supply technician	✓ Annual: $10,500–18,300
CHIEF TECHNICIAN	✓ On-the-job experience	✓ Annual: $12,500–22,000

■ Possess desire to work with equipment, do repetitive procedures, and perform routine cleaning and assembling tasks

■ Possess the ability to be alert and accurate in following set procedures and rules

Tasks

■ Use solutions to scrub and wash surgical instruments, containers, syringes, and equipment

■ Sterilize articles (e.g., instruments, equipment, linens) using the steam autoclave, gas autoclave, or antiseptic solution

■ Prepare packs of supplies, instruments, dressings, and treatment trays; carefully wrap, label, and seal each pack

■ Store and inventory prepared articles, supplies, and equipment

■ Fill requisitions (gathering supplies and equipment as requested) and post charges

■ Check expiration dates on sterilized materials

For more information, write
American Hospital Association
840 North Lake Shore Drive
Chicago, IL 60611

Hospital Cleaners (Housekeepers)/Environmental Services Technicians

Housekeepers are responsible for the cleanliness of the environment (Figure 2–30). Cleanliness helps prevent the spread of infection and creates a more pleasant environment for patients/clients, staff, and visitors.

Hospital cleaners (housekeepers)/environmental service workers have many job opportunities and work in long-term care facilities, acute hospitals, and clinics (Figure 2–31). They have frequent contact with water and cleaning solutions. They walk, stand, and stoop during their shift. They also push and pull equipment, climb on ladders when necessary, and may be exposed to body fluids. Their hours may include shift work and weekend work.

FIGURE 2–30. A housekeeping attendant cleaning public areas, one of housekeeping's many duties.

FIGURE 2–31.

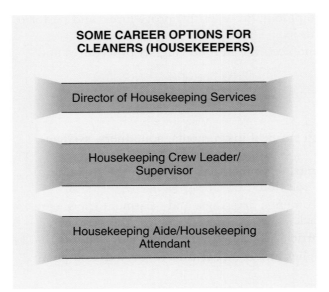

SOME CAREER OPTIONS FOR
CLEANERS (HOUSEKEEPERS)

Director of Housekeeping Services

Housekeeping Crew Leader/
Supervisor

Housekeeping Aide/Housekeeping
Attendant

CAREER BASICS

HOUSEKEEPING WORKERS

	Education and/or Experience Required	Average Income
HOUSEKEEPING AIDE/ ATTENDANT	✓ One to three months on-the-job training ✓ Completion of a vocational education program	✓ Annual: $10,900–18,750
HOUSEKEEPING CREW LEADER/SUPERVISOR	✓ High school diploma or equivalent ✓ Completion of courses in hospital housekeeping and institutional management ✓ One to four months of on-the-job training ✓ Up to two years of experience as a housekeeping attendant ✓ Completion of a vocational education program	✓ Annual: $12,000–23,000
DIRECTOR OF HOUSEKEEPING SERVICES	✓ High school diploma or equivalent ✓ College degree in housekeeping management or completion of courses in housekeeping and institutional management ✓ Experience in the housekeeping department	✓ Annual: $18,000–40,000

Hospital Cleaners/Housekeeping Attendants

Traits

- Possess the ability to perform such tasks as dusting, scouring, and polishing
- Possess a willingness to do routine, repetitive activities
- Possess a preference for working with objects
- Possess an ability to accept supervision while doing repetitive work

Tasks

- Load service cart
- Clean assigned areas (e.g., rooms, offices, laboratories)
- Dust, vacuum, and clean blinds, floors, furniture, and equipment
- Polish floors using a buffing machine
- Wash walls, ceilings, windows
- Empty ashtrays and trash
- Scour sinks, tubs, and mirrors
- Disinfect bedsprings and unit equipment
- Replenish soap and towels
- Replace cubicle curtains and soiled draperies
- Report malfunctioning equipment
- Move furniture, equipment, and supplies and turn mattresses

For more information, write
Institute of Sanitation Management
1710 Drew Street
Clearwater, FL 33515

National Executive Housekeepers Association
204 Business and Professional Building
Second Avenue
Gallipolis, OH 45631

Food Service Department Workers

Food service workers are responsible for providing nutritional care to clients. They plan special and balanced diets. They also distribute menus, prepare food trays, and deliver food to the patients throughout the hospital (Figure 2–32).

Food service workers have many career options and may work in acute care hospitals and in long-term care facilities (Figure 2–33). They generally work 40 hours a week and may work in shifts. The areas might be very warm, with much activity in a relatively small area. Some lifting, reaching, moving of equipment, and occasional bending are required. They walk and stand most of the shift.

Food Service Workers

Traits

- Possess hand and finger dexterity, as well as coordination for handling dishes, trays, and food
- Possess a desire to work in a routine, organized manner, dealing with objects and following specific procedures

FIGURE 2–32.
One of the many duties of a food service worker is preparing meals.

Tasks

■ Prepare and deliver food trays to patients/clients

■ Read color-coded menu cards to determine appropriate items to place on trays

■ Measure food servings according to diet list; prepare individual servings of salad, desserts, sandwiches

FIGURE 2–33.

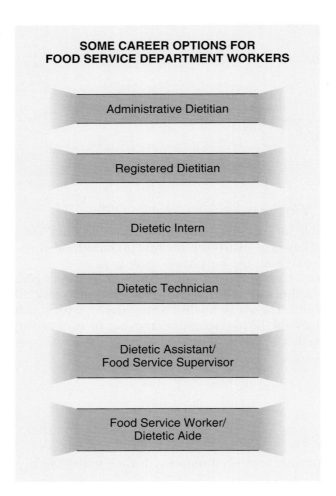

SOME CAREER OPTIONS FOR FOOD SERVICE DEPARTMENT WORKERS

Administrative Dietitian

Registered Dietitian

Dietetic Intern

Dietetic Technician

Dietetic Assistant/ Food Service Supervisor

Food Service Worker/ Dietetic Aide

CAREER BASICS

FOOD SERVICE DEPARTMENT WORKERS

	Education and/or Experience Required	Average Income
FOOD SERVICE WORKER/ DIETETIC AIDE	✓ On-the-job training ✓ Completion of a vocational education program as a food service worker	✓ Annual: $12,000–16,400
DIETETIC TECHNICIAN	✓ Completion of a dietetic technician program in a community college	✓ Annual: $15,000–24,000
DIETETIC INTERN	✓ Bachelor's degree with a major in foods and nutrition or institutional management	✓ Annual: $20,000–31,000
REGISTERED DIETITIAN	✓ Bachelor's degree with a major in foods and nutrition or institutional management ✓ Six- to 12-month internship in a dietary department	✓ Annual: $35,300–45,000
ADMINISTRATIVE DIETITIAN	✓ Must be a registered dietitian ✓ Graduate study credits in institutional or business administration	✓ Annual: $40,000–60,000

■ Prepare foods for soft or liquid diets using a blender
■ Check trays for accuracy and completeness, push food tray carts to client floors, and serve trays to patients (according to hospital policy)
■ Return food tray carts to kitchen
■ Clean work area, wrap silverware, and restock condiments for tray line

For more information, write
American Dietetic Association
216 West Jackson Boulevard, Suite 800
Chicago, IL 60606-6995
http://www.eatright.org

American Home Economics Association
2010 Massachusetts Avenue, NW
Washington, DC 20036

■ ADDITIONAL HEALTH CARE AREAS

There are many other positions in the health care area. You may use the skills that you have learned in Unit 1 to do a career search for other areas that interest you. Here are some suggestions for you to consider in the health-related field:

Dental Occupations

- Dental ceramist

Medical Practitioners

- Chiropractor
- Ophthalmologist
- Optometrist
- Osteopath
- Physician (all specialties)
- Physician's assistant
- Veterinarian

Medical Technologists, Technicians, Assistants, and Aides

- Artificial plastic-eye maker
- Audiometrist
- Cardiopulmonary technician
- Chiropractor
- Contact lens technician
- Cytotechnologist
- Dialysis technician
- Electroencephalographic (EEG) technologist
- Heart-lung machine operator/perfusionist
- Mental health worker
- Mental retardation assistant
- Operating room technician
- Optometric assistant
- Orthopedic technician
- Orthotist
- Physician's assistant
- Prosthetic aide
- Psychiatric aide
- Surgical technician/assistant
- Transporter
- Ultrasound technologist/sonographer
- Veterinarian's assistant

Nursing Occupations

- Licensed psychiatric aide
- Midwife
- Nurse anesthetist
- Nurse practitioner

Therapy and Rehabilitation Occupations

- Alcoholic rehabilitation center attendant
- Audiologist
- Dance therapist
- Kinesiotherapist
- Music therapist
- Recreation therapist
- Speech pathologist

Other Health-Related Occupations

- Clinical engineer and biomedical equipment technician
- Director of volunteer services
- Dispensing optician
- Funeral director
- Grounds maintenance and facilities worker
- Health service administrator
- Insurance clerk
- Medical illustrator
- Medical writer
- Morgue attendant/embalmist
- Nursing home administrator
- Optometrist
- Orthodontist
- Podiatrist
- Prosthetist
- Social service worker
- Speech pathologist
- Transporter

■ SUMMARY

In this unit, you reviewed many health occupations. You learned that each occupation has different tasks and different education requirements. You also learned that different occupations require different traits in the worker. With this information, you can evaluate an occupation before you research it carefully. Use the information in Unit 1 to research any occupational area.

CHAPTER REVIEW *Your link to success*

Thinking Critically: Check Your Understanding

1. **Communication** How does your ability to communicate affect those around you? What are you doing to increase your ability to communicate effectively?

2. **Legal and Ethical** Give an example of each of the following:
   a. Legal considerations that relate to becoming a health care worker **b.** Ethical dilemmas that a health care worker may face

3. **Cultural Competency** Cultures throughout our communities are very different. In the health care environment, we also experience a variety of cultures. Identify the services and departments that require workers to have the ability to interact effectively with people from other cultures. Explain your reasoning.

4. **Case Study** Glenda needs to find a good job as soon as she graduates. She is unsure about how to find the right career. She must earn enough to pay for an apartment, a car, living expenses, and leisure activities. She wants a position that is well respected, provides a clean environment, and offers potential for professional growth. She enjoys working with people and feels really good when she is able to help others. List the steps Glenda should take to help her identify the best career options for her.

Portfolio Connection

The following provides a guideline for creating the structure of your portfolio. When you are done you can add and exchange documents as you complete them. Keeping your file current shows your organizational skills and provides you immediate access to materials that reflect the positive results of your learning. To create your portfolio follow the instructions on Worksheet 7 of your student workbook, you must acquire a three-ring notebook, three-ring pocket inserts and tab dividers. Label each tab with the following:

Portfolio
- Title page
- Table of contents
- Letter of introduction
- Résumé
- Letter(s) of recommendation
- Advanced training or college requirements
- Certificates/licenses
- Skills check-off sheets

- Practical experience evaluation
- Evaluation of paid or unpaid time working in your vocation
- Written reports and assignments in your vocation area
- Final portfolio checklist

Once your portfolio file is organized, it is ready for your work samples. Add work evaluations from current or previous jobs and keep this file in a place that is easy to access.

3 MEDICAL ETHICS AND LAW

Ethical Roles and Responsibilities of a Health Care Worker

Steps to success

1. Complete Vocabulary Worksheet 1 in the Student Workbook.
2. Read this unit.
3. Complete Worksheets 2 through 5 as assigned.
4. When you are confident that you can meet each objective for this unit, ask your instructor for the unit evaluation.

Rationale

Members of the health care team must be aware of their ethical roles and responsibilities. This awareness protects them, the patients, their co-workers, and the facility where they work. Ethical behavior ensures quality patient care, positive work relationships, and a well managed workplace environment.

Objectives

When you have completed this unit, you will be able to do the following:

✓ Match vocabulary words with their correct meanings.
✓ Summarize the code of ethics that every health care worker follows.
✓ Explain why following a code of ethics is important.
✓ Use the value indicators to explain the employee's responsibilities to his or her employer.
✓ Explain how each health care worker affects the health care team.

■ VALUE INDICATORS

Quality health care workers show a commitment to certain values. Health care workers are expected to live by values that show others respect. You show respect by treating others with dignity, demonstrating a spirit of service, performing your duties with excellence, and treating others with fairness/justice. Each person determines how values are reflected in his or her day-to-day actions. An employer describes what values are important and how to reflect them while working. These descriptions are usually found in an employee handbook or policy and procedure book. These values are discussed in many parts of this text. As you read about these values write your thoughts in a diary, describing other attitudes and actions that reflect parts of the four values. The following is a brief description of these key values.

■ *Dignity.* You treat people with dignity when you are honest, truthful, trustworthy, and sincere. You are respectful of others. You always do what is needed to the best of your abilities and you ask for assistance when tasks are beyond your understanding or ability. Dignity is communicated through listening actively, being positive, showing understanding, and respecting all people.

■ *Service.* Service means responding to patients/clients and co-workers with an understanding of their unique needs. You show kindness and patience. Service also means making comments that are positive, courteous, and helpful.

■ *Excellence.* Performance excellence is taking responsibility for yourself, your team's decisions, and the results. You adapt to changing needs by learning new skills, knowledge, and behaviors that encourage continuous improvement. Accepting and seeking feedback help you improve your performance excellence.

■ *Fairness/Justice.* You treat all people with mutual respect and provide the same dignity, service, and performance excellence regardless of the patient's race, beliefs, ethnic background, or financial resources. You also use supplies and available resources effectively to provide **appropriate** care and a safe environment for everyone.

appropriate Suitable, correct.

   Health care workers reveal their core values and qualities in everything that they do. Tables 3–1 and 3–2 outline your responsibilities within each of the key value indicators for health care.

FIGURE 3–1. Good grooming is important.

TABLE 3–1   Code of Ethics

Ethics is a code of conduct representing ideal behavior for a group of people. A health care worker observes the following code of **ethics.**

Dignity	Service	Excellence	Fairness/Justice
Know your limitations. Know what you are trained to do and what you are capable of doing.	*Be a good citizen.* Respond to the needs of others. Demonstrate concern for meeting those needs.	*Be accountable.* Seek out and use feedback from others to learn. Take responsibility for yourself and for your team's actions, decisions, and results.	*Be loyal* to patients/clients, co-workers, and your employer. Always **project** a positive attitude toward the institution where you are employed.
Be sincere. Always be honest and trustworthy in the performance of your duties. Expect your salary in return for your work. Do not solicit gifts or additional money.	*Be caring.* Try to understand the unique needs of others. Respond quickly and effectively to problems that arise while you are working.	*Be informed.* Learn from your experiences. Seek growth and development opportunities for yourself and others.	*Respect the privacy of others.* Always keep privileged information about any personal or private matter **confidential.**
Be well-groomed. ☛ Always clean your uniform, shoes, hair, nails, skin, teeth, and body to prevent the spread of disease-causing bacteria. ☛ Be sure your uniform is free of wrinkles, tears, and runs. All buttons must match. Shoes and laces must be clean and bright. ☛ Wear a name tag. This helps people you work with know you and your title. It is required in most states. ☛ Do not wear excessive jewelry. It harbors bacteria and can cause you or your patients injury. Wedding rings and watches are acceptable. ☛ Never wear perfume or aftershave lotion. They make some people who are ill feel even worse.		*Follow the rules and regulations.* ☛ Read the policy manual. ☛ Read the procedure manual. ☛ Practice Standard Precautions and the Bloodborne Pathogen Rule.	

ethics Social values, conduct, description of what is right and wrong.

project To show or reflect.

confidential Private, personal, restricted, secret.

TABLE 3-2   Responsibilities of an Employee

Employees are required to assume certain responsibilities. The responsibilities that are most important to employers include being dependable, honest, and well-groomed (Figure 3–1); displaying a good attitude; and following the rules and regulations of the organization.

Dignity	Service	Excellence	Fairness/Justice
Communicate effectively. ☛ Express ideas, information, and viewpoints clearly. ☛ Use active listening skills, and seek to understand others. ☛ Create and maintain positive working relationships. ☛ Try to understand and respect differences in people. ☛ Be supportive of others' success when they do well.	*Have a good attitude.* ☛ Be willing to help your co-workers. ☛ Be aware of your body language and facial expressions, and reflect a positive outlook. ☛ Be respectful by changing your behavior when it appears to irritate others. ☛ Work effectively under pressure.	*Be dependable.* ☛ Be on time. ☛ Report in when you arrive. ☛ Report to the person taking care of your assignment prior to leaving your area. ☛ Do your job to the best of your ability. ☛ Call your supervisor ahead of time on those few occasions when you are unable to be at work.	*Be honest.* ☛ Never clock in or out for another person. ☛ Never take anything from the facility that is not yours. ☛ Never say that you have completed a task when you have not. ☛ Work with commitment and enthusiasm to improve the care patients/clients receive.

■ THE TEAM CONCEPT

Quality health care depends on every health care worker's doing his or her part. Each member is an important part of the **interdisciplinary** team. Professionals with different backgrounds, different education, and different interests all work together to provide appropriate quality care.

The registered nurse (RN) **delegates** duties to a team of licensed and unlicensed assistive personnel. The RN determines what tasks the members of the interdisciplinary team are assigned. The RN oversees health care workers from various departments and trains them to provide patient care and effectively delegates by using *the five rights of delegation:*

■ *Right task.* Identifying an appropriate caregiver-patient relationship.

■ *Right circumstances.* Verifying that the correct patient setting and resources are available.

■ *Right person.* Identifying a person who is trained and capable of doing the task.

■ *Right direction/communication.* Providing a clear, short description of the task and clarifying limitations and the expected result.

■ *Right supervision.* Providing appropriate monitoring, assistance, and **feedback.**

All departments are responsible for quality patient care, even if they are not providing hands-on care. For instance, if the medical records department fails to keep

interdisciplinary Involving two or more disciplines.

delegates Gives another person responsibility for doing specific tasks.

feedback Information received as a result of something done or said.

correct files of the patient/client chart, the physician will not have the test results and history needed to provide care. If housekeepers do not clean properly and bacteria are present, patients/clients may acquire additional diseases.

Remember: It is the team effort of all health care workers that provides service to the patient/client!

■ SUMMARY

responsibility One's answerability to an employer in areas such as dependability and honesty.

As a health care worker, you are part of a very important team. You must demonstrate many qualities both in the care of your patients/clients and in your **responsibility** to your employer. Health care workers are expected to conduct themselves in an ethical manner. Ethical behavior protects you, your patients/clients, their families, the staff, and your place of employment. Dignity, service, excellence, and fairness/justice are essential for every health care worker.

| UNIT 2 | Legal Roles and Responsibilities of a Health Care Worker |

*S*teps to success

1. Complete Vocabulary Worksheet 1 in the Student Workbook.
2. Read this unit.
3. Complete Worksheets 2 through 4 as assigned.
4. When you are confident that you can meet each objective for this unit, ask your instructor for the unit evaluation.
5. Complete "Your Link to Success" at the end of this chapter.

Rationale

Health care workers must be aware of their legal responsibilities for the protection of the patients/clients, their co-workers, their employers, and themselves. Health care workers may be brought to trial and held liable if they do not perform their duties in a legal manner.

Objectives

When you have completed this unit, you will be able to do the following:

✓ Match vocabulary words with their correct meanings.
✓ Explain the importance of the Patient's/Client's Bill of Rights.
✓ Explain living will, directive, advanced directive, durable power of attorney, and ombudsman.
✓ List three controls on health care workers.
✓ Explain "scope of practice."
✓ Match legal terms with their correct meanings.
✓ Explain why understanding legal responsibilities is important.
✓ Differentiate between policies and procedures.

■ LEGAL RESPONSIBILITIES

It is important for health care workers to remember that patients/clients have rights that represent not only moral and ethical issues, but also rights legislated by both federal and state governments. It is each health care worker's responsibility to recognize the importance of treating patients/clients with dignity. A list of patient/client rights is meaningless unless the person working with the patient understands and follows them. All health care workers must commit to giving the best possible care. The health care worker is legally bound to provide care as it is stated in the **Patient's/Client's Bill of Rights.** (See the Student Workbook for a copy of the Patient's/Client's Bill of Rights.)

Patient's/Client's Bill of Rights Document written by the American Hospital Association outlining expected patient/client rights while in a hospital.

Living Will, Directive, Advance Directive, Durable Power of Attorney, Ombudsman

For many years, patients/clients were not allowed to make decisions about death with dignity. Today, new laws allow them to have a say in how they want to live their last days.

Living Will

A patient/client may wish to sign a living will. The living will can tell the family and provider: **Do not resuscitate** me or take any measures to keep me alive. The living will protects the patient's/client's right to refuse treatment.

do not resuscitate Do not perform cardiopulmonary resuscitation (CPR).

Directive

A written directive gives the physician consent to follow the patient's/client's wishes. A patient can tell the provider not to use medical intervention and to let death occur naturally. The directive must follow certain rules:

■ A second provider must agree with the diagnosis of a terminal illness.
■ The directive must have been signed at least 14 days after the patient/client was told that he or she has a terminal illness.
■ The directive can be changed at any time by telling the provider.
■ A statement can be signed and dated by the patient/client asking to cancel the directive.

Advance Directive

An advance directive tells the provider and family what to do if the patient/client has a serious illness or injury. The written form tells what kind of treatment the patient/client wants if he or she cannot make his or her own decision; for example,

■ If he or she will be permanently unconscious
■ If prolonging life means being fed through a tube
■ If prolonging life means living in pain
■ If the treatment means always needing a machine, such as a respirator

The advance directive must be witnessed by two adults. They may not be the provider or the provider's employees, facility employees, or anyone who benefits from the death.

Durable Power of Attorney

The Durable Power of Attorney for health care is another type of instruction. It allows the patient/client to name someone to make treatment decisions for him or her. The patient/client can say what kind of treatment he or she wants and when he or she wants treatment stopped. Another type of Durable Power of Attorney allows an appointee to manage the patient's/client's financial affairs.

Ombudsman

An ombudsman is a social worker, nurse, or trained volunteer who makes certain that the patient/client is not abused and that the person's rights are secure.

Controls on Health Care Workers

Licensure, certification, and registration tell what a health care worker may or may not do. They determine the scope of practice for the health care worker. Controls help to improve the quality of care. Although not all health occupations require licensure, certification, or registration, it is important to be aware of these controls.

recognition Acknowledgment as being worthy of approval.

- *Licensure* is given by a governmental agency when a person meets the qualifications for a particular occupation.
- *Certification* is given for **recognition.** If specific guidelines must be met, the certification equals licensure.
- *Registration* is a list of individuals on an official record who meet the qualifications for an occupation (e.g., registered nurse, registered dental assistant).

Legal Terms and Boundaries

Health care workers need to understand how medical-legal problems affect them. Read the following terms. They explain how the health care worker can have a legal problem.

- *Assault* is a threat or an attempt to injure another person. *Example:* A health care worker threatens to hit a patient/client or co-worker.

resultant Resulting from an action.

- *Battery* is the unlawful touching of another person without his or her consent, with or without **resultant** injury. Assault and battery are often charged together because of the successful attempt to injure. *Example:* A health care worker hits a patient/client or co-worker.
- *Informed consent* is the permission granted by a person in his or her right mind who voluntarily gives consent for treatment. Written consent ensures that patients are informed of all risks and complications of the procedure before signing. *Example:* A patient is asked to sign a consent form for certain procedures in the hospital or physician's office. The procedure must not be done without consent.

omission Neglect of duty.

- *Crime* results from performing a forbidden act or from the **omission** of a duty commanded by a public law. This makes the offender liable to punishment by law. *Example:* A health care worker takes a patient/client or co-worker's belongings. Stealing from the workplace is a crime.

defamatory Statement that causes injury to another's reputation.

- *Libel* is writing **defamatory** matter about an individual or group to a third party. *Example:* A newspaper writes damaging information about a local health care institution. The newspaper cannot provide proof of the statement. The paper is charged with libel. What you write in a patient record could be libel if you make a statement such as, "Mr. M. is nasty."

■ *Slander* is a spoken statement of false charges or **misrepresentations** that defame or damage another's reputation. *Example:* A health care worker tells friends that a famous person was treated for a drug overdose when in fact he or she was treated for a serious medical problem.

■ *False imprisonment* is the holding or retaining of a person against his or her will. *Example:* A physician or a health care worker refuses to allow a patient to leave the hospital.

■ *Felony* is a serious crime that carries a penalty of imprisonment for more than one year and possibly the death penalty. *Example:* A health care worker withholds treatment for a terminally ill patient, which causes the patient's premature death.

■ *Invasion of privacy* is a civil wrong that unlawfully makes public knowledge of any private or personal information without the consent of the wronged person. *Example:* A health care worker gives personal information to a newspaper about a patient/client or co-worker.

■ *Malpractice* means "bad practice." It is care that leads to **faulty** practice or neglect. *Example:* A respiratory therapy aide dislikes cleaning equipment, so he **dismantles** each item and places it on the racks as though it were clean. This action leads to a serious infection in a patient/client.

■ *Negligence* is the failure to perform in a reasonably **prudent** manner. *Example:* A health care worker forgets to lock the brakes on a wheelchair, and the patient/client is injured.

■ *Privileged communication* concerns any personal or private information given by a patient/client to medical personnel that is **relevant** to his or her care. *Example:* A health care worker should consider all information in the chart as privileged communication (Figure 3–2).

■ *Reasonable care* is the legal **obligation** of health care workers. They must perform according to the standards of practice expected in their community for comparable workers. *Example:* A laboratory aide draws blood from a patient/client after watching the procedure several times and feeling **competent.** However, she was not taught to do the procedure. Therefore, reasonable care was not exercised.

■ *Sexual harassment* is defined by federal regulations as "unwelcome sexual advances, requests for sexual favors, and other verbal and physical contact of a sexual nature." Innocent remarks, inappropriate pictures, and written material can be perceived as sexual. You can guard against harassment accusations by not making personal remarks or sexual gestures and by not participating in sexually explicit discussions around co-workers. *Example:* A co-worker gets really close and frequently touches another person when talking. The closeness and physical touch may be interpreted as sexual harassment, even if it is innocent.

■ A *will* is a legal **document** that defines the **disposition** of property and takes effect after death. *Example:* A patient/client legally declares who will inherit his or her personal property.

■ Reportable incidents and conditions. The health care worker is obligated to file a confidential report to the county health department when child or adult abuse is suspected. Reports are also required when certain diseases are diagnosed. It is important to check your facility's policy and procedures book for a current listing of reportable diseases and the procedure for reporting abuse.

These definitions and examples provide the knowledge you need to avoid medical-legal problems.

misrepresentations Untruths; lies.

faulty Defective or imperfect.

dismantles Takes apart.

prudent Careful or cautious.

relevant Pertaining to, or having to do with, the patient/client.

obligation Moral responsibility (e.g., to give the best possible patient/client care, to be on time for work).

competent Capable or able to perform a skill or task.

document Written record.

disposition Act of disposing of (e.g., a person desires that his or her monies be given to an organization after his or her death).

FIGURE 3–2. All information about patients/clients is confidential.

Discuss patient information only with your supervisor. Do *not* discuss patient information with

■ Other patients
■ Relatives and friends of the patient
■ Visitors to the hospital
■ Representatives of news media
■ Fellow workers, except when in conference
■ Your own relatives and friends

■ CONFIDENTIALITY

Patient/client information is confidential. *Confidential* means "secret." Health care workers are obligated to protect and keep all patient/client information confidential. A good rule is to discuss a patient/client only when the discussion affects his or her care in some way—for example,

■ When you find candy with the belongings of a diabetic
■ When you find alcohol or medications with the belongings of a patient/client
■ When patients discuss areas of stress in their personal life, such as financial problems or relationship problems

A medical facility, a physician, or a health care worker can be fined, sued, or lose his or her job for sharing *any* information about patients/clients with others, including family members.

■ POLICIES AND PROCEDURES

manual Book with guidelines.

Successful health care workers are familiar with their employer's policies and procedures. Each facility or agency has a policy **manual** that explains the facility's or agency's rules and regulations, including

■ Holiday and vacation policy
■ Insurance and sick leave benefits
■ All other information concerning the operation of that business

A procedure manual explains the step-by-step method of performing tasks, including

■ How to take a temperature
■ How to fill out forms
■ How to package and wrap trays

The facility's policy and procedure manuals are the guidelines that health care workers must follow to do their jobs correctly. Remember your limitations, and do only those procedures that you were taught to do. Always follow your facility's code of ethics. When you follow your facility's policies and procedures, you protect patients, co-workers, your employer, and yourself.

■ SUMMARY

In this unit you learned about legal **boundaries** for health care workers. You also learned that confidentiality is an important part of staying within the legal boundaries. When health care workers perform their duties within these boundaries, they help prevent medical-legal problems. Policies are the guidelines that provide information about facility rules and regulations. Procedures tell you how to complete tasks the way your employer wants them done.

boundaries Legal limits (e.g., you may know how to perform a task, but you may not do it because you are limited by your license, certification, registration, or rules and regulations).

Thinking Critically: Check Your Understanding

1. **Communication** Being an effective communicator involves active listening, honesty, and assertiveness. Think about the last time you had to tell another person something unpleasant. Were your comments constructive or destructive? Explain in writing how you could change destructive comments into constructive ones. Use the health care value indicators to help you decide what and how to send your message.

2. **Legal and Ethical** A co-worker asks you to clock out for him at the end of the shift so he can leave early. Will you do it? Explain the reasoning for your decision. What you will tell your co-worker? Identify which value is in jeopardy.

3. **Cultural Competency** One of the members of your care team is having difficulty understanding directions given by the supervisor. Your co-worker speaks English, but it is her second language, and she frequently misinterprets instructions. How can you treat your co-worker with dignity while helping her understand the instructions?

4. **Patient Education** A patient/client asks about advance directives. Describe how you will respond.

5. **Case Study** Your patient/client did not take time to write a will while he was healthy. Now he is ill and afraid that he is going to die. He is very anxious and worried about how his family will be taken care of when he dies. Explain what steps you can take to resolve this worry and help reduce his anxiety.

6. **Computers** While searching for information in the computer about your patient/client, you see that your co-worker has an appointment with a heart specialist. What legal issues affect how you use this information?

Portfolio Connection

How you express what you value causes positive or negative responses from others. Your manner encourages open and sincere or closed and guarded responses. Your values and the way you express them affect your success in your occupation. The values discussed in this chapter provide basic guidelines for working closely with others in health care. Think about your most common behaviors. List behaviors you exhibit when you are happy and when you are sad. Compare those behaviors with behaviors that reflect the health care values discussed in this chapter. Write a clear explanation of three behaviors you display. Include

■ At least one behavior that best reflects health care values. Describe why the behavior fits the value.

■ At least one behavior that does not reflect health care values. Describe why the behavior does not fit the values.

Develop and describe a plan to change this behavior into a positive value-based action. Follow these guidelines when preparing your report:

- Use 8.5-by-11-inch paper.
- Type, word-process, or write neatly in ink.
- Use correct spelling and grammar.

Include the following in your action plan:

• Negative behavior, with an explanation about what makes it negative or outside the health care values discussed in this chapter • Action that changes the behavior, with an explanation about how it fits the health care values • Evaluation plan, including a time line to determine the final outcome of the action plan.

When your paper is perfect in format and grammar, place it in your portfolio in Section Four, "Written Samples."

4

MEETING YOUR NEEDS AND THE NEEDS OF OTHERS

UNIT 1	Holistic Health

Steps to success

1. Complete Vocabulary Worksheet 1 in the Student Workbook.
2. Read this unit.
3. Complete Worksheets 2 and 3 as assigned.
4. When you are confident that you can meet each objective for this unit, ask your instructor for the unit evaluation.

Rationale

Responsible health care promotes lifestyles that encourage wellness. It is important for the health care worker to understand that mind, body, spirit, and social involvement must be balanced. Understanding wellness promotes good health in the health care worker and in the patient/client.

Objectives

When you have completed this unit, you will be able to do the following:

✓ Define the vocabulary words.
✓ List three parts of holistic health.
✓ Explain wellness and preventive care.
✓ Compare holistic health to disease-oriented care.

■ HEALTH AND WELLNESS

The World Health Organization defines health as follows: "Health is a state of complete physical, mental and social well-being and not merely the absence of disease or **infirmity.**" This definition of health has been expanded with the recent growth and emphasis on **holistic** health. Today we think in terms of the body's working as a unit (mental, physical, social, emotional) to maintain and promote optimum wellness through daily actions. The World Health Organization definition of health gives the impression of perfection; wellness implies feeling good regardless of your infirmity or disease.

    In health care, *holistic* refers to the well-being of the whole person. It is important to meet physical needs and also mental and social needs when giving care. Holistic health care is a part of the wellness approach, which encourages good health. Understanding these needs helps you care for yourself and for your patients/clients.

infirmity Unsound or unhealthy state of being.

holistic Pertaining to the whole; considering all factors.

■ WELLNESS AND PREVENTIVE HEALTH CARE

Wellness and preventive health care emphasize keeping patients well, not waiting until they are ill to provide treatment. Health education is vital to helping clients maintain good health. A holistic approach includes all of the following:

■ *Physical fitness* makes us alert and energetic in activities of daily living. It gives us enough energy to enjoy leisure time and to respond when emergencies arise. It can be achieved through

• Routine physicals • Adequate rest • Good nutrition • Weight control • **Elimination** of waste • **Aerobic** exercise • Immunizations • Well-baby checks • Avoiding substance abuse, including

    • Drugs • Alcohol • Tobacco • Excessive food intake

elimination Process of getting rid of.

aerobic Requiring oxygen.

■ *Mental fitness* allows us to interact effectively with others and to feel balanced. Mentally healthy people

• Self-direct (being the captain of your own ship) • Have a sense of belonging • Trust their own senses and feelings • Accept themselves • Have **self-esteem** • Practice stress management

self-esteem Belief in oneself.

■ *Social well-being* allows us to feel comfortable with others and allows us to accept their behavior, attitudes, and beliefs as well as our own (Figure 4–1). It includes

• Enjoying companionship • Sharing ideas and thoughts • Having a sense of belonging • Showing enthusiasm for life

    Holistic health requires health care workers to promote physical, emotional, and social well-being. For example, a patient experiencing stomach pain may be referred to a psychologist if the physician suspects that the patient is under a lot of emotional stress. The psychologist may refer him to a biofeedback specialist for stress management. This process continues until the client's needs are met in all areas.

FIGURE 4–1. Enjoying companionship, sharing ideas, having a sense of belonging, and showing enthusiasm for life are vital to well-being.

■ JOBS AND PROFESSIONS

- ■ Psychologist
- ■ Psychiatrist
- ■ Social worker (rehabilitation worker)
- ■ Biofeedback specialist
- ■ Physician
- ■ Nurse
- ■ Parish nurse specialist
- ■ Acupressurist
- ■ Acupuncturist

■ SUMMARY

You have learned that the holistic approach to health is important because it includes all aspects of a person's well-being. When we are in balance physically, emotionally, and socially, we experience life in a positive way. The trend in health care is toward wellness and preventive care.

UNIT 2 Understanding Human Needs

Steps to success

1. Complete Vocabulary Worksheet 1 in the Student Workbook.
2. Read this unit.
3. Complete Worksheets 2 through 6 as assigned.
4. When you are confident that you can meet each objective for this unit, ask your instructor for the unit evaluation.

Rationale

Understanding a person's **physiological** and **psychological** needs is essential for every health care worker. Every person has needs that must be satisfied to maintain **stability.** Health care workers must be aware of these needs to maintain their own stability and to meet the needs of patients/clients and co-workers.

Objectives

When you have completed this unit, you will be able to do the following:

✓ Match vocabulary words with their correct meanings.
✓ Name four psychological needs that must be met to maintain stability.
✓ Name four physiological needs that must be met to maintain stability.
✓ Explain five benefits of pet-facilitated therapy.
✓ Match five defense mechanisms with the correct descriptions.
✓ Explain how you use defense mechanisms daily.

■ MEETING THE NEEDS OF PATIENTS/CLIENTS

Physiological Needs

Biological needs are the basic needs for survival. They include food, water, sleep, and elimination. Any one or several of these needs may be threatened by illness. Food and water are often withheld prior to surgery or other **procedures.** Sleep may be interrupted by the change of environment, unfamiliar noises, or **anxiety** when hospitalization is required. Elimination is frequently affected by a change in routine, foods, or medications. Although these changes are temporary, they do affect patients/clients.

   Communication: Explain to new patients/clients about mealtimes, how to request water or snacks, and any special orders for using the bathroom (for example, if they are on intake and output or sharing a bathroom). Always explain expected interruptions in routine as soon as possible. When sleep must be interrupted, inform the patient/client before he or she goes to sleep. It is important to adapt the way you communicate this information to patients/clients in accordance with their age or level of understanding. Show your commitment to treating others with dignity by using effective communication skills. Communicating to patients/clients how their biological needs will be met during their hospitalization helps eliminate fear and anxiety.

physiological Pertaining to normal body functions.

psychological Pertaining to the mind.

stability Ability to maintain a balance, both mentally and physically.

procedures Methods used to accomplish a desired result.

anxiety Upset or distress felt over a real or imagined problem.

therapies Methods of treatment of disease or injury (e.g., physical therapy, radiology, diet, nursing).

Safety needs are the need to feel secure and the need to avoid bodily harm and injury. When patients are ill, they may feel very insecure and frightened. They may be facing outpatient procedures they do not understand, such as injections or **therapies** that are frightening to them. They may be facing hospitalization for the first time and are afraid that they will be hurt or that they will die.

Geriatric clients have these fears, also. They may be entering a nursing home where they will stay for the rest of their lives. They wonder, "What will happen to me? How will I be treated? Will I be safe?"

Communication: Tell your patients/clients how to reach you or your co-workers when they need something. Explain the call system and the intercom. Reassure them when they are feeling unsafe. It is helpful to take a few minutes to sit with a person who is feeling insecure. Your reassuring presence and warm touch may be all he or she needs. Patients/clients entering a new living environment often require verbal reassurance. Always communicate this reassurance so it is understood by patients/clients regardless of their age or level of understanding. Show your commitment to service and treating others with dignity by always doing what you say you are going to do. This helps create a level of trust and builds a sense of security for patients/clients.

sensory Pertaining to the ability to hear, see, feel, smell, and taste.

Sensory *needs* include stimulation of the five senses (hearing, seeing, feeling, smelling, and tasting) as well as intellectual stimulation. When the senses are not stimulated, people lose touch with reality. Patients/clients often experience a loss of at least one of the senses. For example, when an intravenous feeding is necessary, the client may not be allowed to eat. When a patient is unable to eat, the senses of taste and smell are not stimulated. Patients may be unable to read because their sight has become blurred due to illness or medications.

Geriatric patients/clients may have lost one or more of these senses in the aging process. They may have difficulty hearing what you say to them. Their vision may be poor and may cause them to be fearful in a new environment. The loss of taste and smell may affect their appetite. These losses add to their loss of well-being. As a health care worker, you can help relieve these problems by being aware that sensory needs are important.

Communication: Communicating with patients/clients who are experiencing a sensory loss takes patience and imagination. Try some of the following to stimulate your patients. Patients with hearing loss can experience music by touching a speaker while it plays music. They can feel the rhythm vibrate through the speaker. Feeling-impaired patients usually lose feeling in their hands and feet. When it is reasonable, touch their face or arms with things that they want to feel, such as a warm towel. Patients with visual, smell, and taste impairments appreciate your clear description of colors, smells, or flavors in their environment. For example, you might say, "Remember the smell of turkey roasting and fresh bread baking? That's what it smells like today." When working with patients/clients, show your commitment to excellence by being sensitive and remembering to share these sensory stimuli often.

impaired Weakened; deteriorated; not functioning in the usual manner.

Motor activity involves the movement or exercise of the body. If this need is not satisfied, the body will not function properly. Patients may experience a loss in this ability for a variety of reasons. They may be too weak or too sick to exercise, or a limb may be **impaired.**

Geriatric clients may have disorders of the joints that affect mobility. They may also have difficulty with balance. In many cases, they need to use a cane or a walker. Degeneration of the nervous system often causes difficulty with coordination (e.g., getting food on the spoon and into the mouth). These problems only add to their **frustration.** As a health care worker, your awareness that the patient is frustrated helps you do a better job.

frustration Deep, chronic sense of insecurity.

Communication: Patients/clients who are experiencing difficulty moving around require special information. Keep them informed about how to reach you throughout the day. The first time you help move a patient, be sure to explain in detail how you will support and protect him or her. Patients who experience discomfort when changing positions or locations require appropriate pain control, frequent encouragement, and reassurance. Your commitment to service excellence makes an important difference with these patients. Share expected times for changing or moving your patients, and always follow through.

Psychological Needs

Adequacy and *security* are important needs. People must feel that they can handle any situation that arises in their lives. When these needs are not satisfied, depression and anxiety occur. Certainly, when a person is ill, these needs are threatened. Patients frequently lose control of their physical and emotional well-being. They are told what to do, when to do it, and how to do it.

Communication: When patients/clients feel inadequate or out of control, it is important to give them an opportunity to make decisions and choices whenever possible. Ask patients what they want to wear or what time they want to bathe. Allow them to decide to sit on the patio, in the dining room, or in the recreation area. Show your commitment to fairness/justice by providing opportunities for all patients/clients to make personal decisions.

Social approval and *self-esteem* needs must be satisfied. These include recognition and acceptance by other people. When these needs are not satisfied, emotional problems can occur. Self-esteem also includes the feeling that the person is worthwhile in his or her activities. When people become ill, they have a complete change in their routines. They may be responsible for the support of their household, and now they are unable to work. They may feel that they will have difficulty paying their bills or that they could lose their jobs. Your awareness of these concerns helps you understand your patients and lessens their anxieties and fears (Figure 4–2).

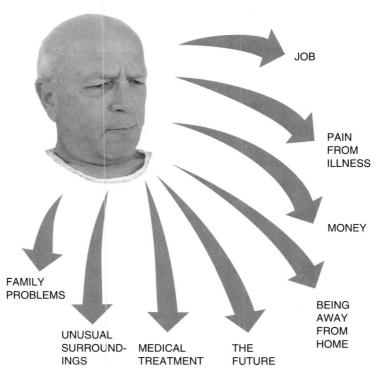

JOB

PAIN FROM ILLNESS

MONEY

BEING AWAY FROM HOME

FAMILY PROBLEMS

UNUSUAL SURROUND-INGS

MEDICAL TREATMENT

THE FUTURE

FIGURE 4–2.
Clients worry about many things when hospitalized.

Communication: It is important for you to be aware of resources available to assist patients/clients. When you recognize feelings of inadequacy in a patient, try to spend extra time with him or her. Use active listening skills and refer the patient to the appropriate resources, or talk to your supervisor. When you care for your patients/clients in this way, it reflects your excellence and service values.

Order and *meaning in life* include an understanding of what is going on in the environment. They help people know what to expect in the future. Illness often brings new and different experiences to patients. They are unable to understand all the tests and treatments. Since this is all new, they do not know what to expect or how to plan for the future. This results in worry and anxiety. It is your knowledge of this need and its possible loss that helps you deal in a more effective way with your patients.

Communication: Tell your patients/clients what to expect before, during, and after procedures. This helps them psychologically prepare for the experience. Patients/clients can also plan and prioritize their current and future needs more realistically when they have a sense of order and meaning. The values of dignity and excellence are evident when you communicate effectively and help your patients/clients meet their psychological needs.

Self-growth is a need for fulfillment beyond basic needs. When this need is not satisfied, the person continues to function but may feel that "something is missing." When clients are ill, they are concerned with meeting their basic needs; self-growth is frequently "put aside" temporarily.

Communication: Patients/clients who experience a long illness or physical changes that limit their abilities may experience a loss of personal growth. Use active listening skills to identify their special interests. Allow them to share the details of these interests. When appropriate, discuss possible options with the care team that will allow the patient/client to experience learning. Your service excellence and commitment to treating others with dignity are a reality when you take action in this way.

Understanding people's physiological and psychological needs helps you be a better health care worker. You are able to recognize the reasons for certain behaviors and respond appropriately to help meet your patients' needs. Always report evidence of all unmet needs to your supervisor. Your supervisor will determine what to include in the next patient care meeting. A plan will be determined concerning how to best meet the patient's/client's need.

■ PET-FACILITATED THERAPY

value Importance, worth.

There is a great deal of interest focused on the **value** of the human-pet bond. Recent studies show that petting or stroking a pet has an immediate effect on the body. Most people studied showed

- A slowing heartbeat
- Deeper breaths
- Fewer abnormal heartbeats
- Lowered blood pressure
- An increased sense of well-being

Over 50 percent of American households have pets in the home, primarily for the companionship that they provide. Research shows that even when people do not respond well to other people, they do respond to pets. They talk to their pets. They care for the needs of their pets. When there is a human-animal bond, the patient often finds new meaning in life. They feel less lonely. They feel needed because their pets are totally dependent on them. They have a reason to get out of the house to buy food for their pets. The pet may be just the friend or responsibility they need to help them feel better or to feel good about themselves. Research also shows that fish swimming gracefully in a pleasant aquarium with swaying plants creates a very relaxing environment that reduces stress.

All of this research has alerted the medical community to methods of providing new ways to promote healthier lifestyles through the companionship of pets. People who are experiencing many changes in their lives may find a pet to be the one unchanging element. Other people may be lonely and find that a pet is a good companion. Yet others may just enjoy the pleasure and presence of a pet.

In some places, pet-facilitated therapy is used as a treatment. Animals are taken into convalescent homes and children's hospitals. Some hospitals have arranged to have a pet live on the premises. Other programs have been developed with the Humane Society, and pets are brought in to visit on a regular basis. Hospitals are certainly only one place where pet-facilitated therapy is successful. It is especially effective in the home. An aging person may feel very depressed and alone. A pet brings new meaning to life. Now there is something that really needs him or her and is affectionate and loving. The same kind of therapy is effective for a sick child.

Pet-facilitated therapy has become a form of treatment. It is successful. When working with your patients, be alert to their needs. Perhaps a pet will meet a need that no other care can.

■ MEETING THE NEEDS OF CO-WORKERS AND OTHER STAFF

Recognizing human needs in your patients/clients makes you a better health care worker. Recognizing human needs in the staff you work with helps make you a successful member of the health care team.

Physiological Needs

When the *biological needs* of every staff member are not met, **friction** may occur. It is important to eat properly and to get adequate sleep. Many disagreements occur when people are irritable and easily upset because they failed to meet their biological needs.

friction Disagreement because of a difference of opinion.

It is important that every member of the staff have their *safety needs* met. They should feel secure and know that bodily harm can be avoided. As a staff member, always follow safety regulations, such as cleaning up spills, reporting damaged equipment, and taking care to protect others. When someone needs help lifting, help the person. This establishes a sense of safety for all the staff and creates a good working environment.

As a fellow staff member, it is important that you realize what the *sensory needs* are. This helps you understand fellow staff members who have sensory impairments. For instance, if a co-worker's hearing or sight is impaired, you need to be aware of this impairment. Your awareness allows you to be patient and to build a good working relationship.

Psychological Needs

Adequacy and *security* are important to all people. Your attitude toward other staff members is either cooperative or disruptive. When staff members work together, they establish a sense of a job well done.

rapport Harmony; a close relationship with another.

Social approval and *self-esteem* can be met in our relationships with our fellow employees. It is important that you develop **rapport** with other staff members. As you work together to create a healthy environment for the patients/clients and the staff, everyone feels accepted and worthwhile.

Order and *meaning* needs are met by the day-to-day activities on the job. If every staff member does his or her share and comes to work when scheduled, these needs are met.

The need for *self-growth* is met as you and the other staff members are able to accomplish your jobs and look toward promotion and new learning.

■ DEFENSE MECHANISMS

All people use defense mechanisms to help them feel more comfortable with themselves and to make their behavior seem reasonable. Defense mechanisms are mental devices that help people cope with various situations. Health care workers who are aware of defense mechanisms better understand themselves, their co-workers, their supervisors, and their patients' behavior. Following are some key defense mechanisms:

■ *Rationalization:* Finding good reasons to replace the real reason for behavior in order to maintain self-esteem. *Example:* Mark did poorly on a test and explained it by saying, "I'd rather be popular than smart."

■ *Compensation:* Substituting one goal for another. *Example:* Mary really wanted to be on the track team but wasn't good enough. Instead, she joined the choir and became a soloist.

■ *Projection:* Placing the blame for your actions on someone or something else because you cannot accept the responsibility. *Example:* "I didn't get a good grade in my health occupations class because the teacher doesn't like me."

aggressiveness Tendency to start fights and quarrels or to attack without reason.

■ *Sublimation:* Redirecting feelings toward a constructive objective. *Example:* You enjoy playing tennis and you use the game to work out **aggressiveness** and **hostility** instead of directing those feelings toward others.

■ *Identification:* **Idolizing** someone you would like to be like. *Example:* Margaret especially admired her music teacher. She began to walk and dress like her.

hostility Unfriendliness; ill will toward another.

idolizing Loving to excess.

When you are aware that everyone uses defense mechanisms, and when you know what they are, you are able to understand your behavior and the behavior of others. As a health care worker, it is important for you to realize that a defense mechanism may be involved in certain behavior. This allows you to give better care. Your knowledge of defense mechanisms also helps you understand the behavior of the people with whom you work.

■ SUMMARY

You have learned that human beings have physiological needs, which include biological needs, safety needs, sensory needs, and motor activity needs. They also have psychological needs, which include the need to feel adequate and secure, to have social approval and self-esteem, to have order and meaning in life, and to experience self-growth. These needs must be met at all times. It is important that we are always aware of these needs in our patients/clients, our co-workers, our supervisors, and ourselves. You have also learned that all people use defense mechanisms to help them feel comfortable inside. These include rationalization, compensation, projection, sublimation, and identification.

UNIT 3 Cultural Competency

Steps to success

1. Read this unit.
2. Complete Worksheets 1 through 5 as assigned.
3. When you are confident that you can meet each objective for this unit, ask your instructor for the unit evaluation.
4. Complete "Your Link to Success" at the end of this chapter.

Rationale

Health care workers **interact** with people from many cultural backgrounds. It is important to know culturally acceptable and effective gestures, terms, and behaviors. This knowledge allows the health care worker to adapt his or her care and communication techniques. The patient/client receives quality care, and the experience is positive.

interact To work together; to have an impact on each other.

Objectives

When you have completed this unit, you will be able to do the following:

✓ Explain how culture influences behavior.
✓ Identify culturally acceptable and effective gestures, terms, and behaviors.
✓ Recognize communication techniques that create a positive exchange of information.
✓ Identify common folk medicine practices.
✓ Compare and contrast cultural differences.
✓ Explain how understanding cultural beliefs affects you as a health care worker.

■ CULTURE AND BEHAVIOR

When caring for and working with people from different cultures, you must understand their cultural background. Understanding allows you to have positive experiences and to communicate effectively. Our understanding and opinions of other cultures develop through our environmental influences. Some environmental influences are

■ People (e.g., parents, friends, and others with whom we come in contact)
■ Places (e.g., home, school, place of worship, workplace)
■ Experiences (e.g., what you see, read, hear, and do and what happens to you)

Because of these influences it is easy to **prejudge** and to form prejudices. Some prejudices include

prejudge To decide or make a decision before having the facts.

■ *Age prejudice.* A person is too old or too young.
■ *National prejudices.* A person comes from a foreign country.

FIGURE 4–3. Motioning with a finger for someone to come.

■ *Physical prejudices.* How the person looks different from you.
■ *Mental prejudice.* A person judges an individual by how smart a person is, how much a person knows, how well a person thinks.
■ *Religious prejudices.* A person's beliefs are different from yours.
■ *Racial prejudice.* A person belongs to a different race than you.

You can control prejudice by learning about others. Here are some suggestions:

■ Keep an open mind.
■ Look for additional information. Why do people think the way they think? (For example, why does someone think people of another culture are lazy or not smart?)
■ Read books, magazines, and newspapers for information.
■ Look at many resources before you form an opinion.
■ Evaluate all the information. Is it true? Is it false?

Now decide what your opinion is.

Our behavior sends a message to others. They receive or understand the message by the way they interpret behavior. When more than one culture is involved, the interpretation of a behavior is often different. For example, to use the motion illustrated in Figure 4–3 to get a person to come is acceptable in the United States. In many other cultures, it is insulting and rude. Learning about communication in other cultures helps the health care worker understand the true meaning of behavior. This information allows you to respond with understanding.

■ GESTURES AND BODY LANGUAGE

Personal Space and Touching

Personal space and touching are defined in different societies as close contact and more distant contact. Personal space is the space needed to feel comfortable when we are with other people. Figures 4–4 to 4–6 show examples of societies where more distant contact is expected.

People in close-contact societies are comfortable with less space between them. There is more touching. It is important to use caution when touching. A touch can easily be misunderstood.

FIGURE 4–4. Two people talking intimately.

FIGURE 4–5. Personal distance.

FIGURE 4–6. People talking socially.

In close-contact societies,

- Men hold hands with men.
- Women hold hands with women.
- Men kiss each other on both cheeks.
- Women kiss each other on both cheeks.

Some close-contact societies are

- Latin America
- Africa
- Indonesia
- Southern Europe
- Mediterranean countries

More-distant societies are

- United States
- Canada
- Great Britain
- Northern Europe

See Figure 4–7.

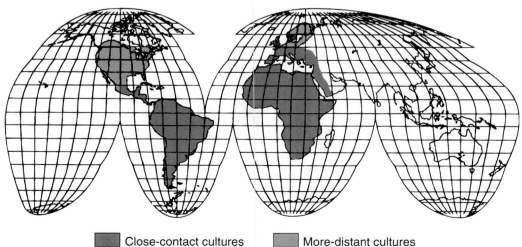

FIGURE 4–7. Regions of the world showing the location of close-contact and more-distant cultures.

■ Close-contact cultures   ■ More-distant cultures

FIGURE 4–8.
Guidelines restricting
touch and physical
closeness in Southeast
Asian cultures.

CAMBODIAN	VIETNAMESE	LAOTIAN
• Only a parent can touch the head of a child. • Members of the opposite sex never touch each other in public, not even brothers and sisters.	• Only the elderly can touch the head of a child.	• It is necessary to ask permission to move near another person.

Some Southeast Asian cultures believe that a person's spirit is on the head. Touching the head is often considered an insult. Figure 4–8 explains who is permitted to touch or not touch the head.

Greetings

Greeting another person is important in all cultures. The way a greeting is given and received often determines how positive or negative the meeting is. Figure 4–9 describes greetings in various cultures.

Hand Gestures

Hand gestures help communicate many things. It is very important to use correct gestures so that others are not offended. Figure 4–10 illustrates gestures that are offensive in other cultures.

Eye Contact

In some cultures, eye contact may indicate that a person is listening, sincere, or honest. In other cultures, direct eye contact is considered to be hostile or disrespectful. Figure 4–11 explains some cultural views about eye contact.

FIGURE 4–9.
Guidelines for greeting
people.

ANGLO-AMERICAN	LATIN-AMERICAN	CAMBODIAN, LAOTIAN	VIETNAMESE	HMONG
Shake hands if desired.	Shake hands or hug.	Do not shake hands. Instead, put hands together at different levels. 1. Equal status—hands must be at chest level. 2. Older person or stranger—hands must be at chin level. 3. Relative or teacher—hands must be at nose level.	Salute by joining both hands and moving them against the chest.	Bow head or shake hands.

SAME GESTURE, SAME MEANING, BUT VERY DIFFERENT CONNOTATIONS

FIGURE 4–10.
Hand gestures.

| | American Culture | | Asian Cultures |

American Culture

OK for "Come here."

Asian Cultures

Absolutely *taboo* for calling a person, even a child. It's the way to call an animal (a dog, in particular), especially when accompanied by a whistle. Considered *very insulting.*

OK for "Come up here."

Never use.
Only an inferior person would be summoned this way. Considered *insulting*, even to a child.

OK to point at someone or something.

OK to point at *something* but not at *someone*. Considered too direct a reference, amounting to confrontation, which the Indo-Chinese avoid by all means.

Slight threat (or warning) when making a point to someone.

Relatively strong threat made by a person of superior rank to an inferior (father to son, teacher to student). This is one step ahead of corporal punishment. (A parent would *never* use this gesture to a girl because it is considered too brutal.)

FIGURE 4–11.
Eye-contact guidelines.

ANGLO–AMERICANS	BLACKS	NAVAJOS	JAPANESE, SOUTHEAST PERSIANS MEXICAN–AMERICANS
Eye contact is important; it indicates interest, honesty, and listening.	Eye contact may not be important. Being in the same room indicates attentiveness.	Direct eye contact is avoided. • Peripheral vision is used. • Direct stares are considered hostile or a way to scold children.	Eye contact is avoided as a form of respect.

■ COMMUNICATING EFFECTIVELY WITH PEOPLE FROM OTHER CULTURES

When speaking with people from other cultures, the tone of your speaking voice is similar in importance to the gestures you use. Speaking tone includes voice quality, volume, and pitch. Voice tones cause positive or negative reactions from others. Clear pronunciations are more easily understood. When speaking to others who are learning English,

- Speak clearly; do not slur words.
- Speak so that they can hear you easily.
- Do not raise your voice or yell.
- Speak in moderate tones.
- Pronounce the entire word; do not draw it out or shorten sounds.
- Summarize often.
- Confirm their understanding.
- Clarify when necessary.
- Do not assume that they understand.

You gain greater interpersonal effectiveness when you strive to understand and respect people of a different culture and viewpoint. Making every effort to understand and to be understood is one way to treat others with dignity.

■ FOLK MEDICINE

traditional Customary beliefs passed from generation to generation.

Folk medicine is a collection of **traditional** beliefs and customs for treating pain or illness. Many who practice folk medicine believe that natural materials, such as herbs, spices, and tree herbs, and spiritual prayers and rituals keep evil spirits away and allow the body to heal.

It is very important to respect the beliefs of other cultures. If you insult the patient, you will be ineffective in providing care. Some caregivers work with their patients' beliefs to create positive relationships. Then they can introduce other suggestions for care.

Learn about the common practices in your clients' cultures. Read magazines and books about other cultures. Ask questions. Learn about ritual healing, folk medicine, and spiritual healing. Keep informed! Your understanding helps the patient get well faster and feel respected. The experience will be positive for both of you.

The following information is an overview of some common folk medicine practices in various cultures. Some practices that cause painful symptoms are not considered abusive because they are based on a belief of the culture.

Armenians

- Give the mother a party one week after a baby is born. The mother is served bread, which she dips into a paste of margarine, sugar, and flour. This is a celebration of the birth of the child.

prohibit To not allow.

- **Prohibit** a menstruating woman from attending church, taking a shower, or eating spicy foods.

Cambodians

■ Use herbs as medicine.

■ Use cupping for headaches. Cupping leaves a round mark on the forehead. A cotton ball saturated in alcohol is placed in a glass and set on fire. After burning for a few seconds, the cotton is discarded. The heated glass is placed upside down over the painful area.

■ Use coining for pain. Oil or ointment is applied to the skin. Then a large coin is used to rub the painful area in one direction until the blood is raised to just below the surface of the skin. This leaves red areas on the skin.

■ Consider the color white to be a sign of bad luck. White indicates mourning and death. Think about a Cambodian's first visit to a caregiver. Is it possible that the white uniform might seem frightening?

Central and South Americans

■ Use herbal home remedies.

■ Teach a menstruating woman not to get her head wet and to avoid eating cucumbers, oranges, lemons, pork, lard, and deer meat.

Chinese

■ Use herbs as medicine.

■ Practice acupuncture and use herbs over puncture sites.

■ Use cupping with heated bamboo.

Hmong and Mien Tribes

■ Perform spiritual ceremonies to please the spirits that cause illness.

■ Use herbal home remedies, including opium.

Iranians

■ Believe that poor health is predetermined (fatalism).

■ Use herbs, foods, rituals, and magic formulas for healing.

■ Believe the "Evil Eye" (a person or animal that causes injury through a look) causes sudden illness.

■ When of the Islamic faith, require washing of the face and hands before prayer.

■ Require periodic baths for cleansing.

Koreans

■ Practice alchemy, a medieval practice of magic and natural herbal remedies.

■ Use acupuncture.

■ Go to hot springs for bath rituals and massage.

■ Use energy and brain stimulants.

FIGURE 4–12.
Terms that describe
health problems.

TERMS	CONDITION
Weak heart	Palpitations, dizziness, faintness, feeling of panic
Weak kidney	Impotence, sexual dysfuntion
Weak nervous system	Headache, malaise, inability to concentrate
Weak stomach or liver	Indigestion
I'm skinny.	Sickliness
Fire, hot	Dark urine, flatulence, constipation
Air/wind, cold	Illness was caused by too much air.

Native Americans
■ Use herbs and spices.
■ Use modern medical practices.
■ Some rely on a shaman (medicine man or woman) to remove pain and evil spirits.

Vietnamese
■ Commonly use herbal medicine.
■ Use cupping for head pain, cough, muscle pain, and motion sickness.
■ Use acupuncture for musculoskeletal problems, visual problems, and other ailments.

Figure 4–12 lists typical terms used by non-English-speaking Asian cultures to describe health problems.

■ SUMMARY

Cultural beliefs are very important to all societies. You give quality care when you take the time to understand and respect patients of other cultures. Your caring about them as individuals will help them improve more quickly. If they are not ill, your caring builds mutual respect for future meetings.

Thinking Critically: Check Your Understanding

1. **Communication** Your on-the-job training takes place in a physician's office. The person you work the closest to is always leaving cupboard doors open. You are afraid that you or someone else will be hurt by walking into these open doors. Describe in writing an effective way to communicate to your co-worker your need to have the cupboard doors closed.

2. **Legal and Ethical** Describe the legal and ethical pros and cons surrounding pet-facilitated therapy in a long-term care facility. (For example, residents might trip over small animals; animals can carry bacteria.)

3. **Cultural Competency** Your patient/client population consists mainly of people from Asia. Describe what you would tell a new employee about appropriate ways to communicate with your patients/clients and understand their needs.

4. **Medical Terminology** Compare and contrast the World Health Organization's definition of *health* with the meaning of *holistic*.

5. **Patient Education** You have a patient/client from Iran. Her family is concerned about leaving her alone during the day, so they admit her to a long-term care facility. She is convinced that she is going to die because her family brought her to the hospital. Describe the basic need that is not met, and explain your reasoning. Develop a plan to satisfy the need for your patient/client.

6. **Case Study** Your co-worker has a loud voice and demonstrates everything with his hands as he talks. You have also seen his gentle manner and tender, caring nature. You observe that some of your Cambodian patients seem to be afraid of him and even back away or avoid being around him. Explain why the Cambodian patients might respond to your co-worker in this manner. Describe what you would do and say to help your co-worker communicate his gentle, caring nature to the Cambodian patients.

Portfolio Connection

Mrs. Summers is an alert, ambulatory, 85-year-old patient. You observe that she argues about everything and with everyone. You cannot remember her ever agreeing to or being willing to do anything. Develop a plan to identify why Mrs. Summers is so argumentative.

Your plan must clearly identify what you would do to involve other people. In your written paper, clearly identify her behavior, what causes it, and what the positive and negative outcomes are for her. Include a proposed solution, a method of evaluation, and a time line. When your paper is perfect in format and grammar, place it in Section Four, "Written Samples."

Your successful completion of this assignment shows your ability to organize, analyze, and evaluate. These skills help you work effectively with the various needs of your patients/clients.

5

EFFECTIVE COMMUNICATIONS

Steps to success

1. Complete Vocabulary Worksheet 1 in the Student Workbook.
2. Read this unit.
3. Complete Worksheets 2 through 4 as assigned.
4. When you are confident that you can meet each objective for this unit, ask your instructor for the unit evaluation.

Rationale

communication Act of exchanging information.

The health care worker should understand that there are many factors in **communication.** A knowledge of the techniques of communication will increase your skills in communicating with co-workers and patients/clients. With this knowledge, you will be able to do a better job and to make good observations about your patients.

Objectives

When you have completed this unit, you will be able to do the following:

✓ Match vocabulary words with their correct meanings.
✓ Explain why communication is important.
✓ Name four elements that influence our relationship with others.
✓ List three barriers to communication.
✓ Identify your communication assertiveness level.

98

✓ List three elements necessary for communication to take place.

✓ Describe three things that a good listener does.

✓ Differentiate between verbal and nonverbal communication.

✓ Demonstrate responding, transferring a caller, and taking a message.

Communication is essential in the exchanging of ideas, feelings, and thoughts. Communication helps us know what the needs of others are and how to meet those needs. There are several kinds of communication. These include words, either written or spoken, **gestures,** facial expressions (frowns, smiles), body posture, touch, and listening. The following discussion has important information to help you become a better communicator with patients, families, co-workers, and supervisors.

gestures Motions of a part of the body to express feelings or emotions (e.g., nodding the head yes or no).

■ ELEMENTS THAT INFLUENCE YOUR RELATIONSHIPS WITH OTHERS

Prejudices

All people form opinions or **biases** as they are growing up. These **prejudices** affect how they feel about other people and how they relate to them. You may have very strong feelings about the backgrounds or the values of your patients or co-workers. Your feelings affect how you communicate. For instance, if you believe that certain people are lazy, overly emotional, or **inferior,** you need to think about your prejudices. When you understand your prejudices and feelings, you have an opportunity to overcome them.

biases Tendencies; prejudices.

prejudices Judgments or opinions formed before the facts are known.

inferior Lower (e.g., one product is inferior in quality to another product).

Frustrations

When you care for and work with others, you may experience **impatience, annoyance,** and probably anger. Perhaps other people do not understand your directions, or they may move too slowly. You feel irritated. These feelings interfere with your ability to communicate. Take time to understand why you feel frustrated. Evaluate the situation, and then try to correct it. It is your responsibility to control your behavior and to understand that patients, families, and co-workers have problems that are the cause of their behavior.

impatience Unwillingness to tolerate.

annoyance Irritation (e.g., to feel irritated with a co-worker or patient).

Attitudes

How you act toward others and how they act toward you affect the quality of communication. If you are disinterested or bored, if you are in a bad mood, if you wish you were someplace else—communication breaks down. However, if you show interest and concern for others, you will experience worthwhile communication, your job will become easier, and you will be more effective.

Life Experiences

People have new experiences every day. These help us know what to expect in day-to-day living. They also help us know how to act in certain situations. This understanding gives health care workers a knowledge of their own behavior and helps them communicate more effectively.

■ BARRIERS TO COMMUNICATION

Recognizing barriers to communication allows you to become an understanding health care worker. The following are three major communication barriers:

labeling Describing a person with a word that limits them (e.g., *lazy, stupid*).

■ ***Labeling.**** Deciding the other person is mean, lazy, a complainer, or difficult causes a breakdown in communication. You do not pay attention to the message being sent. If you listen, you might find out the reason for the behavior.

■ *Sensory impairment.* Deafness or blindness can be a communication barrier. Always evaluate the people you are communicating with to be certain that they do not have a sensory impairment.

■ *Talking too fast.* It is especially important when you are working with elderly people to speak slowly. Communication can break down when the message is delivered too rapidly.

courteous Polite; considerate toward others.

Developing skills in communication helps you become a better health care worker. It is important always to be **courteous** and understanding. Take time to evaluate gestures, facial expressions, and tone of voice in order to understand what is really being said. You may feel frustrated, angry, or irritated, but as a health care worker, it is up to you to attempt to understand and to listen. Hearing accurately and then responding appropriately are essential. Remember to communicate your messages so that they can be understood easily.

■ ELEMENTS OF COMMUNICATION

For communication to take place, there are three essential elements:

convey To say, tell, or express.

■ *A message.* There must be something that you want to **convey** to another person. Perhaps the purpose of the message is to give information or to acquire information. Perhaps there is something you want another person to do.

■ *A sender.* Unless there is someone who wants to send a message, there cannot be communication.

■ *A receiver.* Even if there is a message and a sender, there must be a receiver. If there is no one to receive the message, communication is incomplete.

■ GOOD LISTENING SKILLS

When you think of communication, you may not think of listening. However, listening is a very important element in all communication. If you do not receive the message that is being sent, communication has not taken place. Your understanding of how to be a good listener makes you a better health care worker.

■ *Show interest.* It is important for you to show interest in the person who is sending you a message. If you follow all of the other rules of being a good listener but tune out the message because you are not interested, communication will not take place.

■ *Hear the message.* Health care workers frequently think that they understand what is being said to them when they really do not. It is important to repeat what you believe you heard being said to be certain you heard correctly. It is not necessary to repeat exactly what was said, but check to see if you have understood the general message.

■ *Do not interrupt.* Have you ever tried to send a message and been frustrated by the receiver's interrupting you? Allow the sender to give you the entire message without interruptions. If you need to ask a question to clarify the meaning, be patient and wait until the sender is finished. She or he may give you the information you need without your questions.

Being a good listener takes patience. You need to concentrate on being a good listener until the skills become easy for you. As a health care worker, good listening is an essential skill. Good listening skills also help you follow directions, make good observations of patients, and understand your fellow workers.

■ ASSERTIVE COMMUNICATION

Communicating assertively is an honest and direct way to say what you feel or think. Being assertive allows you to express your feelings and thoughts. You must believe that you have the right to be heard and believed by others. You recognize that it is OK for you and for others to say no when it is appropriate—for example, when you are asked to do something you are not trained to do. It is OK to ask for something you want or need to accomplish a goal or task. This type of open, honest communication shows that you are a genuine person with self-respect and confidence. Assertiveness says that you have an awareness of and respect for others. To communicate strong health care values effectively, it is important for you to be an assertive communicator.

There are three common styles of communication:

■ *Unassertive, or passive, communication* allows others to control the conversation.

■ *Assertive communication* does not take power or authority away from others. It empowers individuals to speak up and be heard.

■ *Aggressive communication* occurs when power is taken away from others and communication breaks down.

Most people communicate in all three of these styles, depending on their feelings or thoughts at the time. Health care workers are more effective when they use assertive communication skills. You can develop your skills over time. Start by rating your preferred communication style on the assertiveness inventory in the Student Workbook, and follow the portfolio directions at the end of this chapter.

■ NONVERBAL COMMUNICATION

Communication also takes place in nonverbal ways. It is not necessary to speak in order to send a message. You send messages with your eye contact, facial expressions, gestures, and touch.

■ *Eye contact.* Making eye contact with the person with whom you are communicating is important. Eye contact lets others know that you are paying attention. When you do not make eye contact, you send others a message that you are not interested or that you wish to avoid them.

■ *Facial expressions.* A smile sends a different message than a frown does. It is possible to say something very kind and still send a message of anger with your eyes. Try to think of an instance when you knew that what was being said was not what was meant. How did you know? The expression on the sender's face probably sent you a different message.

■ *Gestures.* Shrugging your shoulders, turning your back, and leaving the room while someone is talking to you certainly convey a lack of interest in the sender's message. You need not say, "I am not interested," because you have effectively sent that message through your gestures.

■ *Touch.* Touch can convey great caring, warmth, concern, and tenderness. It can also convey anger, rejection, and distaste. Touch is a very important part of your communication. It is important that your nonverbal communication be supportive and positive.

■ VERBAL COMMUNICATION

Verbal communication includes spoken and written messages.

■ *Spoken messages.* When you speak to someone, you send a message. The tone of your voice, the language you use, and the message you send are interpreted by the receiver. Always speak clearly and concisely. This ensures that your message is understood.

■ *Written messages.* You communicate frequently with the written word. You take messages and orders. You may write notes in the patient's/client's chart, and you may need to leave instructions for fellow workers. It is important to spell correctly, use proper grammar, and write in a clear and concise manner.

Telephone Communication

The telephone is an important communication tool between you and your clients/patients. All departments in the health care setting require good telephone communication skills. You may be asked to answer the phone, take a message, or respond to a request. It is very important to follow the rules of good communication for incoming and outgoing calls.

Guidelines for Incoming Calls

1. Answer the phone on the first ring if possible and no later than the third ring.
2. Remember to smile as you answer the phone. The caller may not be able to see your smile but can hear the smile in your tone of voice.
3. Speak clearly.
4. Be courteous.
5. Remember to thank the caller when he or she returns your call.
6. Identify your department or doctor's office (e.g., "Dr. Smith's office.").
7. Identify yourself and give your title (e.g., "This is Monica, nurse assistant.").
8. Give a confident impression by using words such as "may" instead of "can" (e.g., "How may I help you?" not "Can I help you?").
9. Get as much information as possible about why the patient is calling.
10. Use proper etiquette.

    Correct Response

    May I have your name, please?

    Could you repeat that, please?

    How may I help you?

    I'm sorry; I didn't understand.

Wrong Response

What's your name?

What did you say?

What do you want?

Huh?

11. Be patient. Remember that the patient may be apprehensive about calling (e.g., asking about test results).

12. If you are unsure of the proper response, ask for assistance.

13. Before putting a caller on hold, give the caller the option to hold or leave a message.

14. Do not keep a caller on hold for more than 30 seconds. Always check back with callers to see if they want to continue holding.

15. Always read the message back to the caller to ensure that you have the correct information. Check the following:

   a. Spelling of the caller's name b. Phone number and area code c. Date and time of call d. Complete and correct information for the message

16. Allow the caller to hang up first so that you do not miss something he or she may want to add.

Guidelines for Outgoing Calls

1. Prepare any questions that you need to ask before you call.

2. Have all the information that might be asked of you.

3. Do not call to socialize.

Always remember: Use **discretion** with confidential information.

discretion Caution about what one says and does.

Telephone Technique

Answering the Telephone

1. Assemble materials.

   a. Pencil b. Message pad c. Telephone setup d. Directory of other departments

2. Answer the phone on the first ring if possible and no later than the third ring.

3. Identify the physician's office: "Dr. Smith's office."

4. Identify yourself: "This is _____ speaking."

5. Ask who is calling and the reason for the call.

6. Determine an appropriate course of action.

   a. Take a message. b. Take an order. c. Send supplies. d. Refer the call to your supervisor. e. Refer the caller to another department or office.

7. If the call is for another area, use your directory and refer the caller.

8. Take a message.

   a. Record the time and date. b. Write clearly. c. Take the name and telephone number of the caller. (Ask callers to spell their names.) d. Write the message.

      (1) Summarize information. (2) Repeat the message to the caller to be certain that it is correct.

   e. Record the action taken, if any. f. Sign or initial the message.

9. Thank the caller, and ask if there is anything else that you can do for him or her.

10. If not, say good-bye but allow the caller to hang up first so that you do not miss anything that he or she might add.

Putting the Caller on Hold

1. Ask callers if they want to hold or leave a message.
2. Check back with callers at least every 30 seconds.
3. Ask if the caller wants to continue to hold, and let him or her know about how long it will be.
4. Put the call through as soon as possible.
5. End the call pleasantly, and gently hang up the receiver. (Allow the caller to hang up first.)

Leaving a Message

1. State your name and where you're calling from.
2. Leave your phone number, with the area code.
3. Leave the times that you will be available.
4. Remember to use discretion with confidential information.

■ SUMMARY

Communication requires a sender, a receiver, and a message. The message may be verbal or nonverbal, and many factors influence the effectiveness of communication. These factors include prejudices, frustrations, attitudes, and life experiences. Good listening skills are important to ensure successful communication, and an awareness of barriers to good communication is important.

UNIT 2   Charting and Observation

Steps to success

1. Read this unit.
2. Complete Worksheet 1.
3. When you are confident that you can meet each objective for this unit, ask your instructor for the unit evaluation.

Rationale

Observation and documentation of your observations are a key component of health care. Your ability to observe patient/client behavior and symptoms will directly affect their care. Accurate documentation provides information needed to make decisions about their care. It is important that you develop sharp observation, reporting, and documentation skills.

Objectives

When you have completed this unit, you will be able to do the following:

✓ Explain the difference between subjective and objective observations.
✓ Explain which type of reporting allows immediate feedback and action.
✓ List information that must be on all health records.
✓ Apply five general charting guidelines.

■ OBSERVATION

Every health care worker is responsible for observing the patient/client. Even if you are not responsible for charting, you must report your observations to your supervisor. You are responsible for making good observations moment by moment. Your observation skills must be fine-tuned so that you are aware of the patient's mental and physical state. This awareness helps you and your co-workers be more effective.

When interacting with patients and their families, use all of your tools to evaluate the situation. Your tools are four of your five senses: sight, hearing, touch, and smell.

■ *Look* for all visible signs that may indicate a reason for the client's complaint.
■ *Listen* carefully. Don't put thoughts or words into others' minds. Be sure that you understand fully what you are told.
■ *Feel* for changes in the skin, body temperature, abnormal structures, and so on.
■ *Smell* unusual odors, which are often the first clue to a problem (e.g., fruity breath, foul stools).

There are two types of observations:

■ *Subjective observations* cannot be seen. They are ideas, thoughts, or opinions. If you cannot see it, feel it, hear it, or smell it, it is a subjective observation. (The patient complains of pain—you cannot see it, feel it, hear it, or smell it.)
■ *Objective observations* can be seen. If you can see it, feel it, hear it, or smell it, it is an objective observation. (The patient has a cut—you can see it.)

The health care worker must report and document all subjective and objective observations. Any unusual event or change in a patient must be reported verbally to the supervisor and then documented on the client's legal record.

■ REPORTING

Reporting unusual events or any change in behavior or condition is every health care worker's responsibility. Observation of people in a waiting area or a patient care area is important. Verbal reports to a supervisor allow immediate feedback and action when necessary. For example, you must always report changes in blood pressure, breathing, or coloring (e.g., pale, **flushed**) and any indications that a person is in distress. It is also important to report anyone who acts strangely, threateningly, or weakly or appears to be in pain. Do *not* wait for others to report unusual observations. You may prevent a serious situation by reporting your observation in a timely manner.

flushed Showing reddening of the skin.

■ DOCUMENTATION

Documentation is required in all health care settings. Documentation is a record of the patient's progress throughout treatment. Many people may be responsible for documenting information on a single patient/client. This record provides the information needed to allow each health care provider to give the care that best benefits the patient.

All records must contain certain information:

- Client's name
- Client's address
- Diagnosis
- Client's age
- Identification number
- Physician's orders

Depending on the department where the record is kept, other information may be required. Each health care worker who cares for the patient makes a notation on the chart. (Your facility policy tells you if you are required to chart. Even if you do not chart, you must always report your observations.) These notations should contain specific information about the client, including

- Care or treatment given
- Time of treatment
- How the patient tolerated the care or treatment
- Any observations that would be helpful to other health care workers
- Information that the patient has given that would affect treatment

This documentation is admissible in a court of law. This means that anything you write is considered to be true. If you do not write down something that you did for the patient, it is assumed that it was not done. As you can see, it is very important to be accurate and careful when you chart.

Everyone must follow these general guidelines for charting:

- Use ink for record keeping. In some facilities, different colors are used for different shifts.

legible Capable of being read easily.

- Entries must be **legible.** If your writing is difficult to read, you should print.
- If you make an error, do not erase it or scratch it out or cover it up. Draw a single line through the error so that it can still be read. Write "error" next to it, and then place your initials next to the correction (e.g., "~~Patient refused~~ error/KG Patient tolerated procedure well.")
- Entries should be in short phrases. You do not need to write complete sentences. You do not need to use the patient's name because you are writing in the patient's chart. Your entries should be concise, clear, and meaningful.
- All entries that you make are followed by your signature. You sign with your first initial, your last name, and your title.

Hospital Chart

The rules listed above apply to all charting. However, additional charting may be required. This is especially true for the nurse assistant. Each facility has its own policy and procedures for charting. Learn what these are. However, there are some standard types of charting that all nurse assistants are required to do:

■ *Nurses' notes* may be in narrative or checkoff form. These notes state

• What personal care was given • What activities the client participated in • The patient's skin condition • General observations about the client • Any unusual occurrences • Any complaints that the client has • What treatments were given • Any information that is important to the patient's well-being.

■ The *graphic chart* is a record of the patient's vital signs. All graphic charts have time blocks and numbers that relate to temperature, pulse, and respiration. On some graphic charts there is also space for blood pressure, intake and output, bowel movements, and weight (Figure 5–1).

Other parts of the chart include

■ A front sheet with personal information, such as name, address, marital status, place of employment, and admission diagnosis
■ A physical examination and a medical history
■ The daily progress report written by the physician
■ There may be

• A discharge plan • A social worker's report • Treatment records from other departments in the hospital or from specialists

Documentation is a very important responsibility. Learn how to write good records, and always be responsible and careful when you chart.

GRAPHIC CHART

FIGURE 5–1.
Graphic chart with intake and output section.

■ CONFIDENTIALITY

It is important to remember our discussion of confidential information in Chapter 3. When communicating any information concerning the client, remember that it is confidential and is not discussed unless it affects the treatment. The physician and patient will decide if family members or others will share the information.

■ JOBS AND PROFESSIONS

- ■ PBX operator
- ■ Psychologist
- ■ Social worker
- ■ Psychiatrist
- ■ Receptionist
- ■ Speech pathologist

UNIT 3   Computers in Health Care

Steps to success

1. Complete Vocabulary Worksheet 1 in the Student Workbook.
2. Read this unit.
3. Complete Worksheets 2 and 3 as assigned.
4. When you are confident that you can meet each objective for this unit, ask your instructor for the unit evaluation.
5. Complete "Your Link to Success" at the end of this chapter.

Rationale

Computers are essential in health care. Health care agencies use computers in most departments to help save time and improve accuracy. They are used for record keeping, diagnostic tests, education, research, and many other tasks. Health care workers must have a basic understanding of how computers work and how they are used in health care in order to be employable.

Objectives

When you have completed this unit, you will be able to do the following:

✓ Match vocabulary words with their correct meanings.
✓ List and explain how four computerized diagnostic tests help diagnose disease or illness.
✓ State how environmental services use computers.
✓ Describe ways that information services use computers.
✓ Discuss ethics and confidentiality as they relate to computers.

■ COMPUTERS IN GENERAL

During the past 40 years, computer technology has grown at an unbelievable rate. The early computers were made of vacuum tubes and required large, environmentally controlled rooms. They often overheated and became inoperable for many hours. Repairing them was time consuming. Large systems were very expensive, and only the largest organizations were able to afford them. Today's computer technology allows computers to be smaller, more powerful, and less expensive.

■ BASIC COMPUTER COMPONENTS

Computers have basic components that you need to learn in order to understand computer terminology. All computers must allow users to input information, must be able to process information, and must have some way to output information.

Inputting

Several devices are used to input information into a computer. The most common are the keyboard and the light pen. The keyboard looks like a typewriter with a few extra keys. One key plays a very important function. This is the Enter key. When you finish putting your information into the computer, you must signal the computer, "I'm done. Now it's your turn." You do this with the Enter key.

The light pen looks like a pencil, but it is designed to sense the writing on the computer screen. The user selects one of the choices displayed on the screen and moves the light pen across the choice. Then the user presses the Enter key.

Other input devices include keypunch cards, floppy diskettes, and magnetic disks or tapes. These devices are used for both inputting and storing records.

Processing

A computer processes the information that is input and returns the information to the person who input it or to someone in another department. The central processing unit (CPU) is the working unit of the computer. The CPU consists of many electronic components and microchips. The CPU can only process the information it receives; if it receives incorrect information, it processes incorrect information. This is where the phrase "Garbage in, garbage out" comes from. You must be accurate when you enter information.

Outputting

Just as there are several devices for inputting information into a computer, there are several devices for outputting it. The two most common are the monitor and the printer. The health care worker uses both of these devices.

Monitor

A monitor or video screen, also called a *cathode ray tube (CRT)*, looks much like a television screen. As you input information, you can see it on the screen of the monitor. When it is processed, you see the results on the screen. You can also recall stored information to the screen.

Printer

A printer is used to print the processed information on paper. Information printed on paper is called *hard copy* and can be filed with the patient's records.

■ COMPUTERS IN HEALTH CARE

Computers are processors of information. They process large amounts of information at incredible speeds, accurately and consistently. Wherever your career path in the health field takes you, you will do a portion of your work on a computer. Hospitals and medical and dental offices are converting medical records, accounting, and purchasing functions to computers. Some health care agencies have computer diagnostic services where a complete physical examination is analyzed by a computer.

In the hospital, a computer performs many functions. The following are some of the procedures computers assist with:

- Recording physicians' notes and orders
- Charting at bedside
- Ordering or changing diets
- Ordering unit supplies
- Processing charges for nursing care equipment
- Ordering lab work and receiving lab results
- Recording lab results for patient records
- Scheduling x-rays, special tests, and surgeries
- Processing discharges
- Diagnostic testing

In medical and dental offices, computers can be used to schedule appointments, set up a recall system, bill patients, schedule lab work, dial the telephone, manage the security system, and keep the inventory. Computers are an important part of the search for correct specific patient/client data that meets the **HEDIS** requirements. Computerized medical record keeping is becoming a necessary method of monitoring patient/client progress and quality health care.

HEDIS Health Plan Employer Data and Information System; an organization that provides quality care guidelines.

antagonist Something that works against.

homeostasis Constant balance within the body. This balance is maintained by the heartbeat, blood-making mechanisms, electrolytes, and hormone secretions.

invasive Entering the body.

Therapeutic Services

If you choose to enter an occupation in the therapeutic services, you will have opportunities to work with a computer each day. In the pharmacy, drugs are inventoried using a computer. A computer also assists the pharmacist in keeping track of medications that a person receives. The computer can alert the pharmacist when one medication acts as an **antagonist** to another medication or contains a substance that causes an allergic reaction. In physical and occupational therapy, a computer assists paralyzed patients to walk. In respiratory therapy, a computer keeps critically ill patients in **homeostasis.** In emergency services and intensive care areas, computers do direct patient/client monitoring and are programmed to warn health care workers when a potentially dangerous condition occurs.

Diagnostic Services

In diagnostic services, highly sophisticated computers are being used. In the past, surgery and other **invasive** procedures were used to reach a diagnosis. Today, computerized diagnostic equipment helps diagnose many illnesses. Using computerized equipment removes the risks of surgery and reduces the pain and discomfort of invasive tests. Computerized tests include the following:

■ The *CAT scanner* does computerized axial **tomography.** This test allows an organ to be transversely dissected to help find abnormalities (such as tumors) without surgery. A photograph is taken to provide the radiologist and the physician with a permanent record for future use.

tomography X-ray technique that produces film of detailed cross sections of tissue.

■ The *Coulter counter* completes multiple examinations of many blood specimens in seconds.

■ The *electrocardiogram computer* creates pictures on a computer screen. It prints out the electrical activity of the heart. This helps the physician diagnose heart disease correctly.

■ The *magnetic resonance imaging* computer scans the body. The scanner produces a cross-sectional image of the body. This helps the physician find tumors, see the results of medication and treatment, and diagnose the cause of an illness or disease.

■ The *positron emission tomography* (PET) computer is also a scanner. It produces a three-dimensional image that shows an organ or bone from all sides.

■ The *ultrasound imager* computer produces a picture of internal organs, tumors, aneurysms, and other abnormalities. It also produces pictures of the fetus developing in the uterus to help with fetal monitoring. These pictures can be seen on the monitor or can be processed on a photographic film.

Environmental Services

Environmental careers also offer an opportunity to work with computers. Central supply services/central processing services are computerized for reordering inventory and for billing. Supplies are even categorized and identified by bar scanners like those you see in the grocery store.

Information Services

In information services, the computer is used in a variety of ways. Medical records workers manage and process records on computers. With diagnostic-related groupings, the computer is used to help categorize and track patients in the medical system. Health unit coordinators/unit secretaries use the computer to process many of the orders, transmitting requests to other departments.

The growing need to access medical data from patient/client files quickly is forcing health care providers to use computerized information systems. This means that to be employable, every health care worker must know the basics of computer keyboarding.

Contingency Planning

Whenever human beings depend on machines, **contingency** plans need to be made just in case the machine stops functioning. When a computer is not functioning, it is said to be *down*. Downtime can be scheduled to allow a new program to be entered into the computer's memory or to make changes. Downtime can also be unexpected (e.g., due to a power failure or component failure). Hospitals and medical/dental offices have learned that it is important to have an alternative plan if failure occurs. Despite modern technology, you still need to know manual methods of entering orders. The use of computers can make you more efficient in your job. With time, you will learn all of the things the computer can do, and you will

contingency Event that may occur but is not intended or likely to happen.

learn how to do them. Practice is important in learning how to use the computer to its fullest capability.

Ethics and Confidentiality

The health care worker must remember the importance of ethics and confidentiality when using a computer. Computers contain privileged information that must be protected. Keep your identification code or password confidential to protect you and the patient.

■ SUMMARY

In this unit you read that computers are an essential part of health care. All health care services have gained a greater ability to treat, diagnose, and care for patients/clients through computerization. Computers do shut down occasionally, making contingency planning important. The responsible use of computers means that all users must keep information learned about patients/clients confidential. Keeping your identification code or password a secret is also your responsibility.

Your link to success

Thinking Critically:
Check Your Understanding

1. **Cultural Competency** Identify one cultural behavior that creates a barrier to effective communication for you. Create a positive action plan to help you communicate effectively when you experience a behavior that creates a barrier.

2. **Communication** Describe a recent event in which you or someone else did not use good listening skills. Explain what you or the person you observed could have done differently to demonstrate good listening skills in that situation.

3. **Legal and Ethical** Using the value indicators described in Chapter 3 (dignity, service, excellence, and justice), identify which values are ignored when poor listening skills are practiced. Compare and contrast the values conflicts that result when poor listening skills are practiced within each value category.

4. **Patient Education** Explain how you know when patients/clients understand and can do what you have instructed them to do.

5. **Case Study** The licensed nurse you are working with has been waiting all morning for a physician to call her back about a patient. Ten minutes after the nurse leaves the facility for a late lunch, you answer the telephone and it is the physician calling her back. Explain in writing what you will say and do.

Portfolio Connection

The ability to communicate effectively is essential to successful interactions with others. Your decision to develop effective communication skills directly affects your success or failure in the work world. Your experience in a health occupations program is the perfect place to focus on developing assertive communication skills. There are many easy-to-read books on assertiveness training that are helpful in learning about and practicing assertiveness. Go to your local library or resource center, and select and read a book that teaches assertive communication skills.

Identify your most common and least common communication type (unassertive, assertive, aggressive). Think of three recent experiences that demonstrate your use of unassertive or aggressive communication. What caused you to respond the way you did? What could you have done or said that would have made your responses assertive? What was the outcome of the unassertive or aggressive communication?

Explain your answer for all three experiences by writing a short paper. Your explanation must clearly identify the unassertive or aggressive statements or actions, indicate what you would change to create an assertive, effective communication, and compare the expected results with those of the unassertive or aggressive communication.

This assignment helps you evaluate the effectiveness of your most frequently used communication skill and allows you to express it in writing. Assertive written communication skills reflect your ability to communicate effectively in the health care environment. Your ability to demonstrate this skill in your portfolio presents you as an appropriate candidate for higher education or job opportunities. Place this assignment in Section Four, "Written Samples."

6 MEDICAL TERMINOLOGY

Pronunciation, Word Elements, and Terms

Steps to success

1. Read this unit.
2. Complete Worksheets 1, 2, and 3 as assigned in the Student Workbook.
3. When you are confident that you can meet each objective for this unit, ask your instructor for the unit evaluation.

Rationale

Health care workers use medical terminology in their work every day. It is the professional language that helps them communicate effectively and quickly. All caregivers use medical terminology to record orders, write instructions, take notes, and to chart. Health care workers are unable to perform their job if they cannot use and understand medical terminology.

Objectives

When you have completed this unit, you will be able to do the following:

✓ Define roots, prefixes, and suffixes.
✓ Define the word elements listed.
✓ Match medical terms with their correct meanings.
✓ Divide medical terms into elements.
✓ Combine word elements to form medical terms.

■ INTRODUCTION TO MEDICAL TERMINOLOGY

Medical **terminology** can be fun, interesting, and challenging. At first medical terminology may seem hard to learn. However, with practice it becomes easier and easier. You need to learn how to build a medical term, how to pronounce it, and what it means. This unit gives you the tools that you need to learn and understand medical terms.

terminology Specialized terms used in any occupation.

■ PRONUNCIATION

If you have never heard medical terms pronounced, they may seem very difficult. To make it easier for you, the following are some hints to help you pronounce the terms correctly:

■ **ch**   sounds like *k*

Examples: chyme (kīm), cholecystectomy (kō-lē-sis-tek′-ō-me), chronic (kro-nic), chondroid (kon′-droyd)

■ **ps**   sounds like *s*

Examples: psychiatric (sī-ki-a′-trik), pseudomonas (sū-dō-mō′-nas), psychology (sī-kol′-ō-ji), psoriasis (sō-rī′-a-sis)

■ **pn**   sounds like *n*

Examples: pneumonia (nū-mō′-ni-a), pneumatic (nū-mat′-ik)

■ **c**   sounds like a soft *s* when it comes before *e, i,* and *y*

Examples: cycle (sī-kl), cytoplasm (sī′-tō-plazm), cisternal (sis-ter′-nal), centrifuge (sen′ tri-fūj)

■ **g**   sounds like *j* when it comes before *e, i,* and *y*

Examples: giant (jī′-ent), gestation (jes-tā′-shun), generic (jen-er′-ik), gyration (jī-rā′-shun)

■ **i**   sounds like *eye* when added to the end of the word to form a plural

Examples: glomeruli (glō-mer′-ū-lī), villi (vil′-lī), alveoli (al-vē′-ō-lī), bacilli (ba-sil′-lī)

■ FORMING MEDICAL TERMS
FROM WORD ELEMENTS

Medical terms are words that consist of several parts. All medical terms have a word root. Most medical terms have the root word and a prefix, a combining vowel, and a suffix. In some cases, the word has only a prefix or suffix added to the root. When you add different prefixes and suffixes to the word root, you change the meaning of the medical term. The combining vowel makes the word easier to pronounce. You build a large medical term vocabulary when you learn the meanings of word parts and how to combine them (Figure 6–1).

FIGURE 6–1.

Prefix   Root   Root   Suffix

FIGURE 6–2.

Root   Combining   Suffix
             vowel

■ The *word root* is the main part of the word and tells what the word is about. For instance, *cardio* is the root word that means "heart." This is the subject of the word you are going to build.

■ The *prefix* is a word element added to the beginning of a word root. The prefix is added to the root to change the meaning or to make it more specific. The prefix *electro* means "pertaining to electricity."

■ The *suffix* is an element added to the end of the word root that changes or adds to the meaning of the root. The suffix *gram* means "record."

■ The *combining vowel* makes it possible to combine several word roots. It also makes the word easier to pronounce (Figure 6–2).

When all the word elements above are combined, the word is *electrocardiogram* (electr/o/cardi/o/gram). It means "an electrical record of the heart."

The following are some examples of (common) English words (Figure 6–3):

Combining Word Elements

Prefix	Root	Suffix	Word
pre	heat	ing	preheating
	gentle	ness	gentleness
	speed	o/meter	speedometer

Rules for Combining Word Elements

Rules help make medical terminology easier to learn. When everyone uses the rules, there are fewer mistakes. A mistake in combining a word can change its meaning and cause confusion.

Combining Vowels

■ The combining vowel is usually an *o*, for example, *oste/o. Oste* means "bone," and the *o* is the combining vowel. The *o* can be added to join a word root with another word root or a suffix. Sometimes an *i, y,* or *u* is used. Combining vowels make it easier to pronounce the term. For example, *osteomyelitis* is easier to pronounce than *ostemyelitis.*

■ When the suffix begins with one of the vowels *(a,e,i,o,u),* the *o* on the root word is not used. Since *oste/o* ends in *o* and the suffix *-itis* begins with a vowel, the *o* is dropped. The word is *osteitis,* which means "inflammation of the bone."

FIGURE 6–3.

Prefix   Root   Suffix

■ The combining vowel is placed between root words, for example, *osteoporosis* (oste/o/por/osis). Pronounce the word with the combining vowel, and you can tell that it is easier to say than *osteporosis*.

The following words are examples of word elements that have been combined to form a medical term:

aden/o/pathy   disease of the glands

hepat/o/rrhagia   hemorrhage of the liver

poly/arthr/itis   inflammation of many joints

hyster/ectomy   surgical removal of the uterus

hyster/o/salping/ectomy   surgical removal of the uterus and fallopian tubes

oste/o/por/osis   condition of pores in the bone

After you learn the roots, prefixes, and suffixes, you can combine many word parts to form medical terminology. There is always at least one root word, and there may be more than one root word. When you add a prefix or a suffix you create a new word.

Changing Words from Singular to Plural

■ Use the rule for changing words from singular to plural that applies to the language the word comes from; for example, the English word *wavelength* adds an -*s* to become *wavelengths*. Since many medical terms come from Greek or Latin, use the following rules for Greek or Latin words.

■ Add an -*e* to a word ending in -*a*—for example, *axilla* to *axillae*.

■ Drop the -*ax* at the end of a word and add -*aces*—for example, *thorax* to *thoraces*.

■ Change the -*x* to -*g* in a word that ends in -*nx* and add -*es*—for example, *phalanx* to *phalanges*.

■ Drop -*ix* or -*ex* at the end of the word and add -*ices*—for example, *appendix* to *appendices*.

■ Drop the -*y* at the end of a word and add -*ies*—for example, *myringotomy* to *myringotomies*.

■ Drop the -*us* at the end of a word and add an -*i*—for example, *alveolus* to *alveoli*.

■ Drop the -*on* at the end of a word and add an -*a*—for example, *ganglion* to *ganglia*.

■ Drop the -*is* at the end of a word and add -*es*—for example, *metastasis* to *metastases*.

■ Drop the -*um* at the end of a word and add -*a*—for example, *ischium* to *ischia*.

■ Drop the -*ma* at the end of the word and add -*mata*—for example, *stoma* to *stomata*.

When you learn the following word elements, you have the tools to combine hundreds of medical terms. Learn which words are prefixes, which are roots, and which are suffixes. When you know the terms, it is easy to learn the specialized language of a health care worker.

Prefix	Meaning
a, an	without
ab	away from
ad	toward
ante	before
anti	against
bi	both, two
brady	slow
circum	around
con	with
contra	against
diplo	double
dors	back
dys	painful, difficult
ecto	outside
endo	inside, within
epi	upper, above
ex	out from
hemi	half
hyper	excessive, above, more than
hypo	deficient, below, less than
inter	between
intra	inside, within
macro	large
mal	bad
micro	small
mono	one, single
neo	new
ortho	straight
pan	all
para	beside, beyond
peri	around
poly	many
post	behind, after
pre	before, in front of
pro	forward
pseudo	false
retro	backward

Prefix	Meaning
semi	half
sub	below
super	above
supra	above
tachy	rapid
trans	across

Root	Meaning
acro	extremities
aden	gland
angio	vessel (blood)
ankyl	crooked, looped
arterio	artery
arthro	joint
aud, aur	ear, hearing
blepharo	eyelid
brachi	arm
bronchi	bronchial
bucca	cheek
carcin	cancer
cardio	heart
caud	tail
cephal	head
cerebro	brain
cervic	neck
cheil	lip
chole	bile
cholecyst	gallbladder
chondro	cartilage
coccus	round
col	colon
colp	vagina
costo	ribs
cranio	skull
cut	skin
cyan	blue
cysto	bladder, sac
cyt, cyte	cell

Root	Meaning
dacry	tear duct
dactyl	fingers, toes
dent	tooth
derma	skin
dextr	right
duoden	duodenum
edema	swelling
electr	electric
emesis	vomit
enter	intestine
erythro	red
esophag	esophagus
esthesi	feeling
faci	face
fascia	band, fibrous
gastro	stomach
gingiva	gum
gloss	tongue
gyne	woman
hemo	blood
hepat	liver
hydro	water
hystero	uterus, womb
iri	iris (eye)
kerat	cornea, scaly
labia	lip
lacrim	tear
lacto	milk
lapar	abdomen
laryng	larynx
leuko	white
lingua	tongue
lip	fat
lith	stone
lymph	fluid
mamm, mast	breast
melan	black
mening	membrane (pertaining to the covering of the brain or spinal cord)

Root	Meaning
meno, mens	menstruate
myelo	bone marrow
myo	muscle
nares	nose, nostrils
necr	death
nephro	kidney
neuro	nerve
ocul	eye
odont	tooth
oophoro	ovary
ophthal	eye
orchis	testes
osteo	bone
oto	ear, hearing
ovario	ovary
ovi	egg
part	birth, labor
ped, pod	foot
ped	child
phagia	swallow
pharyng	pharynx
phasia	speak
phleb	vein
pleur	pleura of the lung
pneumo	lung
procto	rectum
psycho	mind, soul
pulm	lung
pyelo	pelvis of the kidney
pyo	pus
ren	kidney
rhin	nose
salpingo	tube
semin	seed
soma	body
splen	spleen
spondyl	spine
squam	scaly

Root	Meaning
stoma	mouth
stric	narrowing
therm	heat
thorac	thorax
thrombo	clot
trachi	trachea
vas	vessel
vesic	bladder, sac
viscera	organ

Suffix	Meaning
a, ac	pertaining to
al	like, similar, pertaining to
algia	pain
cele	hernia
cente	puncture
crine	secrete
desis	surgical fixation
ectomy	surgical removal
emia	blood
genesis, genic	source, origin
gram, graph	pictures
ia	a disease; an unhealthy state or condition
ic, ical, is	pertaining to
itis	inflammation
lysis	destruction
malacia	softening
megaly	enlarged
oid	like, similar
ology	study of
oma	tumor
orrhagia	hemorrhage
orrhaphy	suture
orrhea	flow
osis	condition of
ostomy	surgical opening
otomy	incision into
pathy	disease

Suffix	Meaning
penia	deficiency
pexy	fixation
phobia	fear
plasty	surgical repair
plegia	paralysis
ptosis	drooping down
sarcoma	tumor, cancer
sclerosis	hardening
scope	picture, inspection
spasm	contraction
stasis	stoppage
-um	pertaining to
uria	urine
-y	the act of or result of an action

■ SUMMARY

Medical terminology is formed by using three components: prefixes, roots, and suffixes. To make the words easier to pronounce, a combining vowel such as *i, o, y,* or *u* may be used. In this unit, you memorized many word elements to help you be a better-prepared health care worker.

UNIT 2 Medical Abbreviations

Steps to success

1. Complete Vocabulary Worksheet 1 in the Student Workbook.
2. Read this unit.
3. Complete Worksheets 1 through 3 as assigned.
4. When you are confident that you can meet each objective for this unit, ask your instructor for the unit evaluation.
5. Complete the "Your Link to Success" at the end of this chapter.

Rationale

Health care workers use **abbreviations** to convey information about their patients/clients. Abbreviations help save time and **conserve** space on medical documents.

abbreviations Words that have been shortened.

conserve Save (e.g., when you shorten a word to save space).

Objectives

When you have completed this unit, you will be able to do the following:

✓ Recognize and define abbreviations that are commonly used by health care workers.
✓ Replace terms with abbreviations.

■ INTRODUCTION TO ABBREVIATIONS

concisely In a brief manner; to express in a few words.

Abbreviations are the shortened form of words. They are an efficient way of communicating quickly and **concisely** with other health care workers. You must be very careful when you use abbreviations. Always use standard abbreviations. Never make up an abbreviation. Doing so is confusing and will be a problem if a record is used in a legal action, because no one will understand what you wrote. Never use an abbreviation if you are unsure about its meaning. It is better to write the word out so that it is easily understood. Be considerate about when you use an abbreviation. Your patients/clients do not know what the abbreviations mean. For instance, *NPO* posted over the bed means "nothing by mouth." You know what it means, but you should always explain it to your patient/client. The following abbreviations are the most common abbreviations that health care workers use.

Abbreviation	Meaning
abd.	abdomen
a.c.	before meals
ADL	activities of daily living
ad lib	as desired
adm	admission
am/AM	morning (midnight to noon)
amb	ambulate/walk
amt.	amount
approx.	approximately
ax	axillary, armpit
bid/BID	twice a day
bm/BM	bowel movement
B/P	blood pressure
BR, br	bed rest
BRP	bathroom privileges
°C	Celsius degree, centigrade
c̄	with
CA	cancer
cath.	catheter
CBC	complete blood count

Abbreviation	Meaning
cc	cubic centimeters
CCU	coronary care unit
c/o	complains of
CO_2	carbon dioxide
CPR	cardiopulmonary resuscitation
CS	central supply
CVA	cerebrovascular accident/stroke
dc, d/c	discontinue
Del. Rm.	delivery room
Dr.	doctor
dx	diagnosis
ECG/EKG	electrocardiogram
EEG	electroencephalogram
EENT	eye, ear, nose, and throat
ER	emergency room
°F	Fahrenheit degree
ft	foot
fx	fracture
GI	gastrointestinal
GU	genitourinary
Gyn	gynecology
H_2O	water, aqua
hr	hour
hs	bedtime, hour of sleep
ht	height
hyper	above, high
hypo	below, low
ICU	intensive care unit
I & O	intake and output
IV	intravenous
lab	laboratory
liq.	liquid
LPN	licensed practical nurse
LVN	licensed vocational nurse
M.D.	medical doctor
med.	medicine
min.	minute
NA	nurse aide/nursing assistant

Abbreviation	Meaning
ng	nasogastric tube
noct, noc.	night
NPO	nothing by mouth
O_2	oxygen
Ob	obstetrics
OOB/oob	out of bed
OPD	outpatient department
OR	operating room
ord.	orderly
ORTH	orthopedics
O.T.	occupational therapy
pc	after meals
PEDS	pediatrics
per	by, through
pm/PM	afternoon (noon to midnight)
po	by mouth
post	after
postop, PostOp	postoperative
pre	before
preop, PreOp	before surgery
prn	whenever necessary, when required
Pt, pt	patient
P.T.	physical therapy
$\bar{q}$	every
qd	every day
q2h	every 2 hours
q3h	every 3 hours
q4h	every 4 hours
qhs	every night at bedtime
qid, QID	four times a day
qod/QOD	every other day
qs	quantity sufficient
r	rectal
RN	registered nurse
ROM	range of motion
R.R.	recovery room
R_x	prescription or treatment ordered by a physician

Abbreviation	Meaning
s̄	without
sob	short of breath
spec.	specimen
s̄s̄	one half
stat	at once, immediately
surg.	surgery
TID/tid	three times a day
TLC	tender loving care
VS	vital signs
WBC	white blood count
w/c	wheelchair
wt	weight

■ SUMMARY

Health care workers use abbreviations to help communicate quickly and effectively. Abbreviations are the shortened form of words and help reduce the time needed to chart important information. You have learned the most commonly used abbreviations; however, in your work experience you may find other abbreviations that are not listed here.

Thinking Critically: Check Your Understanding

1. **Communication** You have a patient who is complaining of the following symptoms. Write a description of these symptoms using medical terminology so that your supervisor understands what the patient is experiencing. The symptoms include headache, vomiting, stomach pain, and excessive perspiration.

2. **Medical Terminology** Choose ten terms related to body parts. Use different prefixes and suffixes and additional word roots to create several medical terms related to each body part. For example, some terms that use the word *gastr/o* are *gastroenteritis, gastritis, gastralgia, gastrointestinal,* and *gastric ulcer.* After completing the list, look the words up in the dictionary. Check the meaning of each word and your spelling. Also check in the dictionary to see if the words you created are medical terms. Write a short description of each word.

3. **Legal and Ethical** You are in a hurry to finish your charting and cannot remember some of the abbreviations you have learned. You can think of several ways to shorten words that you are using. Should you use an abbreviation that you make up? Explain your answer.

4. **Cultural Competency** You have several co-workers who have English as their second language. They are having a problem learning and understanding medical terminology. What are some suggestions you can make to help them learn this new language?

5. **Patient Education** Your patient is asking you about the sign above her bed. The sign reads, "NPO, ROM tid, and BRP." How do you explain these terms to your patient?

Portfolio Connection

Imagine that you are the instructor of a medical occupation class. You want your students to learn to communicate effectively in the health care environment. Create five assignments for your students to complete. Use the information in the medical terminology and abbreviation units. Look at the objectives in your textbook to guide you in developing what you want your students to accomplish in the assignment. Develop worksheets and evaluations. Provide clear directions for the student. An employer is interested in your ability to use in a meaningful way the new information you have learned. This exercise for your portfolio develops your skills in organizing what you are learning.

MEDICAL MATH

UNIT 1 Math Review

S*teps to success*

1. Complete Worksheet 1, Pretest in the Student Workbook.
2. Read "Introduction to the Math Review" and "numbers," then complete Worksheet 2.
3. Read "Numbers" starting on p. 132 through "Subtraction" and complete Worksheet 3.
4. Read "Multiplication" and complete Worksheet 4.
5. Read "Division" and complete Worksheet 5.
6. Read "Decimals, Percentages, and Fractions" and complete Worksheet 6.
7. When you are confident that you can meet each objective for this unit, ask your instructor for the unit evaluation.

Rationale

Health care workers are required to perform simple math calculations when doing various tasks. Knowing basic math concepts and when to apply them is essential for all health care workers. Knowing how to add, subtract, convert standard figures into metric figures, calculate percentages, and manipulate fractions is a part of your responsibility when working in the health care field.

Objectives

When you have completed this unit, you will be able to do the following:

✓ Add and subtract whole numbers, decimals, and percentages.
✓ Multiply and divide whole numbers, fractions, mixed numbers, decimals, and percentages.
✓ Convert
  • Decimals to percentages
  • Percentages to decimals

■ INTRODUCTION TO THE MATH REVIEW

Some students have not used math for a long time. This unit review will help you accurately apply basic math concepts and skills necessary to your success as a health care worker. Take the pretest in the Student Workbook. If you pass it with 100 percent, skip this unit. If you do not get 100 percent, read through this unit and complete all workbook assignments.

■ NUMBERS

Numbers are expressed in different forms.

■ Whole numbers
■ Nonwhole numbers
■ Mixed numbers
■ Percentages

Numbers with more than one digit are defined by their place value. The number 7777 is given the following values:

This number is described by saying "seven thousand, seven hundred seventy-seven." Numbers are written with a comma placed to the left of every third digit. The number 7777 is properly written "7,777." The number 22222 is given the following place values:

It is written "22,222" and described as "twenty-two thousand, two hundred twenty-two."

Numbers indicating less than a whole number are placed to the right of a decimal. The number 7,777.255 is given the following place values:

It is written "7,777.255" and described as "seven thousand, seven hundred seventy-seven and two hundred and fifty-five thousandths."

Whole Numbers

Whole numbers are the counting numbers and zero. Whole numbers do not contain decimals or fractions. *Examples:* 1, 2, 3, 10, 15, 18, 0. Ignore zeros before whole numbers. *Example:* 025 → Ø25 and is written 25.

Nonwhole Numbers

Nonwhole numbers are numbers with decimals. *Examples:* 7,777.255, 12.25, 5.9

Mixed Numbers

Mixed numbers are whole numbers and a fraction. *Examples:* 12¼ or 45¾.

Percentages

The word *percent* means "by the hundred"; 100 percent = the whole or all of something. The symbol for percent is %. *Example:* Four turtles = 100% or all of the turtles present. When one turtle is sold, ¼ (one-fourth) or 25% of them are gone and ¾ (three-fourths) or 75% are left.

One turtle or 25% of the turtles are sold.

Three turtles or 75% of the turtles are left.

■ ADDITION

Adding is the totaling of two or more whole numbers. For example, 2 computers in the reception area + 3 computers in accounting = a total of 5 computers in the office. To add, place numbers in columns. Put a line under the last number in the column. Add all the numbers above the line and write the total or sum of the numbers below the line. *Examples:*

	2		34
	+3		+ 4
Total	5	Total	38

When adding more than one column of numbers, always keep the numbers in each column in a line under each other. This helps you add the correct numbers together. Always start adding numbers in the right column first.

Example:

11 + 234 + 10 + 4 is written like this:

```
   11
  234
   10
+   4
 259
```

When figuring numbers that total more than 10 in a column, it is necessary to carry numbers to the left of the column being added. In the example below, the first column of 1 + 4 + 0 + 9 = 14. In the total, the number to the left of the 4 is 1. Move or carry the 1 to the column at the left and add it to the top number of that column (8), then add the remaining numbers in the column, 1 + 8 + 8 + 1 = 18. The number to the left of the 8 is 1. Move or carry the 1 to the column at the left and add it to the top number of that column (3), then add the remaining numbers in the column, 1 + 3 = 4. The total is 484. (See example 1 that follows.)

Example 1:

= 14; leave the 4 in the total row and carry the 1 to the top of column at the left.

= 18; leave the 8 in the total row and carry the 1 to top of the column at the left.

= 4; place the 4 in the total row of the column added.

Example 2:

= 14; leave the 4 in the total row, carry the 1 to the top of column at the left.

= 35; leave the 5 in the total row, carry the 3 to the top of column at the left.

= 12; leave the 2 in the column you're working in at the total row, carry the 1 to the column at the left. (Since there is no number above the total line, write the 1 in the total column.)

■ SUBTRACTION

Subtraction is the opposite of addition. Subtracting numbers means taking a number away from another number. Simple subtraction problems are written in the following way:

$$\begin{array}{r} 84 \\ -23 \\ \hline \boxed{61} \end{array} \quad \text{or} \quad 84 - 23 = \boxed{61} \qquad \begin{array}{r} 136 \\ -\ 12 \\ \hline \boxed{124} \end{array} \quad \text{or} \quad 136 - 12 = \boxed{124}$$

Check your answer by adding the answer to the number subtracted. If your answer is correct, your total will equal the number at the top of your problem. Examples:

$$\begin{array}{r} 84 \text{ \tiny check} \\ - \boxed{\begin{array}{c} 23 \\ +61 \end{array}} \\ \text{Total} \quad \boxed{= 84} \end{array} \quad \text{or } 23 + 61 = \boxed{84} \qquad \begin{array}{r} 136 \text{ \tiny check} \\ - \boxed{\begin{array}{c} 12 \\ +124 \end{array}} \\ \boxed{= 136} \end{array} \quad \text{or } 12 + 124 = \boxed{136}$$

Subtracting by Borrowing Numbers

Borrow a number from the column to the left. This allows a larger number, such as 8, to be subtracted from 5. See the following examples to help you understand.

$$\begin{array}{r} {}^2\cancel{3}{}^1 5 \\ -1\ 8 \\ \hline \boxed{1\ 7} \end{array}$$ 5 becomes 15 when 1 is borrowed from the 3; 3 becomes 2.

$$\begin{array}{r} {}^1\cancel{2}{}^{16}\cancel{7}{}^1 2 \\ -1\ 9\ 5 \\ \hline \boxed{\cancel{0}\ 7\ 7} \end{array}$$ 2 becomes 12 when 1 is borrowed from the 7; 7 becomes 6 because you borrowed 1; 6 becomes 16 when 1 is borrowed from the 2; 2 becomes 1.

■ MULTIPLICATION

Multiplication is a quick, easy way to add. For example, $9 + 9 + 9 = 27$, but an easier process is $3 \times 9 = 27$. Adding large numbers is bulky and takes a lot of time. Multiplication is much easier.

To multiply numbers easily, memorize the multiplication table. Memorizing this table allows you to calculate numbers quickly and without difficulty. You probably already know most of the multiplication facts. Review the table below and test yourself by completing Worksheet 1, pretest in your Workbook. For instructions on how to read a multiplication table see Worksheet 4 in your Workbook.

Multiplication Table

	1	2	3	4	5	6	7	8	9	10
1	1	2	3	4	5	6	7	8	9	10
2	2	4	6	8	10	12	14	16	18	20
3	3	6	9	12	15	18	21	24	27	30
4	4	8	12	16	20	24	28	32	36	40
5	5	10	15	20	25	30	35	40	45	50
6	6	12	18	24	30	36	42	48	54	60
7	7	14	21	28	35	42	49	56	63	70
8	8	16	24	32	40	48	56	64	72	80
9	9	18	27	36	45	54	63	72	81	90
10	10	20	30	40	50	60	70	80	90	100

The following symbols are used to indicate multiplication: $\times$, $\cdot$, ()(), or *. These symbols are used in writing problems. *Examples:*

$$\begin{array}{r} 8 \\ \times\ 9 \\ \hline 72 \end{array} \quad \text{or } 8 \times 9 = 72 \quad \text{or } 8 \cdot 9 = 72 \quad \text{or } (8)(9) = 72 \quad \text{or } 8 * 9 = 72$$

Using calculators is helpful when figuring complicated calculations; however, you are responsible for knowing how to calculate numbers without a calculator. Most of the calculations in your work are simple and easy to figure without the use of a calculator. Do not use a calculator to work through your worksheets. Use your mind, not a calculator.

Long Multiplication

When you are multiplying numbers with more than one digit, it is sometimes necessary to carry and add. See the following examples to review these steps.

The next problem does not require carrying numbers. It does require multiplying and adding.

A.
```
      5 2
  ×  3 2
  1 0 4
```
$2 \times 2 = 4$; place 4 in first column, below 2 and 2.

$2 \times 5 = 10$; place 0 in column under the 5 and 3 and place 1 in column at left.

B.
```
        5 2
    ×  3 2
    1 0 4
+ 1 5 6
```
$3 \times 2 = 6$; place 6 in column under the 5, 3, and 0.

$3 \times 5 = 15$; place 5 in column under 1 and place 1 in column at left.

C.
```
        5 2
    ×  3 2
    1 0 4
+ 1 5 6
  1 6 6 4    Answer
```
Add together, keeping each number in the correct column.

This problem requires carrying, adding, and multiplying:

A.
```
  ¹8 ¹9 8
  ×  5 6 2
  1 7 9 6
```
$2 \times 8 = 16$; place the 6 in the first column and carry the 1 to top of column at left. $2 \times 9 = 18 + 1$ [that was carried] $= 19$; place the 9 in column under 9 and 6 and carry the 1 to top of column at left. $2 \times 8 = 16 + 1$ [that was carried] $= 17$; place 7 in column under 8 and 5 and place 1 in column at left of 7.

B.
```
   ⁵8 ⁴9 8
  ×  5 6 2
    1 7 9 6
  5 3 8 8
```
$6 \times 8 = 48$; place the 8 in column under 9, 6, and 9 and carry the 4 to top of column at left. $6 \times 9 = 54 + 4$ [that was carried] $= 58$; place the 8 in column under 8, 5, 7 and carry the 5 to top of column at left. $6 \times 8 = 48 + 5$ [that was carried] $= 53$; place 3 in column under 1 and place 5 in column at left next to the 3.

C.
```
      ⁴8 ⁴9 8
     ×  5 6 2
        1 7 9 6
      5 3 8 8
  4 4 9 0
```
$5 \times 8 = 40$; place 0 in column below 8, 5, 7, and 8 and carry the 4 to top of column at left. $5 \times 9 = 45 + 4$ [that was carried] $= 49$; place 9 below 1 and 3. Carry the 4 to top of column at the left. $5 \times 8 = 40 + 4$ [that was carried] $= 44$; place 4 below 5 and place 4 next to 4 in column at the left.

D.
```
            8 9 8
        ×  5 6 2
      ¹1 ¹7 9 6
    ¹5 3 8 8
+ ¹4 4 9 0
  5 0 4 6 7 6   Answer
```
Add together, keeping each number in the correct column.

■ DIVISION

Division is the opposite of multiplication. Knowing the multiplication table is essential when dividing. As a health care worker, you may divide to determine costs per item or to determine the amount of items used daily. Here is a simple example: A medical office budget allows $600 a year for magazines. You are responsible for selecting and ordering the magazines. As you survey appropriate magazine subscriptions, you determine that the average annual cost is $35 per magazine. To determine how many subscriptions you can purchase, you divide $35 into $600. This problem is written as follows:

$600 \div 35$, or $35\overline{)600}$

$35\overline{)600}$ 17 magazine subscriptions

To understand how 17 magazine subscriptions can be purchased for $600, review the following division skills:

Dividing three-digit numbers by one-digit numbers:

$812 \div 4$ Divide hundreds   Divide tens   Divide ones

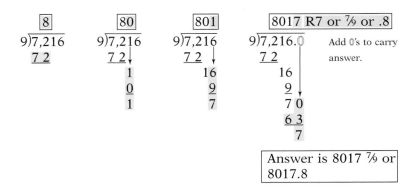

Dividing four-digit numbers by one-digit numbers:

$7{,}216 \div 9$

Answer is 8017 ⅞ or 8017.8

As shown in the example, *R* stands for *remainder*. The remainder is what is left over that is less than a whole. A remainder is usually expressed as a fraction or a decimal.

■ DECIMALS, PERCENTAGES, AND FRACTIONS

Numbers to the left of a decimal are whole numbers. Numbers to the right of a decimal are less than one.

Dividing *decimals* by whole numbers:

$24.5 \div 4 = 4\overline{)24.5}$ Place the decimal point in the answer directly above the decimal point in the dividend.

$$
\begin{array}{r} 6. \\ 4\overline{)24.5} \\ \underline{24} \end{array}
\qquad
\begin{array}{r} 6.1 \\ 4\overline{)24.5} \\ \underline{24} \\ 5 \\ \underline{4} \\ 1 \end{array}
\qquad
\begin{array}{r} 6.125 \\ 4\overline{)24.500} \\ \underline{24} \\ 5 \\ \underline{4} \\ 10 \\ \underline{8} \\ 20 \\ \underline{20} \end{array}
$$

Add 0's to carry answer.

Numbers to the right of a decimal point indicate less than one whole. For example 1.5 is the same as $1\frac{1}{2}$. *Examples:*

Decimal		Percentage		Fraction(s)
.10	=	10%	=	$^{10}/_{100}$ or $^{1}/_{10}$
.25	=	25%	=	$^{25}/_{100}$ or $^{1}/_{4}$
6.25	=	625%	=	$6^{25}/_{100}$ or $6^{1}/_{4}$

Change a decimal number into a percentage by moving the decimal two places to the right. *Examples:*

0.5 = 0.5 0. = 50%

30.0 = 30.0 0. = 3000%

.04 = .0 4. = 4%

To change a percentage into a decimal number, replace the % sign with a decimal and move the decimal two spaces to the left.

To find the percentage of a number, first change the percentage to a decimal. Then multiply that decimal by the number. *Examples:*

15% of 63 change 15% to .15 then multiply .15 × 63 = 9.45

9.45 is 15% of 63

20% of 100 change 20% to .20 then multiply .20 × 100 = 20

20 is 20% of 100

■ SUMMARY

In this unit, you reviewed the skills for adding, subtracting, multiplying, and dividing whole numbers, nonwhole numbers, mixed numbers, fractions, and percentages. You also practiced converting percentages, decimals, and fractions.

UNIT 2   The Metric System

S*teps to success*

1. Read this unit.
2. Complete Worksheets 1 through 3 in the Student Workbook as assigned.
3. When you are confident that you can meet each objective for this unit, ask your instructor for the unit evaluation.

Rationale

The health care worker is expected to measure and calculate weights, heights, and volume in metric units of measure. Understanding how to convert standard and metric units of measure helps you work in a variety of health care settings.

Objectives

When you have completed this unit, you will be able to do the following:

✓ Match vocabulary words with their correct meanings.
✓ State the metric unit of measure used to determine length, distance, weight, and volume.
✓ Use metric terms to express 100 and 1,000 units of measure.
✓ Use metric terms to express 0.1, 0.01, and 0.001 units of measure.
✓ List four basic rules to follow when using the metric system.
✓ Identify metric measures of length and volume.
✓ Convert ounces to cubic centimeters/milliliters, pounds to kilograms, and ounces to grams.

■ USING THE METRIC SYSTEM

The health care industry uses the metric system for measuring. The metric system is used by 90 percent of the world and is known as the International System of Units. Table 7–1 will help you learn the metric terms, their abbreviations, and what they measure. Each metric unit in this table is a single unit of measure. Table 7–2 explains terms used when *more than one* unit of measure (meter, gram, liter) is being measured. Following are examples of more than one unit:

TABLE 7–1   Metric Terms, Their Abbreviations, and What They Measure

Term	Abbreviation	Measures	In Place of:
meter	m	length	inch, foot, yard, mile
gram	g	weight	ounce, pound
liter	L*	volume	fluid ounce, cup, pint, quart, gallon

*Capital L is commonly used to prevent confusion of lowercase letter l and the number 1.

TABLE 7-2   Metric Terms, Their Abbreviations, and What They Measure

Term	Abbreviation	What It Measures
kilo	k	1,000 units
hecto	h	100 units

■ Measures of weight

• 1 hectogram = 100 grams • 1.5 hectograms = 150 grams • 1 kilogram = 1,000 grams • 1.5 kilograms = 1,500 grams

■ Measures of length

• 1 hectometer = 100 meters • 1.5 hectometers = 150 meters • 1 kilometer = 1,000 meters • 1.5 kilometers = 1,500 meters

Table 7–3 explains terms used when *less than one* unit of measure is being measured. Following are examples of less than one unit:

■ Measures of length

• 1 decimeter (dm) = 1/10 or 0.1 of a meter • 1 centimeter (cm) = 1/100 or 0.01 of a meter • 1 millimeter (mm) = 1/1000 or 0.001 of a meter

■ Measures of volume

• 1 deciliter (dL) = 1/10 or 0.1 of a liter • 1 milliliter (mL) = 1/1000 or 0.001 of a liter

There are four basic rules to follow when using the metric system.

decimal A number containing a decimal point.

■ Numbers indicating less than one unit are always written in **decimal** form, *not* as fractions. *Example:* 1/10 = 0.1 or 1/100 = 0.01 or 1/1000 = 0.001

■ When writing decimals, if there is no number before the decimal, it will always be a 0. *Example:* .1 is 0.1, .5 is 0.5, .75 is 0.75.

■ Abbreviations for metric terms are never plural; they are always written in singular form. *Examples:* grams is g, not gs, and liters is L, not Ls. Always capitalize the abbreviation L for liter to reduce confusing the lowercase l with the number 1.

■ Leave a space between the number and the abbreviation, as shown in the following examples: 8 g, 0.1 dm.

TABLE 7-3   Metric Terms, Their Abbreviations, and What They Measure

Term	Abbreviation	What It Measures
deci	d	1/10 or 0.1 unit
centi	c	1/100 or 0.01 unit
milli	m	1/1000 or 0.001 unit

FIGURE 7–1. Comparison of standard and metric units of length.

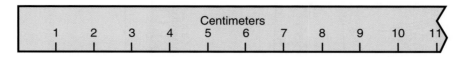

■ USING THE METRIC SYSTEM TO MEASURE

Meters, Centimeters, and Millimeters

A meter stick can be used to measure length in the following units:

- ■ centimeters (cm) (Figure 7–1)
- ■ millimeters (mm)
- ■ meters (m)

One meter is slightly more than 3 feet.

Liters, Milliliters, and Cubic Centimeters

- ■ A liter (L) is slightly larger than a quart.
- ■ A milliliter (mL) is 1/1000 of a liter.
- ■ Cubic centimeters (cc) are interchangeable with mL.

Scales can be used to measure weight in grams, hectograms, and kilograms.

Celsius (C) and Centigrade

The metric measure of heat is Celsius or centigrade, which are the same. More information can be found in the unit explaining vital signs (see page 226).

■ CHANGING STANDARD MEASURES TO METRIC MEASURES

It is easy to change liquid or volume measurement by multiplying 30 cc/mL times the number of ounces (Table 7–4).

TABLE 7–4 Changing Ounces to Milliliters and Cubic Centimeters	
1 oz medicine	$1 \times 30 = 30$ mL = 30 cc
8 oz water	$8 \times 30 = 240$ mL = 240 cc
6 oz soup	$6 \times 30 = 180$ mL = 180 cc
4 oz juice	$4 \times 30 = 120$ mL = 120 cc
12 oz soda pop	$12 \times 30 = 360$ mL = 360 cc

FIGURE 7–2 Various measuring devices for fluid ounces and cubic centimeters.

Measuring cup   **Baby's bottle**   **Graduate**

- They are all calibrated.
- They are made of metal, glass, or plastic.
- They are used for measuring liquids in cubic centimeters (cc).
- They are used for measuring liquids in ounces (oz).
- The measuring cup is used to measure liquids in the home.
- The baby's bottle is used to measure liquids in the home.
- The calibrated graduate is used to measure fluid in the health care institution.

Health care workers use various types of measuring devices to measure liquid (Figure 7–2).

To change measurements of mass or weight, compare pounds with kilograms and grams with ounces. One pound equals 0.45 kilogram; 1 kilogram equals 2.2 lb (Table 7–5).

■ To change pounds to kilograms, multiply the number of pounds by 0.45.
■ To change kilograms to pounds, multiply the number of kilograms by 2.2

One ounce (oz) equals 30 grams (g). To change ounces to grams, multiply 30 × the number of ounces. To change grams to ounces, divide 30 into the number of ounces (see Table 7–6).

There are practice questions in your Student Workbook to help you learn the metric system.

■ SUMMARY

We have discussed the basic units of measure in the metric system. These include meters, grams, and liters. When the prefix *kilo* is used before a basic unit of measure, it multiplies the unit 1,000 times. When *hecto* is used, it increases the basic unit by 100 times. We have also discussed how less than one unit is expressed by

TABLE 7–5.   Changing Pounds to Kilograms and Kilograms to Pounds
110 lb changed to kilograms: 110 × 0.45 = 49.5 kg
200 lb changed to kg: 200 × 0.45 = 91 kg
50 kg changed to lb: 50 × 2.2 = 110 lb
91 kg changed to lb: 91 × 2.2 = 200 lb

TABLE 7–6   Changing Ounces to Grams
1 oz changed to grams: 1 × 30 = 30 g
8 oz changed to grams: 8 × 30 = 240 g

using prefixes of *deci,* 1/10 of a unit; *centi,* 1/100 of a unit; and *milli,* 1/1000 of a unit. You have learned four basic rules to follow when using the metric system, methods of converting standard units to metric units, and various ways to measure.

UNIT 3   The 24-Hour Clock/Military Time

Steps to success

1. Read this unit.
2. Complete Worksheet 1 in the Student Workbook as assigned.
3. When you are confident that you can meet each objective for this unit, ask your instructor for the unit evaluation.
4. Complete "Your Link to Success" at the end of this chapter.

Rationale

Medical facilities frequently use the 24-hour clock system. The 24-hour clock clearly states time and eliminates confusion when documenting information. A health care worker is required to understand and interpret time in every health care setting.

Objectives

When you have completed this unit, you will be able to do the following:

✓ Recognize time on a 24-hour clock.
✓ Express **24-hour time/military time** verbally and in writing.
✓ Convert **Greenwich time** to 24-hour time.

■ INTRODUCTION TO THE 24-HOUR CLOCK/MILITARY TIME

In the health care setting, it is important that time be stated in a clear, concise manner. All medical records are legal documents. Time indicates when treatment, medication, and other activities are done and how long procedures or incidents last. A 24-hour clock eliminates the confusion between A.M. (12 midnight to 12 noon) and P.M. (12 noon to 12 midnight) hours. It provides a clear, concise record for recording medical services. The military services were the first to use a 24-hour clock; therefore, the 24-hour system is often referred to as *military time.* Table 7–7

24-hour time/military time Method of telling time by counting each hour consecutively for 24 hours (i.e., . . . 11, 12, 13, . . .).

Greenwich time Standard time, a 12-hour clock.

TABLE 7–7	Comparison of Greenwich and 24-Hour/Military Time		
Greenwich	**Military**	**Greenwich**	**Military**
1:00 A.M.	0100	1:00 P.M.	1300
2:00 A.M.	0200	2:00 P.M.	1400
3:00 A.M.	0300	3:00 P.M.	1500
4:00 A.M.	0400	4:00 P.M.	1600
5:00 A.M.	0500	5:00 P.M.	1700
6:00 A.M.	0600	6:00 P.M.	1800
7:00 A.M.	0700	7:00 P.M.	1900
8:00 A.M.	0800	8:00 P.M.	2000
9:00 A.M.	0900	9:00 P.M.	2100
10:00 A.M.	1000	10:00 P.M.	2200
11:00 A.M.	1100	11:00 P.M.	2300
12:00 noon	1200	12:00 P.M./ midnight	2400/ 0000

FIGURE 7–3.
24-hour clock: military time.

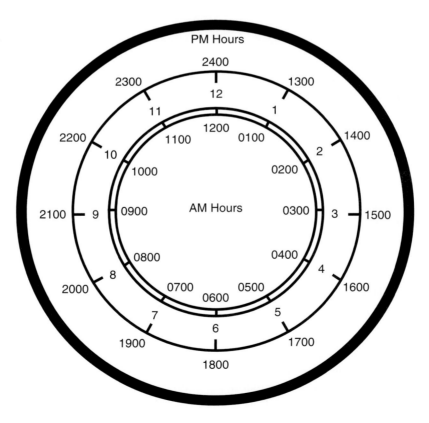

shows you the difference in expressing Greenwich and military time (see also Figure 7–3).

Military time is always expressed in four digits, and no colons are used to separate hours and minutes. Always use a 0 to complete the four-digit number (for example, 0100 instead of 100). When expressing military time, remember to state it in hundreds: for example, zero one hundred hours (0100) is 1:00 A.M.; eleven hundred hours (1100) is 11:00 A.M.; twenty-three hundred hours (2300) is 11:00 P.M.

It is easy to remember that morning hours are 0100 to 1200 hours. The afternoon and nighttime hours can be added to the 1200 hours of noon. For example:

■ To determine how 5:00 P.M. is expressed in military time, add 1200 and 0500 (1200 + 0500 = 1700 hours).

■ To determine how 12 midnight is expressed in military time, add 1200 and 1200 = 2400 hours.

Table 7–7 will help you understand the relationship between Greenwich time and military time.

■ SUMMARY

In this unit, you learned the relationship between Greenwich time and military time and how to determine the time of day using a 24-hour clock. You also learned that the 24-hour clock eliminates confusion between A.M. and P.M. hours.

Thinking Critically: Check Your Understanding

1. **Communication** Health care workers are expected to communicate effectively with co-workers, patients, and their families. In the United States, standard units of measure are common, and metric units of measure are less common. Patients or their families may be expected to measure or calculate their medicine, fluid intake, or output. It is essential to explain how to do this in terms they understand. Write instructions to a 75-year-old patient explaining the difference between ounces and cubic centimeters. Your instructions must describe how to measure and calculate the patient's 24-hour fluid intake and output and how to fill in a 24-hour I & O sheet.

2. **Medical Terminology** Create a one-page story using five new terms you learned in this chapter.

3. **Computers** Computers are used in every area of the medical field. Identify ways computers are used to help diagnose and treat medical conditions. Give one example of how computers determine a diagnosis and possible treatment.

4. **Medical Math** The metric system is used in calculating weights and measures appropriately in the medical profession. Describe the equivalents of a meter, gram, and liter, and define *kilo, hecto, deci, centi,* and *milli.*

Portfolio Connection

It is time to review your vocational choices once again. This assignment leads you through a cost analysis of schools and associations that can help develop your knowledge and skills.

Review the outcome of your career search from Chapter 2. Write down any new vocational areas of interest you have identified since completing your original career search. Answer the questions in Chapter 2, Unit 1 Worksheets 3 and 4 in your Student Workbook concerning any new areas of vocational interest. Compare your answers to these questions with your values on Worksheet 1 and satisfaction on Worksheet 2 in Chapter 2. Review the vocations that seem best for you at this time.

Research private and public schools for higher education in your vocational choice. Create a spreadsheet that clearly compares costs for each school, using the following criteria:

■ Entrance requirements
■ Tuition (costs must be compared equally, that is, semester to semester, quarter to quarter, or hours to hours)
■ Books (number of books and the cost for new and used books)
■ Supplies and materials (list and compare like items)
■ Uniforms (identify all required uniform parts, e.g., shoes, name tag)

- Housing
- Transportation (type of transportation, round-trip miles)
- Miscellaneous
- Financial aid resources (eligibility criteria, amount of dollars available, repayment requirements, and interest rates)

This assignment shows your ability to organize data into an easy-to-read, usable document. Use this process to guide future research and cost comparisons. Repeat this assignment as you approach the time for finalizing your decision concerning your professional development.

8 YOUR BODY AND HOW IT FUNCTIONS

UNIT 1	Overview of the Body

Steps to success

1. Complete Vocabulary Worksheet 1 in the Student Workbook.
2. Read this unit.
3. Complete Worksheets 2 through 5 as assigned.
4. When you are confident that you can meet each objective for this unit, ask your instructor for the unit evaluation.

structure Form in which the body is made.

functions Action or work of tissues, organs, or body parts (e.g., the heart's function is to pump blood).

cell Smallest structural unit in the body that is capable of independent functioning.

tissues Group of cells of the same type that act together to perform a specific function.

Rationale

The health care worker assists people who are ill, injured, or seeking a healthy lifestyle. Understanding the body's **structure** and **functions** provides the health care worker with the basic knowledge necessary to help each person reach his or her goal.

Objectives

When you have completed this unit, you will be able to do the following:

✓ Match vocabulary words with their correct meanings.
✓ List seven **cell** functions.
✓ Identify three main parts of the cell and explain their functions.
✓ Describe the relationship between cells, **tissues,** organs, and systems of the body.
✓ Identify terms relating to the body.
✓ Label a diagram of the body cavities.
✓ Explain why health care workers must have a basic knowledge of body structures and how they function.

146

FIGURE 8–1. Basic cell.

Nucleus

Cytoplasm

Cell membrane

■ INTRODUCTION TO THE BODY

The Cell

The cell is the building block of the body. Cells are **microscopic.** This means that they are so small they can only be seen with the aid of a microscope. The body is made up of millions of cells. Every cell is programmed to do a specific job that allows the body to function. Each cell reproduces, grows, and repairs itself, uses oxygen and **nutrients,** digests food for energy, eliminates waste, produces heat and energy, and is able to move around. The structure of the cell has three main parts (Figure 8–1):

■ The **nucleus** regulates the activity of the cell and has an important role in the **reproduction** of the cell.
■ The **cytoplasm** is a jellylike liquid where the activities of the cell occur.
■ The **cell membrane** is the outer covering of the cell that keeps the cytoplasm contained. The cell membrane also allows matter to flow in and out of the cell.

Tissues

The body is made up of specialized groups of cells. These groups of cells form tissues. These tissues have a specific job. There are five primary kinds of tissue in the body: nerve (Figure 8–2), **epithelial** (Figure 8–3), connective (Figure 8–4), blood (Figure 8–5), and muscle (Figure 8–6).

Organs

Organs are made up of specialized tissues that allow each part of an organ to perform its own specific function. Several different types of tissues make up an entire organ. For example, the heart is an organ made up of **connective tissue,** cardiac tissue, and nerve tissue. These three types of tissue work together in the heart, causing the heart to beat and pump blood throughout the body.

microscopic Too small to be seen by the eye but large enough to be seen through a microscope.

nutrients Food.

nucleus The part of a cell that is vital for its growth, metabolism, reproduction, and transmitted characteristics.

reproduction Process that takes place in animals to create offspring.

cytoplasm All of the substance of a cell other than the nucleus.

cell membrane Thin, soft layer of tissue that surrounds the cell and holds it together.

epithelial Pertaining to covering of the internal and external organs of the body.

connective tissue Tissue specialized to bind together and support other tissues.

NERVE TISSUE

Neuron

FIGURE 8–2. Nerve tissue receives stimuli and responds to stimuli.

FIGURE 8-3.
Epithelial tissue forms
the outer skin and lines
body cavities and pas-
sages to the outside of
the body.

EPITHELIAL TISSUE

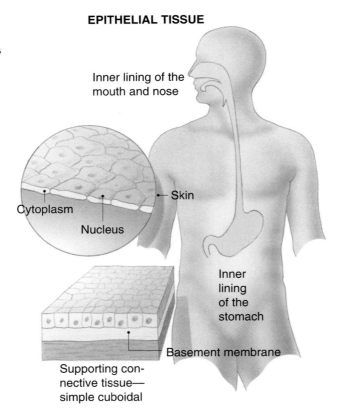

Inner lining of the
mouth and nose

Cytoplasm

Nucleus

Skin

Inner
lining
of the
stomach

Basement membrane

Supporting con-
nective tissue—
simple cuboidal

**CONNECTIVE
TISSUE**

Connective
tissue in bones

Bony (osseous)
tissue

FIGURE 8-4. Bone and connective tissue
form the skeletal system.

White blood
cells

Red blood
cells

Platelets

Lymph cells

BLOOD CELLS

FIGURE 8-5. Blood tissue
moves through the circulatory
system delivering nourishment,
electrolytes, hormones, vitamins, antibodies, heat, and
oxygen to all body tissues.

FIGURE 8–6.
Muscle tissue makes all body movement possible.

Skeletal muscle tissue

Smooth muscle tissue

Cardiac muscle tissue

MUSCLE TISSUE

Muscle fibers

Cross section of muscle

Systems

A system is a group of organs working together to perform a certain function. The body is **composed** of several systems. In the next units of this chapter, we discuss the following:

- Skeletal system
- Muscular system
- Circulatory system
- Lymphatic system
- Respiratory system
- Digestive system
- Urinary system
- Glandular systems
- Nervous system
- Reproductive system
- Integumentary system

composed Formed by putting many parts together.

It is important to understand the unique structure and functioning of the body. You need to learn that *cells* combine to form tissues, *tissues* combine to form organs, *organs* combine to form systems, and *systems* combine to form the human body (Figure 8–7).

Directions of the Body

To document information about patients, use terms that specify regions or directions of the body; for example, to identify locations of pain or injury, write: 1 cm laceration on the right **anterior** forearm, **distal** to the elbow (Figure 8–8).

The body directions are shown in Figure 8–9. Here are the most common:

- *Cranial:* located near the head.
- *Superior:* above or in a higher position. The head is superior to the torso.

anterior Located in the front; opposite of posterior (e.g., the abdominal wall is anterior to the back).

distal Farthest from the point of attachment.

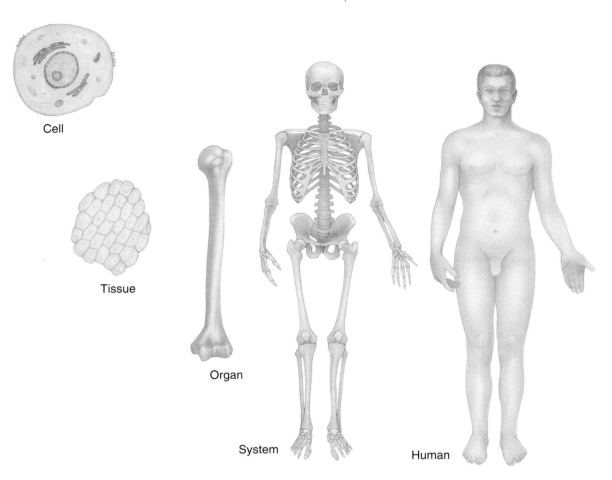

FIGURE 8–7. Combination of cells, tissues, organs, and systems forms the body.

posterior Behind, to the rear, toward the back (e.g., the heel is posterior to the toes).

sacral region The area where the sacrum is located; forms the tail end of the spinal column.

- ▪ *Inferior:* below, lower. The knee is inferior to the thigh.
- ▪ *Ventral* or *anterior:* located near the surface or in front of the body.
- ▪ *Dorsal* or **posterior:** located to the back of the body.
- ▪ *Medial:* near the center or midline of the body. Think of the midline as dividing the body in half with a left and a right side.
- ▪ *Lateral:* away from the midline.
- ▪ *Proximal:* nearest the point of attachment.
- ▪ *Distal:* farthest from the point of attachment or the midline.
- ▪ *Caudal:* located near the **sacral region.**

FIGURE 8–8. To identify the location of this laceration, write: 1 cm laceration on the right anterior forearm, distal to the elbow.

FIGURE 8–9.
Directions of the human body.

Cavities of the Body

The cavities of the body (Figure 8–10) are another way to identify location of pain or injury.

Dorsal Cavities—Located to the Back of the Body

- ■ *Cranial cavity:* houses the brain
- ■ *Spinal cavity:* encloses the spinal cord

Ventral Cavities—Located Toward the Front of the Body

- ■ *Thoracic cavity:* contains the following:

- • Heart • Lungs • Large blood **vessels**

- ■ *Abdominal cavity:* contains the following:

- • Stomach • Most of intestines • Kidneys • Liver • Gallbladder • Pancreas • Spleen

- ■ *Pelvic cavity:* contains the following:

- • Urinary bladder • Rectum • Parts of the reproductive system

vessels Tubes that carry fluid in the body.

FIGURE 8–10.
Body cavities.

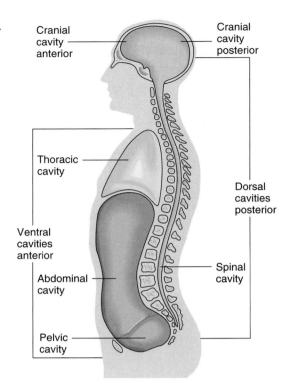

Cranial cavity anterior

Cranial cavity posterior

Thoracic cavity

Dorsal cavities posterior

Ventral cavities anterior

Spinal cavity

Abdominal cavity

Pelvic cavity

MEDICAL TERMINOLOGY

- **aplasia**   failure of any part of the body to develop naturally
- **endogenous** anything occurring within the body
- **exogenous** anything occurring outside the body
- **induration** hardened tissue
- **infarct**   tissue that has lost blood supply and died
- **interlobar** between lobes
- **intervisceral** between two organs

- **intralobar** within a lobe
- **necrosis**   condition of dead or decaying tissue
- **peristalsis** progressive wavelike movement that occurs in some of the tubes of the body (e.g., intestines, esophagus)
- **plasma**   liquid part of the blood and lymph
- **symptom**   any noticeable change in the body or its function
- **visceratonic** lack of normal tone in an organ

tone Firmness or tightness.

■ JOBS AND PROFESSIONS

- ■ Medical doctor (M.D.)
- ■ Microbiologist
- ■ Pathologist
- ■ Registered nurse (RN)
- ■ Nurse practitioner (NP)

- ■ Licensed vocational nurse (LVN)
- ■ Licensed practical nurse (LPN)
- ■ Nursing assistant (NA)
- ■ Orderly

UNIT 2 | The Skeletal System

S*teps to success*

1. Complete Vocabulary Worksheet 1 in the Student Workbook.
2. Read this unit.
3. Complete Worksheets 2 through 5 as assigned.
4. When you are confident that you can meet each objective for this unit, ask your instructor for the unit evaluation.

Objectives

When you have completed this unit, you will be able to do the following:

✓ Match vocabulary words with their correct meanings.
✓ Label a diagram of major bones in the body.
✓ Select from a list the functions of bones.
✓ Name the long, short, flat, and irregular bones of the body.
✓ Identify immovable, slightly movable, and freely movable joints of the body.
✓ Identify common disorders of the skeletal system.
✓ Label a diagram of four types of bone fractures.
✓ Explain why a health care worker must have a basic knowledge of the skeletal system and how it functions.

■ INTRODUCTION TO THE SKELETAL SYSTEM

Structure of the Bone

The skeletal system (Figure 8–11) is made up of bone tissue (**osseous** tissue) (see Figure 8–4). Bones have their own system of blood vessels and nerves which allows **circulation** to occur within the bone.

The **components** of bone change from conception to old age. In the first month after **conception,** an **embryo**'s skeletal framework is made up of **cartilage.** In the second and third months after conception, you can see calcium deposits in the bone. Throughout life, calcium continues to form in the bone structure, causing the bone to become hard. For example, a small child's bone is more **flexible** than the bone of a 30-year-old. The added calcium makes the bones of the 30-year-old harder, less flexible, and more **brittle.** A 60-year-old may lose calcium from the bone. This makes the bone **porous** so that it breaks easily.

Functions of the Bone

Bones perform many functions. Some of these are

■ To serve as a framework for the body, giving the body structure and support.
■ To protect internal structures, such as the brain and spinal cord.
■ To act as a storage area for calcium. This calcium is used in the blood if the diet does not provide enough calcium.

osseous Bonelike.

circulation Continuous one-way movement of blood through the heart and blood vessels to all parts of the body.

components Parts or elements of a whole, an ingredient.

conception Occurs when the male sperm fertilizes the female ovum and a new organism begins to develop.

embryo Living human being during the first eight weeks of development in the uterus.

cartilage Tough connective tissue; forms pads at end of bones, is found in the nasal septum and external ear, and forms the major portion of the embryonic skeleton.

flexible Able to bend easily.

brittle Fragile, easy to break.

porous Filled with tiny holes.

FIGURE 8–11. The human skeleton is made of bone tissue. There are 206 bones in the body.

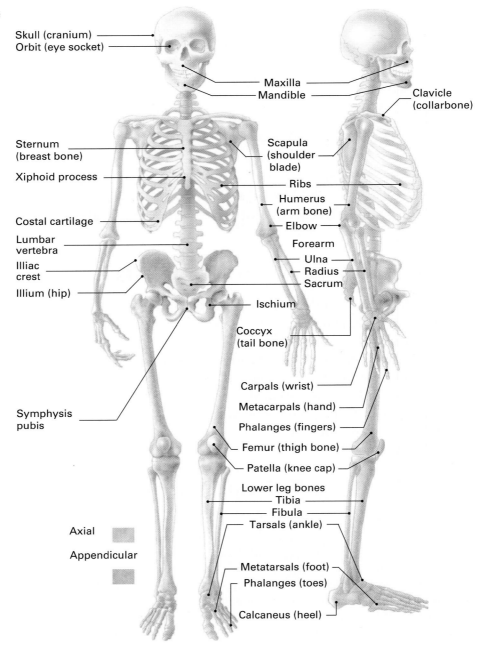

Skull (cranium)
Orbit (eye socket)
Maxilla
Mandible
Clavicle (collarbone)
Sternum (breast bone)
Scapula (shoulder blade)
Xiphoid process
Ribs
Humerus (arm bone)
Costal cartilage
Elbow
Forearm
Lumbar vertebra
Ulna
Illiac crest
Radius
Sacrum
Illium (hip)
Ischium
Coccyx (tail bone)
Symphysis pubis
Carpals (wrist)
Metacarpals (hand)
Phalanges (fingers)
Femur (thigh bone)
Patella (knee cap)
Lower leg bones
Tibia
Fibula
Tarsals (ankle)
Axial
Appendicular
Metatarsals (foot)
Phalanges (toes)
Calcaneus (heel)

■ To produce blood cells. The red bone marrow produces most of the red blood cells.

■ To allow flexibility when muscles move them.

Types of Bones

There are four types of bones:

■ *Long bones* (bones that are longer than their width)

• Humerus • Radius • Ulna • Femur • Tibia • Fibula

■ *Short bones* (length and width are nearly equal)

• Wrist and hand • Ankle and feet

■ *Flat bones* (two layers of bone divided by a narrow span)

• Skull • Sternum • Ribs • Shoulder blade

■ *Irregular bones* (bones that do not fit into the shapes of the other three groups)

• Face • Spine • Hip

Groups of Bones

The human skeleton is divided into two groups of bones. The **axial** skeleton includes 80 bones (see Figure 8–11). These are found in the

• Skull • Vertebrae • Ribs and sternum

The **appendicular** skeleton includes 126 bones (see Figure 8–11). These bones are found in the

• Arms • Hands • Legs • Feet • Pelvis

axial Pertaining to the central structures of the body (e.g., vertebrae, skull, ribs, and sternum).

appendicular Pertaining to any body part added to the axis (e.g., arms and legs are attached to the axis of the body).

Joints

The point where two bones meet is a joint. Joints are divided into three main groups, depending on the amount of movement permitted. These groups are

■ *Immovable joints*

• Cranium (suture joints)

■ *Slightly movable joints*

• Vertebral discs • Symphysis pubis • Sacroiliac joints

■ *Freely movable joints*

• Shoulder joint • Elbow, wrist, and finger joints • Knee and ankle joints

Ligaments

Ligaments connect to bone and hold bones together. Joints are formed where the bones meet.

■ COMMON DISORDERS OF THE SKELETAL SYSTEM

■ *Arthritis* is an inflammation of the joints.

■ *Degenerative joint diseases* cause changes in the structure of a joint. These changes usually occur in older people.

■ *Fracture* is a break in a bone. The different types of fractures are shown in Figure 8–12:

• *Simple fracture* occurs when the bone is broken but the skin is not broken.
• *Compound fracture* occurs when the bone is broken and **penetrates** the skin.
• *Comminuted fracture* occurs when the bone breaks and there are bone fragments in the tissue.

penetrates Enters or passes through (e.g., a fractured bone passes through the skin).

FIGURE 8–12.
Types of bone fractures.

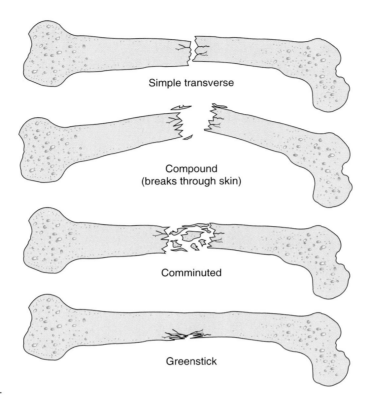

Simple transverse

Compound
(breaks through skin)

Comminuted

Greenstick

concave Curved inward, depressed; dented.

spontaneous Occurring naturally without apparent cause.

calcify To harden by forming calcium deposits.

lateral Relating to the sides or side of.

fixation Repair or fix.

• *Greenstick fracture* occurs when the bone is bent and splits, causing an incomplete break. This kind of break is most common in children.

■ *Kyphosis* is an abnormal posterior curve of the spine (hunchback).

■ *Lordosis* is an excessive **concave** (inward) curvature of the spine (swayback).

■ *Osteomyelitis* is an infection of the bone that is usually caused by a blood-borne pathogen that infects the bone and/or the bone marrow.

■ *Osteoporosis* occurs when the bone becomes porous, causing it to break easily. This disorder occurs more frequently in women after menopause and is often the cause of **spontaneous** fractures in elderly women.

■ *Rickets* occur when the bones do not **calcify** sufficiently, and they remain soft. This is caused by lack of calcium and phosphorus.

■ *Scoliosis* is a **lateral** (to the side) curvature of the spine.

MEDICAL TERMINOLOGY

• arthrodesis	surgical fixation of a joint	• costochondral	pertaining to a rib and its cartilage
• caudocephalad	from tail or coccyx to head	• craniomalacia	softening of the skull bones
• cephalalgia	pain in the head, headache	• craniosclerosis	thickening of the skull bones
• cephalocentesis	surgical puncture of the head	• dactyledema	excess fluid in the fingers and toes
• cerebrotomy	incision into the brain	• dactylology	representing words by signs made with the fingers (sign language)
• chondroma	tumor consisting of cartilage		

• dactylus	toe or finger	• osteoplasty	plastic repair of the bone
• ilio	pertaining to the ilium and femur	• osteosarcoma	malignant tumor of the bone
• lumbosacral	pertaining to the lumbar vertebrae and the sacrum	• osteotomy	incision into a bone
• myelitis	inflammation of the spinal cord	• phalanx	finger or toe bone
• osteomalacia	softening of the bone	• prosthesis	artificial organ or part of the body

■ JOBS AND PROFESSIONS

■ Orthopedist
■ Orthopedic technician

■ Cast technician
■ Prosthetist

UNIT 3   The Muscular System

Steps to success

1. Complete Vocabulary Worksheet 1 in the Student Workbook.
2. Read this unit.
3. Complete Worksheets 2 through 6 as assigned.
4. When you are confident that you can meet each objective for this unit, ask your instructor for the unit evaluation.

Objectives

When you have completed this unit, you will be able to do the following:

✓ Match vocabulary words with their correct meanings.
✓ Explain the difference between muscle and bone functions.
✓ List three major functions of the muscles.
✓ Match common disorders of the muscular system with their descriptions.
✓ Match basic muscle movements to their correct names.
✓ Label a diagram of the muscular system.
✓ Describe how muscles provide support and movement.
✓ Explain why the health care worker's understanding of the muscular system is important.

■ INTRODUCTION TO THE MUSCULAR SYSTEM

The muscles of the body make all movement possible. Muscles move body parts, allowing for proper functioning, such as heartbeat, breathing, **digestion** of food,

digestion Process of breaking down food mechanically and chemically.

and movement of the body from place to place. The next sections help you understand how muscles work.

Muscle Function

elastic Easily
stretched.

Muscles are made up of **elastic** fibers. These fibers are like a rubber band that lengthens and shortens. The main functions of muscles are to

• Produce heat • Produce movement • Maintain posture

Types of Muscle

There are two kinds of muscle:

contract To shorten,
to draw together;
muscles shorten
when you flex a body
part.

■ *Voluntary muscle* that you **contract** when you want to move (e.g., skeletal muscles; see Figure 8–13). You control these muscles; the movement is not automatic.
■ *Involuntary muscles,* which contract automatically (e.g., stomach, intestine, and heart). The heart pumps blood automatically. The stomach digests food automatically. You cannot tell the heart or stomach to start or stop.

Tendons

Tendons connect muscles to bones. When the muscle moves, it moves the tendon and bone.

Types of Muscle Tissue

Muscle tissue is classified into three categories:

voluntary Under the
control of the person
(e.g., you voluntarily
raise your arm; it
does not rise auto-
matically).

involuntary Not
under control (e.g.,
muscle twitching).

■ *Skeletal muscles* or *striated muscles* are **voluntary** muscles (see Figures 8–6 and 8–13). These muscles provide movement of the body.
■ *Visceral muscles* or *smooth muscles* form the walls of the internal organs of the body (e.g., digestive tract, respiratory passage, and walls of blood vessels). They are **involuntary** muscles (see Figure 8–6).
■ *Cardiac muscle* forms the wall of the heart. This muscle circulates the blood (see Figure 8–6).

Basic Movements of the Skeletal Muscle

There are six basic movements of skeletal muscles:

axis A center point
that can be rotated
around.

■ *Adduct:* moving a body part toward the midline (Figure 8–14a)
■ *Abduct:* moving a body part away from the midline (Figure 8–14b)
■ *Extend:* straightening a body part by moving it away from the body (Figure 8–15)
■ *Flex:* bending a body part toward the body (Figure 8–15)
■ *Rotate:* turning a body part on its **axis**
■ *Open and close openings:* like the anus; called sphincters

Frontalis
Temporalis
Orbicularis Oculi

Masseter
Orbicularis Oris

Sternocleidomastoid
Trapezius (upper back
and neck)

Deltoid
(shoulder)

Pectoralis
(chest)

Triceps
Serratus
Anterior
Biceps
Lattisimus
Dorsi (back)

Rectus
Abdominis (abs)

Exterior
Oblique

Sartorius

Rectus Femoris
(quads)

Vastus Lateralis

Vastus Medialis

Gastrocnemius
(calf)

Tibialis Anterior
(shin)

Gluteus
Maximus
(gluts)

Bicep
Femoralis
(hamstring)

Achilles
tendon

FIGURE 8–13. Skeletal muscular system.

FIGURE 8–14.
(a) Adduction;
(b) abduction.

(a)   (b)

FIGURE 8–15. Extension and flexion.

Triceps contracted
Biceps relaxed

Triceps relaxed
Biceps contracted

Extension

Flexion

Extension   Flexion

FIGURE 6–15. Extension and flexion.

■ COMMON DISORDERS OF THE MUSCULAR SYSTEM

trauma Damage to the body caused by an injury, wound, or shock; mental trauma occurs from emotional shock.

deteriorates Breaks down.

■ *Fibrositis* is inflammation of connective tissue.
■ *Muscle strain* is a **trauma** to the muscle, usually caused by a violent contraction.
■ *Muscular dystrophy* is a disease that progressively **deteriorates** muscle tissue.
■ *Myalgia* means muscle pain.
■ *Torn muscle* is a tear of the muscle tissue, usually caused by extreme trauma to the muscle.

MEDICAL TERMINOLOGY

• **myasthenia**   muscle weakness

• **myocardium**   heart muscle or cardiac muscle

• **myocele**   muscular protrusion (bulging or sticking out) through a muscle

• **myocelialgia**   pain of the abdominal muscle

• **myogenic**   beginning in the muscle

• **myography**   record of muscle contractions

• **myoid**   resembling muscle

• **myoma**   tumor containing muscle tissue

• **myomelanosis**	**abnormal darkening of muscle tissue**	• **myothermic**	**pertaining to a rise in muscle temperature**
• **myoparesis**	**weakness or partial paralysis of a muscle**	• **tenorrhaphy**	**suturing of a tendon**
• **myosclerosis**	**hardening of a muscle**	• **tenositis**	**inflammation of a tendon**

■ JOBS AND PROFESSIONS

- ■ Myologist
- ■ Physical therapist
- ■ Sports medicine assistant
- ■ Tenotomist

UNIT 4 The Circulatory System

*S*teps to success

1. Complete Vocabulary Worksheet 1 in the Student Workbook.
2. Read this unit.
3. Complete Worksheets 2 through 5 as assigned.
4. When you are confident that you can meet each objective for this unit, ask your instructor for the unit evaluation.

Objectives

When you have completed this unit, you will be able to do the following:

✓ Match vocabulary words with their correct meanings.
✓ Name the major organs of the circulatory system.
✓ Label a diagram of the heart and blood vessels.
✓ Recognize functions of the circulatory system.
✓ Identify the common disorders of the circulatory system.
✓ List the parts of the circulatory system through which blood flows.
✓ Describe how the circulatory system supports life.
✓ Explain why the health care worker's understanding of the circulatory system is important.

■ INTRODUCTION TO THE CIRCULATORY SYSTEM

Circulation is the continuous one-way movement of blood throughout the body. All of the systems and organs depend on the circulatory system. Arteries carry blood with **oxygen** and nutrients to each cell, and veins carry away the cell's

oxygen Element in the atmosphere that is essential for maintaining life.

waste products Elements that are unfit for the body's use and are eliminated from the body.

adequate Enough, sufficient.

oxygenated Contain oxygen.

unoxygenated Lacking oxygen.

carbon dioxide A gas, heavier than air; a waste product from the body.

primarily For the most part; chiefly.

waste products. If the circulation is not **adequate,** cells die. When the cells die, tissues begin to die, and the organs stop working properly. This may cause an entire system to stop functioning.

Kinds of Blood Vessels

■ *Arteries* carry blood from the lower chambers of the heart (ventricles) to all parts of the body. Arteries carry **oxygenated** blood, with the exception of the pulmonary artery. The *pulmonary artery* carries **unoxygenated** blood.

■ *Arterioles* are small arteries that connect arteries with capillaries.

■ *Capillaries* have very thin walls that allow nutrients, oxygen, and **carbon dioxide** to move in and out of the blood (see Figure 8–16).

■ *Venules* are small veins that connect veins with capillaries.

■ *Veins* carry blood from all the different parts of the body and return it to the heart. Veins carry unoxygenated blood, with the exception of the pulmonary vein. The pulmonary vein carries oxygenated blood. Veins have valves that aid in returning blood to the heart.

The Heart

The heart is the pump that forces blood throughout the body (see Table 8–1). The outside of the heart is made **primarily** of muscle, and the inside is divided into four hollow chambers (see Figure 8–17). The heart wall is made of three different layers of tissue.

■ *Endocardium* is the smooth inside lining of the heart.

■ *Myocardium* is the thickest layer and is made up of muscle.

■ *Pericardium* is a double membrane that lines the outside of the heart.

The inside of the heart is divided into four parts or chambers:

■ The *right atrium* receives unoxygenated blood from the veins.

■ The *right ventricle* receives blood from the right atrium and pumps it to the lungs through the pulmonary artery.

■ The *left atrium* receives oxygenated blood from the lungs and pumps it into the left ventricle.

■ The *left ventricle* pumps blood into the aorta, which is the largest artery in the body. The aorta delivers the blood throughout the body.

FIGURE 8–16. Blood vessels and capillary bed of the body.

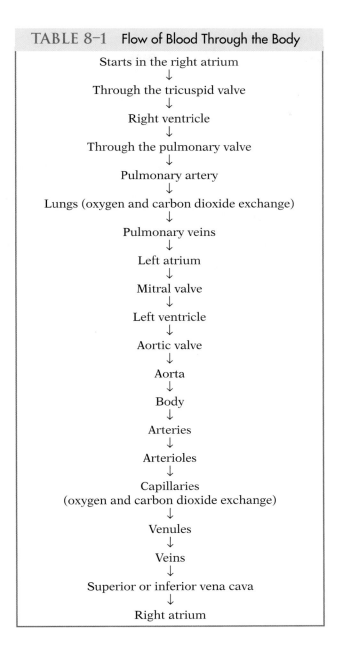

TABLE 8-1   Flow of Blood Through the Body

Starts in the right atrium
↓
Through the tricuspid valve
↓
Right ventricle
↓
Through the pulmonary valve
↓
Pulmonary artery
↓
Lungs (oxygen and carbon dioxide exchange)
↓
Pulmonary veins
↓
Left atrium
↓
Mitral valve
↓
Left ventricle
↓
Aortic valve
↓
Aorta
↓
Body
↓
Arteries
↓
Arterioles
↓
Capillaries
(oxygen and carbon dioxide exchange)
↓
Venules
↓
Veins
↓
Superior or inferior vena cava
↓
Right atrium

Valves separate the chambers in the heart from the vessels leaving the heart.

■ The *tricuspid* valve is between the right atrium and right ventricle. It closes when the right ventricle pumps blood out of the heart. This keeps the blood from flowing back into the right atrium.

■ The *pulmonary semilunar* valve lies between the right ventricle and the pulmonary artery. It closes after all the blood from the right ventricle has been pushed into the pulmonary artery. When the valve closes, it stops blood from flowing back into the ventricle.

■ The *mitral* (bicuspid) valve is found between the left atrium and the left ventricle. It closes to prevent blood from flowing back into the left atrium when the left ventricle contracts.

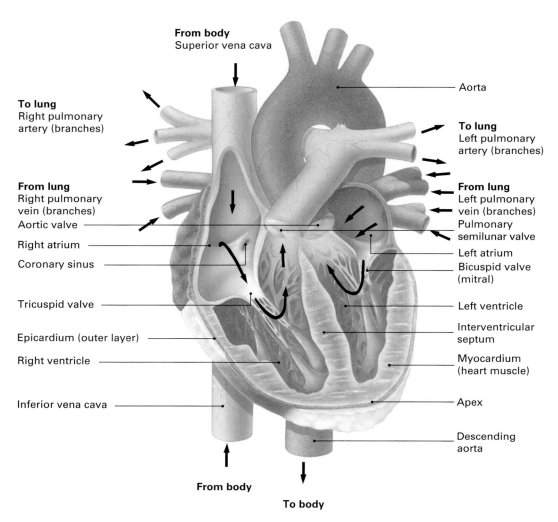

From body
Superior vena cava

To lung
Right pulmonary
artery (branches)

From lung
Right pulmonary
vein (branches)

Aortic valve

Right atrium

Coronary sinus

Tricuspid valve

Epicardium (outer layer)

Right ventricle

Inferior vena cava

Aorta

To lung
Left pulmonary
artery (branches)

From lung
Left pulmonary
vein (branches)
Pulmonary
semilunar valve

Left atrium

Bicuspid valve
(mitral)

Left ventricle

Interventricular
septum

Myocardium
(heart muscle)

Apex

Descending
aorta

From body

To body

FIGURE 8–17. Cross section of the heart.

■ The *aortic semilunar* valve is located between the left ventricle and the aorta. It stops blood from returning to the left ventricle after it has been forced into the aorta.

■ COMMON DISORDERS OF THE CIRCULATORY SYSTEM

■ An *aneurysm* is a weakened section in the wall of a blood vessel. Aneurysms are often found on the aorta. An aortic aneurysm that ruptures usually causes immediate death.

■ *Arteriosclerosis* is present when the walls of the arteries become thick and harden. This causes a loss of elasticity of the vessels. Less blood is able to flow through the artery because the opening is small. This is a disease commonly found in geriatric patients.

■ *Varicose veins* are enlarged veins that are not efficient in returning the blood to the heart. Varicose veins can occur anywhere in the body but most often are found in the lower **extremities.**

extremities Arms, legs, hands, and feet.

■ *Myocardial infarction (M.I.)* or *heart attack* occurs when the coronary arteries of the heart are blocked. This blockage can be due to arteriosclerosis. An M.I. can also be caused by a blood clot, which is called *coronary thrombosis.*

■ *Heart murmur* is a sound that indicates a faulty heart valve that does not close completely, allowing blood to flow back into the chamber it just left. It happens most often in the tricuspid or mitral valves.

■ *Endocarditis* is an inflammation of the inside lining of the heart. This condition usually affects the valves of the heart.

■ *Myocarditis* is an inflammation of the heart muscle.

■ *Pericarditis* is an inflammation of the outer lining of the heart.

■ *Congenital heart disease* includes **abnormalities** of the heart present since birth.

■ *Hypertension,* high blood pressure, places increased strain on the entire circulatory system. Although hypertension may be found in any age group, it is more common as people age.

abnormalities
Things that are not usual, that differ from the standard (e.g., congenital heart disease means that the heart is different from a normal heart).

MEDICAL TERMINOLOGY

• angiocele	hernia of a blood vessel	• embolus	blood clot in the circulatory system
• bradycardia	abnormally slow heart rate	• endocarditis	inflammation of the inside of the heart
• cardiogenic	beginning within the heart		
• cardiopulmonary	pertaining to the heart and lungs	• erythrocytosis	disease of red blood cells
• cardioscope	instrument used to examine the inside of the heart	• hemostasis	stoppage of blood flow
		• hyperemia	excess of blood in any part of the body
• cardiovascular	pertaining to the heart and blood vessels	• hypertension	high blood pressure
• carditis	inflammation of the heart muscle	• intravenous	IV, within a vein
• cyanosis	bluish discoloration of the skin	• leukocyte	white blood cell
• ecchymosis	bruised condition	• leukopenia	deficiency of white blood cells
• ectopic	pertaining to an abnormal position	• thrombus	blood clot that obstructs circulation
• electrocardiogram	ECG/EKG, a tracing of heart activity		

■ JOBS AND PROFESSIONS

■ Internist

■ Cardiologist

■ Cardiopulmonary technician

■ ECG/EKG technician

■ Echocardiogram technician

UNIT 5 | The Lymphatic System

Steps to success

1. Complete Vocabulary Worksheet 1 in the Student Workbook.
2. Read this unit.
3. Complete Worksheets 2 and 3 as assigned.
4. When you are confident that you can meet each objective for this unit, ask your instructor for the unit evaluation.

Objectives

When you have completed this unit, you will be able to do the following:

✓ Match vocabulary words with their correct meanings.
✓ Describe the general functions of the lymphatic system.
✓ Describe what lymph is.
✓ Match lymph vessels and organs to their function.
✓ Explain the difference between an antigen and an antibody.
✓ Identify common disorders of the lymphatic system.
✓ Describe how the lymphatic system helps provide immunity.

■ INTRODUCTION TO THE LYMPHATIC SYSTEM

The lymphatic system is an important part of the body's defense against disease. It filters out organisms that cause disease, produces white blood cells, and makes antibodies. It also drains excess fluids and protein so that tissues do not swell up. The lymphatic system and the circulatory system have structures that are joined together by a capillary system. The lymphatic system is made up of the lymph capillaries, lymph vessels, lymph nodes, spleen, tonsils, thymus, lacteals, thoracic duct, right lymphatic duct, and the cisterna chyli.

Kinds of Lymphatic System Vessels and Organs

interstitial Space between tissues.

■ *Lymph capillaries* are tubes that reach into the **interstitial** spaces of most body tissues. The capillaries have very thin walls that allow tissue fluids to move into them. When the fluid moves into the capillary, it is called lymph. The lymph contains waste products and foreign bodies from the cells. The lymph passes from the capillaries to the lymph vessels.

■ *Lymph vessels* are similar to veins. Muscle contractions help move the lymph from the tissues to the lymphatic trunks. Valves prevent backflow of the lymph. The lymphatic trunks receive the lymph from the body. The lymph from the lymphatic trunks empties into the veins and becomes part of the blood **plasma.**

plasma Watery, colorless fluid containing leukocytes, erythrocytes, and platelets.

■ *Lymph nodes* lie along the lymph vessels. They are located in the neck, armpit, chest, abdomen, elbows, groin, and knees (see Figure 8–18). They filter out bacte-

FIGURE 8–18.
Lymph nodes in torso.

ria and other waste products from the lymph as it moves toward the lymphatic trunks. They also produce **lymphocytes,** which help the body defend itself against microorganisms.

lymphocytes Type of white cell.

■ *Tonsils* are masses of lymph tissue that are exposed to the outside. They filter tissue fluid, not lymph. They may filter so many bacteria that the pathogens overwhelm the tonsil. The tonsils then become infected.

■ The *spleen* is behind the stomach. It filters microorganisms and waste products from the blood. The spleen makes lymphocytes and **monocytes** to help the body defend itself against microorganisms. The spleen also stores red blood cells and destroys worn-out red blood cells.

monocytes Large single-nucleus white cell.

■ The *thymus* is in front of the aorta and behind the upper part of the sternum. It is lymphatic tissue that stores lymphocytes that work with the lymphatic system to defend the body.

■ The *lacteals* pick up digested fats from the small intestine.

■ The *cisterna chyli* stores purified lymph before it empties into the bloodstream.

■ *Thoracic duct* is the common trunk of all lymphatic vessels in the body except those on the right side.

■ *Right lymphatic* duct is the vessel that carries lymph from the right side of the head, neck, thorax, lung, upper right limb, right side of the heart, and the diaphragmatic surface of the liver.

The Lymphatic System and Immunity

The lymphatic system helps the body remove substances that are harmful. These substances may be microorganisms or other foreign bodies. The foreign body is called an **antigen.** Examples of antigens are poisons, splinters, and microorganisms. When these enter the body, the body responds by producing **antibodies.** The antibodies attack the antigen. This process is called the *immune response.*

antigen Foreign matter that causes the body to produce antibodies.

antibodies Substances made by the body to produce immunity to an antigen.

Immune Response

phagocytes Cell that surrounds, eats, and digests microorganisms and cellular waste.

The immune system has many specialized cells. Two types of white blood cells are lymphocytes and **phagocytes.** Phagocytes circulate through the body and eat diseased and dead cells. Other types of white cells surround foreign bodies and destroy them. All of the white blood cells are important in protecting the body. Some things which tell you that the immune system is working are fever, inflammation, and pus. When these are present, you know that the immune system is responding to protect the body.

■ COMMON DISORDERS OF THE LYMPHATIC SYSTEM

parasitic Pertaining to an organism that lives in or on another organism, taking nourishment from it.

■ *Elephantiasis* is a condition caused by a **parasitic** worm. The worm blocks the lymphatic vessels and causes edema and swelling.

■ *Hodgkin's disease* is a chronic disease in which the lymph nodes enlarge. It is seen mostly in young men.

■ *Lymphadenitis* is an inflammation of a lymph node.

■ *Lymphatitis* occurs when the lymph system is inflamed.

■ *Lymphedema* is edema caused by the obstruction of the lymphatics.

■ *Tonsillitis* is an infection of the tonsils. This is caused by the large amounts of microorganisms the tonsilar lymph tissue is filtering.

MEDICAL TERMINOLOGY

• asplenia	absence of a spleen
• lymphadenectomy	surgical removal of the lymph nodes
• lymphadenopathy	enlargement of the lymph nodes
• lymphocytopenia	an abnormally low number of lymphocytes in the blood
• lymphocytosis	abnormally high number of lymphocytes in the blood
• lymphoma	tumor made up of lymphatic tissue
• lymphosarcoma	cancer in the lymphatic tissue
• splenectomy	surgical removal of the spleen
• splenitis	inflammation of the spleen
• splenomegaly	abnormal enlargement of the spleen
• splenorrhexis	rupture of the spleen
• splenotomy	incision into the spleen
• thymectomy	surgical removal of the thymus gland
• thymitis	inflammation of the thymus gland

■ JOBS AND PROFESSIONS

■ Immunologist

■ Immunology technologist

UNIT 6   The Respiratory System

S*teps to success*

1. Complete Vocabulary Worksheet 1 in the Student Workbook.
2. Read this unit.
3. Complete Worksheets 2 through 4 as assigned.
4. When you are confident that you can meet each objective for this unit, ask your instructor for the unit evaluation.

Objectives

When you have completed this unit, you will be able to do the following:

✓ Match vocabulary words with their correct meanings.
✓ Label major organs of the respiratory system on a diagram.
✓ Describe the flow of oxygen through the body.
✓ Identify common disorders of the respiratory system.
✓ Describe how the respiratory system supports life.
✓ Explain why the health care worker's understanding of the respiratory system is important.

■ INTRODUCTION TO THE RESPIRATORY SYSTEM

Respiration is breathing. Breathing is necessary to supply life-giving oxygen to each cell in the body and to remove the waste products of each cell. The cell's gaseous waste product is called *carbon dioxide.*

Oxygen enters the body when air is pulled in through the mouth and nose. This process is called **inspiration/inhalation. Expiration/exhalation** occurs when the body forces air out of the lungs. This is the body's way of eliminating the cells' gaseous waste (carbon dioxide).

inspiration/inhalation Process of breathing in air during respiration.

expiration/exhalation Process of forcing air out of the body during respiration.

Structure of the Respiratory System

See Figure 8–19 and Table 8–2.

■ The *nasal cavity* (nose) is where air enters the body. The nasal cavity is the preferred passage for air to enter the body. The nasal lining helps stop dust particles and pathogens. If dust and pathogens enter the lungs, the chance for infection is increased.

■ The *oral cavity* (mouth) is where air enters the body when the nasal passage is blocked or when a person breathes through the mouth.

■ The *pharynx* (throat) is the passageway that air enters after leaving the nose and mouth.

FIGURE 8–19.
Respiratory system.

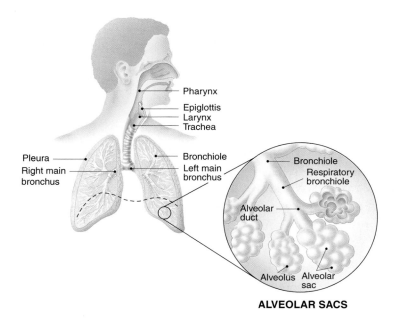

ALVEOLAR SACS

■ The *epiglottis* is a flap that closes when food or water is swallowed. When it closes, it covers the opening of the trachea that leads to the lungs. This prevents food and water from entering the lungs.

pouch Small bag or sac.

■ The *larynx* (voice box) is located just below the epiglottis. It is a **pouch** containing a cordlike framework that creates voice sounds.

■ The *trachea* (windpipe) is the passageway between the pharynx and the lungs.

■ The *bronchi* are air passageways that connect to the trachea. The trachea divides into two main branches, the bronchial tubes, that lead into the right and left lungs. The bronchial tubes are lined with hairlike objects called **cilia.**

cilia Hairlike projections that move rhythmically.

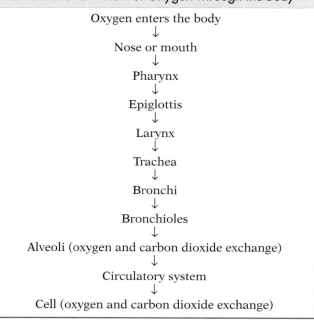

TABLE 8–2   Flow of Oxygen Through the Body

Oxygen enters the body
↓
Nose or mouth
↓
Pharynx
↓
Epiglottis
↓
Larynx
↓
Trachea
↓
Bronchi
↓
Bronchioles
↓
Alveoli (oxygen and carbon dioxide exchange)
↓
Circulatory system
↓
Cell (oxygen and carbon dioxide exchange)

The cilia help move mucus, which catches dust and pathogens, up and out of the lungs.

■ The *bronchioles* are the smallest subdivisions of the bronchi.

■ The *alveoli* (air sacs) are at the end of each bronchiole. The alveoli are covered with capillaries that absorb oxygen into the blood. Carbon dioxide is forced out of the blood into the alveoli (carbon dioxide and oxygen exchange). Once the carbon dioxide has been released into the alveoli, it can be exhaled from the body.

■ The *diaphragm* is the muscular wall that divides the chest cavity from the abdominal cavity. To begin inspiration, the diaphragm moves down, creating a vacuum that pulls air into the lungs. When the diaphragm relaxes and moves upward again, air is exhaled (forced out) from the lungs.

■ COMMON DISORDERS OF THE RESPIRATORY SYSTEM

■ *Upper respiratory infection (URI)* is any infection of the trachea, larynx, throat, or nose.

■ *Emphysema* is a leading cause of death. In emphysema, the alveoli become stretched out and are not able to push the carbon dioxide and other **pollutants** out of the lungs.

pollutants Things that contaminate the air (e.g., smoke, smog).

■ *Pneumonia* is an inflammation of the lungs that is usually caused by bacteria, viruses, or an irritation by chemicals.

■ *Tuberculosis* is an infectious disease caused by the Tubercle bacillus. The Tubercle bacillus is difficult to destroy. The bacillus can be carried around in the air by dust particles for long periods of time. When they are inhaled into the respiratory system, the bacillus may become active and destroy tissue. The proper treatment causes the bacillus to become inactive. This keeps it from multiplying and from doing more damage to tissues.

■ *Lung cancer* is a growth of **malignant** tissue in the lungs that destroys tissues. When tissue is destroyed or the passageways are blocked, less oxygen is able to reach the blood. This causes the entire body to be deprived of oxygen.

malignant Cancerous.

■ *Hay fever* is a reaction to plants, dust, or certain foods. Hay fever causes watery drainage from the eyes and nose. Occasionally, hay fever progresses to asthma.

■ *Asthma* causes the bronchial tube walls to spasm. These spasms narrow the passageways. With the passageways narrowed, it is difficult to exhale, and the patient feels as if he or she is suffocating.

MEDICAL TERMINOLOGY

• apnea	absence of breathing
• bronchiectasis	dilation of the bronchi
• bronchitis	inflammation of the bronchial tubes
• dyspnea	difficult or painful breathing
• E.E.N.T.	abbreviation for "eye, ear, nose, throat"

• epistaxis	nosebleed
• hypoxia	lack of oxygen
• intercostal	between the ribs
• laryngitis	inflammation of the larynx
• nares	nostrils

- **pharyngospasm**   spasmodic contraction of the pharynx
- **pleurocentesis**   surgical puncture of the pleura
- **pneumonolysis**   breakdown of lung tissue
- **pneumothoracic**   pertaining to the lungs and chest
- **pulmonary edema**   fluid, swelling of the lungs
- **rales**   rattling or bubbling sounds in the chest
- **rhinoplasty**   plastic repair of the nose

- **rhinorrhea**   running nose
- **sublingual**   beneath the tongue
- **tachypnea**   rapid breathing
- **thoracotomy**   incision into the chest
- **trachelosis**   any condition of the neck
- **tracheostomy**   opening into the trachea
- **U.R.I.**   abbreviation for upper respiratory infection

■ JOBS AND PROFESSIONS

- ■ Pulmonologist
- ■ Respiratory therapist
- ■ Thoracic surgeon
- ■ Otologist

- ■ Pulmonary technician
- ■ Oxygen technician
- ■ Otorhinolaryngologist

UNIT 7   The Digestive System

Steps to success

1. Complete Vocabulary Worksheet 1 in the Student Workbook.
2. Read this unit.
3. Complete Worksheets 2 through 5 as assigned.
4. When you are confident that you can meet each objective for this unit, ask your instructor for the unit evaluation.

Objectives

When you have completed this unit, you will be able to do the following:

✓ Match vocabulary words with their correct meanings.
✓ Label a diagram of the digestive system and its accessory organs.
✓ Explain the functions of the digestive system.
✓ Recognize the function of organs associated with the digestive system.
✓ Match common disorders of the digestive system with their descriptions.
✓ Describe how the digestive system absorbs nutrients.
✓ Explain why the health care worker's understanding of the digestive system is important.

■ INTRODUCTION TO THE DIGESTIVE SYSTEM

In this unit, we discuss the body's processing of food. This process prepares nutrients so that they can be used by each cell. Body cells cannot absorb nutrients from food. Food must be changed into a substance that the body cells can use. This process of changing food into a usable substance is known as *digestion*. Once digestion occurs, nutrients move into the bloodstream. This transfer of nutrients into the blood is called **absorption.** Digestion and absorption are the two main functions of the digestive system.

Digestive Organs

The digestive system is a very long muscular tube that begins at the mouth and ends at the **anus.** This tube, called the **alimentary canal,** is made up of many parts (Figure 8–20).

■ The *mouth* (oral cavity) is where food enters the body. The digestive process begins with the mechanical breakdown (the chewing, mashing, and grinding of food by the teeth).
■ The *salivary glands* are located under the tongue, near the jawbone, and at the back of the throat. The purpose of the salivary glands is to produce a

absorption Passage of a substance through a body surface into body fluids and tissues (e.g., nutrients from digested food pass through the wall of the small intestine into the blood).

anus Outlet from which the body expels solid waste.

alimentary canal Long muscular tube beginning at the mouth and ending at the anus.

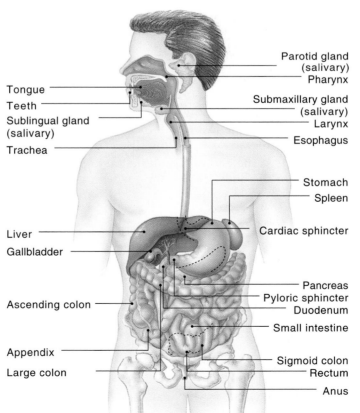

FIGURE 8–20. The digestive system is also called the alimentary canal.

Parotid gland (salivary)
Pharynx
Tongue
Submaxillary gland (salivary)
Teeth
Larynx
Sublingual gland (salivary)
Esophagus
Trachea
Stomach
Spleen
Cardiac sphincter
Liver
Gallbladder
Pancreas
Pyloric sphincter
Duodenum
Ascending colon
Small intestine
Appendix
Sigmoid colon
Rectum
Large colon
Anus

secretion Producing and expelling a special substance (e.g., sebaceous glands secrete oil; salivary glands secrete saliva).

peristalsis Progressive, wavelike motion that occurs involuntarily in hollow tubes of the body.

sphincter Circular muscle that allows the opening and closing of a body part (e.g., anus, pylorus).

chyme Creamy semifluid mixture of food and digestive juices.

minute Exceptionally small.

villi Tiny projections.

feces Solid waste that is evacuated from the body through the anus.

evacuated Emptied out.

secretion that dissolves food and coats food with a mucus that allows it to pass through the esophagus more easily.

■ The *pharynx* (throat) is located at the back of the oral cavity and is a passageway for food.

■ The *epiglottis* is a flap that covers the trachea when food or water is swallowed. By covering the trachea, the epiglottis keeps food and water out of the lungs.

■ The *esophagus* receives food and water from the pharynx. Food is moved through the esophagus by a rhythmic wavelike motion called **peristalsis.**

■ The *cardiac* **sphincter** is a ring of muscle fibers located where the esophagus and stomach join. This muscle keeps stomach contents from moving up into the esophagus.

■ The *stomach* is an enlarged part of the alimentary canal that receives food and water from the esophagus. The stomach holds food until digestive juices have chemically broken down the food particles into **chyme.** Chyme is a creamy semifluid mixture of food and digestive juices.

■ The *pyloric sphincter* is a ringlike muscle found at the far end of the stomach. Its main purpose is to keep food in the stomach long enough to become chyme.

■ The *small intestine* is attached to the stomach at the pyloric sphincter. The small intestine is about 20 feet long. The first 10 to 12 inches of the small intestine are called the *duodenum.* The duodenum receives juices from the pancreas, liver, and gallbladder, which aid in further chemical breakdown of the chyme. This final chemical breakdown is the completion of digestion. The small intestine is the portion of the alimentary canal where most absorption takes place. The lining of the small intestine contains many **minute** projections called **villi.** Each villus contains capillaries that absorb nutrients from the food we eat (Figure 8–21). Those food substances that are not absorbed are moved through the 20 feet of the small intestine by peristalsis to the large intestine.

■ The *large intestine* is attached to the small intestine and receives food substances that are of little value to the body. The large intestine absorbs water, mineral salts, and vitamins. It secretes (discharges) mucus to aid in the movement of **feces** through the intestine.

■ The *rectum* is the last 6 to 8 inches of the alimentary canal. It serves as a storage area for feces.

■ The *anus* is the end of the alimentary canal. It is where fecal material is **evacuated** from the body.

FIGURE 8–21. Villi in the lining of the small intestine.

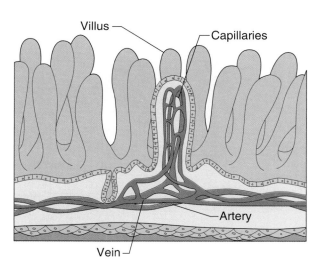

■ COMMON DISORDERS OF THE DIGESTIVE SYSTEM

■ *Constipation* is the infrequent, difficult **defecation** of fecal material.

■ *Diarrhea* is an abnormally frequent watery bowel movement.

■ *Enteritis* is inflammation of the intestines. It causes abdominal cramping and **diarrhea.**

■ *Gastritis ulcer* is an open sore in the stomach, causing pain and sometimes internal bleeding.

■ *Gastritis* is inflammation of the stomach lining. It causes **epigastric** pain, indigestion, and burning in the stomach area.

■ *Gastroenteritis* is inflammation of the stomach lining and intestines. It causes vomiting, abdominal cramping, and diarrhea.

defecation The pushing of solid material from the bowel.

diarrhea Passage of watery stool at frequent intervals.

epigastric Pertaining to the area over the pit of the stomach.

■ THE ACCESSORY STRUCTURES

The accessory structures of the digestive system assist in the process of digestion. These structures are the liver, the gallbladder, and the pancreas.

■ The *liver*, the largest gland in the body, has many functions. Some of these functions are

• Production of bile • Removal of poisons that have been absorbed in the small intestines • Storage of vitamins • Production of heparin, which prevents blood from clotting • Production of antibodies, which act against infection and foreign matter

■ The *gallbladder*, a muscular sac, stores the bile that the liver produces. When chyme reaches the duodenum, the gallbladder squeezes bile into the duodenum to aid in chemical breakdown of the chyme.

■ The *pancreas* produces pancreatic juices that also aid in the chemical breakdown of food. It also manufactures **insulin,** which regulates the amount of sugar used by the tissues.

insulin Hormone secreted by the pancreas; essential for maintaining the correct blood sugar level.

■ COMMON DISORDERS OF THE ACCESSORY STRUCTURES

■ *Hepatitis* is an inflammation of the liver. It is caused by a virus or a poison.

■ *Cirrhosis* occurs when the cells of the liver become damaged, and scarring prevents the liver and other systems from functioning.

■ *Cholelithiasis* is the presence of a stone in the gallbladder.

■ *Pancreatitis* is the inflammation of the pancreas that is caused by an overproduction of its own pancreatic juices.

MEDICAL TERMINOLOGY

• anorexia   lack of appetite

• antacid   without acid

• buccolingual   pertaining to the cheek and tongue

• cholecyst   gallbladder

• cholelithotomy incision for the removal of a gallstone

- **colitis**   inflammation of the colon
- **colostomy**   opening into the colon
- **dysphagia**   difficult or painful swallowing
- **emesis**   vomiting
- **emetic**   substance that induces vomiting
- **enterocele**   hernia involving the intestine
- **enterocyst**   cyst of the intestinal wall
- **enterohepatic**   pertaining to the intestines and the liver
- **gastrointestinal**   GI, pertaining to the stomach and intestines

- **gastrophrenic**   pertaining to the stomach and diaphragm
- **gastrosis**   condition affecting the stomach
- **hepatopathy**   any disease of the liver
- **hepatoptosis**   liver dropping downward
- **metabolism**   process by which food is changed into energy for the body's use
- **splenomegaly**   enlargement of the spleen

■ JOBS AND PROFESSIONS

- ■ Dietary aide
- ■ Gastroenterologist
- ■ Dietitian
- ■ Hepatologist

UNIT 8   The Urinary System

Steps to success

1. Complete Vocabulary Worksheet 1 in the Student Workbook.
2. Read this unit.
3. Complete Worksheets 2 through 4 as assigned.
4. When you are confident that you can meet each objective for this unit, ask your instructor for the unit evaluation.

Objectives

When you have completed this unit, you will be able to do the following:

✓ Match vocabulary words with their correct meanings.
✓ Label a diagram of the urinary system.
✓ Identify the function of organs in the urinary system.
✓ Match common disorders of the urinary system with their descriptions.
✓ Describe how the urinary system removes liquid waste and eliminates it from the body.
✓ Explain why the health care worker's understanding of the urinary system is important.

■ INTRODUCTION TO THE URINARY SYSTEM

The urinary system rids the body of liquid waste and assists in the regulation of water and chemical balance. Its functions include

■ The excretion of urine, a liquid waste produced in the body

■ The maintenance of water balance; water balance occurs when the intake of water equals the output of water

■ Regulation of the chemical balance or acid-base balance of the body; the body must maintain a balance of acids and bases in order to function properly

These functions are accomplished by the organs of the urinary system (Figure 8–22).

Structure of the Urinary System

Two kidneys are located at the back of the upper abdomen. Their primary function is to filter (remove) waste products from the blood. Each kidney has the following structure (see Figure 8–23).

■ The *capsule* is the sac surrounding the kidney.

■ The *cortex* is the outer part of the kidney.

■ The *medulla* is the inner part of the kidney.

■ The **nephron** is the chief filtering **mechanism** of the kidney. Part of the nephron is in the cortex, and part of it is in the medulla. The nephron is made up of

• A tiny twisted tube called the *convoluted tubule* • A cuplike capsule called *Bowman's capsule* • A cluster of capillaries in Bowman's capsule called the *glomerulus*

nephron Functional part of the kidney that filters liquid waste.

mechanism Process or a series of steps that achieve a result.

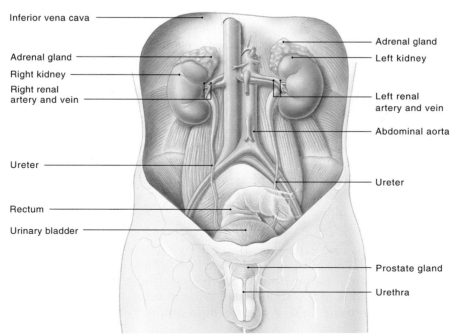

Inferior vena cava

Adrenal gland

Right kidney

Right renal artery and vein

Ureter

Rectum

Urinary bladder

Adrenal gland

Left kidney

Left renal artery and vein

Abdominal aorta

Ureter

Prostate gland

Urethra

FIGURE 8–22. The urinary system removes liquid waste from the body.

FIGURE 8–23.
Cross section of a
kidney.

SECTIONED KIDNEY

Cortex

Medulla
(pyramid)

Papilla

Calyx

Pelvis

Renal
column

Ureter

Renal
capsule

■ The *ureters* are tubes that carry urine (liquid waste) from the kidneys to the urinary bladder.

■ The *urinary bladder* is a muscular sac that expands to hold urine received from the kidneys.

■ The *urethra* is a tube extending from the urinary bladder to the outside of the body. This allows for the excretion of urine.

■ COMMON DISORDERS OF THE URINARY SYSTEM

edema Swelling; abnormal or excessive collection of fluid in the tissues. Usually, the swelling is in the hands, ankles, legs, or abdomen.

obstruction Blockage or clogging.

dialysis Process of removing waste from body fluids.

infuses Flows into the body by gravity (e.g., IV drips through a tube into the body).

peritoneal cavity Area of the body containing the liver, stomach, intestines, kidneys, urinary bladder, and reproductive organs.

■ *Nephritis* is an inflammation of the kidney due to infection or arteriosclerosis. A symptom of nephritis is **edema,** a collection of fluid in the tissues that causes swelling.

■ *Uremia,* an accumulation of urine substances in the blood, occurs when the nephron is unable to completely filter out waste from the blood.

■ *Hydronephrosis* is an expanded *renal pelvis.* This is normally caused by an **obstruction** (kidney stone, tumor) that keeps urine from flowing down the ureter.

■ *Renal calculi* are kidney stones that develop when the liquid waste from the blood becomes solid.

■ *Cystitis* is an inflammation of the urinary bladder due to infection. The bladder is susceptible to infection because bacteria can easily travel up the urethra to infect the bladder.

■ *Urethritis* is an inflammation of the urethra or the glands of the urethra. The urethra is susceptible to infection because it is open to the outside of the body.

■ *Kidney failure* occurs when the nephron of the kidney is unable to filter liquid waste from the blood. A common treatment for kidney failure is the use of **dialysis,** a means of filtering waste products from the blood. There are two methods of dialysis:

• *Hemodialysis* circulates the blood through a machine that filters out the waste and returns the clean blood to the body. • *Peritoneal dialysis* carefully **infuses** sterile fluids into the **peritoneal cavity** and then drains the fluid from the cavity. While the fluid is in the abdomen, waste products are chemically drawn out of tissues and into the fluid. When the fluid drains from the abdomen, the waste is also removed.

MEDICAL TERMINOLOGY

• calculi	stones	• nephrostomy	an artificial opening into the kidney
• cystitis	inflammation of the bladder	• pyelectasis	dilation of the renal pelvis
• cystoscopy	inspection of the bladder	• pyelitis	inflammation of the pelvis of the kidney
• diuresis	passage of abnormally large amounts of urine	• pyelolithotomy	removal of kidney stone
• glycouria	sugar in the urine	• pyelometry	measurement of the kidney's pelvis
• hematuria	blood in the urine	• renal	pertaining to the kidney
• nephralgia	renal pain	• renal colic	severe pain in the kidney
• nephric	pertaining to the kidney	• uremia	condition in which blood contains toxins usually excreted from the kidneys
• nephroid	resembling a kidney		
• nephrolithotripsy	crushing of kidney stones		
• nephropexy	surgical attachment of a floating kidney	• ureteropyelitis	inflammation of the kidney pelvis and the ureter
• nephrorrhagia	renal hemorrhage	• urethrism	irritability or spasm of the urethra

■ JOBS AND PROFESSIONS

- ■ Urologist
- ■ Nephrologist
- ■ Dialysis technician

UNIT 9   The Glandular Systems

Steps to success

1. Complete Vocabulary Worksheet 1 in the Student Workbook.
2. Read this unit.
3. Complete Worksheets 2 through 4 as assigned.
4. When you are confident that you can meet each objective for this unit, ask your instructor for the unit evaluation.

Objectives

When you have completed this unit, you will be able to do the following:

✓ Match vocabulary words with their correct meanings.
✓ Label endocrine glands on a diagram.
✓ Identify functions of the endocrine glands.

✓ Identify common disorders of the endocrine glands.
✓ Explain the difference between the endocrine and exocrine glands.
✓ Describe the effects of the endocrine glands on the body.
✓ Explain why the health care worker's understanding of the glandular systems is important.

metabolism The body's process of using food to make energy and use nutrients.

excreted Thrown off or eliminated as waste material.

sebaceous Pertaining to fatty secretions.

lacrimal Pertaining to tears.

■ INTRODUCTION TO THE GLANDULAR SYSTEMS

The glands of the body (Figure 8–24) make substances that help regulate the body processes of growth, **metabolism,** muscle contraction, and many other processes. Glands are divided into two categories. These are the exocrine and endocrine glands.

■ *Exocrine glands* have ducts that carry substances to organs, body parts, or the outside of the body. The substance made by the gland is **excreted** and is deposited in the organ or body part. *Examples:*

• Digestive juices from the salivary glands, pancreas, and gallbladder • Milk from the female mammary glands • Moisture from the sweat glands • Sebum (oil) from the **sebaceous** glands • Tears from the **lacrimal** glands

FIGURE 8–24.
The glandular systems provide substances that help regulate body processes.

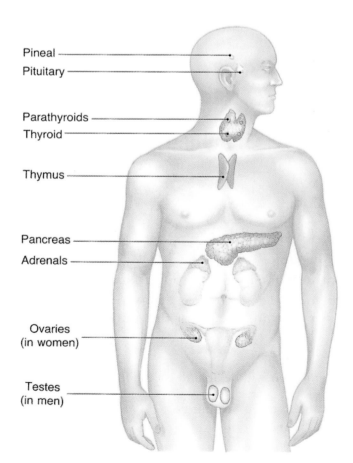

Pineal
Pituitary
Parathyroids
Thyroid
Thymus
Pancreas
Adrenals
Ovaries (in women)
Testes (in men)

TABLE 8–3　Endocrine Glands, Hormones, and Their Functions

Gland	Hormone	Function
Pituitary	TSH (thyrotropic hormone), ACTH (adrenocorticotrophic hormone), FSH (follicle-stimulating hormone), LH (luteinizing hormone), oxytocin, prolactin, and somatotropic hormone	Controls other glands; stimulates growth
Thyroid	Thyroxin	Controls rate of metabolism
Parathyroid	Parathyroid hormone	Regulates calcium and phosphorus metabolism
Pancreas	Insulin from islands of Langerhans	Essential for utilization of glucose
Ovaries	Estrogen and progesterone	Development and maintenance of female reproductive organs
Testes	Testosterone	Development and maintenance of male reproductive organs
Adrenal medulla	Adrenalin	Prepares the body for fight or flight
Adrenal cortex	Corticoids	Aids body in coping with stress or infection

■ *Endocrine glands* are glands without ducts. They secrete **hormones** directly into the bloodstream. The secretions from these glands are separated into two main groups:

• *External secretions* (excretions) are fluids that are carried to a nearby organ or to the outside of the body. • *Internal secretions* are hormones that are carried to all parts of the body through the blood and lymph systems. The endocrine glands that secrete hormones are included in Table 8–3.

hormones Protein substances secreted by an endocrine gland directly into the blood.

■ COMMON DISORDERS OF THE GLANDULAR SYSTEMS

■ *Hypothyroidism* is decreased production of the thyroid secretion.

■ *Hyperthyroidism* is increased production of the thyroid secretion.

■ *Addison's disease* is an insufficient amount of hormones from the adrenal glands.

■ *Diabetes mellitus* is too much sugar in the blood, usually the result of the pancreas failing to produce insulin.

■ *Hypoglycemia* is too little sugar in the blood, usually caused by the excessive production of insulin in the pancreas.

MEDICAL TERMINOLOGY

• acromegaly	enlargement of bones of the extremities
• adenectomy	removal of any gland
• adenoidectomy	removal of the adenoids
• adrenogenic	originating in the adrenals
• dwarfism	condition of being abnormally small
• endocrine	ductless; to secrete within

• endocrinotherapy	treatment with endocrine preparation	• parathyrotoxicosis	poisonous condition of the parathyroid
• exocrine	to secrete through a duct	• pinealoma	tumor of the pineal gland
• goiter	enlarged thyroid gland	• pituitarigenic	originating in the pituitary
• goitrogens	any substance that causes a goiter	• pituitarism	any disorder of the pituitary gland
• lymphocytopenia	deficiency of lymph cells	• thyroadenitis	inflammation of the thyroid gland
• pancreatolysis	breakdown of the pancreas		

■ JOBS AND PROFESSIONS
■ Endocrinologist

UNIT 10   The Nervous System

Steps to success

1. Complete Vocabulary Worksheet 1 in the Student Workbook.
2. Read this unit.
3. Complete Worksheets 2 through 6 as assigned.
4. When you are confident that you can meet each objective for this unit, ask your instructor for the unit evaluation.

Objectives

When you have completed this unit, you will be able to do the following:

✓ Match vocabulary words with their correct meanings.
✓ Match and select the functions of various parts of the nervous system.
✓ Label diagrams of the eye and ear.
✓ Match common disorders of the nervous system with their correct names.
✓ Describe the influence of the nervous system on the body.
✓ Explain why the health care worker's understanding of the nervous system is important.

■ INTRODUCTION TO THE NERVOUS SYSTEM

stimuli Elements in the external or internal environment that are strong enough to set up a nervous impulse.

The nervous system is a delicate system of nerve cells (Figure 8–25) linked together to receive **stimuli** and to respond to stimuli.

■ Stimuli are anything that cause a reaction (response) (e.g., when your hand touches a hot object or when something flies into your eye).

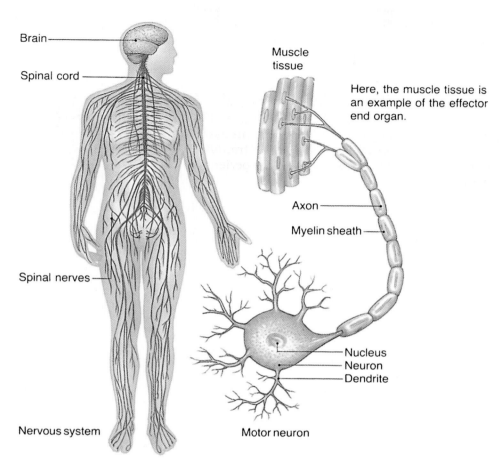

FIGURE 8–25.
Central and peripheral nervous systems; neuron (nerve cell).

■ Response is the reaction to the stimuli (e.g., moving your hand when it touches something hot or tears in the eye when something flies into it).

   The nervous system is divided into two parts: the central nervous system and the **peripheral** nervous system.

   The *central nervous system (CNS)* includes the brain and the spinal cord (see Figure 8–25). Nerves of the spinal cord carry messages to and from the brain. The brain has three main parts:

peripheral Situated away from a central structure.

■ The *cerebrum* processes thought having to do with memory and learning. It controls voluntary movements and sense interpretation.
■ The *cerebellum* coordinates muscle activity and balance so that muscles function smoothly.
■ The *medulla* controls breathing, heartbeat, circulatory action, and digestive movements.

   The *peripheral nervous system* includes the nerves and **ganglia** outside the brain and spinal cord. There are

■ Twelve pairs of cranial nerves
■ Thirty-one pairs of spinal nerves
■ Various nerve branches in body organs

ganglia Mass of nerve tissue composed of nerve cell bodies. Ganglia lie outside the brain and spinal cord.

All parts of the central and peripheral nervous systems work together to relay messages to the brain. Each message is carried to the correct area of the brain by its specialized **neuron** or nerve cell (see Figure 8–25).

Each specialized neuron leads into a passage that delivers the message or stimuli to the brain or the spinal cord. The areas in the spinal cord that can receive messages cause an action or response to stimuli that does not require interpretation. The stimuli that are received by the brain are interpreted and cause a response. This response can occur any place in the body but is most easily recognized in the sense organs. For example, sound waves are received by the ears; light rays are received by the eyes; the nose and tongue respond to smell and taste; and the nerve endings throughout the body respond to pressure, heat, cold, pain, and touch.

The following are the sensory organs of the body.

The Eye

The eye provides vision (Figure 8–26). It is a ball-shaped organ located in the eye orbit of the skull.

Protection for the Eye

■ The lids and eyelashes aid in protecting the eye.
■ Tears from the lacrimal **duct** help wash away foreign matter.

Coats of the Eye

■ The *sclera,* or the white of the eye, is the outer lining. The front portion of the sclera is clear and is called the *cornea.*
■ The *choroid,* the second coating, is heavily **pigmented** to keep light rays from **scattering.**

neuron Nerve; includes the cell and the long fiber coming from the cell.

duct Narrow, round tube that carries secretions from a gland.

pigmented Colored; relating to various parts of the body (e.g., iris of the eye, lips, moles, freckles).

scattering Spreading in many directions, dispersing.

FIGURE 8–26.
Cross section of the eye and external eye.

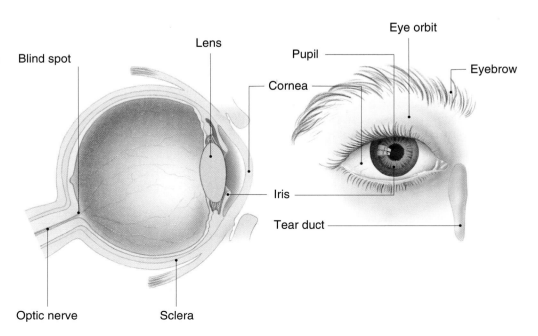

Blind spot · Lens · Cornea · Pupil · Eye orbit · Eyebrow · Iris · Tear duct · Optic nerve · Sclera

■ The *retina,* the innermost coating of the eye, houses the mechanisms that sense vision.

■ The *optic nerve,* located at the back of the eye, receives a picture and sends it to the brain for interpretation.

The Ear

The ear provides hearing and **equilibrium** (Figure 8–27). The ear can be divided into three main parts:

■ The *external ear* includes the following:

• *Auricle,* or outside projection • *External auditory canal* • *Tympanic membrane* or eardrum, which separates the external and middle ear

■ The *middle ear* is an air space that contains three bones or **ossicles.** These bones **amplify** sound waves received by the tympanic membrane.

■ The *inner ear* contains the semicircular canals, which transmit sound waves received from the middle ear to the nerves that allow us to **translate** sound.

equilibrium State of balance.

ossicles Three small bones in the middle ear: incus, stapes, and malleus.

amplify To increase or elevate a sound (e.g., the ossicles of the ear amplify sound waves).

translate To make understandable.

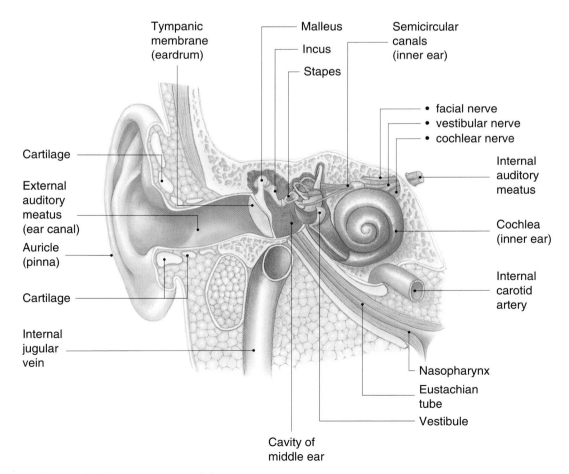

FIGURE 8–27. Cross section of the ear.

Organs of Taste and Smell

Sense of Taste

receptors Nerves that respond to stimuli.

Taste is sensed by **receptors** in the tongue called *taste buds*. The taste buds sense four main tastes:

• Sweet • Sour • Salty • Bitter

Sense of Smell

Receptors that receive smells are located high in the upper part of the nasal cavity called the *olfactory epithelium*. The *olfactory nerve* sends the smell to the brain for interpretation.

General Senses

General senses are found throughout the body. These general senses are different from the special senses of sight, hearing, taste, and smell; they are not limited to specific areas of the body (Figure 8–28).

Pressure Sense

subcutaneous Beneath the skin.

Pressure is sensed by the pressure receptors in the **subcutaneous** tissue layer beneath the skin.

Temperature Sense

Heat and cold are sensed by receptors that respond only to heat or cold and send messages through nerves to the brain.

Sense of Touch

Touch is sensed by receptors called *tactile corpuscles*. These receptors are found in the dermis layer of skin. They are very close together in the fingertips and the toes and also in the tip of the tongue.

FIGURE 8–28.
General senses: heat, cold, touch, pressure, pain.

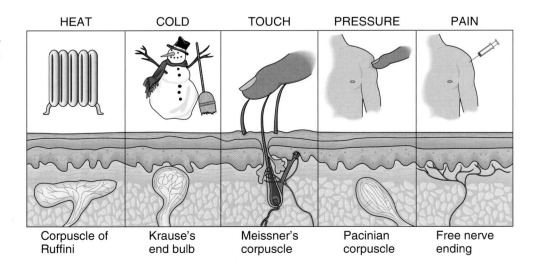

HEAT	COLD	TOUCH	PRESSURE	PAIN
Corpuscle of Ruffini	Krause's end bulb	Meissner's corpuscle	Pacinian corpuscle	Free nerve ending

Sense of Pain

Pain is the most important protective sense because it tells us that something is wrong in the body. Pain receptors are found in the

• Skin • Muscles • Joints • Internal organs

These receptors are nerve fibers that send messages of pain to the brain when parts of the body are injured.

■ COMMON DISORDERS OF THE NERVOUS SYSTEM

■ *Neuritis* is the inflammation of a nerve caused by injury, malnutrition, alcoholism, or toxic poison.

■ *Shingles* or *herpes zoster* is caused by a virus. Many blisters appear on the skin over nerve routes and cause a great deal of pain. The blisters usually disappear in about a week, but the pain may recur for years after.

■ *Conjunctivitis* is an inflammation of the eyelid lining caused from bacteria or an irritation from dirt in the eye.

■ *Cataract* formation occurs when the lens of the eye loses its transparency. Light is less able to reach the inner eye. Cataracts are the most common cause of blindness and a very common ailment in the geriatric patient.

■ *Glaucoma* occurs when there is high pressure within the eye, causing the optic nerve to deteriorate. Glaucoma appears frequently as a person ages.

■ *Otosclerosis* causes deafness because the bones in the ear change and sounds are not transmitted properly.

MEDICAL TERMINOLOGY

• audiometer	instrument to measure hearing	• lacrimal	pertaining to tear ducts
• blepharitis	inflammation of the eyelid	• ophthalmologist	specialist in the study of the eye
• blepharorrhaphy	suturing the eyelid	• otitismedia	inflammation of the middle ear
• cerebrocular	pertaining to the brain and eyes	• otoneurology	study of the ear and neural disorders
• dacryadenitis	inflammation of a tear duct		
• gustation	sense of taste	• otoplasty	plastic repair of cartilage of the ear
• iridocele	hernia of the iris of the eye	• otorrhea	purulent discharge from the ear
• iridoplegia	paralysis of the iris of the eye		

■ JOBS AND PROFESSIONS

■ Neurologist
■ Ophthalmologist
■ Otologist
■ Otorhinolaryngologist

UNIT 11   The Reproductive System

Steps to success

1. Complete Vocabulary Worksheet 1 in the Student Workbook.
2. Read this unit.
3. Complete Worksheets 2 through 5 as assigned.
4. When you are confident that you can meet each objective for this unit, ask your instructor for the unit evaluation.

Objectives

When you have completed this unit, you will be able to do the following:

✓ Match vocabulary words with their correct meanings.
✓ Label a diagram of the male and female reproductive systems.
✓ Match the various organs in the reproductive systems with their functions.
✓ Match common disorders of the reproductive system with their descriptions.
✓ Describe how the reproductive system affects the body.
✓ Explain why the health care worker's understanding of the reproductive system is important.

■ INTRODUCTION TO THE REPRODUCTIVE SYSTEM

Reproduction occurs in all species. Tiny one-celled organisms divide or separate by themselves to reproduce. Most animals require a male and female, each with their own special cells that unite to reproduce. The male and female reproductive systems have several characteristics in common. They are gonads, tubes that carry secretions, and exocrine glands.

■ *Gonads* (endocrine glands) or sex glands in the male are called *testes,* and they produce sperm. In the female they are called *ovaries,* and they produce ova.

sex cells Cells that allow reproduction to occur.

■ The *tubes* form passageways for the **sex cells,** sperm and ova.
■ *Exocrine glands* aid in the reproductive process.

The Female Reproductive System

fetus Infant developing in the uterus after the first three months until birth.

The main function of the female reproductive system is to produce the ovum for fertilization and to house a developing **fetus.** Reproduction occurs when the male and female sex cells unite within the female. After the union of these cells, they grow for 9 months or 40 weeks and develop into a new individual. Look at Figure 8–29 to identify parts of the female reproductive system.

estrogen Female hormone.

■ *Female gonads,* the ovaries, are small oval-shaped structures that produce the female sex cells or *ova* and the hormone called **estrogen.** Approximately every 28

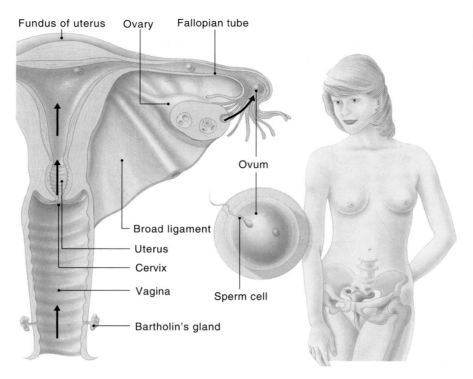

FIGURE 8–29.
Cross section of the female reproductive system.

days an ovum **matures** and is forced from the ovary and received by the fallopian tube.

■ *Fallopian tubes* are muscular tubes about 5 inches long. The tubes do not connect to the ovaries. When the **ovum** is forced from the ovary into the peritoneal cavity, it floats in the peritoneal fluid. At the end of each fallopian tube, fingerlike projections called fimbriae create a current that sweeps the ovum into the tube. Once inside the tube, the ovum is swept forward by small cilia and by peristalsis. The ovum takes about 5 days to move through the fallopian tube and is then deposited into the uterus.

■ The *uterus*, a pear-shaped organ, is attached to the fallopian tubes. While the ovum is maturing, the uterus begins to build an interlining called the **endometrium.** If the ovum is not fertilized in the fallopian tube, it deteriorates shortly after entering the uterus. The endometrium then deteriorates, causing bleeding or **menstruation.** The main function of the uterus is to house and nourish the fertilized ovum until delivery of a fully developed fetus.

■ The *vagina* is a muscular tube that houses the neck of the uterus or *cervix.* This tube extends approximately 3 inches to the outside of the body. The vagina is known as the birth canal.

The Male Reproductive System

■ *Male gonads* or *testes* are found outside the body, between the legs, in a sac called the *scrotum.* The testes produce the male sex cell or **spermatozoa** (or *sperm*) and the hormone **testosterone.** The *penis* is the primary male sex organ. It lies anterior to the testes (Figure 8–30).

■ The *epididymis* is a 20-foot-long tube that is coiled inside the scrotal sac. Sperm are stored here until they mature and are able to move by themselves. As the epididymis extends upward, it becomes the vas deferens.

matures Becomes fully developed.

ovum Female reproductive cell that when fertilized by the male develops into a new organism.

endometrium Interlining of the uterus.

menstruation Cyclic deterioration of the endometrium.

spermatozoa Male sex cells.

testosterone Male hormone.

FIGURE 8–30.
Cross section of the male reproductive system.

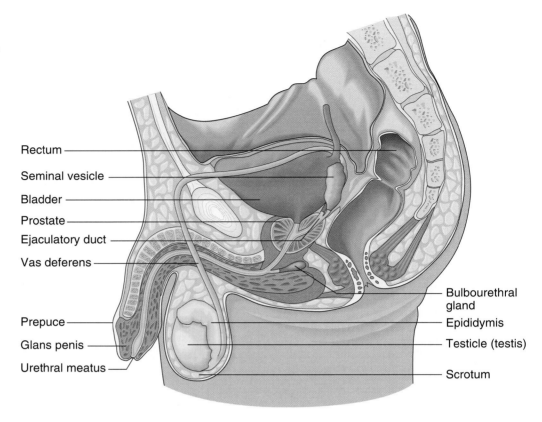

Rectum

Seminal vesicle

Bladder

Prostate

Ejaculatory duct

Vas deferens

Prepuce

Glans penis

Urethral meatus

Bulbourethral gland

Epididymis

Testicle (testis)

Scrotum

■ The *vas deferens,* the spermatic cord, extends through the abdominal wall and curves over and behind the urinary bladder. It functions as a passageway for sperm.

■ *Seminal vesicles* are outpouchings at the end of the vas deferens. They produce a thick yellow secretion that adds to the volume of **semen** and nourishes the sperm.

■ The *prostate gland,* located just below the urinary bladder, produces a secretion that maintains mobility of sperm. The *ejaculatory duct* carries sperm from the junction of the vas deferens and the seminal vesicles through the prostate gland and connects to the urethra.

■ The *urethra* is a small passage for urine and sperm, and leads from the urinary bladder through the prostate gland and the penis to the outside of the body.

semen Fluid from the testes, seminal vesicles, prostate gland, and bulbourethral glands. Contains water, mucin, proteins, salts, and sperm.

■ COMMON DISORDERS OF THE REPRODUCTIVE SYSTEM

■ *Amenorrhea* is the absence of menstruation in women.

■ *Leukorrhea* is a nonbloody vaginal discharge usually caused by an infection.

■ *Fibroid tumors* are very common in women over the age of 50. They are usually benign and produce no symptoms.

■ *Sexually transmitted diseases (STDs)* affect both male and female. The most common sexually transmitted diseases are

• *Acquired immune deficiency syndrome* (AIDS), a contagious disease that causes severe illness and results in death. It infects the body when the **AIDS** virus enters the blood of a person from the blood or body fluids of a carrier. It is most commonly transmitted by sexual contact or contaminated needles. It is characterized by swollen lymph glands, diarrhea, abnormal or unusual bleeding, fungal infection of the mouth and throat, loss of memory, fatigue, extreme weight loss, and constant cough. All or some of these symptoms may be present. There is no successful treatment at this time. • *Chlamydia,* a contagious disease characterized by purulent discharge from the urethra in the male or the vagina in the female. • *Gonorrhea,* a contagious disease characterized by a purulent discharge from the urethra. Gonorrhea can be cured with early treatment by antibiotics. • *Syphilis,* a contagious disease characterized by lesions. Lesions may not appear for many months after exposure; therefore, the disease may go untreated. Syphilis lesions can appear on any organ of the body and may cause severe damage. Antibiotics are a successful treatment. • *Venereal herpes,* a contagious disease characterized by recurrent lesions appearing in the genital region and the mucosa of the mouth. There is no successful treatment available at this time.

■ *Cryptorchidism* means "hidden testes." This disorder occurs when one or both testes fail to descend into the scrotum.

■ *Orchitis* is an inflammation of the testes.

■ *Phimosis* refers to a tightness of the foreskin over the end of the penis.

MEDICAL TERMINOLOGY

• amenorrhea	scant or no menstruation	• mammectomy	surgical removal of breast tissue
• cervicitis	inflammation of the cervix	• mastalgia	pain in the breast
• colpectasis	dilation of the vagina	• menorrhagia	excessive menstrual flow
• colpoplasty	plastic surgery on the vagina	• metrorrhexis	rupture of the uterus
• dysmenorrhea	painful or difficult menstruation	• oophorocystectomy	removal of an ovarian cyst
• ectopic pregnancy	pregnancy outside the uterus	• orchiopexy	fixation of the testes in the scrotum
• gonorrhea	flow from the genitals caused by infection	• orchioplasty	plastic surgery of the testes
• gynecomastia	abnormal enlargement of one or both breasts in men	• orchitis	inflammation of the testes
• hysterectomy	removal of uterus	• prenatal	occurring before birth
• hystersalpingo-oophorectomy	removal of the uterus, fallopian tubes, and ovaries	• postnatal	occurring after birth
• insemination	injection of semen into the female reproductive system	• sterile	unable to produce young
• lactation	secretion of milk from the breast	• tubal ligation	procedure in which fallopian tubes are blocked
• leukorrhea	whitish vaginal discharge	• vasectomy	procedure for male sterilization

■ JOBS AND PROFESSIONS

■ Embryologist

■ Gynecologist

■ Midwife

■ Obstetrician

UNIT 12   The Integumentary System

S*teps to success*

1. Complete Vocabulary Worksheet 1 in the Student Workbook.
2. Read this unit.
3. Complete Worksheets 1 and 2 as assigned.
4. When you are confident that you can meet each objective for this unit, ask your instructor for the unit evaluation.
5. Complete "Your Link to Success" at the end of this chapter.

Objectives

When you have completed this unit, you will be able to do the following:

✓ Match vocabulary words with their correct meanings.
✓ Label a diagram of a cross section of skin.
✓ List the five main functions of skin.
✓ Identify three main layers of the skin.
✓ Match common disorders of the integumentary system with their descriptions.
✓ Describe how the integumentary system protects the body.
✓ Explain why the health care worker's understanding of the integumentary system is important.

■ INTRODUCTION TO THE INTEGUMENTARY SYSTEM

The skin is the body's largest organ and is the body's first line of defense against infection. It contains several kinds of tissue, including epithelial, connective, and nerve tissues. It also contains sweat and oil glands. The combination of these tissues and glands works together as the integumentary system (Figure 8–31). The main functions of the skin are to

■ Protect the underlying body parts from injury and the invasion of pathogens
■ Regulate body temperature by controlling the loss of body heat
■ Eliminate wastes through perspiration
■ Store energy in the form of fat and vitamins
■ Sense touch, heat, cold, pain, and pressure through receptors

Structure of the Skin

epidermis Outer layer of skin.

Skin is made up of three main layers of tissue.

sloughed Discarded; separated from (e.g., to shed dead cells, as from the outer skin).

■ The **epidermis** is the outermost layer and has no blood vessels. These cells are constantly **sloughed** off.

■ The *dermis* is just beneath the epidermis and contains many blood vessels. New cells are continually forming to replace those lost from the epidermis.

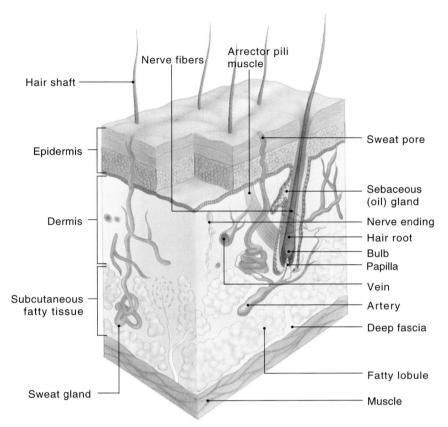

FIGURE 8–31.
Cross section of the integumentary system (skin).

Hair shaft

Nerve fibers

Arrector pili muscle

Epidermis

Dermis

Subcutaneous fatty tissue

Sweat gland

Sweat pore

Sebaceous (oil) gland

Nerve ending

Hair root

Bulb

Papilla

Vein

Artery

Deep fascia

Fatty lobule

Muscle

■ *Subcutaneous* means "under the skin," and this layer connects the skin to muscle.

■ COMMON DISORDERS OF THE INTEGUMENTARY SYSTEM

■ *Dermatosis* refers to any skin condition.

■ *Eczema* appears as reddened areas on the surface of the skin. These reddened areas often itch and appear unsightly.

■ *Athlete's foot* is caused by a fungus. It usually involves the toes and the soles of the feet but is occasionally found on the hands.

■ *Boils* are caused by bacteria entering the hair follicles or sebaceous glands.

■ *Skin cancer* is a rapid growth of cells on the skin that can invade blood vessels, lymph glands, and connecting ducts. Skin cancers can be cured if treated early. If they are left untreated, they can cause death. This type of cancer is easy to prevent by applying sunscreen and avoiding excessive exposure to the sun.

MEDICAL TERMINOLOGY

• acne	inflammation of the sebaceous gland	• ceroma	tumor of waxy appearance
• alopecia	baldness	• debridement	removal of dead tissue
• ceraceous	waxlike in appearance	• dermatitis	inflammation of the skin

- **desquamation** shedding skin in scales, sheets
- **erythema** redness of the skin
- **keloid** excessive scarring, resembling a tumor
- **keratoderma** scaly skin
- **keratogenesis** formation of scaly skin
- **pustule** elevation of skin filled with pus
- **scleraderma** hardened, thickened skin
- **sebaceous** pertaining to oily, fatty matter from the sebaceous gland
- **sebolith** stone in a sebaceous gland
- **seborrhea** excessive discharge of sebum
- **squamous** platelike, scaly
- **urticaria** itching wheals on the derma, hives

■ JOBS AND PROFESSIONS

■ Dermatologist

■ SUMMARY

You have learned that the cell is the building block of the body. Cells form tissues, which form organs. The organs of the body form the systems. All of these components must work together to keep the body in homeostasis (balance). You have also learned about some of the disorders that affect the body. This knowledge helps you take better care of your health and better care of your patients.

Your link to success

Thinking Critically:
Check Your Understanding

1. **Communication** Explain how you think that your understanding of the body systems helps you communicate with patients/clients and co-workers. Your patient/client asks you to explain how the muscles in her upper arm cause the forearm to move. Write how you can communicate this information to a child under six, an adult over eighty, and a teenager.

2. **Medical Terminology** Every cell, tissue, organ, and system in the body has medical terminology related to it. The best way to learn terminology is to learn word parts. If you know that a word part is a prefix, a root, or a suffix, it helps you combine the words correctly. For instance, the prefix *endo-* does not make sense if added to the end of a word root *cardi/o*, which would be *cardiendo*. The same is true if you added the suffix *-ic* to the beginning of *cardi/o*, which would be *iccardio*. Use the roots *gastr/o*, *cardi/o*, *oste/o*, and *nephr/o* to make ten new terms using prefixes, suffixes, and additional roots. Look up each word in the dictionary. Write the words on an index card with their correct spelling and definition.

3. **Legal and Ethical** A patient's doctor just told him that he has a serious problem in the gastrointestinal system. The doctor thinks that it is probably a malignant tumor. The patient asks you what you know about his condition. What is your responsibility in this case?

4. **Computers** Computers offer many opportunities for learning and for accessing information. They are also used to diagnose disorders of the various body systems. Identify as many computerized tests as you can. Create a list by writing the full name of each test and the name of the computerized equipment used to perform the test.

5. **Case Study** Mr. Jones is admitted to the hospital. His reports say that he has severe retinopathy, erythemia over the right lateral tibia, cyanosis of the oncus of distal metatarsals, and edema over the calcaneus of the right foot. He also has hyperthemia and nausea that is causing frequent emesis. Write these symptoms in terms that a non-medical person can understand.

Portfolio Connection

Employers look for health care workers who have knowledge of the body and body systems. Assistive personnel work in many different departments and must be able to recognize problems and report them correctly to a supervisor. Complete the following exercise and put it in your portfolio for review in the future: Identify one body system disorder. Research the objective and subjective symptoms that result from this disorder. Explain your findings in a typed or neatly written paper.

9 HUMAN GROWTH AND DEVELOPMENT

Steps to success

1. Complete Vocabulary Worksheet 1 in the Student Workbook.
2. Read this unit.
3. Complete Worksheets 2 through 6 as assigned.
4. When you are confident that you can meet each objective for this unit, ask your instructor for the unit evaluation.

Rationale

continuum Progression from start (birth) to finish (death).

Health care workers provide care for all age groups. It is important to understand the emotional and physical stages of the life **continuum.** This knowledge assists you in recognizing normal and abnormal development and behavior. This awareness of life's stages allows you to be an effective health care worker.

Objectives

When you have completed this unit, you will be able to do the following:

✓ Match vocabulary words with their correct meanings.
✓ Identify three stages of development between conception and birth.
✓ List four common developments of growth in the first year of life and the age at which they usually occur.
adolescent Pertaining to the period of life between childhood and maturity.
✓ Define and describe characteristics of **adolescent** development.
✓ Interview a person between the ages of 50 and 80.
✓ Compare your life experiences to each stage described in this chapter.

196

✓ Design a bulletin board representing one stage of growth and development, including age-specific communication requirements.

■ DEVELOPMENT AND BEHAVIOR

People experience many physical and emotional changes over a lifetime. These changes are part of the normal growth and development process. In this unit, we discuss the stages of development and behavior from conception through the life continuum.

Conception or fertilization occurs when a male sperm and a female ovum combine. This combination causes the single-cell ovum to divide into many cells. This stage of development is called a **zygote.** Within five weeks, the rapidly multiplying cells duplicate into an embryo.

zygote Any cell formed by the coming together of two reproductive (sex) cells.

■ Five weeks after conception, the embryo is about the size of a grain of rice.
■ Six weeks after conception, the nervous system, eyes, and ears are visible.

Fetal and Infant Stage

At 12 weeks or 3 months after conception, the embryo has grown to about 2½ inches (6 cm) long. It is now called a fetus. Babies are born 38 to 40 weeks after conception. The following are stages of average development and behavior.

■ *6 weeks.*   Baby first begins to smile.
■ *10 weeks.*   Infant has the ability to roll from a **prone** to a **supine** position.
■ *4 to 6 months.*   Infant raises head and shoulders while in a supine position. *Communication:* Hold, cuddle, and speak to infants frequently. Talking to infants helps them recognize sounds and make associations. It is helpful to talk slowly and clearly when holding, feeding, or bathing infants at this age. Sudden, strange noise may cause fear. Comfort infants by speaking in a soothing tone and touch them gently to communicate your presence and reassurance.

prone Lying on the stomach.

supine Lying on the back.

■ *6 to 8 months.*   Infant sits without being supported; eye color may change.
■ *8 to 12 months.*   Attempts to feed self and begins to crawl, stand, and take steps. As infants become toddlers, expect frequent falls while they are learning to walk. Provide a safe environment free of sharp edges and, if possible, keep them on carpeting instead of cement or tile flooring. *Communication:* Distract or move infants when they are headed for trouble. Use simple terms to warn them: "Hot!" "Hurt," or "Tastes bad." Always praise good behavior.
■ *1 year.   Communication:* Understands simple conversation or commands. Most 12-month-olds can say four or five clear words. Children who are spoken to with clear word pronunciation (not baby talk) develop clearer speech. Learning and experimenting absorbs most of their waking hours. Show them what is expected, resist saying a constant "No," and be patient.

Toddler Stage (18 Months to 3 Years of Age)

■ *18 months.*   Walks alone, feeds itself, and stacks objects. *Communication:* "Mine" becomes a favorite claim. Communicate clear limits about acceptable and unacceptable behavior. Reinforce good behavior. Playing easy games and reading simple stories help develop vocabulary. Time spent in this way provides opportunity to share in positive, nurturing experiences.

■ *20 to 24 months.*   Begins bowel and bladder control. Experiences exploration and a feeling of security. *Communication:* Vocabulary increases rapidly at this age. Pronunciation may take time to develop; your patience allows normal speech development. Resist trying to correct pronunciation too frequently. Listen carefully and confirm your understanding of the child's words.

■ *3 to 4 years.*   *Communication:* Talks in simple complete sentences. Begins to think of other children as equals. May be shy and unwilling to explore.

Preschool and Elementary Age (3 to 8 Years of Age)

■ *4 to 5 years.*   Dresses and undresses with little assistance. Experiences a span of emotional growth.

coordination State of harmonized action, such as eye and hand coordination.

■ *5 to 6 years.*   Eye and body **coordination** improves. The child is able to hop, skip, and draw figures. Awareness of the ability to choose one action over another is present. Child begins to feel guilt and shame.

■ *6 to 8 years.*   Physical skills continue to improve. Children start school. They begin to look for reasons that explain why they believe certain things. They also compare themselves with others. About age 7, they experience emotional withdrawal or shyness.

■ *Communication with children 3 to 8:*   Children at this age require frequent reassurance and truthful, caring conversation. Keep discussions short and easy to understand, allowing time for the child to say everything he wants to say. Acceptance of what the child says is important, and positive reflection of her words provides the support necessary to help the child overcome shyness and withdrawal.

Communication during medical care—toddlers and children of early elementary age: Refer to the child by her favorite name (name, nickname, or special term the family uses). Use the same words the family uses for toileting. Do not blame or scold if toileting accidents occur. Explain in simple terms what is happening to and around the child. Answer his questions honestly and in understandable terms for his level. When possible spend time with the child, talking and playing simple games. Taking time to communicate and enjoy activities with each child is important in creating a positive sense of well-being during medical care.

Preteen Years or Preadolescent Years

■ *8 to 13 years.*   Physical growth rate increases, and adult sexual characteristics become noticeable. Girls begin menstruation. Boys develop more hair on their faces and bodies, and the voice deepens. Preteens look to their friends for acceptance and approval rather than to their parents. Children ages 8 to 12 experience emotional security; 13-year-olds feel insecure and shy. *Communication:* Children 8 to 12 years old do best when you listen to them and give them a chance to express themselves. Use positive responses to indicate that you hear what they are saying. It is also important to explain clearly the differences between acceptable and unacceptable behavior. Acknowledge positive actions and discuss why other behaviors are not appropriate. Thirteen-year-olds often require increased words of reassurance and encouragement to overcome feelings of insecurity and shyness.

Adolescent or Teenage Years

■ *13 to 18 years.*   The teens are the years between childhood and adulthood. The teenager strives for independence. They also experience puberty, a dramatic sexual development caused by increased hormone production of certain glands.

(Girls may start puberty by 11 years; boys usually start at 13 years.) Puberty is a time of both physical and emotional adjustment. *Communication:* Adolescents need others to listen and reflect their words back to them. This type of communication allows teenagers to hear what they are thinking and gain increased understanding of themselves. Respect their privacy. Question personal behavior and habits only when it is pertinent to their health and well-being.

Communication during medical care—adolescents: Be sensitive to their fear even when they act fearless. Honestly explain all procedures at their level of understanding and communicate a desire to honor their privacy. When possible, discuss their areas of interest and participate in activities (e.g., cards, games) with them to provide an increased sense of well-being.

Young Adulthood

■ *18 to 20 years.* People become more independent. As they mature, they begin to seek ways of contributing to society.

Adulthood

■ *20 to 30 years.* This is the beginning of adulthood, when people attempt to build a firm, safe foundation for the future. There is a strong desire to do the right thing. Patterns of living are set during this **decade,** such as

decade Period of 10 years.

• Helper patterns (rescuing others) • Leadership patterns (taking charge, organizing) • Passive patterns (acting without influence, not taking an active part in things)

These are just a few simple patterns people may fall into; there are many other patterns.

■ *30 to 40 years.* In this decade, people often feel confined by the guidelines that they established for themselves in their 20s. This confined feeling often leads to restructuring of work, family, and social habits. Through this change, people develop more freedom and a new view of self.

■ *40 to 50 years.* People often evaluate the first part of their life. They make decisions about future directions. Many find themselves adjusting basic values and their emphasis toward life. This time of adjustment is often referred to as "midlife crisis" or the "deadline decade." *Communication:* Women develop assertiveness. Men become more tender and make stronger commitments to ethical issues.

■ *50 to 60 years.* These are the years when people experience a sense of comfort, an acceptance of life, and a new warmth and mellowing. Privacy becomes important, and friends become more cherished. Truth and sincerity become more valued. Renewal of earlier hobbies and interests often sparks new energy and enthusiasm.

■ *60 to 70 years.* These are the years in which people look forward to retirement. For some people there is a gradual change in their work lives. Others prefer full retirement. The additional hours away from work can now be filled with interests or hobbies. This newfound time often allows people to complete lifelong projects or desires. *Communication:* Sharing of one's self with others aids in maintaining a sense of self-worth. Listening and sharing interest in stories and experiences as they are relayed is a way for younger people to learn and to show gratitude for the mentorship of people of this age.

■ *70 and older.*   After the 70s, people continue their daily life in the same adult patterns. The effect of aging on the body is discussed in Unit 2 of this chapter. If the body loses its resilience and functions become impaired, the individual's lifestyle may change. It is important to note that of the increasing geriatric population, only 5 percent require in-patient health care. The remaining 95 percent are **viable,** active seniors.

viable Capable of living.

Communication with adults of any age: Show positive interest in adults' conversation, and interpret and respond to their body language. Use words that are understandable and meaningful to each individual's level. Express your desire to protect people's privacy; resist questioning personal behaviors and habits unless they are pertinent to the person's health and well-being.

Communication during medical care—adults of all ages: Be aware of the impact medical care is having on each person. Be sensitive to fears; honestly explain procedures and expected outcomes. When speaking about a patient, *always* go to areas away from the patient's view and hearing. Your behavior must communicate dignity toward others—be aware of your body language and verbal tone. Thoughtfully communicate by being aware of when words are helpful and when to be silent and present with a simple touch.

■ SUMMARY

In this unit, you have learned about development from conception throughout the life continuum. You have also become aware of emotional and behavioral experiences and communication issues related to each decade of life.

UNIT 2   Aging and Role Change

*S*teps to success

1. Complete Vocabulary Worksheet 1 in the Student Workbook.
2. Read this unit.
3. Complete Worksheets 2 through 4 as assigned.
4. When you are confident that you can meet each objective for this unit, ask your instructor for the unit evaluation.

Rationale

The population of people over the age of 65 is expanding. Most people over 65 are active, and they adapt well to change. They continue to enjoy physical activities such as tennis, biking, and skiing. Only 5 percent are in long-term care. To care adequately for senior citizens with health problems, health care workers must be aware of the emotional and physical changes that occur during the aging process. Understanding these changes allows the health care worker to assist the aging person in adapting more easily to new roles and ability levels.

Objectives

When you have completed this unit, you will be able to do the following:

✓ Match vocabulary words with their correct meanings.
✓ Identify six body systems and the common physical changes that occur with aging.
✓ Identify basic human needs that are met through work, **environment,** socialization, and family relationships.
✓ Write an "action plan" to assist another person cope with changes caused by aging.

environment Surroundings we live in. Environmental disease can occur in any area around us (e.g., hospital, restaurants, public places, home, school).

■ PHYSICAL CHANGES OF AGING

The process of aging begins in every person at the moment of birth. Aging is a very natural process, and the health care worker needs to be aware of the physical changes that take place. Understanding these changes helps you be patient and less frustrated with others.

Nervous System

■ The *brain* experiences changes in a number of nerve cells and in the brain mass. Elderly people frequently suffer from arteriosclerosis, which causes a decrease in blood flow and oxygen to the brain. This often results in confusion, which is misunderstood and may be very annoying to the health care worker.

■ *Vision* begins to change with aging:

• Small print, small items, and things at a distance are more difficult to see.
• More light is needed to see things clearly. • Night driving may become difficult. • **Adaptation** to light is more difficult. The eyes take longer to adjust to changes from dark to light and from light to dark. • Diseases may occur:

adaptation Changing to work better.

> • *Cataract:* clouding of the normally transparent lenses of the eye • *Glaucoma:* intraocular pressure causes damage to the optic disks and hardening of the eyeball

■ *Hearing* changes become noticeable in the 60s:

• High-frequency sounds such as a telephone or doorbell may not be heard.
• Loss of understanding of consonants and vowel sounds may result in a person complaining that others mumble or speak too softly.

■ *Taste, smell,* and *touch* senses decline with age.

• The elderly may not smell gases, spoiled food, or body odor. • Taste buds decline 50 percent, and food enjoyment is reduced. • Elderly people may request extra salt and sugar because they cannot taste well. • Touch and **reflexes** change. The ability to respond to stimuli is decreased. The elderly may burn themselves or hold an ice tray too long and damage tissue or take longer to respond to the directions you give.

reflexes Result when a nerve is stimulated and an involuntary action occurs (e.g., touch a hot stove, and the muscles react involuntarily to move the fingers away).

Musculoskeletal System

■ Osteoarthritis is an inflammation of the joints and causes pain and slowing down of movement.

stamina Body's strength or energy.

■ Osteoporosis is caused by a loss of calcium in the bone. This is found more in women after menopause, when the bones may become very brittle. They may fracture with very little stress.

■ With reduced **stamina,** the elderly are often less active, which results in the muscles becoming smaller. The elderly generally slow down, which may cause the health care worker to feel impatient.

Respiratory and Circulatory System

alveolar-capillary Pertaining to air sacs in the lungs.

■ The lungs become less elastic, and the **alveolar-capillary** membrane thickens. This makes oxygen exchange more difficult.

■ The rib cage does not expand as much.

■ The heart becomes less efficient, and the arteries may become narrowed and clogged. The systolic pressure may rise and result in high blood pressure.

■ The heart also becomes a less efficient pump. Heart disease is the number one cause of death in older people. Among these diseases are

• Congestive heart failure • Cardiac arrhythmias • Ischemic heart disease
• Hypertensive heart disease

Gastrointestinal System

constipation Infrequent or difficult emptying of the bowel.

■ Many elderly patients/clients experience **constipation.**

■ Loss of teeth may interfere with chewing.

■ The liver is important in metabolism. With age, the liver loses up to 20 percent of its weight. This is not serious, because the liver can be effective at 50 percent capacity. However, the liver becomes less effective in metabolizing drugs. Older people must be monitored carefully and be alert to drug side effects.

Urinary System

retention Keeping elements within the body that are normally eliminated (e.g., waste products such as urine and feces).

■ The bladder holds less urine as a person ages. This may cause an urgent and frequent need to urinate.

■ Bladder infections may occur from **retention** of urine in the bladder. This results in urinary urgency and urinary discomfort.

Your awareness of these changes helps you be patient and understanding. These physical changes often cause frustration in your patient and in you. Remember that these changes occur because the body is aging. Listen and reflect understanding. Explain procedures in understandable terms.

■ ROLE CHANGES IN THE AGING

Because aging persons are experiencing physical and emotional changes, they need understanding and patience. They want to continue as a part of society, and they need to feel human dignity.

All people have basic needs that are met through the roles they have throughout their life span.

■ *Work role.*   The work a person does gives a sense of independence, security, and self-esteem. When occupational identity is lost through retirement or physical disability, these needs must be met in some other way.

■ *Family relationships.*   Being a member of a family meets our needs for emotional warmth, intimacy, and identity. When members of the family begin to leave or die, the person may be left without a means of filling these basic needs. To adapt to these losses, people need help in directing their interests and energies in other areas. Some of these may include social activities, volunteer work, or membership in organizations.

■ *Social roles.*   Social contacts fill a person's need for interaction with others. Through social contacts, the person feels respected and admired. As the years pass, friends move away or die, and personal relationships change. These losses may cause people to feel that they are no longer socially important. It is very important that the aging person take part in developing new social contacts. Senior centers, churches, and other organizations are available to help meet this need. Becoming involved helps fill the need for interaction with other human beings.

■ *Environment.*   The home a person lives in is a place where he or she can be in control, where he or she has a feeling of belonging. As aging occurs, it may become necessary to change environments. The home may become a financial burden, or it may be physically impossible to remain there. The elderly may move into their children's home, a nursing home, or a room of their own. This change may be very frightening, and the need for control in their environment is threatened.

As a health care worker, your understanding of these changes helps you develop the necessary skills to work with elderly clients. Human beings have a great ability to adjust to changes in their life roles. Acceptance of their needs allows you to be patient and understanding as you care for them.

■ SUMMARY

As people age, physical changes occur in the body. These changes affect many body systems. When these changes occur, elderly patients experience frustration with their conditions. The health care worker has an important role in helping the elderly patient understand and accept changes.

There are many role changes that occur in aging persons. They may no longer have the identity that their work gave them. They may lose a spouse or other important family members, leaving them lonely. Often, their social role changes as they are less involved in activities. They may find it difficult to develop new friendships. They may have to leave the home where they have their roots and move to a strange place. Awareness of these changes helps the health care worker work effectively with elderly patients.

UNIT 3   Disabilities and Role Changes

Steps to success

1. Complete Vocabulary Worksheet 1 in the Student Workbook.
2. Read this unit.
3. Complete Worksheets 2 and 3 as assigned.
4. When you are confident that you can meet each objective for this unit, ask your instructor for the unit evaluation.

Rationale

adapt To change, to become suitable, to adjust.

Physical disabilities can affect any age group. When a disability, injury, or illness changes a person's lifestyle, he or she must **adapt** to these changes. This is often difficult and causes frustration and depression. As a health care worker, you need to understand these changes. When you understand such changes, you are more effective, and you can be a positive influence as these patients/clients begin to adapt.

Objectives

When you have completed this unit, you will be able to do the following:

✓ Match vocabulary words with their correct meanings.
✓ Define *health*.
✓ List three examples of activities of daily living (ADL).
✓ Define assistive/adaptive devices.
✓ Identify ways to encourage independence.
✓ List eight **birth defects.**
✓ List ten **debilitating** illnesses.
✓ Identify seven common changes that occur following the loss of body functions.
✓ State the goal of rehabilitation.
✓ Select a disability and summarize your feelings and expectations concerning
  ✓ What you think it would be like to live with that disability
  ✓ The type of care you would expect
  ✓ The way others respond to the disability

birth defects Defects present at birth.

debilitating Causing weakness or impairment.

■ DEFINITION OF HEALTH

The World Health Organization defines health as "a state of complete physical, mental, and social well-being and not merely the absence of disease or infirmity." As a health care worker, you strive to help patients/clients reach their highest potential.

■ IMPORTANCE OF INDEPENDENCE

When a person is ill or injured, they often have limitations. These limitations usually affect their activities of daily living. The activities include

• Bathing • Combing hair • Going to the bathroom • Dressing • Eating • Brushing teeth • Communicating effectively

Some patients/clients can do these activities with little or no help. Others need a lot of help. The goal is to allow each person to be as independent as he or she possibly can be. Always encourage a patient to try an activity. (For example, the person may be able to put toothpaste on the brush but needs your help to brush the teeth.) You can encourage the client by being patient and positive and by letting him or her make choices. This helps the patient/client feel more independent and increases feelings of well-being and self-respect. There are many assistive/adaptive devices available (Figure 9–1). Computers are effective assistive/adaptive devices

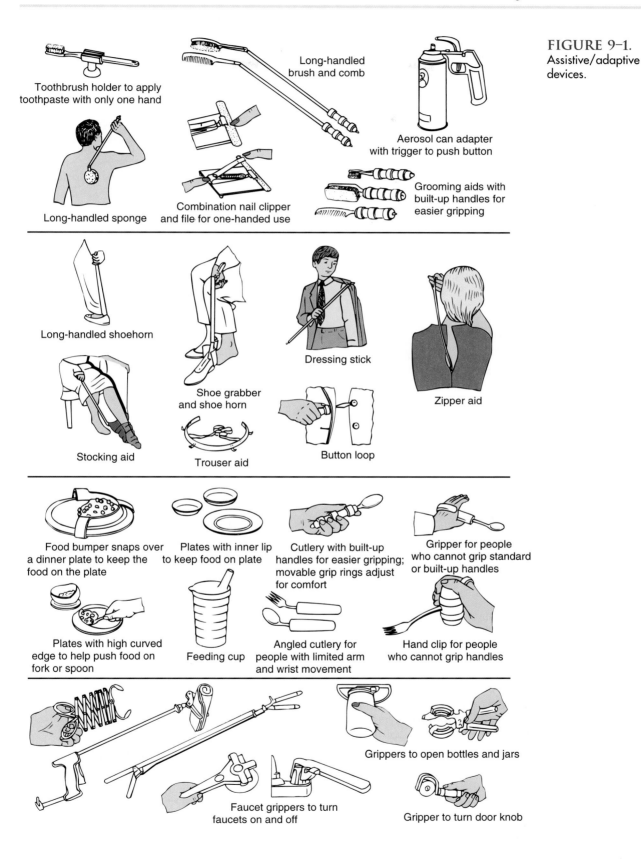

FIGURE 9–1.
Assistive/adaptive devices.

Toothbrush holder to apply toothpaste with only one hand

Long-handled brush and comb

Aerosol can adapter with trigger to push button

Long-handled sponge

Combination nail clipper and file for one-handed use

Grooming aids with built-up handles for easier gripping

Long-handled shoehorn

Shoe grabber and shoe horn

Dressing stick

Zipper aid

Stocking aid

Trouser aid

Button loop

Food bumper snaps over a dinner plate to keep the food on the plate

Plates with inner lip to keep food on plate

Cutlery with built-up handles for easier gripping; movable grip rings adjust for comfort

Gripper for people who cannot grip standard or built-up handles

Plates with high curved edge to help push food on fork or spoon

Feeding cup

Angled cutlery for people with limited arm and wrist movement

Hand clip for people who cannot grip handles

Grippers to open bottles and jars

Faucet grippers to turn faucets on and off

Gripper to turn door knob

for children and adults with physical disabilities. People who cannot hold a pencil or speak can use computers with special enhancements to communicate. Individualized computer programs are created to guide learning. Computers with e-mail and Internet capabilities provide opportunities for people with disabilities to interact with the outside world. The computer enables people with certain disabilities to communicate their needs, thoughts, desires, and intelligence to their parents and caregivers. These devices help the patient be more independent and self-sufficient. They help clients

• Eat • Reach objects • Complete personal care • Dress and button clothing • Communicate

■ PHYSICAL DISABILITIES

Physical disabilities may be caused by a birth defect, a debilitating illness, or an injury. Understanding these disabilities helps you give better care to your patients.

Birth Defect

syndrome A number of symptoms occurring together.

Babies who are born with a physical defect, inherited **syndrome,** or other problems have a birth defect. As a health care worker, you need to recognize these defects in order to give good care and be supportive to family members. Common birth defects include the following.

■ *Cerebral palsy* is a motor function disorder that is caused by a brain defect or lesion present at birth or shortly after. Some of the identifying characteristics include the following:

• Spastic hemiplegia • Seizures • Some degree of mental retardation in some people • Impaired vision, speech, and hearing • Stiff, awkward movements

embryonic Pertaining to the embryo.

■ *Cleft lip and/or cleft palate* occurs when fusion of the palate and/or lip does not take place during **embryonic** development. This can usually be observed. However, a partial cleft may not be observable. Some of the characteristics are

• An inability to suck or nurse • Crying when the child tries to nurse • Fluid coming out of the nose

■ *Down syndrome* is characterized by varying degrees of mental retardation and multiple defects. Other identifying characteristics include the following:

• Typical face appearance with a mongoloid slant to the eyes • Depressed nasal bridge • Low-set ears • Large, protruding tongue • Short, broad hands with a simian crease and stubby fingers • Broad, stubby feet with wide spaces between the first and second toes • Being prone to respiratory infections, visual problems, abnormalities in tooth development

neurological Pertaining to the nervous system.

■ *Epilepsy* is caused by a group of **neurological** disorders that may be birth defects but can occur later in life due to cerebral trauma, intracranial infection, brain tumor, **intoxication,** or chemical imbalance. Some characteristics are

intoxication State of poisoning or becoming poisoned.

• Recurrent **episodes** of convulsive seizures • Sensory disturbances • Abnormal behavior • Loss of consciousness

episodes Events in a series.

■ *Hydrocephaly* occurs when there is an overproduction or underabsorption of cerebrospinal fluid. It may cause an increase in the size of the head, depending on the onset and whether the cranial sutures have closed. If the sutures have not closed, the cranium expands. If the sutures have closed, the pressure in the brain is increased. Some characteristics are

• Globe-shaped head • Flat nose bridge • Eyes pushed downward and out, becoming widely spread • Mild to severe retardation

■ *Sickle-cell anemia* is a **hereditary** disease that is most common among the black population. The red blood cell is crescent shaped (sickle shaped) and carries an abnormal hemoglobin. Some of the characteristics are

• Severe joint pain • Thrombosis • Fever • Chronic anemia

■ *Spinal bifida cystica* is a developmental defect. A hernial sac containing the meninges, spinal cord, or both protrudes at the end of the vertebral column. This sac is easily ruptured, causing such problems as

• Leakage of spinal fluid • Risk of meningeal infection (infected lining of the brain) • Severe neurological **dysfunction** (nervous system is not working normally) • Paralysis • Muscle weakness • Retardation

■ *Tay-Sachs syndrome* is also an inherited disease, caused by an **enzyme deficiency.** It occurs primarily in families of Eastern European Jewish origin. The major problems are difficult breathing and decreased exchange of oxygen and carbon dioxide.

Debilitating Illness

Debilitating illness may occur at any age. Depending on the severity of the disease, physical changes may be minimal or very extensive. The following are some common illnesses.

■ *Acquired immune deficiency syndrome (AIDS)* is caused by a virus that reduces the immune system's ability to respond to **opportunistic infections.** Common opportunistic infections that result from AIDS include pneumocystis pneumonia, candidiasis, cryptococcoses, and herpes. Cancers that may develop are Kaposi's sarcoma and lymphomas.

■ *Alzheimer's disease* affects men and women in later middle life and causes confusion, memory failure, **disorientation,** and many other problems.

■ *Arteriosclerosis* is hardening of the arteries, which reduces the elasticity of the arterial walls. This causes an increase in blood pressure.

■ *Atherosclerosis* occurs when **lipid-**containing material collects on the inside surfaces of the blood vessels. This inhibits the flow of blood.

■ *Cancer* occurs anywhere in the body. It is characterized by an uncontrolled growth of cells.

■ *Cardiovascular disease* refers to many abnormal heart and circulatory conditions. Some of these are rheumatic heart disease, enlarged heart tissue, damage to the heart, and hypertension.

■ *Cystic fibrosis* is an inherited disorder of the exocrine glands that causes an excessive amount of thick mucus. This occurs especially in the respiratory system, frequently causing respiratory disease.

■ *Emphysema* is an abnormal condition of the pulmonary system in which the alveoli are damaged. A major cause of chronic emphysema is cigarette smoking.

■ *Leukemia* is the rapid and abnormal growth of leukocytes in the blood-forming organs (bone marrow, spleen, and lymph nodes).

■ *Multiple sclerosis* is a **progressive** disease that affects the nerve fibers of the brain and spinal cord. It generally begins in young adulthood and continues

hereditary Passed from parent to child.

dysfunction Impaired or abnormal functioning.

enzyme Substance that causes a change to occur in other substances.

deficiency Shortage (e.g., a deficient diet causes the body to function poorly because it is missing an important element).

opportunistic infections Infections that occur when the immune system is weakened. Common organisms that the body normally resists cause infection.

disorientation State of being confused about time, place, and identity of persons and objects.

arteriosclerosis Condition of hardening of the arteries.

lipid Fat.

progressive Moving forward, following steps toward an end product.

throughout life. It causes muscle weakness, visual disturbances, and dizziness. It affects the whole body, including emotional stability.

■ *Parkinson's disease* is a slowly progressive, degenerative, neurological disorder. Symptoms include tremors, shuffling gait, masklike face, forward flexion of the trunk, muscle rigidity, and weakness.

Injury

Injuries may occur at any age and cause many different disabilities. Some of the most common are

coma Deep sleep; unconscious state for a long period of time.

amputation Removal of a body part.

■ Spinal cord injuries, which may cause paralysis
■ Stroke, which may cause paralysis, brain dysfunction, speech impairments, and/or loss of memory
■ Head injuries, which may cause **coma,** loss of memory, and/or paralysis
■ **Amputation** of a limb

■ ROLE CHANGES IN THE DISABLED

When people experience a lengthy disability, they require understanding and patience. The disabled need to remain a productive part of society and to maintain a sense of well-being. The health care worker can be a positive influence on patients/clients during the period of adjustment and rehabilitation.

People who lose a body part or a part of their body functions experience the same stages of loss as do people with a terminal illness. These are denial, rage and anger, bargaining, depression, and acceptance. Many people who suddenly find themselves disabled are dependent on others for many of their daily needs. Being dependent often leads to feelings of not being in control. Physical losses can cause various body functions to be impaired.

Loss of body function often means that changes may occur in the following:

■ Communication skills
■ Sensory awareness
■ Ability to think and comprehend
■ Ability to move
■ Elimination of waste products
■ Eating
■ Sexual activity

Loss of physical functions may cause emotional stability to change. The areas of emotional insecurity usually focus around the following:

• Self-esteem • Self-confidence • Self-image

Physical impairments that lead to emotional changes may also create a sense of loss concerning the following:

• Ability to develop relationships with others • Ability to earn a living • Ability to be a useful member of society

The health care worker helps patients/clients reach their goals by being understanding and knowledgeable about the process involved in acceptance of a disability and rehabilitation.

Rehabilitation

When physical changes occur, the goal of rehabilitation is to help the patient/client return to the highest level of functioning possible. Rehabilitation promotes a healthy return to a productive lifestyle. There are many rehabilitation areas involved in this process. The most common are as follows:

■ Physical therapy restores the body to normal functioning when possible.
■ Occupational therapy restores the ability to be involved in purposeful activity.
■ Speech therapy restores the ability to communicate effectively.
■ Psychotherapy changes inappropriate behavior patterns, improves interpersonal relationships, and resolves inner conflicts.

There are several groups available to aid the client and family during the recovery and rehabilitation period. These groups, called *support groups,* are organized to help patients and family members cope with changes during this period. Examples of groups are

■ Breast cancer support groups
■ Ostomy support group
■ Vital Options—a support group for young adults with cancer

You can locate groups in your area by contacting the social services department at hospitals, community centers, and organizations oriented to health care.

■ SUMMARY

Physical disabilities, injury, and debilitating illness can occur from birth to old age. There are many different types of disabilities. Some of these are caused by accident, heredity, injury, or illness. When any of these are present, the patient may be frustrated or depressed. As a health care worker, you are responsible for the care and support of these patients. It is important to understand their illness and to be familiar with assistive/adaptive devices and support organizations that are available to help patients and their families.

UNIT 4   Psychological Stages in the Terminally Ill

Steps to success

1. Complete Vocabulary Worksheet 1 in the Student Workbook.
2. Read this unit.
3. Complete Worksheets 2 and 3 as assigned.
4. When you are confident that you can meet each objective for this unit, ask your instructor for the unit evaluation.
5. Complete "Your Link to Success" at the end of this chapter.

Rationale

As a health care worker, you come in contact with clients who are terminally ill. Your knowledge of the psychological stages experienced by the terminally ill gives you an understanding of their behavior.

Objectives

When you have completed this unit, you will be able to do the following:

✓ Match vocabulary words with their correct meanings.
✓ Match the psychological stages of a long terminal illness with their names.
✓ Identify and discuss your feelings about terminal illness.
✓ Explain the **philosophy** of hospice care.

philosophy Theory; a general principle used for a specific purpose.

■ TERMINAL ILLNESS

Patients/clients who have an illness that cannot be cured are terminally ill. They are expected to die. When the patients learn of their illness, they usually pass through five different psychological stages (Figure 9–2).

■ *Stage one: Shock and denial.*   People find it very difficult to believe that they are really going to die. "No, not me!" During this stage they feel very lonely and **isolated.** *Communication:* If they can discuss these feelings and talk about their **impending** death, they are able to move into the next stage. You may be the only health care worker available to listen to their feelings.

isolated Limited in contact with others.

impending About to happen.

■ *Stage two: Rage and anger.*   No matter how much kindness you have shown, your client may become very insulting; there might be many complaints about everything you do. You may be tempted to leave them to their anger. *Communication:* If you realize it is not a personal attack, you will be able to listen and to understand that the anger is not directed at you. It is directed at the injustice of the situation. Be a good listener. When patients have exhausted their anger, they will move out of the anger stage.

■ *Stage three: Bargaining.*   Although they now admit to themselves that they are dying, the clients try to prolong their life with bargaining. For example, they

FIGURE 9–2.
Stages of dying.

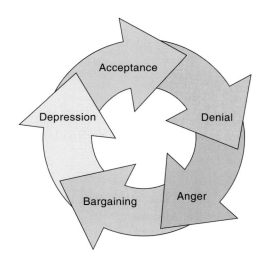

might say, "Just let me live until my children are independent." *Communication:* Listen and reflect what is said, express your understanding, and be aware of your voice tone and body language. Be aware of times when your presence in silence is helpful and when words are not helpful.

■ *Stage four: Depression.*   Your patients may refuse to talk to you or even look at you. They are experiencing great sadness, for they are losing everyone and everything. *Communication:* Although they may not want to be bothered with friends or visitors, your touch is very important. Your understanding of their feelings of loss enables them to move into the last stage.

■ *Stage five: Acceptance.*   At last your clients can accept their death. This is a time when your presence lets them know you will not desert them. *Communication:* They may want to discuss their death. Your willingness to be available will help your patients in a very difficult time.

Friends and family often experience the same stages when someone they love and care about is terminally ill. As a health care worker, you need to be understanding. Family and friends may experience the following stages:

■ *Shock and denial.*   They may continue to make plans for the future that include the dying person.

■ *Rage and anger.*   They may be irritable and angry and say unkind things occasionally.

■ *Bargaining.*   They may ask the physician to keep the patient/client alive for a special occasion.

■ *Depression.*   They feel extreme sadness and even despair.

■ *Acceptance.*   They finally accept that death is going to occur. They may ask you to recommend someone for them to talk to.

■ HOSPICE CARE

In many communities, hospice care is available for the terminally ill. The hospice philosophy is to help the terminally ill patient/client live each day to the fullest. This care is provided in the home or in a hospice facility. Patients are kept comfortable and free from pain. When the time for death comes, they are allowed to die peacefully. An important service of hospice is family involvement. Families are counseled and helped to accept the impending death of a loved one. Following the death, the family has continuing support for at least a year. This support helps make the grieving period more tolerable.

You are an important member of the health care team. Your insight into the patient/client and his or her family and friends provides valuable information to decision makers concerning the care process. This knowledge of what your patients/clients may experience helps you meet their needs.

■ JOBS AND PROFESSIONS

■ Gerontologist
■ Hospice worker
■ Nurse assistant/orderly in long-term care facility
■ Ambulatory care clinics
■ Assistive personnel

■ SUMMARY

Most health care workers come in contact with terminally ill patients/clients and are involved in the care of a dying person. The terminally ill patient usually experiences five psychological stages: denial, anger, bargaining, depression, and acceptance. Patients who are terminally ill have an opportunity to choose a hospice for the final days of their illness.

Your link to success

Thinking Critically: Check Your Understanding

1. **Communication** Describe at least five examples of situations with disabled patients/clients. Explain ways to communicate that you value their dignity and need for fairness and justice.

2. **Legal and Ethical** An elderly husband and wife decide to live in a long-term care facility so that their family won't worry about them. Upon admission, the wife is placed in room 125, and the husband is placed next door in room 126. They ask to share the same room, but the admitting clerk explains that the facility policy doesn't allow men and women to stay in the same room. Describe your remarks to the family and how you would respond to the admitting clerk or your supervisor.

3. **Cultural Competency** A female patient/client of Asian heritage refuses to eat her food until it is room temperature. She frequently does not get to eat because her tray is collected and returned to the kitchen before she thinks it is the right temperature. Describe what you would do to help this patient/client.

4. **Patient Education** A 55-year-old male patient is recovering from a stroke. He is a high school principal and has always been able to take care of himself. His right hand and leg are paralyzed. Each day he is increasingly frustrated because he is unable to bathe or dress himself. Describe devices that could help reduce his frustration. Explain what you would say and do to educate him in the use of assistive/adaptive devices.

5. **Case Study** A 30-year-old woman suffered a head injury, which left her unable to speak. Her daily care provides a bath, clean clothes, and food. People around her rarely speak to her. She stays in her room and looks out the window most of the time. Compare and differentiate between her day and yours. Make specific recommendations that could assist in moving this person toward health as described by the World Health Organization. Explain how your recommendations would change this client's health status.

6. **Computers** Patients/clients with disabilities are using computers to communicate and be productive citizens as they live with their disability. Do research on ways computers can be adapted to meet the needs of disabled individuals and write a report explaining what you have learned. Look for *assistive technology, alternative input mechanisms, alternative output mechanisms,* and *computer use with handicapped or disabled children.*

Portfolio Connection

Working with people who are ill causes unfamiliar feelings and experiences. Your ability to identify your feelings and understand how you react to those feelings helps you carry on and continue to care for others. Select a disability described in this chapter.

Imagine that you are diagnosed with this disability. Identify your fears, feelings, and expectations. Explain what each day would be like, what type of care you would need, how others would respond to you, and how you would respond to others.

Your explanation must clearly identify your self-evaluation and new insights about disabilities and behaviors, and must show how you would approach others with disabilities. This assignment helps you investigate your feelings and identify possible behaviors of patients who live with disabilities. Including this assignment in your portfolio gives you easy access to it for review during your training. Comparing assignments throughout your training shows how your experiences have brought about change in your thinking.

NUTRITION

10

UNIT 1 Basic Nutrition

Steps to success

1. Complete Vocabulary Worksheet 1 in the Student Workbook.
2. Read this unit.
3. Complete Worksheets 2 through 4 as assigned.
4. When you are confident that you can meet each objective for this unit, ask your instructor for the unit evaluation.

Rationale

vitality Ability of an organism to go on living.

Health care workers must maintain good health in order to be efficient in their work. When you eat the proper foods, you have the energy and **vitality** to function effectively. Patients must have a healthy diet to maintain or to restore good health. Your knowledge of a balanced diet helps you understand how good nutrition maintains good health for yourself and your patients/clients.

Objectives

When you have completed this unit, you will be able to do the following.

✓ Match vocabulary words with their correct meanings.
✓ Name the four functions of food.
✓ Name the five basic nutrients and explain how they maintain body function.
✓ Explain the food pyramid.
✓ Compare your diet with the recommendations in the pyramid.

■ INTRODUCTION TO BASIC NUTRITION

resistance Ability of the body to protect itself from disease.

Good nutrition promotes a healthier body and mind. It also aids in **resistance** to illness. When we eat a healthy diet, our energy and vitality are increased. The right foods speed the healing process and help a person feel better and sleep better.

Your patients/clients are all from different cultural and religious backgrounds. Each culture and religion has dietary differences. Appetites, food budget, cultural food preferences, and religious restrictions influence some of these differences. You and your patients need the same basic nutrients provided by a balanced, healthy diet. The health care worker must understand about foods and their effect on the body in order to assess his or her own diet and the patient's diet.

The Function of Food

When food is taken into the body, it is used in many different ways. The right combination of nutrients work together in the body to

- Provide heat
- Promote growth
- Repair tissue
- **Regulate** body processes

regulate To control or adjust.

Basic Nutrients

Nutrients are chemical compounds found in food. When the food we eat enters the digestive tract, it is changed into a simple form and absorbed into the blood. The blood carries these nutrients to body cells, where they are used to maintain body functions. Table 10–1 lists the basic nutrients.

Water is essential to the body. It carries nutrients to the body cells and carries waste products away from the body cells. It also lubricates the joints and helps regulate body temperature and body processes.

proteins Complex compound found in plant and animal tissues, essential for heat, energy, and growth.

Fiber

Fiber adds bulk to the diet and helps prevent bowel and colon diseases. Fiber also helps prevent constipation. The diet many people eat is high in protein, fats, and carbohydrates but very low in fiber. To keep the bowel healthy, a person should eat

minerals Inorganic elements that occur in nature; essential to every cell.

vitamins Group of substances necessary for normal functioning and maintenance of health.

essential Necessary (e.g., certain food elements are necessary for the body's functions).

TABLE 10–1 Basic Nutrients	
Proteins (See Figure 10–1)	Builds and renews body tissues Provides heat energy
Carbohydrates (See Figure 10–2)	Provides the basic source of energy for body heat and body activities
Fats (See Figure 10–3)	Provides fatty acids for normal growth and development Provides energy Carries vitamins A and D to the cells
Minerals (See Figure 10–4)	Regulate the activity of the heart, nerves, and muscles Build and renew teeth, bones, and other tissues
Vitamins (See Figure 10–5)	Are **essential** for normal metabolism, growth, and body development

PROTEINS

FIGURE 10–1.
Proteins.

CARBOHYDRATES

FIGURE 10–2.
Carbohydrates.

FATS

FIGURE 10–3. Fats.

several servings of fiber each day. Fiber is found in greens, kale, cabbage, celery, vegetable salads, raw and cooked fruits, whole-grain food, and cereals.

Good nutrition enhances your appearance and increases your stamina. It is important to plan meals and snacks that include all of the basic nutrients each day.

Calories

Food is the source of energy for our bodies. The body metabolizes food nutrients to create energy. As the body creates energy, it produces heat. Energy is required to ensure that all of the body systems function. The amount of energy created by the food we eat is measured in **calories.** Calorie needs vary from person to person. A large, active man needs more calories than a smaller, inactive man does. The number of calories we eat and the amount of exercise we do balance weight. If we eat more calories than we burn, we gain weight. If we burn more calories than we eat, we lose weight. When a patient is inactive and feels ill, she may not want to eat. It is your responsibility to encourage her to take in enough calories to produce the energy needed to heal the body.

calories Units of measurement of the fuel value of food.

The Food Pyramid

Good nutrition and a healthy diet help maintain good health. The U.S. Department of Agriculture (USDA) has provided the food pyramid (Figure 10–6) as a guideline. The "eating right" pyramid focuses on low-fat foods, such as grains, pasta, vegetables, fruits, nonfat dairy products, and lean meats. The pyramid illustrates the

Calcium

Milk and milk products, except butter; most dark green vegetables; canned salmon.

Iron

Eggs, meat, especially liver and kidney; deep yellow and dark green vegetables; potatoes, dried fruits, whole-grain products; enriched flour, bread, and breakfast cereals.

Iodine

Fish (obtained from the sea), some plant foods grown in soils containing iodine; table salt fortified with iodine (iodized).

FIGURE 10–4. Minerals are calcium, iron, and iodine.

A

One form of Vitamin A is yellow and one form is colorless. Apricots, cantaloupe, milk, cheese, eggs, meat organs (especially liver and kidney), fortified margarine, butter, fish-liver oils, dark green and deep yellow vegetables.

B Complex
B₁ (Thiamine)

Whole-grain and enriched grain products; meats (especially pork, liver, and kidney); dry beans and peas.

B₂ (Riboflavin)

Milk, cheese, eggs, meat (especially liver and kidney), whole-grain and enriched grain products, dark green vegetables.

B₁₂

Liver, other organ meats, cheese, eggs, milk.

C (Ascorbic Acid)

Fresh, raw citrus fruits and vegetables—oranges, grapefruit, cantaloupe, strawberries, tomatoes, raw onions, cabbage, green and sweet red peppers, dark green vegetables.

D

Provided by Vitamin D fortification of certain foods, such as milk and margarine. Also fish-liver oils and eggs. Sunshine is also a source of Vitamin D.

Niacin

Liver, meat, fish, poultry, eggs, peanuts; dark green vegetables, whole-grain and enriched cereal products.

FIGURE 10–5. Vitamins include A, B complex, B1, B2, B12, C, D, and niacin.

recommended daily portions of each food group. Follow these guidelines for yourself and your patients/clients. The food choices of all cultures fit into these guidelines when you plan carefully.

How Poor Nutrition Affects the Body

When we do not supply our bodies with the proper nutrients, many things can go wrong. We lose stamina and vitality. An unhealthy diet often results in illness and disease. The following are a few of the problems that poor nutrition can cause.

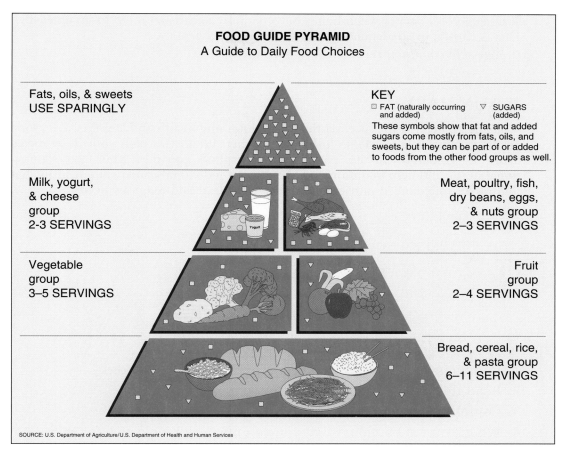

FOOD GUIDE PYRAMID
A Guide to Daily Food Choices

Fats, oils, & sweets
USE SPARINGLY

KEY
□ FAT (naturally occurring
  and added)   ▽ SUGARS
                        (added)
These symbols show that fat and added
sugars come mostly from fats, oils, and
sweets, but they can be part of or added
to foods from the other food groups as well.

Milk, yogurt,
& cheese
group
2-3 SERVINGS

Meat, poultry, fish,
dry beans, eggs,
& nuts group
2–3 SERVINGS

Vegetable
group
3–5 SERVINGS

Fruit
group
2–4 SERVINGS

Bread, cereal, rice,
& pasta group
6–11 SERVINGS

SOURCE: U.S. Department of Agriculture/U.S. Department of Health and Human Services

FIGURE 10–6. The "eating right" pyramid.

■ *Anemia,* a decreased number of red blood cells or a decreased amount of **hemoglobin,** results in

• Tiredness • Dyspnea (shortness of breath) on exertion • Headache • Insomnia (inability to sleep) • Paleness • Indigestion • Rapid heartbeat

■ *Anorexia nervosa* occurs when a person refuses to eat or drastically reduces his or her intake of food. This is related to an emotional disturbance about image (e.g., a person who is very underweight sees herself or himself as overweight). Anorexia nervosa is seen primarily in teenage girls. It results in

• Amenorrhea • Skeleton-like appearance

■ *Bulimia* occurs when a person experiences intervals of food craving and **bingeing** and then **purging.** The side effects are the same as those of anorexia and result in depression.

■ *Constipation* is the infrequent, difficult defecation of fecal material. It is commonly caused by lack of activity and by not eating enough vegetables, fruit, or water.

■ *Dull hair and eyes* are symptoms of poor diet.

■ *Mental slowdown* can occur when nutrition is poor.

■ ***Obesity*** occurs when a person takes in more calories than the body uses. This results in increasing amounts of fatty tissue.

hemoglobin Complex chemical in the blood; carries oxygen and carbon dioxide.

bingeing Eating excessively.

purging Causing oneself to vomit.

obesity Extreme fatness; abnormal amount of fat on the body.

■ *Osteoporosis* occurs when bones become porous, causing them to break easily. This is caused by inadequate calcium intake or absorption.

■ *Poor skin condition* results from poor nutrition.

■ SUMMARY

A balanced, healthy diet is essential for maintaining health and stamina. Everyone needs certain basic nutrients in his or her diet. When you plan your daily meals using the guidelines in the "eating right" pyramid, you meet your body's nutritional needs and help maintain good health. All individuals must eat a healthy diet that provides balanced nutrients and meets cultural and religious needs.

UNIT 2   Therapeutic Diets

Steps to success

1. Complete Vocabulary Worksheet 1 in the Student Workbook.
2. Read this unit.
3. Complete Worksheet 2 as assigned.
4. When you are confident that you can meet each objective for this unit, ask your instructor for the unit evaluation.
5. Complete "Your Link to Success" at the end of this chapter.

Rationale

Some patients/clients have illnesses that require special diets. Therapeutic diets are diets that modify a patient's normal diet in order to treat an illness. Understanding why the diet has been changed helps you encourage clients to eat the food prepared for them. When you are knowledgeable about their diet, you are able to explain how important it is to their recovery.

Objectives

When you have completed this unit, you will be able to do the following.

✓ Match vocabulary words with their correct meaning.
✓ List three factors that influence food habits.
✓ Select a correct therapeutic diet for physical disorders.

■ INTRODUCTION TO THERAPEUTIC DIETS

It is especially important to remember the factors that influence food habits for patients who are on a therapeutic diet. Always respect the patient's personal attitudes and preferences, nationality, race, and religious needs. A therapeutic diet is often very different from the foods the patient normally eats. Your understanding of the reason for the diet and your patients' special needs helps ease their concerns. The dietitian will talk with the patient and try to adapt a therapeutic diet to meet a patient's nutritional and personal needs. An example of a special or personal need is religious restrictions.

Many religions of the world follow specific dietary laws. These guidelines are very important to clients. The stress caused by breaking the law when clients are on a therapeutic diet may cause added worry. Always be respectful of the dietary requests that your clients make, and report their requests to your supervisor. Ask your clients what diet they normally follow. If there is a problem with the diet, report it to your supervisor, who will talk with the dietitian. Table 10–2 lists a few of the restrictions that you may observe.

Purposes of Therapeutic Diets

Therapeutic diets are given to

- Regulate the amount of food in **metabolic** disorders
- Prevent or restrict edema by restricting sodium intake
- Assist body organs to regain and/or maintain normal function
- Aid in digestion by avoiding foods that irritate the digestive tract
- Increase or decrease body weight by adding or eliminating calories

metabolic Pertaining to the total of all the physical and chemical changes that take place in living organisms and cells.

Types of Therapeutic Diets

Table 10–3 describes the various types of therapeutic diets and their purposes.

The physician may order other diets. Always check the diet that has been ordered for the patient/client. If you have any question about it, ask the person in charge. Correct diets are essential in maintaining good health, and only those foods allowed should be served.

TABLE 10–2   Religious Dietary Restrictions

Christian Science Church of Latter-Day Saints (Mormons) Conservative Protestants	Avoid alcohol, coffee, tea.
Greek Orthodox	No meat or dairy products on fast days.
Muslim (Moslem)	No alcohol, pork, or pork products.
Orthodox Jewish	No shellfish, pork, or nonkosher meats. No serving milk and milk products with meat. No eating leavened bread during Passover. Abstain from eating on specific fast days.
Roman Catholic	No meat one hour before Communion, Ash Wednesday, and Good Friday. Abstain from eating on other specific fast days.
Buddhist	Generally vegetarian.
Hindu	Generally vegetarian.

deficient Lacking something (e.g., a deficient diet causes the body to function poorly because it is missing an important element).

gastrointestinal Pertaining to the stomach and intestine.

colitis Inflammation of the colon.

ileitis Inflammation of the ileum (the lower three-fifths of the small intestine).

diabetes mellitus Condition that develops when the body cannot change sugar into energy; there is an insufficient amount of insulin, leading to an increased amount of sugar in the blood.

TABLE 10–3 Some Therapeutic Diets and Their Purposes

Type of Diet	Purpose of Diet	Description
Clear liquid Nutritionally inadequate	Replaces fluids lost from vomiting, diarrhea, surgery	Plain gelatin, ginger ale, tea, coffee (no cream), fruit or apple juice (no pulp), fat-free broth
Full liquid May be **deficient** in iron	Trouble chewing or swallowing, **gastrointestinal** disturbances	All clear liquids, fruit or vegetable juices, strained soup, custard, ice cream, sherbet, milk, cream, eggs, buttermilk, carbonated beverages, eggs, cocoa, eggnog
Soft Nutritionally inadequate	For patients who have trouble chewing, postsurgically	Foods that are soft in consistency, such as fish, ground beef, broth, pureed vegetables, strained cream soup, tender cooked vegetables, fruit juices, cooked fruit, refined cereals, pasta, sherbet, ices, ice cream, custard, plain cookies, angel food cake, tea, coffee, cocoa, carbonated beverages, cheese, cottage cheese
Bland Nutritionally adequate	Soothes gastrointestinal tract, avoids irritation in ulcers, **colitis**	Foods low in fiber and connective tissue that are mild flavored and easy to digest, such as pear (tender, broiled, boiled), prune juice, applesauce, custard, pudding, ice cream, plain cookies, sponge cake, decaffeinated coffee, milk, cheese, yogurt
Restricted residue Nutritionally adequate	Reduces normal work of the intestine, in cases of rectal diseases, colitis, **ileitis**	Foods low in fiber and low in bulk, such as milk, buttermilk, cottage cheese, butter, margarine, eggs (not fried), tender poultry, fish, lamb, ground beef (broiled, boiled, baked), broth, refined bread, cereals, pasta, gelatin, angel food or sponge cake, mild-flavored cooked vegetables, lettuce, vegetable and fruit juice, applesauce, canned fruit, citrus fruit without membranes
Low carbohydrate (diabetic) Nutritionally adequate	Matches food intake with insulin uptake and nutritional requirements, used for patients with hyperinsulism and **diabetes mellitus**	Foods that supply enough protein, fat, and carbohydrate to maintain health and activities; requires a balance of carbohydrates, protein, and fat to meet the individual need of the patient; restricts sugar, cookies, pies, candies, etc.

Type of Diet	Purpose of Diet	Description
Low fat Deficient in fat-**soluble** vitamins	For patients with gallbladder and liver disease, obesity, and heart conditions	Foods high in carbohydrates and proteins; all fats are limited; skim milk, buttermilk, cottage cheese, lean fish, poultry, meats, fat-free soup broths, cooked vegetables, lettuce, fruit juice, bananas, citrus fruits, gelatin, angel food cake, coffee, tea, carbonated beverages, jelly, honey as desired
Low cholesterol Nutritionally adequate	Regulates amount of cholesterol in the blood for patients with coronary disease and **atherosclerosis**	Foods low in fat, such as lean muscle meat, fish, poultry without skin or fat, skim milk, vegetables, fruits
Low calorie (800–2,000 cal) Nutritionally adequate	Reduces number of calories for overweight patients and for clients with arthritis or cardiac conditions	Foods low in fats and calories: skim milk, buttermilk, lean meats, clear soup, vegetables, fresh fruit, coffee, tea, herbs, onions, garlic
High calorie (2,000 cal+) Nutritionally adequate	For persons 10 percent or more below desired weight; for patients with **anorexia nervosa** and hyperthyroidism	All foods with nutritionally balanced proteins, carbohydrates, fats, vitamins, minerals
Low sodium Nutritionally adequate	Reduces salt intake for patients with kidney disease, cardiovascular disorders, edema, and **hypertension**	Natural foods prepared without salt, such as fresh fruits, fresh vegetables, foods without salt added
High protein Nutritionally adequate	For children and adolescents needing additional protein for growth; during pregnancy, **lactation;** postsurgically; during illnesses resulting from protein loss	Foods high in protein, such as milk, cheese, eggs, lean meats, fish, and poultry; fruit, cereals, vegetables

soluble Able to break down or dissolve in liquid.

atherosclerosis Condition of hardening of the arteries due to fat deposits that narrow the space blood flows through.

anorexia nervosa Loss of appetite with serious weight loss; considered a mental disorder.

hypertension High blood pressure.

lactation Body's process of producing milk to feed newborns.

■ SUMMARY

There are many factors that influence food habits. Some of these factors are personal attitudes, nationality, race, and religious restrictions. A health care worker must be aware of these factors in order to help the patient/client adapt to therapeutic diets.

The therapeutic diet is prescribed for various ailments. It is important to understand why the diet was prescribed and how it helps in regaining a healthier state. The health care worker should be aware of the foods allowed and not allowed in therapeutic diets and serve only proper foods to his or her patients.

Thinking Critically: Check Your Understanding

1. **Communication** Your little brother's third-grade school class is studying nutrition. The teacher knows that you are a health care worker and has asked you to talk to the students about the USDA food pyramid. Write an outline of your presentation. Design handouts and bulletin board materials for third graders. Write on index cards what you plan to say to the class. Practice giving your talk to the members of your health care class. Give your instructor your outline, copies of handouts and bulletin board materials, and your index cards.

2. **Medical Terminology** Gastroesophageal reflux disease (GERD) is a common disease. The symptoms may be very mild or serious. Heartburn, regurgitation, and dysphagia are common symptoms. Patients with GERD modify their diet and lifestyle and use antacids. If they have problems at night, they can elevate the head of the bed to help reduce reflux of stomach acids. Look up and write the definitions for the following words: *heartburn, regurgitation, dysphagia, reflux,* and *antacids*.

3. **Medical Math** Your patient/client is on a therapeutic diet. It is your responsibility to keep a record of all of her intake and output. At the end of the day, she has taken in 1,200 ounces of fluid, and her output is 925 ounces of fluid. How many cc has she taken in? How many cc has she put out?

4. **Case Study** Mrs. Cohen, an Orthodox Jew, has been in St. Andrews Nursing Home for several years. This evening the staff in the kitchen sent her a dinner with mashed potatoes, pork roast, green beans, and custard. She is very upset and is crying: She is hungry but does not want to eat, because of her dietary restrictions. You know that the staff in the kitchen is new. What steps can you take to remedy this problem?

Portfolio Connection

When you care for patients, it is important to know if they are eating a healthy diet. Therapeutic diets do not always meet the standards of a healthy diet.

Choose an illness that requires a therapeutic diet. Write a paragraph about the illness. Explain the symptoms, how the body is affected, and the treatment. Use the food pyramid as a guide to evaluating the therapeutic diet required. Describe in what ways the diet is nutritionally healthy or deficient.

Place this exercise in your portfolio to help you review the food pyramid, healthy diets, and therapeutic diets.

MEASURING VITAL SIGNS

11

UNIT 1   Temperature, Pulse, and Respiration

Steps to success

1. Complete Vocabulary Worksheet 1 in the Student Workbook.
2. Read in this unit.
3. Complete Worksheets 2 through 4 as assigned.
4. When you are confident that you can meet each objective for this unit, ask your instructor for the unit evaluation.

Rationale

Important indicators of your patient's health status are known as *vital signs*. Vital signs give you information about breathing, body temperature, and the heart. They are a good indication of how well the body systems are functioning. As a health care worker, you need to observe patients whenever you are near them. Your knowledge of vital signs and how to measure them helps you know when to report that a patient is having problems.

Objectives

When you have completed this unit, you will be able to do the following:

✓ Match vocabulary words with their correct meanings.
✓ Define *vital signs*.
✓ List fourteen factors that influence body temperature.
✓ Name the most common site at which to measure a temperature.
✓ Match the normal temperature to the site where it is measured.
✓ Measure temperature with a glass thermometer.

oral Referring to the mouth.

rectal Referring to the far end of the large intestine just above the anus.

axillary Referring to the armpit.

✓ Demonstrate how to measure **oral, rectal,** and **axillary** temperature.
✓ Define *pulse*.
✓ Explain pulse oximetry.
✓ Identify sites where pulse may be counted.
✓ Identify a normal adult pulse rate and a common method for counting a pulse.
✓ List six factors that influence the pulse rate.
✓ Demonstrate counting and recording a radial pulse accurately.
✓ Recognize two parts of a respiration.
✓ Relate types of abnormal respirations to their correct name.
✓ Select eight factors that affect respiration.
✓ Explain the importance of not being obvious when counting respirations.
✓ Demonstrate how to count and record respirations accurately.
✓ Explain the importance of each vital sign.

■ INTRODUCTION TO VITAL SIGNS

blood pressure Highest and lowest pressure against the walls of blood vessels.

Vital signs include body temperature, pulse, respiration rates, and **blood pressure.** Vital signs are the indicators that tell you how the body is functioning. Pulse oximetry is another important indicator of body functioning. When vital signs are within normal limits, the body is considered to be in homeostasis. When the vital signs are not within normal limits, it is an indication that something is wrong. It is important to be accurate when you measure vital signs and to record the results very carefully and accurately. Other health care workers depend on this information when making decisions about the patient's treatment. In this unit, you learn how to measure body temperature and count the pulse rate and respiratory rate. Together these measurements are referred to as **TPR.** Unit 2 teaches you to measure blood pressure.

TPR Stands for "temperature, pulse, respiration."

■ TEMPERATURE

oxidation The mixing together of oxygen and another element.

Temperature is the measure of body heat. Heat is produced in the body by the muscles and glands and by the **oxidation** of food. Heat is lost from the body by respiration, perspiration, and **excretion.** The balance between the heat produced and the heat lost is the body temperature.

excretion Process of eliminating waste material.

Factors That Influence Temperature

Increase Temperature	Decrease Temperature
Exercise	Sleep
Digestion of food	Fasting
Increased environmental temperature	Exposure to cold
Illness	Certain illnesses
Infection	Decreased muscle activity
Excitement	Mouth breathing
Anxiety	Depression

FIGURE 11–1.
Three types of tips or bulbs on glass thermometers. *Note:* Thermometers used to take rectal temperatures should not also be used to take oral temperatures.

Thermometers

The thermometer is the instrument used to measure temperature. There are several types of thermometers: glass thermometers, aural thermometers, chemically treated paper or plastic thermometers, and electronic/digital thermometers.

Glass Thermometers (Clinical/Mercury)

A glass thermometer is a hollow glass tube with **calibration** lines on it. At one end of the thermometer is a bulb that is filled with mercury. The mercury is heat sensitive and rises up the hollow tube when exposed to heat. This enables you to read the client's temperature. There are three types of tips or bulbs on glass thermometers (Figure 11–1).

calibration Standard measure (e.g., each line on a thermometer or a ruler is a calibration).

Aural Thermometers

A tympanic membrane sensor measures body temperature. It is accurate, easy to use, and safe. It is especially effective for babies and children.

Chemically Treated Paper or Plastic Thermometers

This type of thermometer is read by noting the color it changes to. It is disposed of after one use.

Electronic/Digital Thermometers

This thermometer has a probe that you cover with a protective, disposable shield (Figure 11–2). The temperature is measured and registered on a screen. Electronic thermometers are quick and easy to use. There are various types of electronic equipment available. Always follow the manufacturer's instructions.

FIGURE 11–2.
Electronic/digital thermometers.

Procedure

Using an Electronic Thermometer

ALERT: Follow Standard Precautions.

1. Wash hands.
2. Assemble equipment.*
   a. Plastic thermometer covers
   b. Electronic thermometer with appropriate probe (blue for oral, red for rectal)
3. Identify patient/client.
4. Explain procedure to patient.
5. Place plastic thermometer cover over probe.
6. Insert probe in proper position to measure body temperature (blue-tipped probe under tongue or in axilla, red-tipped probe in rectum).

7. Hold probe in place for 15 seconds.
8. Buzzer will ring when body temperature is displayed on electronic thermometer.
9. Remove plastic sheath and discard.
10. Record temperature. (Report elevated temperature to a supervisor.)
11. Position client for comfort.
12. Wash hands.
13. Return electronic thermometer to its storage place.
14. Report any unusual observation immediately.

*Wear gloves for measuring rectal temperatures. Follow facility policy for measuring oral temperature.

How to Read a Glass Thermometer

1. Hold the thermometer at eye level. Rotate the thermometer until you can see the column of mercury.
2. Look at the lines on the scale at the upper side of the column of mercury. Each long line represents a whole degree. There are four short lines between each of the long lines. The short lines represent $\frac{2}{10}$ (0.2) of a degree. Only even numbers are shown on a Fahrenheit clinical thermometer (see Figure 11–3) (e.g., 96°, 98°, 100°).
3. If the mercury ends at one of the short lines, look to see which long line is just before it. This tells you the degree of temperature. Then add $\frac{2}{10}$ for each short line.
4. Read a Celsius thermometer the same way. Each long line represents a degree. Each short line represents $\frac{1}{10}$ (0.1) of a degree (see Figure 11–3).

Celsius Measure of heat; in medicine, a Celsius thermometer is sometimes used to measure body heat. Also called centigrade.

Fahrenheit Measure of heat; in medicine a Fahrenheit thermometer is often used to measure body heat.

You may be asked to change a temperature from **Celsius** to **Fahrenheit** or from Fahrenheit to centigrade. If you need to make these changes, use the information in Table 11–1.

Sites to Take Body Temperature

Oral

The simplest and most common, convenient, and comfortable site to take a temperature is the oral cavity, unless you use the aural thermometer. The average normal oral temperature is 98.6°F or 37°C. Use the oral or aural cavity whenever possible and when the patient has

- Diarrhea • Rectal surgery • Fecal impaction

Fahrenheit

Mercury

Bulb

Calibrations

94 6 8 ↑ 100 2 4 6 8 110

Stem

6 8 ↑ 100

Normal body temperature is 98.6 degrees Fahrenheit and is written 98.6° F.

Celsius

Mercury

Bulb

35 36 ↑ 38 39 40 41 42 43

Stem

36 ↑ 38

Normal body temperature is 37 degrees centigrade (Celsius) and is written 37° C.

FIGURE 11–3.
Average normal temperatures shown on Fahrenheit and Celsius thermometers.

TABLE 11–1	Fahrenheit and Celsius Comparison
Fahrenheit	**Celsius/Centigrade**
32	0
95	35
96	35.5
96.8	36
97.8	36.5
98.6	37
99.6	37.5
100.4	38
101.2	38.4
102.2	39
103	39.4
104	40
105	40.5
105.8	41
106.8	41.5

Procedure

Measuring an Oral Temperature

ALERT: Follow Standard Precautions.

1. Wash hands.
2. Assemble equipment.*
   a. Clean oral thermometer
   b. Alcohol wipes
   c. Watch with second hand
   d. Disposable thermometer cover
3. Identify patient/client.
4. Explain what you are going to do.
5. Remove thermometer from container and apply disposable cover.
6. Check reading—94°F or 35°C.
7. Ask patient if he or she has been smoking, eating, or drinking. If yes, wait 10 minutes before taking temperature.
8. Place thermometer under tongue.
9. Instruct client to hold with closed lips.
10. Leave in mouth for 5 minutes.
11. Remove from mouth.
12. Remove and discard disposable cover and wipe thermometer from stem to tip.
13. Read thermometer correctly.

14. Wash thermometer in cool water.
15. Put thermometer away.
16. Wash hands.
17. Record temperature correctly on pad.
18. Report any unusual observation immediately.

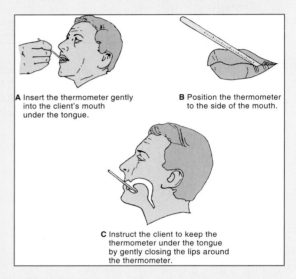

A Insert the thermometer gently into the client's mouth under the tongue.

B Position the thermometer to the side of the mouth.

C Instruct the client to keep the thermometer under the tongue by gently closing the lips around the thermometer.

*Follow facility policy for wearing gloves.

Rectal

The most accurate temperature reading is taken in the rectum. The normal rectal temperature is 99.6°F or 38°C. Rectal temperature is taken when patients/clients

- Are under 6 years old
- Have difficulty breathing
- Are extremely weak
- Are confused, unconscious, or senile
- Are being given oxygen
- Experience partial paralysis of the face caused by a stroke or accident

Aural

The aural temperature is also accurate, easy to use, and appropriate for the patients listed above. To measure an aural temperature, a probe is positioned in the aural canal of the ear. A normal aural temperature is 98.6°F or 37°C.

Procedure

Measuring a Rectal Temperature

ALERT: Follow Standard Precautions.

1. Wash hands.
2. Assemble equipment.
    a. Clean rectal thermometer
    b. Alcohol wipes
    c. Watch
    d. Lubricant
    e. Disposable nonsterile gloves
    f. Disposable thermometer cover
3. Identify patient/client.
4. Explain what you are going to do.
5. Put on gloves.
6. Remove thermometer from container and apply disposable cover.
7. Check reading—94°F or 35°C.
8. Screen patient.
9. Lower backrest on bed.
10. Put lubricant on tissue and apply to bulb end of thermometer.
11. Separate buttocks.
12. Insert thermometer 1½ inches into rectum.
13. Hold in place 3 to 5 minutes.
14. Remove thermometer.
15. Remove and discard disposable cover and wipe thermometer from stem to tip.
16. Read thermometer correctly.
17. Wash thermometer in cool water.
18. Put thermometer away.
19. Remove and discard gloves.
20. Wash hands.
21. Record temperature correctly on pad.
22. Report any unusual observation immediately.

Axillary

The least accurate temperature is taken in the armpit. The normal temperature for this site is 97.6°F or 36.4°C. Use this site only when the temperature cannot be taken orally, aurally, or rectally. Always report a temperature that is above normal to your supervisor.

MEDICAL TERMINOLOGY

- **afebrile**   temperature is within normal range
- **febrile**   temperature is elevated
- **hypothermia** temperature is below normal
- **pyrexia**   above normal temperature
- **pyrogenic** any substance that produces fever

Procedure

Measuring an Axillary Temperature

ALERT: Follow Standard Precautions.

1. Wash hands.
2. Assemble equipment.
   a. Clean thermometer
   b. Alcohol wipes
   c. Watch with second hand
   d. Disposable thermometer cover
3. Identify patient/client.
4. Explain what you are going to do.
5. Remove thermometer from container and apply disposable cover.
6. Check reading—94°F or 35°C.
7. Place thermometer in axillary.
8. Leave in place for 10 minutes.
9. Remove thermometer.
10. Remove and discard disposable cover and wipe thermometer from stem to tip.
11. Read thermometer correctly.
12. Wash thermometer in cool water.
13. Put thermometer away.
14. Wash hands.
15. Record temperature correctly on pad.
16. Report any unusual observation immediately.

■ PULSE

The pulse rate indicates the number of times the heart beats in 1 minute. It is an important vital sign because it indicates how well the blood is circulating through the body. When you feel the pulse, you are feeling the pressure of the blood against the wall of the artery as the heart contracts and relaxes (Figure 11–4).

FIGURE 11–4. The pulse measures the rate of the heartbeat.

Factors That Affect Pulse Rate

Increase Pulse Rate	Decrease Pulse Rate
Exercise	High level of aerobic fitness
Illness	Overmedicated (e.g., digitalis)
Anxiety	Depression
Medication	Medication
Shock	

Location of Pulse Points

When you count the pulse, place your fingers over an artery and squeeze gently against the bone. Figure 11–5 shows the location on the arteries where the pulse may be taken. The pulse rate should be the same at all pulse sites.

Pulse Characteristics

Just counting the beats is not enough. You must also note the

■ *Rate.*   Number of pulse beats per minute.
■ *Rhythm.*   Is the pulse regular? Steady? Or does it skip beats?
■ *Arrhythmia.*   Does the pulse have uneven intervals between pulses or heartbeats?

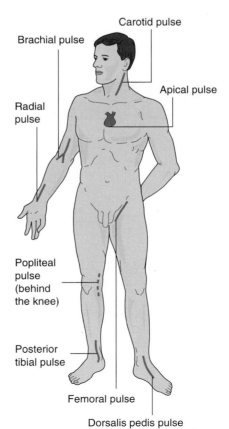

FIGURE 11–5.
Pulse points of the body.

TABLE 11–2	Normal Pulse Rates
Age	**Rate**
Before birth	140–150
At birth	90–160
First year of life	115–130
Childhood years	80–115
Adult	60–80

bounding Leaping, strong, or forceful (e.g., a very strong pulse is a bounding pulse).

hemorrhage Large amount of bleeding.

■ *Force of the beat* (volume).   Is it weak, thready, or **bounding?** Always report a heartbeat below 60 or over 100.

Pulse Rate

Pulse rate is generally increased with exercise, age, emotional excitement, **hemorrhage,** or elevated temperature. Drugs can increase or decrease the heart rate. When the rate is over 100 beats per minute, it is called *tachycardia*. When the rate is below 60 beats per minute, it is called *bradycardia*. When the rate is irregular, it is called *arrhythmia*. When you record the pulse rate, always report to your supervisor anything that is abnormal. This includes rate (see Table 11–2), rhythm, and force.

Radial Pulse

The radial pulse is the most common site for counting the pulse rate. Always count the pulse for one full minute. This prevents missing any abnormalities.

Procedure

Counting a Radial Pulse

1. Wash hands.
2. Assemble equipment.
    a. Watch with second hand
    b. Pad and pencil
3. Identify patient/client.
4. Explain what you are going to do.
5. Place fingers on radial artery—do not use thumb.
6. Count pulse (number of pulsations) for 1 minute.
7. Record pulse rate on pad immediately.
8. Wash hands.
9. Record pulse rate on chart.
10. Report any unusual observation immediately.

Apical Pulse

You may be asked to count an apical pulse. This is the pulse counted at the **apex** of the heart. Count an apical pulse rate when the heart is too weak to transmit a pulse that you can feel along the arteries. Count the apical heartbeat by placing the stethoscope 2 to 3 inches to the left of the sternum, just below the nipple on the chest.

apex Pointed end of something (e.g., the pointed end of the heart is called the apex of the heart).

Procedure

Counting an Apical Pulse

1. Assemble equipment—stethoscope.
2. Wash hands.
3. Tell patient/client what you are going to do.
4. Uncover left side of patient's chest.
5. Locate apex of heart by placing fingertips on client's chest below left nipple at about the fifth intercostal space.
6. Place stethoscope over apical region and listen for heart sounds.
7. Count the beats for 1 minute; note rate, rhythm, and strength of beat.
8. Record pulse rate on pad.
9. Wash hands.
10. Record apical pulse rate on chart.
11. Report any unusual observation immediately.

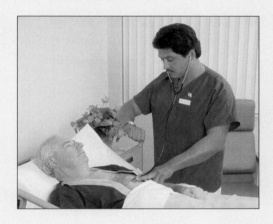

■ PULSE OXIMETRY

The pulse oximeter is an electronic device that determines oxygen (O_2) concentration in the hemoglobin of the arterial blood. When the O_2 concentration in the hemoglobin falls below 90 percent, the tissues do not have enough oxygen to function. Measuring with the oximeter allows monitoring of cardiac and respiratory patients whose blood O_2 content is an important indicator of their condition. The oximeter has light beams that pass through the tissues. The O_2 content and pulse rate are read and displayed on a monitor. Low concentrations of O_2 or a slow or rapid pulse rate cause an alarm to sound. The sensor is attached to a finger or earlobe, the forehead, the nose, or a toe. The sensor is sensitive to movement, light, and dark nail polish. Do not place a sensor over a break in the skin, a swollen area, or an area where the circulation is poor. To chart the O_2 measurement correctly, use the abbreviation SpO_2. This indicates saturation (S), pulse (p), and oxygen (O_2).

MEDICAL TERMINOLOGY

- **arrhythmia**   absence of rhythm
- **bradycardia** abnormally slow heartbeat
- **pulsation**   rhythmic beat
- **tachycardia** abnormally fast heartbeat

■ RESPIRATION

Respiration is the process of taking oxygen (O_2) into the body and expelling carbon dioxide (CO_2) from the body. One inspiration (breathing in) and one expiration (breathing out) are considered as one *respiration* (Figure 11–6). When you count a patient's respiration, you do not want the patient to be aware of what you are doing. If the patient realizes that you are counting respirations, he may not breathe normally. Count the pulse rate and respirations while you are taking the temperature. When you finish counting the pulse, count the respiration rate.

Factors That Affect Respiration

Increase Respiration	Decrease Respiration
Exercise	Relaxation
Anxiety	Depression
Respiratory disease	Head injury
Medication	Medication
Pain	
Heart disease (e.g., congestive heart failure)	

Respiratory Characteristics

Age influences respiration. The rate of newborns may be 40 respirations per minute. The normal adult rate is 14 to 18 respirations per minute. Always note the following:

- ■ *Rate.*   What is the number of respirations per minute?
- ■ *Rhythm.*   Are the respirations regular or irregular?

FIGURE 11–6.
Breathing in once (inspiration) and breathing out once (expiration) make up one respiration.

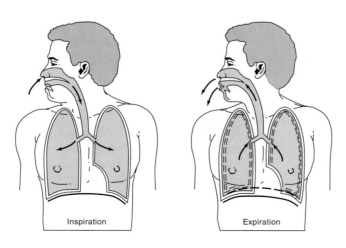

Inspiration   Expiration

■ *Dyspnea.* Is breathing difficult?

■ *Apnea.* Has breathing stopped?

■ *Cheynes-Stokes.* Are there periods of labored respirations followed by apnea?

■ *Rales.* Can you hear bubbling or rattling sounds caused by mucus in the air passages?

Always report any unusual or abnormal respirations to your supervisor.

Procedure

Counting Respirations

1. Wash hands.
2. Assemble equipment.
   a. Watch with second hand
   b. Pad and pencil
3. Identify patient/client.
4. Do not explain what you are going to do.
5. Relax fingers on pulse point.
6. Observe rise and fall of chest.
7. Count respirations for 1 minute.
8. Note regularity and depth.
9. Wash hands.
10. Record respiratory rate accurately.
11. Report any unusual observation immediately.

MEDICAL TERMINOLOGY

- **apnea**   **not breathing**
- **pneascope device for measuring movement of respiration**

- **tachypnea abnormally fast respirations**

■ RECORDING VITAL SIGNS

Always write the temperature, pulse, and respiration in the same order:

T	P	R
98.6	72	16

Since all health care workers write vital signs in the same way, you do not need to put the T P R above the figures. Write 98.6/72/16 for an oral temperature. Put an ® next to a rectal temperature (e.g., 99.6®) and an *AX* next to an axillary temperature (e.g., 97.6AX). Some facilities may have a policy and procedure requiring a

T next to the aural temperature (e.g., 98.6T). These symbols tell other health care workers where you measured the temperature and ensure accuracy. *Always report abnormal or unusual vital signs to your supervisor.*

Taking vital signs may seem routine, but the information is important to the well-being of the patient. Careful recording of vital signs is essential for the protection of the patient.

■ SUMMARY

You have learned that vital signs are important indicators of the body's condition. Three of these vital signs are temperature, pulse, and respiration. There are many factors that influence TPR in the body, and it is important to be aware of them. You have learned the steps for taking temperature, pulse, and respiration, and you know how to recognize a normal TPR and an abnormal TPR. You may also be responsible for accurate measurement of O_2 in the blood. This information is essential in giving good client care and in recognizing problems with your personal health.

UNIT 2   Blood Pressure

Steps to success

1. Complete Vocabulary Worksheet 1 in the Student Workbook.
2. Read this unit.
3. Complete Worksheets 2 and 3 as assigned.
4. When you are confident that you can meet each objective for this unit, ask your instructor for the unit evaluation.
5. Complete "Your Link to Success" at the end of this chapter.

Rationale

You have learned that temperature, pulse, and respiration are signs that indicate whether or not the body is functioning within normal limits. Blood pressure is the fourth vital sign. Measuring the patient's blood pressure gives you a complete picture of his or her vital signs. A complete record of all vital signs helps in the diagnosis and treatment of the patient.

Objectives

When you have completed this unit, you will be able to do the following:

✓ Match vocabulary words with their correct meanings.
✓ Define *blood pressure*.
✓ Match descriptions of systolic and diastolic blood pressure.
✓ List four factors that increase blood pressure.
✓ List four factors that can reduce blood pressure.
✓ State the normal range of blood pressure.

✓ Demonstrate how to measure and record a blood pressure accurately.

✓ Explain how vital signs provide information about the patient's health.

■ BLOOD PRESSURE

Blood pressure is the force of the blood pushing against the walls of the blood vessels. The *systolic* pressure is the greatest force exerted on the walls of the arteries by the heart. This pressure is exerted when the heart is contracting. You hear the first beat when contraction occurs. The *diastolic* pressure is the least force exerted on the walls of the arteries by the heart. This pressure occurs as the heart relaxes between contractions. When the heart relaxes, there is no sound (beat). Blood pressure depends on the volume of blood in the circulating system, the force of the heartbeat, and the condition of the arteries. When arteries lose their elasticity, they give more resistance, and the blood pressure increases.

Factors That Affect Blood Pressure

Increase Blood Pressure	Decrease Blood Pressure
Loss of elasticity in the arteries	Hemorrhage
Exercise	Inactivity
Eating	Fasting
Stimulants (e.g., medication, coffee)	Suppressant (e.g., medications that cause blood pressure to lower)
Anxiety	Depression

millimeters Measure of length.

systolic pressure Highest pressure against blood vessels. Represented by first heart sound or beat heard when taking a blood pressure.

Normal Blood Pressure

The normal blood pressure range is between 90 and 140 **millimeters** (mm) mercury for the **systolic pressure.** For the **diastolic pressure,** it is between 60 and 90 millimeters (mm) of mercury. When you record a blood pressure, it is written

$$120/80 = \frac{120 \text{ systolic}}{80 \text{ diastolic}}$$

When the blood pressure is above the normal range, it is called hypertension, or high blood pressure. Hypertension is called the silent killer. It is a disease that is **asymptomatic** in most cases. This condition is discovered only when the patient/client has his blood pressure measured. Heredity plays a major role in patients who develop hypertension. Some of the effects are stroke, kidney problems, changes in the retina, and heart disease. When the blood pressure is below the normal range, it is called **hypotension.**

diastolic pressure Lowest pressure against the blood vessels of the body. It is measured between contractions.

asymptomatic Without visible symptoms.

hypotension Low blood pressure.

apparatus Equipment needed to perform a task (e.g., blood pressure apparatus includes a blood pressure cuff and a stethoscope).

Blood Pressure Apparatus

Blood pressure is measured with an instrument called a **sphygmomanometer.** In the word *sphygmomanometer,*

■ *Sphygmo:* refers to pulse

■ *Mano:* refers to pressure

■ *Meter:* refers to measure

sphygmomanometer Measuring device used to measure the pressure against the arteries of the body.

Most health care workers refer to the sphygmomanometer as a BP cuff or blood pressure cuff. There are different kinds of blood pressure apparatus:

obsolete Out of date.

■ Mercury (This type is not seen often. In many places it is **obsolete.**) (Figure 11–7a)
■ Aneroid (Figure 11–7b)
■ Electronic/digital (Figure 11–8)

gauge Standard scale for measurement.

The mercury and aneroid apparatuses have a **gauge.** The gauge is marked with a series of long and short lines. The long lines are at 10-mm (millimeter) intervals. The short lines are between the long lines. These lines indicate 2 mm (millimeters)

FIGURE 11–7A.
Mercury sphygmomanometer.

FIGURE 11–7B.
Aneroid sphygmomanometer.

FIGURE 11–8. Digital sphygmomanometer and pulse monitor. Place index finger into finger cuff and follow directions to acquire pulse rate and blood pressure.

Ear pieces

Diaphragm

FIGURE 11–9. Stethoscope.

each. When you measure a blood pressure, you must do two things at one time. You listen to the heartbeat as it pulses through the artery. You also watch the gauge in order to take a reading.

The blood pressure cuff is a cloth-covered rubber bladder that fills with air as the bulb is squeezed. When the cuff is **inflated** around the arm, it stops the flow of blood. As the pressure is relieved, the flow returns and you hear a beat. This is the systolic pressure. As the cuff continues to deflate, you hear last a beat and then silence. The last beat you hear is the diastolic pressure.

inflated To swell or fill up with air.

Stethoscope

When you listen to pulse sounds, you use a stethoscope (see Figure 11–9). A stethoscope picks up sound when it is placed against the body. The stethoscope has earpieces, a spring to help keep the earpieces in the ears, flexible rubber tubing that carries sound, and a bell or diaphragm that magnifies sound.

■ PALPATING BLOOD PRESSURE

You may be asked to take a blood pressure by first palpating (feeling) the radial pulse. This allows you to determine the correct inflation pressure when inflating the cuff.

MEDICAL TERMINOLOGY

- **diastolic**   least force of pressure exerted against the walls of the arteries
- **hypertension** high blood pressure
- **hypotension** low blood pressure

- **stethoscope** instrument used to amplify sound
- **systolic**   greatest force of pressure exerted against the walls of the arteries

Procedure

Measuring Blood Pressure

1. Wash hands.
2. Assemble equipment.
   a. Alcohol wipes
   b. Sphygmomanometer
   c. Stethoscope
   d. Pad and pencil
3. Identify patient/client.
4. Explain what you are going to do.
5. Support patient's arm on firm surface.
6. Apply cuff correctly. (Refer to steps 4 and 5 in procedure "Palpating a Blood Pressure" on page 243.)
7. Clean earpieces on stethoscope.
8. Place earpieces in ears.
9. Locate brachial artery.
10. Tighten thumbscrew on valve.
11. Hold stethoscope in place.
12. Inflate cuff to 170 mm.
13. Open valve; if systolic sound is heard immediately, reinflate cuff to 30 mm Hg above systolic sound.
14. Note systolic at first beat.
15. Note diastolic.
16. Open valve and release air.
17. Record time and blood pressure reading correctly on pad.
18. Wash hands.
19. Wash earpieces on stethoscope.
20. Put equipment away.
21. Record blood pressure in chart.
22. Report any unusual observation immediately.

Procedure

Palpating a Blood Pressure

1. Wash hands.
2. Tell patient/client what you are going to do.
3. Support patient's arm palm side up on a firm surface.
4. Roll up sleeve above elbow, being careful that it is not too tight.
5. Wrap wide part of cuff around client's arm directly over brachial artery. Lower edge of cuff should be 1 or 2 inches above bend of elbow.
6. Find radial pulse with your fingertips.
7. Inflate cuff until you can no longer feel radial pulse, and continue to inflate another 30 mm of mercury.
8. Open valve and slowly deflate cuff until you feel first beat of radial pulse again.
9. Observe mercury or dial reading. This is the palpatory systolic pressure. It is recorded, for example, as B/P 130 (P).
10. Deflate cuff rapidly and squeeze out all the air.
11. Using your first and second fingers, locate brachial artery. You will feel it pulsating. Place

bell or diaphragm of stethoscope directly over artery. You will not hear the pulsation.
12. Tighten thumbscrew of valve to close it.
13. Hold stethoscope in place and inflate cuff until the dial points to about 20 mm above the palpated B/P.
14. Open valve counterclockwise. Let air out slowly until you hear first beat.
15. At this first sound, note reading on manometer. This is the systolic pressure.
16. Continue to release air slowly. Note number on the indicator at which you hear last beat or the sound changes to a dull beat. This is the diastolic pressure.
17. Open valve and release all the air.
18. Remove cuff.
19. Record time and blood pressure.
20. Report any unusual observation immediately.

■ SUMMARY

Blood pressure is the fourth vital sign. Many factors influence blood pressure, and an abnormal blood pressure may indicate a serious condition. It is important to be accurate in following the step-by-step instructions for taking a blood pressure, to record the blood pressure of your patient, and to report any abnormalities immediately.

Thinking Critically: Check Your Understanding

1. **Communication** You are assigned a patient and you need to take vital signs. Mr. Marks is an elderly man and seems very agitated and upset. You know that his agitation affects his vital signs. What verbal and nonverbal communication skills can you use to help reduce his upset? Write a brief description of how to help Mr. Marks relax so that you can take accurate vital signs.

2. **Medical Terminology** Define the following medical terms and explain why they are important when taking vital signs: arrhythmia, atypical, aural, axially, centigrade (Celsius), diastole, dyspnea, Fahrenheit, homeostasis, hypertension, hypoxia, hypothalamus, pyrexia, systole, rales, rhonchi, thready, and tympanic membrane.

3. **Patient Education** You are asked to teach Mrs. Ames how to take her daughter's vital signs. Her teenage daughter has an infection that requires that her vital signs be measured every four hours. Mrs. Ames has never taken TPR or blood pressure before. Demonstrate how to teach Mrs. Ames these skills.

4. **Medical Math** Refer to the medical math chapter of your text if you do not remember how to make conversions from Fahrenheit to centigrade (Celsius) and centigrade to Fahrenheit. Write the steps that you take to make each of the following conversions: 98.4F to centigrade; 105.6F to centigrade; 36C to Fahrenheit; 40.2C to Fahrenheit.

5. **Case Study** Mr. Ames is on oxygen and cannot breath comfortably when you remove his oxygen mask. It is time to take his vital signs. He has a severe infection and an accurate temperature is extremely important. What is the correct location for taking his temperature? Explain why? What information is appropriate to give Mr. Ames before you take his temperature?

Portfolio Connection

As a health care worker you are expected to observe clients for their state of health. You are obligated to report any unusual or abnormal signs or symptoms. Write the following in report form. This report demonstrates your evaluating, observing, and reporting skills. Your patient has an elevated blood pressure of 210/140. Does this blood pressure cause concern? What is the medical term for this blood pressure? What are the possible causes? What can you observe about the patient that is important in your report to your supervisor? Should you report this blood pressure immediately or wait until you report at the end of your shift? What are the key things that you must report? Place the report in your portfolio notebook behind the tab marked "Written Reports and Assignments" in your vocational area.

CONTROLLING INFECTION

12

UNIT 1 The Nature of Microorganisms

Steps to success

1. Complete Vocabulary Worksheet 1 in the Student Workbook.
2. Read this unit.
3. Complete Worksheets 2 and 3 as assigned.
4. When you are confident that you can meet each objective for this unit, ask your instructor for the unit evaluation.

Rationale

Microorganisms are all around us, but we cannot see them. There are both good and bad microorganisms. To help prevent the spread of infection and disease, you must be aware of microorganisms and how they are spread.

Objectives

When you have completed this unit, you will be able to do the following:

✓ Match vocabulary words with their correct meanings.
✓ Define *pathogen* and *nonpathogen*.
✓ List six conditions affecting the growth of bacteria.
✓ List three ways that microorganisms cause illness.
✓ List five ways that microorganisms spread.
✓ List five ways to prevent the spread of microorganisms.
✓ Explain generalized and localized infection.
✓ Explain the difference in signs and symptoms of generalized and localized infections.

■ INTRODUCTION TO MICROORGANISMS

We are surrounded by tiny microorganisms. They are in the air we breathe, on our skin, in our food, and on everything we touch. You cannot see the organisms without a microscope because they are so small (Figure 12–1). Some of these organisms cause illness, infection, or disease. Others are good organisms that help keep a balance in the environment and in the body.

For microorganisms to live, they must have certain elements in their environment. Some organisms require oxygen in order to survive. These are called *aerobic*. Others live in an environment without oxygen. These are called **anaerobic.** Most microorganisms that cause illness like warm temperatures—about the temperature of the body. All organisms need moisture, and most prefer a dark area to grow in (see Figure 12–2). Microorganisms also need food to survive. Some organisms that live on dead matter or tissues are called **saprophytes.** Other organisms use living matter or tissues and are called **parasites** (see Figure 12–2).

Nonpathogenic Organisms

There are many microorganisms that are not **pathogenic.** These organisms are "good" and they are used in different ways: to make buttermilk, to ferment grain for producing alcoholic beverages, to make bread rise, and many other ways. These organisms also **decompose** organic materials in nature. In the body, these organisms work in the digestive system to break down food elements that the body cannot use. This forms feces. **Nonpathogenic** microorganisms also help control the growth of pathogenic organisms.

Pathogenic Organisms

When organisms leave their normal environment in the body and move into other areas, they become pathogens. A common example is *Escherichia coli*, or *E. coli*. *E. coli* lives in the colon and breaks down waste products. *E. coli* can contaminate beef during butchering when organisms from the colon come in contact with meat that is sold to the public. If the contaminated meat is not cooked properly, people who eat it become infected with *E. coli*. This type of *E. coli* infection may cause death. When *E. coli* moves into the urinary tract, it causes infection. It causes **urethritis** and **cystitis,** or it may move into the kidneys, causing serious problems.

Because pathogenic organisms cause disease, health care workers must be aware of the different kinds of organisms. There are several kinds of disease-causing microorganisms: bacteria, viruses, protozoa, fungi, and **rickettsiae.**

anaerobic Able to grow and function without oxygen.

saprophytes Organisms that live on dead organic matter.

parasites Organisms obtaining nourishment from other organisms they are living in or on.

pathogenic Disease causing.

decompose To decay; to break down.

nonpathogenic Not causing disease.

urethritis Inflammation of the urethra.

cystitis Inflammation of the urinary bladder.

rickettsiae Parasitic microorganisms that live on another living organism and cause disease.

FIGURE 12–1. A microscope is needed to see microorganisms.

Micro organisms

Microscope   Organisms

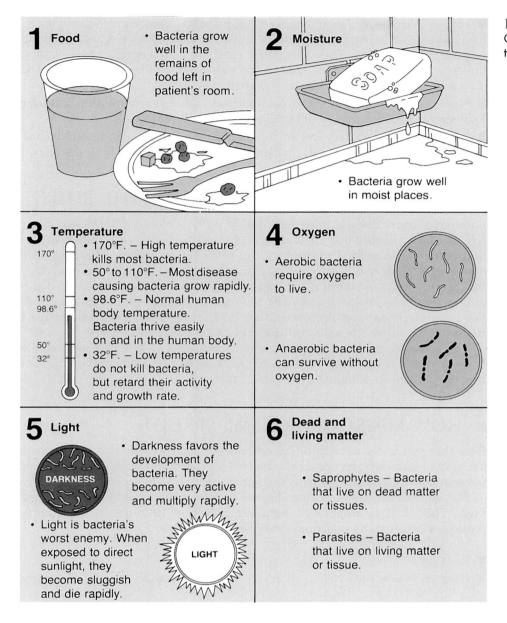

FIGURE 12–2.
Conditions affecting the growth of bacteria.

1 Food
• Bacteria grow well in the remains of food left in patient's room.

2 Moisture
• Bacteria grow well in moist places.

3 Temperature
170°
110°
98.6°
50°
32°
• 170°F. – High temperature kills most bacteria.
• 50° to 110°F. – Most disease causing bacteria grow rapidly.
• 98.6°F. – Normal human body temperature. Bacteria thrive easily on and in the human body.
• 32°F. – Low temperatures do not kill bacteria, but retard their activity and growth rate.

4 Oxygen
• Aerobic bacteria require oxygen to live.
• Anaerobic bacteria can survive without oxygen.

5 Light
DARKNESS
LIGHT
• Darkness favors the development of bacteria. They become very active and multiply rapidly.
• Light is bacteria's worst enemy. When exposed to direct sunlight, they become sluggish and die rapidly.

6 Dead and living matter
• Saprophytes – Bacteria that live on dead matter or tissues.
• Parasites – Bacteria that live on living matter or tissue.

■ *Bacteria.* Bacteria are responsible for many diseases. For example, strep throat is caused by streptococci, staph infection is caused by staphylococci, and syphilis is caused by **spirochetes.** These are only a few of the diseases that bacteria cause.

Staphylococcus and streptococcus are organisms that are always present in health care environments. Staphylococcus (staph) infections can have a serious impact on patients/clients, staff, and families. An uncontrolled or untreated staph infection in a newborn nursery, for example, can cause infants to die. People who have a stressed immune system have trouble fighting a staph infection and may die. Hospital stays are prolonged because of staph infections. Staph is usually the cause of pimples or boils found on the skin. All drainage from a pimple or boil should be handled according to Standard Precautions so as to prevent the spread of infection. Patients with staph infections are always treated with Standard Precautions.

spirochetes Slender, coil-shaped organisms.

■ *Viruses.* Viruses are even smaller than bacteria. They cannot grow until they have taken over a living cell. Viruses cause the common cold and many upper respiratory infections. They also cause smallpox, chickenpox, measles, mumps, influenza, and fever blisters. One of the most serious diseases is AIDS. These are only a few of the illnesses caused by viruses.

■ *Protozoa.* Protozoa are larger than viruses but also grow within a **host** cell. They cause trichomonas, amebic dysentery, and malaria.

■ *Fungi.* Fungi are a very low form of plant life. Fungi include molds and yeasts. They can cause athlete's foot, thrush, vaginitis, and serious lung diseases.

host The organism from which a microorganism takes nourishment. The microorganism gives nothing in return and causes disease or illness.

■ HOW MICROORGANISMS AFFECT THE BODY

Pathogens cause disease in several different ways. Some microorganisms produce **toxins** that affect the body. For instance, staphylococcus produces an **enterotoxin** that is the cause of food poisoning. The toxin causes fatigue, diarrhea, and vomiting. The tetanus bacilli produce a toxin that enters the bloodstream and attacks the central nervous system, causing severe damage and frequently death. Some microorganisms invade living cells and destroy them; this is called *cell invasion.* For example, there is a protozoan that invades the red blood cells of the host. As the protozoa grow, the cells rupture and cause chills and fever.

The presence of some microorganisms causes a violent *allergic reaction* in the body. A runny nose, watery eyes, and sneezing can be caused by the presence of a microorganism to which the host is allergic.

toxins Poisonous substances.

enterotoxin Poisonous substance that is produced in, or originates in, the contents of the intestine.

■ HOW MICROORGANISMS SPREAD

Now that you know something about microorganisms, you need to know how they are spread and how they enter the body. This helps you protect yourself and others from infection. Microorganisms are spread from one place to another in five ways.

For microorganisms to cause disease or infection, they must have a **susceptible** host. This host is unable to fight off infection because its resistance to the pathogen is low. Low resistance may be caused by

susceptible Capable of being affected or infected (e.g., body can be attacked by microorganisms and become ill).

- Poor diet
- Fatigue, inadequate rest
- Stress
- Poor health

Direct Contact

Direct contact occurs when the organisms are transmitted directly from one person to another. Examples include actual physical contact, sexual contact, direct contact with an open area on the body, and breathing in the pathogen directly from an infected person.

Indirect Contact

Indirect contact occurs when an organism is transferred from one object to another. Examples include **contaminated** substances such as foods, air, soil, feces, clothing, and equipment. To prevent the spread of microorganisms by indirect contact:

contaminated Soiled, unclean, not suitable for use.

- Do not, without proper protection, touch objects used by someone who has an infection.
- Hold contaminated linen, belongings, or other items away from your uniform.

Airborne

Some microorganisms are carried in the air. Coughing and sneezing project droplets into the air, and these droplets are carried on air currents until they find a place to land. The droplets cling to hair, uniforms, and medical equipment, or they fall on the floor. As you move from place to place, you may spread these organisms. Examples of illnesses caused by this route are influenza, chickenpox, and wound infections.

To prevent the spread of airborne microorganisms:

■ Keep your hair short or tied back so that it does not swing around, spreading microorganisms.

■ Cover your mouth and nose when you sneeze. Always wash your hands after coughing or sneezing, or you will spread germs to whatever you touch.

■ Do not wear your uniform outside the facility. If you wear your uniform home, put it in the wash immediately to prevent spreading germs.

■ When something is dropped on the floor, consider it contaminated. *Do not use it.*

■ Do not hold patients'/clients' linens against your uniform.

■ Stay home when you are sick with an acute respiratory infection.

Oral Route

Microorganisms also enter the body through water, contaminated food, dirty hands, and from other contaminated objects. Examples of illnesses caused by this route are food poisoning, polio, hepatitis, salmonellosis, and typhoid fever. To prevent the oral route spread of microorganisms, it is essential to

■ Wash your hands before eating or handling food. Wash your hands thoroughly and correctly after using the toilet. You must wash your hands every time you go to the bathroom.

■ Always wash your hands before helping patients/clients.

■ Refrigerate food properly. Microorganisms can grow on food that is not refrigerated.

■ Dispose of wound drainage in a proper way.

Insects and Pests

Microorganisms are spread by insects and pests. The organisms are picked up from contaminated areas and carried to water, food, and people. Examples of illnesses caused by this route are bubonic plague, malaria, and amoebic dysentery.

To prevent the spread of microorganisms by insects and pests, it is important to

■ Keep all flies and insects out of the environment.

■ Report insects or pests immediately.

■ PROTECTION FROM MICROORGANISMS

Standard Precautions and Transmission-based Precautions were created to provide guidelines that prevent the spread of microorganisms. These guidelines are described in Unit 3 of this chapter. Read them carefully and follow them whenever infectious microorganisms are present.

■ SIGNS AND SYMPTOMS OF INFECTION

generalized Affecting all of the body.

localized Affecting one area of the body.

An infection may be **generalized** or it may be **localized.** If the infection is generalized, there is usually headache, fatigue, fever, and increased pulse and respiration. There may also be vomiting and/or diarrhea. If the infection is localized, you can see and feel one or more of the following: redness, swelling, heat, and/or drainage. There is usually pain at the site of the infection.

■ SUMMARY

We are surrounded by microorganisms. They are in the air we breathe, on our skin, in our food, and on everything we touch. Some microorganisms are pathogens; others are nonpathogens. Pathogens include some bacteria, viruses, protozoa, fungi, and rickettsiae. Since pathogens cause illness, it is important to understand how they are spread and how they can be controlled. Learning the signs and symptoms of infection will help you provide better patient care.

It is the responsibility of every health care worker to help in the prevention of the spread of infection. Every year thousands of patients/clients have extended stays in the hospital because they have acquired an infection while hospitalized. It is vital that all health care workers practice good techniques to prevent the spread of infection.

UNIT 2   Asepsis

S*teps to success*

1. Complete Vocabulary Worksheet 1 in the Student Workbook.
2. Read this unit.
3. Complete Worksheets 2 and 3 as assigned.
4. When you are confident that you can meet each objective for this unit, ask your instructor for the unit evaluation.

aseptic technique Methods used to make the environment, the worker, and the patient as germ-free as possible.

Standard Precautions Guidelines designed to reduce the risk of transmission of microorganisms from recognized and unrecognized sources of infection in the hospital.

Rationale

The environment of the health care worker contains larger numbers of microorganisms than do most other environments. The health care worker must acquire the knowledge and skills required to restrict the spread of pathogenic microorganisms. The health care worker who practices good **aseptic technique** and follows **Standard Precautions** protects patients/clients, co-workers, and the community from infection.

Objectives

When you have completed this unit, you will be able to do the following:

✓ Define *medical asepsis.*
✓ Match terms related to medical asepsis with their correct meanings.

✓ List five aseptic techniques.
✓ Demonstrate appropriate handwashing techniques.
✓ Explain the difference between *bactericidal* and *bacteriostatic*.
✓ List four reasons why asepsis is important.

■ INTRODUCTION TO ASEPSIS

Health care facilities are filled with people who are ill. Some of their illnesses are caused by body dysfunction; other people are ill because of infections or injury. Health care environments are constantly filled with pathogenic microorganisms carried in by patients, visitors, and staff. This constant presence of pathogens requires the staff to wage an all-out battle against these organisms. This battle is waged by the continual use of medical asepsis. *Medical asepsis* means to destroy the environment that allows pathogens to live, breed, and spread. Medical asepsis is accomplished by using *aseptic technique.*

Aseptic technique is very important when you are working with patients. The practice of aseptic technique helps to prevent the following:

■ Cross infection, which is caused by infecting the patient with a new microorganism from another patient or health care worker
■ Reinfection with the same microorganism that caused the original illness
■ Self-inoculation by the patient's own organisms, such as *E. coli* from the intestines entering the urethra
■ An illness passing from the patient to the health care worker or from the health care worker to the patient

Aseptic technique includes

■ Employees being clean and neat
■ Proper handling of all equipment
■ Using sterile procedure when necessary
■ Using proper cleaning solutions: *bacteriostatic* solutions, which slow or stop the growth of bacteria, or *bactericidal* solutions, which kill bacteria
■ Proper handwashing
■ Following Standard Precautions

The health care team must strive toward achieving an aseptic environment to reduce the infection rate in the health care setting.

■ STANDARD PRECAUTIONS

Special precautions are necessary to lower the risk of **transmitting** pathogens from person to person. In 1985, health care isolation practices in the United States changed to defend against the increased risk of exposure to Hepatitis B virus (HBV) and human immunodeficiency virus (HIV). For the first time, all blood and body fluids were treated as infected substances. The Occupational Safety and Health Administration (OSHA) of the U.S. Department of Labor established mandatory guidelines published in the Occupational Exposure to Bloodborne Pathogens: Final Rule. These guidelines ensure that all employers provide personal protective equipment to employees at risk of exposure to body fluids. In 1992,

transmitting Causing to go from one person to another person.

TABLE 12–1 Standard Precaution Guidelines	
Protective Equipment	**When to Use Personal Protective Equipment (PPE)**
Gloves (See procedure for removing gloves on page 260.)	Wear when in contact with • Any body fluid • Nonintact skin and mucous membrane Wear when your hands are chapped, when a rash is present, or when you have open sores present.
Nonpermeable gowns or aprons (See procedure for removing and discarding gowns on page 260.)	Wear during procedures that are likely to expose you to • Any body fluid • Nonintact skin and mucous membrane
Mask and protective eyewear or face shield	Wear when • Body fluid droplets or splashes are likely. • Patients are coughing a lot.
Special masks and eyewear that seal close to face	Wear when assisting with procedures that cause body tissues to be aerosolized (e.g., laser treatments).
Handwashing (See procedure on page 254.)	Wash hands before putting on and after removing gloves and before and after working with each patient with his or her equipment, or both.
Shared equipment— multiple-use patient care equipment (e.g., blood pressure cuff, stethoscope, aural thermometer)	Remove all equipment for cleaning immediately upon contact with • Any body fluid • Nonintact skin and mucous membrane

OSHA increased its mandate to employers, insisting that training and immunization be provided to all employees within 10 days of hire. This means that employees at risk for exposure to body fluids must

■ Be offered Hepatitis B vaccine (HBV) at no charge
■ Be trained to use the appropriate protective equipment to prevent exposure to body fluids
■ Receive an annual update and review

nosocomial Infection acquired while in a health care setting, such as a hospital.

In 1996, the Center for Disease Control (CDC) expanded the bloodborne pathogen guidelines to assist in the prevention of **nosocomial** infections. These expanded guidelines are known as Standard Precautions. Standard Precautions are appropriate for all patients/clients receiving care or service in a health care environment regardless of their diagnosis. Standard Precautions provide protection from contact with blood, mucous membranes, nonintact skin, and all body fluids. Body fluids include the following:

■ Blood
■ Tissue specimens
■ Vaginal secretions

- **Cerebrospinal fluid**
- **Pericardial fluid**
- **Interstitial fluid**
- Body fluids containing visible blood
- Semen
- **Amniotic fluid**
- **Pleural fluid**
- **Peritoneal fluid**

Infection with HBV and HIV occur through

- Direct injection of infected blood or a contaminated needle that punctures the skin.
- Contact of infected body fluids with mucous membranes such as the eye or inside of the mouth.
- Sexual contact.
- Pregnancy. When the mother is infected, the infection is transferred to the newborn infant.

The risk of being infected in the health care setting is high. It is important for you to treat everyone as though he or she were infected. If you provide hands-on care to patients, you must follow all Standard Precaution guidelines (see Table 12–1) to protect yourself and others. Make it a habit to follow each step in the Standard Precaution guidelines.

■ CONTROLLING THE SPREAD OF INFECTION

Skin and hair cannot be **sterilized,** because any solutions or procedures that kill microorganisms are harmful to skin. You use a bacteriostatic solution for cleaning skin. Bacteriocidal solutions are used on equipment. This method of controlling the spread of infection is called **disinfection.** A 10 percent solution of household bleach can be used to disinfect items that tolerate exposure to mild bleach solution.

CAUTION Never use bleach on any item that will be put into the body or with any other product (e.g., cleansers, sprays).

Sterilization is the process of killing all microorganisms, even spores (bacteria with a protective hard shell around them). Spores are killed when they are **exposed** to steam under pressure at a high temperature. **Autoclaves** are used to produce steam. Gas autoclaves and chemical baths are used to sterilize equipment that would be damaged by steam. Items needing sterilization are those that are put into the body or around an open wound.

Handwashing is the most effective way to reduce the spread of microorganisms. Many infections contracted while in the medical setting can be traced back to poor handwashing technique or no handwashing. To prevent infecting yourself and others, *always wash your hands* before and after eating, handling objects or equipment, doing procedures, and working with patients.

---

cerebrospinal fluid Liquid that flows through and around brain tissue.

pericardial fluid Liquid that surrounds the heart.

interstitial fluid Liquid that fills the space between most of the cells of the body.

amniotic fluid Liquid that surrounds the fetus during pregnancy.

pleural fluid Liquid that surrounds the lungs.

peritoneal fluid Liquid in the peritoneal cavity.

sterilized Made free from all living microorganisms.

disinfection Process of freeing from microorganisms by physical or chemical means.

exposed Left unprotected.

autoclaves Sterilizers that use steam under pressure to kill all forms of bacteria on fomites (objects that pathogens live on and can transfer infection).

Procedure

Handwashing

1. Turn on water.

2. Regulate temperature.
3. Wet hands, fingers pointed downward.
4. Apply soap to hands and wrists.

5. Rub hands in circular motion.

6. Interlace fingers, rub back and forth (add water when necessary to keep moist).
7. Use a nailbrush. If none is available, rub fingernails on palms of hand.
8. Rinse with fingers pointed down.

9. Dry hands with paper towel.
10. Turn off faucet with paper towel.
11. Leave area clean and neat.

■ SUMMARY

In this unit, we have discussed the importance of infection control. The effective health care worker always strives to provide an aseptic environment by following aseptic technique procedures and Standard Precautions.

Asepsis is the method used to destroy the environment that allows pathogens to live, breed, and spread. Major factors in the control of microorganisms are

- ■ Handwashing
- ■ Disinfection
- ■ Sterilization
- ■ Standard Precautions

UNIT 3   Standard Precautions

Steps to success

1. Complete Vocabulary Worksheet 1 in the Student Workbook.
2. Read this unit.
3. Complete Worksheets 2 and 3 as assigned.
4. When you are confident that you can meet each objective for this unit, ask your instructor for the unit evaluation.
5. Complete "Your Link to Success" at the end of this chapter.

Rationale

As a health care worker, you are exposed to patients/clients, equipment, and supplies that are contaminated with pathogens. An estimated 2,400,000 hospital-acquired infections occur in the United States each year. It is possible that these infections cause 30,000 deaths a year. Use the techniques taught in this chapter to protect yourself and others and help prevent the spread of infection to patients/clients, co-workers, and the community.

Objectives

When you have completed this unit, you will be able to do the following:

✓ Name two primary levels of precautions identified in the guidelines developed by the Center for Disease Control (CDC).
✓ Identify three types of Transmission-Based Precautions.
✓ Demonstrate the correct procedure for entering and leaving an area where Transmission-Based Precautions are followed.
✓ Differentiate between Standard Precautions and Transmission-Based Precautions.

■ INTRODUCTION TO STANDARD PRECAUTIONS

The 1996 guidelines from the CDC established the need for two levels of protection.

■ *Standard Precautions:* the primary strategy for successful hospital-acquired (nosocomial) infection control. Standard Precautions are appropriate for all patients/clients receiving care or service in a health care environment, regardless of their diagnosis. This precaution provides protection from contact with blood, mucous membranes, nonintact skin, and all body fluids.

■ *Transmission-Based Precautions:* for the care of known or suspected patients infected with pathogens spread by

airborne Particles that float in the air.

• **Airborne** or **droplet** transmission • Contact with dry skin or contaminated surfaces

droplet A small drop of fluid.

Transmission-Based Precautions are used in addition to Standard Precautions. There are three types of Transmission-Based Precautions (see Table 12–2):

microns Units equaling one millionth of a meter.

■ *Airborne Precautions* reduce the spread of airborne droplet nuclei (5 **microns** or smaller in size) or dust particles containing the pathogen.

■ *Droplet Precautions* reduce the risk of transmission by contact of the mucous membranes of the eye, nose, or mouth with large-particle droplets.

■ *Contact Precautions* reduce the risk of transmission through direct or indirect contact.

Follow the guidelines shown in Table 12–2 when working with patients/clients in any of the Transmission-Based Precaution environments. See Figures 12–3 and 12–4 for more information.

Transmission-Based Precaution Rooms

See Figures 12–3 and 12–4 for illustrations of appropriate precautions within the room. When entering or leaving a Transmission-Based Precaution room, follow the specific directions on the precaution card at the door of the room. The

TABLE 12–2   Transmission-Based Precautions

Airborne	Droplet	Contact
Standard Precautions	Standard Precautions	Standard Precautions
Private room with specific ventilation criteria	Private room or room with another patient with same microorganism	Private room or room with another patient with the same microorganism
Keep the room door closed.		
Wear respiratory protection.	Wear a mask when working within 3 feet of the patient.	
Wash hands before entering the room. Wash hands before leaving the room and after leaving.	Wash hands before entering the room. Wash hands before leaving the room and after leaving.	Wash hands before entering the room. Wear gloves when entering the room. Remove gloves before leaving. Wash hands. Wear a clean nonsterile gown when entering the room and expecting contact with the patient or with contaminated surfaces.

Transmission-Based Precautions

AIRBORNE PRECAUTIONS
(droplets smaller than 5 microns in size)
Visitors – Report to Nurses' Station
Before Entering Room

1. Masks are indicated.
2. Gowns are indicated only if needed to prevent gross contamination of clothing.
3. Gloves are indicated per Standard Precautions (for contact with blood or body fluids).
4. Hands must be washed after touching the patient or potentially contaminated articles and before taking care of another patient.
5. Articles should be discarded, cleaned, or sent for decontamination and reprocessing.

DROPLET PRECAUTIONS
(droplets larger than 5 microns in size)
Visitors – Report to Nurses' Station
Before Entering Room

1. Masks are indicated for those who come within 3 feet of the patient.
2. Gowns are not indicated.
3. Gloves are indicated per Standard Precautions (for contact with blood or body fluids).
4. Hands must be washed after touching the patient or potentially contaminated articles and before taking care of another patient.
5. Articles contaminated with infective material should be discarded or bagged and labeled before being sent for decontamination and reprocessing.

FIGURE 12–3. Transmission-Based Precautions

257

FIGURE 12–4.
Contact precautions.

CONTACT PRECAUTIONS

Dirty-linen hamper
(lined with bag)

Garbage can
(lined with
plastic bag)

Patient's Room
(should be private,
but not absolutely necessary)

Waste basket
(lined with plastic bag)

Sink

Isolation sign on door

Isolation cart

Gowns
Gloves
Masks
Plastic bags
Laundry bags

Hall

Clean area

Dirty area

CONTACT PRECAUTIONS
Visitors – Report to Nurses' Station
Before Entering Room

1. **Masks** are not indicated.
2. **Gowns** are indicated if soiling is likely.
3. **Gloves** are indicated for touching infective material.
4. **Hands must be washed after touching the patient or potentially contaminated articles and before taking care of another patient.**
5. **Articles** contaminated with infective material should be discarded or bagged and labeled before being sent for decontamination and reprocessing.

A private room is indicated for Contact Precautions if patient hygiene is poor. A patient with poor hygiene does not wash hands after touching infective material, contaminates the environment with infective material, or shares contaminated articles with other patients. In general, patients infected with the same organism may share a room.

following procedure guides you through the steps in applying and removing personal protective equipment. Each medical environment determines the specific order in which to apply each item. Always follow your organization's policy and procedure.

*P*rocedure

Transmission-Based Precautions: Applying Personal Protective Equipment

1. Assemble equipment.
2. Wash hands.
3. Put on cap, covering all of hair.
4. Put on mask.
   a. Unfold.
   b. Cover mouth and nose.
   c. Tie top string at back of head.
   d. Tie lower string at back of neck.

c. Overlap gown edges.
d. Tie at waist.
e. Make sure that uniform is completely covered.

5. Put on gown.
   a. Put opening in back.
   b. Tie bow at back of neck.

Procedure box continued

6. Put on gloves.

   a. Do not tear or puncture.
   b. Cover cuff of gown with top of glove.

Removal of Mask, Gown, and Gloves

1. Untie waist tie.
2. Remove gloves.
3. Wash hands.
4. Untie neck tie.
5. Remove gown.
   a. Cross arms, pull forward inside out.
   b. Roll gown, put in dirty hamper marked "Toxic Waste" or "Hazardous Waste" inside room.
6. Wash hands.
7. Remove cap.
8. Remove mask and discard.

9. Wash hands.
10. Use paper towel to turn off faucet.

11. Use paper towel to open door.
12. Discard towel inside room.
13. Wash hands.

■ TRANSMISSION-BASED PRECAUTIONS

Transmission-Based Precautions may be difficult for patients/clients. They are alone most of the time. Visitors must wear personal protective wear. Hugs or touching may not be allowed. The health care worker cannot stay and visit because there is other work to do. This may cause the patient to feel angry, depressed, and frustrated. Take as much time as you can to listen to the client's feelings and concerns. Encourage communication and be supportive. If the patient seems unusually upset, report it to your supervisor.

■ SUMMARY

In this unit, you learned about Standard Precautions and Transmission-Based Precautions. Follow Standard Precautions when working with all patients and follow Transmission-Based Precautions when airborne infection is present and when in contact with pathogenic items. Your careful use of these precautions prevents transmission of infectious agents that cause disease and illness in yourself and others.

Thinking Critically:
Check Your Understanding

1. **Communication** You are assigned Mrs. Maldonado, a difficult client to care for. She is still in Transmission-Based, Contact Precautions after three weeks of care. Your experience with her tells you that she is irritable and unhappy about everything. Write a recommendation about how to communicate with Mrs. Maldonado in a new way that demonstrates dignity and justice.

2. **Patient Education** Your patient/client is newly diagnosed with Hepatitis B. You notice on several occasions that he does not wash his hands after going to the bathroom. Write an explanation of how to educate him on the importance of handwashing to protect his family and others. Your method of educating must clearly convey a tone of respect for his dignity.

3. **Computers** Advances in medicine are continually changing the way health care workers protect themselves and treat infections. Explain how computers help keep the medical community informed about the latest medical progress. Describe ways you can access this information if you do not own a computer.

4. **Medical Math** Airborne Precautions are required when a pathogen 5 microns or smaller is present in the air. It is difficult to imagine how small 5 microns is. Use a ruler with centimeter markings to draw a line 1 mm long to help you picture the size. Calculate the number of microns in a millimeter and show your calculations on paper. Can you draw how long 5 microns is in comparison to 1 mm?

5. **Case Study** Mr. Ramsey is in Transmission-Based Precautions. He is extra quiet today, and his eyes are red and puffy. You think something is wrong, but you are behind in your work. What do you think is wrong? How will you see to it that Mr. Ramsey's psychosocial and physical needs are cared for and still get your work done?

Portfolio Connection

The medical community is constantly finding new information about how microorganisms affect our lives. This constant flow of new information makes it necessary to research how new findings affect us.

Conduct research and write a research paper about a microorganism. Select a microorganism from those mentioned in this chapter or from another source. Explain how the microorganism affects society and describe its shape, size, color, and pattern of growth. Describe its nature (aerobic or anaerobic), its effect on the body, and the physical symptoms it causes.

Use a standard report format on 8.5-by-11-inch paper, typed double spaced or neatly written in ink. When this assignment is perfect in format, grammar, and spelling, place it in your portfolio behind the section labeled "Written Reports and Assignments."

Your ability to formulate an organized research paper shows employers or colleges that you are able to organize, analyze, evaluate, and communicate information effectively.

13 PATIENT AND EMPLOYEE SAFETY

UNIT 1 — General Safety and Injury and Illness Prevention

Steps to success

1. Complete Vocabulary Worksheet 1 in the Student Workbook.
2. Read this unit.
3. Complete Worksheets 2 through 7 as assigned.
4. When you are confident that you can meet each objective for this unit, ask your instructor for the unit evaluation.

Rationale

A health care worker is responsible for maintaining a safe environment. You must know your employer's policies and procedures and be able to respond quickly to prevent injury. Your employer is also obligated to provide a safe environment by supplying equipment that protects against injury. The Occupational Safety and Health Administration (OSHA) of the U.S. Department of Labor determines, develops, and monitors safe practices for each industry. The Joint Commission on Accreditation of Health Care Organizations (JCAHO) establishes guidelines for the operation of health care facilities. They conduct accreditation surveys that endorse OSHA standards. JCAHO audits look for policy and procedures that follow OSHA guidelines. Health care agencies strive to achieve excellence by meeting OSHA and JCAHO standards. Keeping you and those served by your health care agency safe is a priority for your employer. If you or your employer fails to provide appropriate safety for all, OSHA will penalize your employer with a large fine or lock the doors of the facility until the safety violation is corrected. If you are at fault for not providing safe conditions, you could lose your job.

Objectives

When you have completed this unit, you will be able to do the following:

✓ Match vocabulary words to their correct meanings.

✓ Define *OSHA* and explain the agency's role in safety.

✓ Differentiate between IIPP, hazard communication, and exposure control.

✓ Name places to find information about hazards in a facility.

✓ Explain the health care worker's role in maintaining a safe workplace.

✓ Discuss the employer's role in maintaining a safe workplace.

✓ Identify fourteen general safety rules.

✓ Summarize the importance of safety in a health care environment.

■ OSHA STANDARDS

The Occupational Safety and Health Administration (OSHA) is part of the U.S. Department of Labor. OSHA establishes the guidelines for a safe work environment for all employers and their employees. The OSHA standards say that employees have the "right to know" what hazards are present in their environment. OSHA regulations require employers to train and offer immunization to high-risk employees in the first 10 days of a new job. A committed partnership between the employer and employee is necessary to provide a safe environment for everyone. This unit explains the three areas with which health care agencies and facilities must **comply.** They are the

■ Injury and Illness Prevention Program

■ Hazard Communication Program

■ Exposure Control Plan

■ Ergonomic Program

comply To follow directions, do what you are asked to do.

Ergonomic Program

Employers are changing the work environment to meet the expected OSHA **ergonomic** standard. You spend a large portion of your day in the work environment. You should be comfortable, use good posture, and learn the exercises to prevent getting stiff and sore. The safety officer where you work will help you adjust your environment to accomplish this. If you sit in a workstation during the day, your chair, desk, and computer must be adjusted to fit your needs. There are exercises in your Student Workbook to help you evaluate your work environment to ensure that you are in good alignment as you work. This prevents physical problems caused by improper working conditions.

ergonomic Related to the study of the work environment.

Injury and Illness Prevention Program

The Injury and Illness Prevention Program (IIPP) **mandates** that every employer establish, **implement,** and maintain an effective IIPP.

As a student or employee, you are responsible for

■ Knowing who is responsible in the facility for the IIPP.

■ Practicing policy and procedures that ensure safe and healthy work practices.

■ Understanding the communication system used to keep you informed of

• Hazards • Personal protective equipment (PPE) • Knowing how you learn about hazards on the work site

mandates Commands, orders.

implement To accomplish; make it work.

■ Knowing what hazards are present and how to prevent injury from them.

■ Knowing to whom to report an injury or illness during work hours and what documentation to complete.

■ Knowing where the safety bulletin board (or communication book) is in your facility. You are responsible for reading all items posted each month.

Your school or employer will test you for signs of tuberculosis (TB). Exposure to tuberculosis is determined by a TB skin test. If your TB test indicates exposure, additional tests will be necessary. You will also be offered Hepatitis B vaccine. This vaccine protects you from getting Hepatitis B while working in the health care environment.

Hazard Communication Program

The Hazard Communication Program mandates that employers inform employees of

■ Chemicals or hazards in the environment
■ Where chemicals or hazards are stored and used
■ How to interpret chemical labels and hazard signs
■ Methods and equipment for cleaning chemical spills
■ Personal protection equipment and its storage location
■ The hazard communication system

As a student or employee you are responsible for knowing

■ What chemicals or hazards are in your work area
■ Where the chemicals or hazards are stored or used
■ How to read and interpret container signs and labels
■ What to do when a chemical or **biohazard** spills
■ What personal protective equipment (PPE) to wear when working with or around chemicals and biohazards
■ Your facility's system for informing you of hazards in the work area

biohazard Substance that has potential to transmit disease.

Hazard Categories

The way that harm is caused determines the hazard category.

■ *Physical hazards* cause harm when a chemical is mixed with another chemical, causing a reaction. When a chemical reacts with another substance or because of temperature change, it creates a new chemical. For example: Clorox mixed with ammonia creates a harmful gas.
■ *Health hazards* have the potential to harm a healthy body. For example, acid burns and destroys skin.

Material Safety Data Sheets (MSDSs)

Product manufacturers prepare material safety data sheet (MSDS) forms to provide the information needed to handle chemicals safely. Employers must make the MSDSs available to employees. Figure 13–1 identifies the type of information discussed on the MSDS.

MATERIAL SAFETY DATA SHEET
I   Product Identification

COMPANY NAME: Calgon Vestal Laboratories

ADDRESS: 5035 Manchester Avenue   Nights: 314-802-2000

            St. Louis, Missouri 63110   CHEMTREC: (800) 424-9300

PRODUCT NAME: Klenzyme   Product No.:   1103

SYNONYMS: Medical Apparatus and Instrument Presoak

II   Hazardous Ingredients of Mixtures

Material	(CAS#)	% by Wt.	TLV	PEL
Subtilisins (Proteolytic enzymes)	(9014-01-1)	<5	.06ppb	N/A
Sodium tetraborate, decahydrate	(1303-96-4)	<5	5mg/m3	10mg/m3

III   Physical Data

Vapor Pressure, mmHg: N/A   Vapor Density (Air=1) 60–90 F: Undeterm.

Evaporation Rate (ether=1): N/A   % Volatile by wt: N/A

Solubility in H_2O: Complete   pH @ Undiluted Solution: N/A

Freezing Point F: N/A   pH as Distributed: 7.5–8.0

Boiling Point F: >212F   Appearance: Amber liquid

Specific Gravity H_2O=1 @ 25C: 1.08   Odor: Typical, mild odor

IV   Fire and Explosion

Flash Point F: N/A   Flammable Limits: N/A

Extinguishing Media: Not flammable. In event of fire, use water fog, CO_2, and dry chemical.

Special Fire Fighting Procedures: No special requirements given. As with any chemical fire, proper cautions should be taken, such as wearing a self-contained breathing apparatus.

Unusual Fire and Explosion Hazards: None known

V   Reactivity Data

Stability-Conditions to avoid: Stable

Incompatibility: None known

Hazardous Decomposition Products: Propionaldehyde, CO, CO_2 in fire situations.

Conditions Contributing to Hazardous Polymerization: Will not occur.

VI   Health Hazard Data

Effects of Overexposure (Medical Conditions Aggravated/Target Organ Effects)

A. *Acute* (Primary Route of Exposure)

    Eyes & Skin: Upon contact, mildly irritating to eyes. Prolonged or repeated contact may irritate skin.

    Inhalation: Spray mists or dusts from dried residues may result in respiratory irritation, coughing and/or difficulty in breathing.

    Ingestion: May cause upset to gastrointestinal tract.

B. *Subchronic, Chronic, Other:*   Subtilisins chronic exposure to dusts showed allergic sensitization with respiratory allergic reactions within minutes or delayed up to 24 hours.

VII   Emergency and First Aid Procedures

Eyes: Immediately flush eyes with plenty of water for at least 15 minutes. See a physician.

Skin: Immediately wash with soap and plenty of water for at least 15 minutes while removing contaminated clothing. If irritation develops, seek medical aid.

Inhalation: Remove to fresh air. If not breathing, give artificial respiration. If breathing difficult, give oxygen if available. Seek medical aid and report all inhalation exposures to health and safety personnel.

Ingestion: Do not induce vomiting. Give water to dilute. Call a physician. Never give anything by mouth to an unconscious person.

FIGURE 13–1. Example of an MSDS form *(continued on next page).*

VIII   Spill or Leak Procedures

Spill Management: Contain spill and absorb material with an inert substance. Collect waste in suitable container.

Waste Disposal Methods: Dispose of in accordance with local, state, and federal regulations.

IX   Protection Information/Control Measures

Respiratory: Not required under normal use.

Eye: Safety glasses

Glove: Rubber

Other Clothing and Equipment: Clothes sufficient to avoid contact.

Ventilation: Local exhaust.

X   Special Precautions

Precautions to be taken in Handling and Storing: Avoid exposure to high temperature or humidity. Wash hands thoroughly after use. Keep container closed when not in use.

Additional Information: Read and observe all labeled precautions.

Prepared by: R.C. Jente   Revision Date: 08/24/96

Seller makes no warranty, expressed or implied, concerning the use of this product other than indicated on the label.

Buyer assumes all risks of use and/or handling of this material when such use and/or handling is contrary to label instructions.

While Seller believes that the information contained herein is accurate, such information is offered solely for its customers' consideration and verification under their specific use conditions. This information is not to be deemed a warranty or representation of any kind for which Seller assumes legal responsibility.

FIGURE 13–1. Example of an MSDS form *(continued).*

The Hazard Communication Program explains how the employer plans to keep people safe when chemicals are present. The communication system must explain

■ What hazards are present and where they are stored and used.

■ What precautions to take when hazardous products are present. These precautions include

• Wearing appropriate personal protective equipment (PPE) • Proper room ventilation • Keeping flammable products away from flames or other heat sources

■ How to use potentially hazardous products safely.

■ Proper cleanup and disposal of hazardous products.

■ First aid if exposure occurs.

■ How to label containers with a chemical, by always including

• Product name • Chemicals in the product • Precautions for use of the product

As a student or employee you are responsible for knowing where hazard communications are kept and how to access them. You find hazard information on manufacturer's literature. You may receive memorandums from your employer alerting you to new hazards in the environment. Most facilities keep hazard communications

■ In safety policy and procedure manuals

■ In material safety data sheet (MSDS) books

■ On the safety bulletin board
■ On product labels
■ On signs

Exposure Control Program

An exposure control plan provides steps to reduce employee or student exposure to bloodborne pathogens. The plan includes the following:

■ Determining the possibility of exposure under each position description
■ Developing a schedule and method for ensuring that the plan is enforced
■ Postexposure evaluation

See the Occupational Exposure to Blood-borne Pathogens: Final Rule and Standard Precautions in Units 2 and 3 of Chapter 12 for more specific protective guidelines under the Exposure Control Program.

■ GENERAL SAFETY

Safety is everyone's responsibility. There are rules that are important to all health care workers. To be a safe worker and to protect yourself, co-workers, and patients/clients, learn the rules listed here.

■ *Walk! Never run in hallways.* If you run, you may fall and injure yourself. You can collide with another person or object. You can injure someone else, or you might create panic.

■ *Walk on the right-hand side of the hall not more than two* **abreast.** It is important to leave hallways open so that there are no traffic jams. In an emergency, a traffic jam can cause a delay and make the difference between life and death.

abreast Side by side.

■ *Use handrails when using the stairs.* This prevents falling and injuring yourself.

■ *Watch out for swinging doors.* Be certain that someone is not on the other side of a swinging door. You might injure yourself or someone else (see Figure 13–2).

FIGURE 13-2.
Watch for swinging doors!

horseplay Rowdy behavior; acting inappropriately in a work environment.

■ ***Horseplay*** *is not tolerated.* It is disturbing to others, may lead to accidents, causes confusion, and shows a lack of respect for patients and personnel.

■ *Always check labels.* Never use anything from containers that are not labeled. Using the wrong contents can cause injury or death to a patient. Using the wrong contents may also damage or ruin equipment.

■ *Wipe up spills and place litter in containers.* A wet floor can cause someone to slip and fall. If there is litter on the floor, someone may trip and be seriously injured.

■ *Follow instructions carefully.* If you do not understand instructions or do not know how to do a task, always ask for instructions. If you do something incorrectly, you may cause a serious problem.

■ *Report any injury to yourself or others to your supervisor immediately.* Reporting an injury ensures treatment for the injured without delay and correction of the potential hazard.

frayed Worn away or tattered (e.g., electrical cords may be worn, causing wires to be exposed).

■ *Do not use electrical cords that are **frayed** or damaged.* Frayed or damaged cords can cause **shocks,** burns, or fire.

■ *Report a shock you receive from electrical equipment to your supervisor.* This prevents fire or a shock to someone else.

■ *Do not use **malfunctioning** equipment.* It is dangerous and may cause serious injury to you or someone else.

shocks Convulsion of muscles and extreme stimulation of nerves when an electric current passes through the body.

■ *Report unsafe conditions to your supervisor immediately.* Safety is everyone's business. Be aware of your environment. Watch for unsafe conditions.

■ Follow Standard Precaution guidelines.

malfunctioning Not working as it is supposed to.

■ SUMMARY

Safety is the responsibility of all health care workers. OSHA is very strict about enforcement of regulations that keep the work environment safe.

UNIT 2   Patient Safety

Steps to success

1. Read this unit.
2. Complete Worksheet 1 in the Student Workbook.
3. When you are confident that you can meet each objective for this unit, ask your instructor for the unit evaluation.

Rationale

Health care workers are responsible for the safety of patients/clients. If you do not follow Standard Precautions and basic safety precautions, patients can be seriously injured. Accidents involving clients are reduced if simple safety measures are followed. In this unit, we explain rules to follow when using ambulation devices, transporting devices, postural supports, and side rails.

Objectives

When you have completed this unit, you will be able to do the following:

✓ Explain how to use ambulation devices, transporting devices, postural supports, and side rails safely.
✓ Match descriptions and principles associated with ambulation devices, transporting devices, postural supports, and side rails.
✓ Explain the importance of safety measures.
✓ Follow safe practice guidelines when caring for patients/clients.

■ IDENTIFYING THE PATIENT

When you work directly with a patient, you must identify him or her to avoid a mistake. Errors are avoided if you follow these *important* steps:

■ Check with the nurse's station for the right room number.
■ Check the requisition or physician's order, which has the patient's name on it, against the patient's identification band.
■ In ambulatory care, confirm chart name and information with each client.

■ AMBULATION DEVICES

Ambulation devices are devices used to assist in walking. The most common devices in the health care setting are canes, crutches, and walkers (see Figure 19–1, page 511). These devices give the patient/client additional support and aid in balancing while walking or standing.

Safe Practice Guidelines When Using Ambulation Devices

It is essential that all devices be in good condition, because patients/clients depend on these items.

■ Devices must always be structurally safe, without dents or cracks. For example, wood crutches are unsafe if the wood is split or cracked. A loose joint in a walker allows it to wobble or break, and the patient can fall.
■ Areas touching the ground must be covered with rubber tips to prevent slipping.
■ The devices must always be clean and free of blood or body fluids.

■ TRANSPORTING DEVICES

Transporting devices include equipment used to move patients from one place to another. The most common transporting devices are wheelchairs and gurneys. Gurneys and wheelchairs make it easy to move patients who are unable to walk. Follow these basic principles to ensure the patient's safety (see Figure 13–3, page 270).

Back a wheelchair over indented or raised doorways, such as an elevator or any ridges on the floor.

Always back a patient in a wheelchair or a gurney down a hill.

Never leave a patient on a gurney unattended.

Always back the patient on a gurney headfirst into an elevator.

Always secure straps or put side rails up on a gurney.

Always lock the brakes except when you are moving.
Lock brakes when when moving the patient on or off a gurney.

FIGURE 13–3. Principles in the use of gurneys and wheelchairs.

Safe Practice Guidelines When Using Gurneys and Wheelchairs

■ Always lock the brakes except when you are moving.

■ Back a wheelchair over indented or raised doorways, such as an elevator or any ridges on the floor.

■ Always back a client in a wheelchair or a gurney down a hill.

■ Always secure straps or put side rails up on a gurney.

■ Lock brakes when moving the client on or off a gurney.

■ Always back the patient on a gurney headfirst into an elevator.

■ Never leave a patient on a gurney unattended.

■ Always keep the gurney free of blood and body fluids.

■ POSTURAL SUPPORTS

Postural supports are devices that **restrict** a patient's movement. This type of restriction is necessary only when the patient's safety is in jeopardy. Occasionally, patients become disoriented due to a change of environment or as a response to medication. When this occurs, postural supports are used to keep clients safe. Postural supports are more common in long-term care facilities. *Example:* A confused patient may not realize that he is too weak to walk to the bathroom without falling. Use a postural support to remind clients to call for assistance when they need to get out of bed. There are many types of supports. The most common are vest supports, wrist supports, and ankle supports. When you use postural supports, certain principles must be observed. (See Chapter 15, page 405.)

restrict To keep within limits; to confine.

Safe Practice Guidelines When Using Postural Supports

■ A physician's order is required by law.

■ Never use a postural support on a patient in a chair or bed without wheels.

■ Clients requiring postural supports must be checked frequently. The support must be released or loosened every 2 hours.

■ Use a half-bow knot to secure the support.

■ Leave at least two fingers' ease between the patient's skin and the support so his or her circulation is not restricted.

■ Never secure supports to side rails; always attach to the framework of a bed or gurney.

■ Secure the half-bow knot out of the client's reach.

■ Discard supports that have touched blood or body fluids, following Standard Precautions.

■ SIDE RAILS

Use side rails on bedsides and gurneys (stretchers) to keep clients from falling. In the hospital, falls from beds are the most common cause of injury. The use of side rails helps reduce the number of falls. Side rails aid in turning or moving patients who are heavily medicated. Patients use them to help lift or turn themselves, and they prevent the patient from falling out of bed.

Safe Practice Guidelines When Using Side Rails

■ Side rails are always in place at night. If clients refuse to have them in place, a release must be signed relieving the facility of responsibility.

■ Small children, heavily medicated patients, and confused or restless patients require side rails at all times.

■ Side rails must be locked securely. Patients often lean on rails for support. If they are not secure, the patient can fall.

■ Precautions must be taken when side rails are put up or down. Tubing and the client's legs and arms must be in a safe position.

■ If the side rails are up when you begin a procedure, be certain they are up when you leave the room.

■ Side rails should always be clean and free of blood or body fluids.

■ SUMMARY

By following each of the simple principles discussed in this unit, you provide safe conditions for your patients/clients. You have learned to identify the patient to prevent errors and to keep your patients safe when using ambulation devices, transporting devices, postural supports, and side rails.

UNIT 3   Disaster Preparedness

*S*teps to success

1. Read this unit.
2. Complete Worksheet 1 in the Student Workbook.
3. When you are confident that you can meet each objective for this unit, ask your instructor for the unit evaluation.

Rationale

Disasters can occur anywhere and at any moment. As a health care worker, you are expected to respond quickly according to your agency disaster plan. You must be familiar with the practices that are detailed in that plan and be able to follow them if a disaster occurs. A disaster is anything that causes damage and injury to a group of people. Examples are flood, earthquake, tornado, explosion, and fire. Be alert to emergency equipment, exits, and the disaster plan. They provide the essentials necessary to respond effectively in a disaster.

Objectives

When you have completed this unit, you will be able to do the following:

✓ Define vocabulary words.
✓ Identify what you are responsible for knowing and doing when a disaster occurs.

✓ List the three elements required to start a fire.
✓ Explain four ways to prevent fires.
✓ Summarize all safety requirements that protect the employee/student, patient, and employer.

■ DISASTER PLAN

Your facility is required to have a disaster plan. You are responsible for knowing the plan and responding when a disaster occurs. To be prepared, you need to know the following:

■ The floor plan of your facility
■ The nearest exit route
■ The location of alarms and fire extinguishers
■ How to use alarms and fire extinguishers
■ Your role as a health care worker when a disaster occurs

The following are some basic rules to remember when a disaster strikes:

■ Assess the situation; count to 10 to calm yourself.
■ Be sure that you are not in danger. (Placing yourself in danger only makes the situation worse.)
■ Remove those who are in immediate danger, if it is safe to do so.
■ Notify others of the emergency according to facility policy.
■ Use stairs, *not* the elevator.

    Fire is often the result of a disaster. It is your responsibility to be alert to causes of fire and act to prevent fire when possible.

■ FIRE CAUSES AND PREVENTION

There are three elements that must be present before a fire can start (Figure 13–4a):

• Oxygen • Heat • Fuel

    Most fires can be prevented if everyone is **observant** and careful. The following are some ways you can help prevent fires:

observant Quick to see and understand.

■ Provide ashtrays for smokers. Never empty ashtrays into wastebaskets or containers that can burn. Ashtrays must be emptied into separate containers. Smoking is restricted to designated areas.

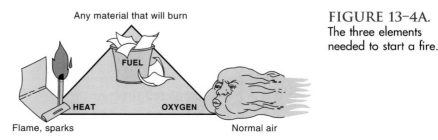

Any material that will burn

FUEL

HEAT   OXYGEN

Flame, sparks   Normal air

FIGURE 13–4A.
The three elements needed to start a fire.

FIGURE 13–4B.
Misuses of electricity.

Using lightweight electrical cord with heavily powered equipment

Defective outlets

Overloading circuits with too many electrical cords

Frayed wires

■ Check electrical equipment for proper functioning and frayed electrical cord. If there is any problem, report it immediately (see Figure 13–4b).

■ When using flammable liquids, take only the amount needed to complete the task. You would spill only the amount you poured, not the whole container. Keep flammable liquids in a container approved by the Underwriters' Laboratories.

■ Post a No Smoking sign when oxygen is in use in an area. If the oxygen is in a **cylinder,** strap the cylinder securely on a cart or stand.

cylinder Long, narrow, circular container.

potential Possible.

■ SUMMARY

Disaster preparedness is everyone's responsibility. Each person is responsible for responding to a disaster and being alert to **potential** hazards.

There are three elements required to start a fire: oxygen, heat, and fuel. There are at least four ways to help prevent fires. These include following the rules for smoking, checking for frayed electrical cords and malfunctioning equipment, careful handling of flammable liquids, and following proper oxygen procedures.

Know the disaster plan of your agency or facility. Move patients to safety if they are in danger. Know where to find the fire extinguishers and which exits to use. Do not use an elevator. Be calm. Do not panic!

UNIT 4   Principles of Body Mechanics

Steps to success

1. Read this unit.
2. Complete Worksheet 1 in the Student Workbook.
3. When you are confident that you can meet each objective for this unit, ask your instructor for the unit evaluation.

Rationale

As a health care worker, you lift, move, and carry many different objects and patients. It is important to use your body correctly to prevent both fatigue and injury. If you injure yourself, you then become ineffective in your job.

Objectives

When you have completed this unit, you will be able to do the following:

✓ Define vocabulary words.
✓ Define *body mechanics*.

✓ List six rules of correct body mechanics.

✓ List six principles of body mechanics.

✓ Demonstrate correct lifting and moving of objects.

■ BODY MECHANICS

Health care workers move, lift, and carry all types of equipment and supplies. They also help position or move patients. When you use proper body mechanics, you save energy, prevent muscle strain, and increase your **efficiency.** Body mechanics is the coordination of body alignment, balance, and movement. When you use your body and your muscles properly, you are practicing good body mechanics.

efficiency Ability to accomplish a job with the least possible difficulty.

Principles of Body Mechanics

1. Stoop. Do not bend.

   • Stand close to the object. • Create a base of support by placing your feet wide apart. • Place one foot slightly forward. • Bend at your hips and knees with your back straight, lower your body, and bring your hands down to the object. • Use the large muscles in your legs to return to a standing position.

2. Lift firmly and smoothly after you size up the load.

   • If you cannot easily pull the object to you (i.e., the load is too heavy), *get help!* • Grasp the load firmly. • Lift by using the large muscles of your legs (see Figure 13–5). • Keep the load close to your body. • Do not twist your body (see Figure 13–6). • To change direction, shift your feet in the direction you want to go.

FIGURE 13–5. Use large muscles of legs when lifting, and keep your back straight.

FIGURE 13–6. Do not twist your body when lifting—turn it.

gravity Natural force or pull toward the earth. In the body, the center of gravity is usually the center of the body.

crouch To stoop, using the large muscles of the legs to help maintain balance.

3. Always use the center of **gravity** when carrying a load.

• Keep your back as straight as possible. • Keep the weight of the load close to the body and centered over your hips. • Put the load down by bending at the hips and knees. Keep your back straight and the load close to your body. • If the load is too heavy, *get help!* • When two or more people carry the load, assign one person as the leader so that he or she can give commands.

4. Pulling: Push or pull rather than lift the load.

• Place your feet apart with one foot slightly forward. Keep close to the object you are moving. • Grasp the object firmly, close to its center of gravity. • **Crouch;** lean away from the object. • Pull by straightening your legs. Keep your back straight. • Walk backwards. Your leg muscles should do all the work.

5. Pushing: Push or pull rather than lift the load.

• Stand close to the object to be moved. • Crouch down with your feet apart. • Bend your elbows and put your hands on the load at chest level. • Lean forward with your chest and shoulders near the object. • Keep your back straight. • Push with your legs.

6. Reaching: Carefully evaluate the distance.

• Always use a stool or a ladder to reach objects that are too high. • Stand close to the object. • If you are standing on the floor, place your feet wide apart, one foot slightly forward. • Maintain good body alignment. Move close to the object. Do not reach to the point of straining. • When reaching for an object that is above your head, grip it with your palms up, and lower it. Keep it close to your body on the way down.

■ SUMMARY

In this unit, you learned that by following basic principles, you prevent fatigue and injury.

There are six important rules to remember when following the basic principles of body mechanics.

Six Rules to Remember

■ Keep your back straight.

■ Bend at the hips and knees.

■ Keep feet approximately 6 to 8 inches apart to provide a wide base of support.

■ Use the strongest muscles of your legs.

■ Do not twist your body.

■ Use the weight of your body to help push or pull.

When you learn to lift and move correctly, you protect yourself and others from injury.

UNIT 5 First Aid

S teps to success

1. Read this unit.
2. Complete Worksheet 1 in the Student Workbook.
3. Complete Worksheets 2 through 8 as assigned.
4. Practice and demonstrate all procedures.
5. When you are confident that you can meet each objective for this unit, ask your instructor for the unit evaluation.
6. Complete "Your Link to Success" at the end of this chapter.

Rationale

In or out of the clinical setting, the health care worker is expected to respond quickly and effectively when there is a sudden illness or injury. As a health care worker you are responsible for seeking information and becoming competent in first-aid skills. This knowledge enables you to be a well-prepared and effective health care worker.

Objectives

When you have completed this unit, you will be able to do the following:

✓ Match vocabulary words with their correct meanings.

✓ Demonstrate the procedures for:

• Mouth-to-mouth breathing

- Obstructed airway
- Serious wounds
- Preventing shock
- **Splints**
- Slings
- Bandaging

splints Firm object used to support an unstable body part.

■ INTRODUCTION TO FIRST AID

This unit is an overview of commonly used first-aid techniques. The authors of this book strongly advise that everyone attend a basic first-aid class and a heart saver or **cardiopulmonary** resuscitation (CPR) class in order to become proficient. These classes are given by the American Red Cross and the American Heart Association. Appropriate first aid can save a life and prevent a permanent disability. Most situations requiring first aid need prompt, **definitive** action. To gain understanding and a high skill level, you need supervised practice for each of the procedures listed.

First aid is the emergency care given to a victim of an accident or a sudden illness. This treatment is required immediately and continues as needed until advanced medical care is available.

cardiopulmonary Having to do with the heart and lungs.

definitive Clear, without question, exacting (e.g., when giving emergency care, each treatment should be done in a definitive manner).

■ GENERAL PRINCIPLES OF FIRST AID

1. Never panic; always remain calm. Unfortunately, this statement is easier said than done. Here are some basic rules that help you remain calm:

   • Take a few slow, deep breaths. • Survey the surrounding area and ensure that it is safe before approaching. • Determine what resources are available and what is needed.

2. Evaluate the situation by

   • Checking the victim's level of consciousness • Opening the victim's airway • Checking for breathing • Checking circulation, including pulse and bleeding

3. Determine if the victim is in a safe environment, free from danger.

4. Determine **priorities** of treatment (i.e., decide which condition requires the most immediate care).

   • Urgent care is required in life-threatening situations, such as stopped breathing, heart attack, shock, serious wounds, poisoning, burns. • A victim may need first aid, but the situation may not be life threatening. Non-life-threatening conditions include **fracture** of an arm or leg and a minor **contusion** or **laceration.**

5. Decide how to provide the care that is needed.

6. Call or send for help as soon as possible.

priorities Those things that are most important.

fracture Broken bone.

contusion Condition in which the skin is bruised, swollen, and painful, but is not broken.

laceration Wound or a tear of the skin.

■ LIFE-THREATENING SITUATIONS

The following situations are considered life threatening and require emergency medical care. Most cities have an emergency medical system (EMS) that responds immediately with emergency care providers. The most common number used to alert the EMS system is 911.

*P*rocedure

Rescue Breathing

ALERT: Follow Standard Precautions.

1. **Put on disposable gloves.**
2. **Check for consciousness** by shaking victim's shoulder gently and asking if he or she is OK. If there is no response, activate **EMS** system.
3. **Open airway** by placing one hand at victim's chin and the other hand on victim's forehead; gently lift chin by supporting jawbone with fingertips and lifting upward to open mouth. (Do not put pressure on throat; this may block airway.) This is called the *head tilt/chin lift*.
4. **Check for breathing** by placing your ear near victim's mouth and nose. Turn your head so that you can see his or her chest. **Look** to see if chest is rising or falling. **Listen** for breathing. **Feel** for air from victim's mouth or nose on your cheek. If breathing is *not* present:
5. **Ventilate.** Place a pocket mask over mouth and nose. Put apex (point) over bridge of nose and

base between lip and chin. Give two breaths (1½ to 2 seconds per breath) through the one-way valve. Allow lungs to empty between each breath. (If dentures obstruct the airway, remove them.) If air does *not* inflate lungs: **Retilt head** to ensure an open airway and repeat the two breaths. Watch for chest to rise, allow for exhalation between breaths. (If lungs still do not inflate, treat victim for an obstructed airway; see the Obstructed Airway procedures.)

6. **Check carotid pulse.**
7. If breathing is absent and pulse is present, **keep the airway open** and give one breath to victim every 5 seconds. If there is no pulse, cardiopulmonary resuscitation (CPR) is needed to circulate oxygenated blood through body. To learn CPR, take a course given by a qualified instructor approved by American Heart Association or American Red Cross.

Step 2.

Step 3.

Step 4.

Step 5.

Airway Breathing (or Closed/Obstructed Airway, Stopped or Not Breathing)

Oxygen is necessary for brain cells to live. Permanent brain damage can occur if oxygen is not present for 4 to 6 minutes. You have only a few minutes to save the life of a person who has stopped breathing.

Obstructed Airway

abdominal thrust
Forceful thrust on the abdomen, between the sternum and the navel, in an upward motion toward the head.

Heimlich maneuver
Forceful upward thrust on the abdomen, between the sternum and the navel.

An obstructed airway occurs when an object blocks the airway leading to the lungs. This occurs when a piece of food or other object lodges in the back of the throat or in the windpipe. Early detection of an airway obstruction is important in determining your plan of action. There are two types of obstructions:

■ *Partial obstruction* occurs when some air can be exchanged. There may be *good air exchange* when the victim coughs forcefully or wheezes between coughs. *Do not* interfere with the victim's attempt to cough the object out. If there is *poor air exchange* and the victim

Procedure

Obstructed Airway in a Conscious Victim

ALERT: Follow Standard Precautions.

When signs of choking are present:

1. Ask "Are you choking?" Observe victim for coughing or wheezing. *Do not interfere* if good air exchange is present.
2. Give **abdominal thrust** or perform **Heimlich maneuver.** Stand in back of victim; put your

arms around victim's waist. Make a fist with one hand and put your thumb between breastbone and navel. Take your other hand and grasp fist; pull into victim's abdomen with quick upward thrust. Repeat separate, rapid inward and upward thrusts until airway is cleared or patient becomes unconscious. (Use chest thrusts for a pregnant or obese victim.)

• Becomes weak • Has an ineffective cough • Has a crowing or high-pitched noise during inhalation • Has increased difficulty breathing • Turns bluish around the mouth and fingernails

Treat the victim for complete airway obstruction (conscious victim).

■ *Complete obstruction* occurs when there is no air exchange or there is poor air exchange. The signs of complete obstruction are present when the victim

• Is suddenly unable to breathe, cough, or speak • Clutches neck (see photograph in procedure box on page 280) • Is struggling to breathe

When you observe these signs, follow the procedure for obstructed airway.

Procedure

Obstructed Airway in an Unconscious Victim

ALERT: Follow Standard Precautions.

If the victim becomes unconscious:

1. **Activate the EMS system.**
2. **Put on disposable gloves.**
3. **Open airway.** Place one hand at victim's chin and the other hand on victim's forehead; gently tip head back. Lift chin in head tilt/chin lift position.
4. **Attempt to ventilate.** Open the airway and ventilate through a pocket face mask with a

one-way valve. If no air enters, retilt head and try to ventilate again. If air enters, give two breaths and continue rescue breathing. If air does not inflate lungs, give abdominal thrusts.

5. **Abdominal thrust.** Straddle victim's legs and place heel of your hand between breastbone and navel. Then push quickly and sharply straight upward and inward up to five times.

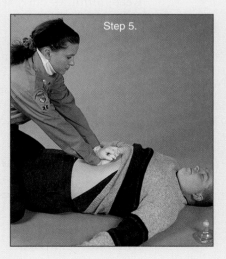

Procedure box continued

6. **Finger sweep.** On an unconscious victim, use the finger sweep to remove objects from the mouth that are, one hopes, loosened during the abdominal thrusts. Use your index finger to sweep from one side of the mouth to the back of the throat and out the other side of the mouth. Be careful not to push the object deeper into the throat.

Step 6.

7. **Attempt to ventilate** using pocket face mask again. If lungs do not inflate, repeat entire procedure. Reposition head and attempt to ventilate again, then do up to five abdominal thrusts; sweep mouth; attempt to breathe for victim again, and repeat until the airway is clear and air enters. Give two breaths and follow steps 6 and 7 of Rescue Breathing.

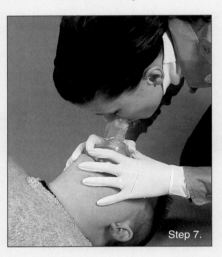

Step 7.

Heart Attack

The first two hours after the onset of a heart attack are the highest-risk period. Recognition of early warning signs alerts you to an impending heart attack. Early warning signs are

■ Squeezing feeling in the chest ("feels like a band around my chest"), pressure, or tightness ("feels like an elephant is sitting on my chest")
■ Persistent discomfort that spreads to shoulders, arms, neck, jaw, or across the chest
■ Sweating, nausea, vomiting, shortness of breath, or feeling faint

When one or all of these signs are present, call for advanced life support systems (doctor or paramedics). If signs continue, the heart and breathing may stop, and CPR will become necessary.

Serious Wounds

spurts To force out in a burst; to squirt.

Serious wounds are life threatening because heavy bleeding is frequently present. Bleeding that pulsates or **spurts** with each heartbeat is from an artery. The victim will bleed to death if the bleeding is not controlled. Venous bleeding is also serious and must be controlled. An open wound allowing a constant flow of blood from a

Procedure

Stopped Breathing in an Infant

ALERT: Follow Standard Precautions.

1. Put on disposable gloves.
2. **Check for consciousness.** Shake baby's shoulders gently and speak baby's name. If no response, shout for help.

3. **Open airway.** Use head tilt/chin lift method. Do not overtilt head or neck.

4. **Check for breathing.** Look, listen, and feel.

If not breathing:

5. Place an infant-sized barrier device on the infant's face.* Ventilate through the one-way valve

and give rescue breathing. Give two slow breaths using only air in your cheeks. (Too much air may overinflate an infant's lungs.) Watch for chest to rise and allow chest to fall or deflate between each breath. If air does not inflate lungs:

6. Retip head to ensure open airway. Repeat the two breaths. If lungs still do not inflate, treat infant for an obstructed airway.

If lungs do inflate:

7. **Keep airway open,** and give one breath to infant every 3 seconds. After 1 minute activate EMS.
8. **Check pulse.** Place three fingers over brachial pulse. The baby's heart may have stopped. In this event, only cardiopulmonary resuscitation (CPR) will help to circulate oxygenated blood throughout the body. CPR can be learned by taking a course offered by an instructor who is certified by the American Heart Association or the American Red Cross. We strongly recommend your involvement in such a program.

*Adult-size pocket face masks can be adapted by inverting (reversing) them. See manufacturer's guidelines.

---

vein can also cause death. The open area is susceptible to infection and needs to be covered.

To stop bleeding and minimize infection, apply direct pressure. Sterile gauze pads/gauze **dressings** are very effective. If gauze dressings are not available, use a piece of clean cloth, a handkerchief, or toweling. Even though the cloth is not sterile, it aids in controlling the bleeding.

dressings Gauze pads that are used to cover a wound.

Procedure

Obstructed Airway in a Conscious Infant

ALERT: Follow Standard Precautions.

1. Put on disposable gloves
2. Observe to determine infant's ability to cry, cough, or breathe. If there is no evidence of air exchange, shout for help.
3. Give five back blows. Place infant face down, supporting head and neck and tilting infant so that the head is lower than rest of body. Give five firm hits with heel of your hand over backbone and between shoulder blades.

4. Give five chest thrusts by turning infant on its back with head lower than rest of body. Using two to three fingers, push five times on midsternum, which is about one finger's width below nipple line at midchest.

5. Continue procedure until obstruction is clear or infant becomes unconscious.

Procedure

Obstructed Airway in an Unconscious Infant

ALERT: Follow Standard Precautions.

Follow steps 1 to 4 above, then . . .

5. If second rescuer is available, instruct him or her to activate EMS system.
6. **Attempt to see the obstruction.** Open infant's mouth. Place your thumb over infant's tongue, and lift jaw by grasping jawbone with your fingers. If object *is* visible, use your little finger to hook it and sweep it from the mouth; then attempt to ventilate. If object is *not* visible:

7. Try to ventilate as described on page 283. If lungs do not inflate, reposition head and try to ventilate again.

8. If air still does not enter, repeat from step 6.

Procedure box continued

9. Repeat five back blows; then

10. Repeat five chest thrusts.

11. Open mouth to attempt to see object. Sweep mouth if object is visible. If not visible:

12. Continue procedure until obstruction is expelled. If the obstruction is not relieved after 1 minute, activate EMS system.

13. Once the airway is clear, ventilate once every 3 seconds.

NOTE Carry disposable gloves. Always wear them when contacting body fluids and follow standard precautions.

How to Treat Serious Wounds

1. Follow the procedure for *preventing shock* (page 287).

2. Apply *direct pressure* over the wound.

3. *Elevate* the wounded area if you do not think there are broken bones (see Figure 13–7).

If direct pressure does not control bleeding:

1. Apply pressure to the appropriate *pressure point* above the wound (see Figure 13–8).

FIGURE 13–7.
Combine elevation and direct pressure to treat serious wounds.

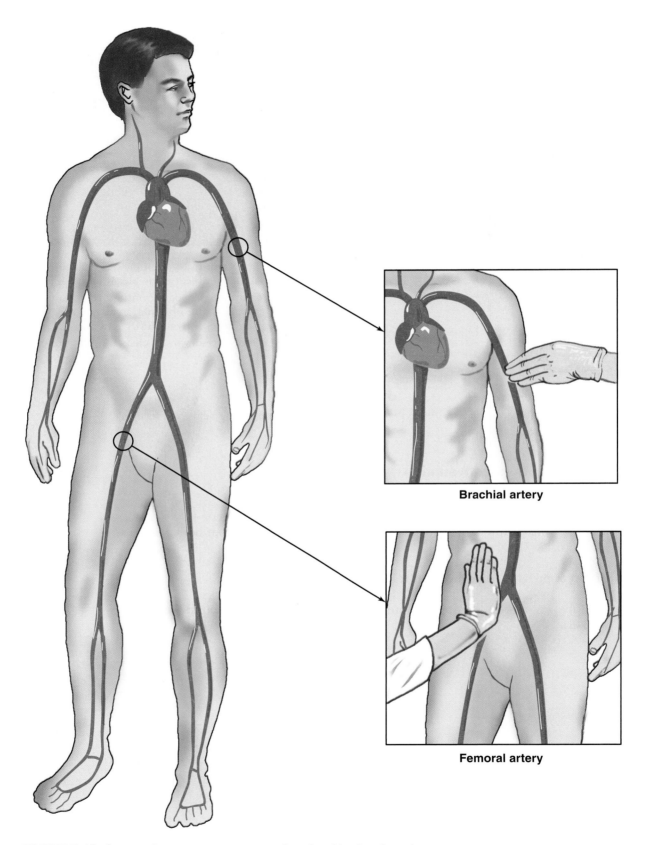

Brachial artery

Femoral artery

FIGURE 13–8. Use of pressure points to control profuse bleeding from the upper extremity, lower extremity, and neck.

2. Continue to apply direct pressure to the wound. Do not remove bandages when they are **saturated.** Apply dry dressings over the saturated bandage.

3. *When bleeding is under control,* gradually release pressure at the pressure point. Keep applying direct pressure to the wound.

4. *Call or send for help* as soon as possible.

saturated Soaked; filled to capacity.

Shock

Shock is life threatening. Shock is usually caused by major body fluid or blood loss. If it is due to major blood loss, body cells and organs are deprived of oxygen, which is carried by the blood. Shock slows body functions and keeps the major organs from functioning normally. Anyone with a serious injury should seek advanced medical care immediately. A victim can be treated appropriately for an injury yet die from shock because of the fluid or blood and oxygen loss. Treat every victim for a life-threatening injury until it is under control; then follow the procedure to prevent shock.

Procedure

Preventing Shock

ALERT: Follow Standard Precautions.

1. Put on disposable gloves.
2. Provide *comfort* and *quiet.*
3. Keep victim *calm.*
4. Keep victim *lying down* on back if possible. *Elevate feet and arms.* Do not elevate an unsplinted arm or leg that is fractured.
5. If victim is vomiting, bleeding from mouth, or feels like vomiting, position victim on side.

6. If person has a *head injury, neck injury,* or *breathing problem,* feet should *not* be elevated.
7. Maintain *normal body temperature* by covering with blanket.
8. Provide oxygen as soon as possible if you have the training and equipment to do so; otherwise, call immediately for someone who does.

Poisoning

Poisoning often causes sudden collapse, vomiting, and difficult breathing. If these symptoms are present, the victim may have taken poison. Poisoning can occur in various ways—for example, **ingestion,** breathing in a poisonous substance, absorption through the skin or by injection, insect or animal bites, or a sting puncturing the skin. Look for items near the victim that may be the source of poisoning, such as an empty container or a needle. Follow the procedure for a *conscious* victim:

ingestion By mouth.

Procedure

Treating a Conscious Poison Victim

ALERT: Follow Standard Precautions.

1. Put on disposable gloves.
2. Give victim water or milk to dilute the poison.
3. Try to locate poison container (try to identify source of poisoning); **do not waste time.**
4. Call 911 to get an ambulance* as soon as possible; then call the nearest poison center, hospital, or physician. (Directions on poison containers and for ingested substances are *not* always correct.) When you call, state that you have a poisoning emergency. If you have the container, be prepared to read ingredients.
5. Be alert for breathing problems. If breathing stops, you will perform mouth-to-mask (rescue breathing) resuscitation as discussed at beginning of unit.
6. Follow procedure for preventing shock.

*Ambulance personnel can communicate directly with the hospital and the poison control center. They can start lifesaving procedures with special equipment and poison treatment medications.

An *unconscious victim* who is suffering from poisoning may be convulsing and vomiting. Follow the procedure for an unconscious poison victim.

Procedure

Treating an Unconscious Poison Victim

ALERT: Follow Standard Precautions.

1. Put on disposable gloves.
2. Do *not* give any fluids.
3. Position victim on his or her side in a safe place.
4. Try to identify the poison source; **do not waste time.**
5. Call 911 to get an ambulance* as soon as possible; then call the nearest poison center, hospital, or physician.
6. Be alert for breathing problems.
7. Follow procedure for preventing shock.

*Ambulance personnel can communicate directly with the hospital and the poison control center. They can start lifesaving procedures with special equipment and poison treatment medications.

Burns

The seriousness of a burn is determined by the degree or depth of the burn (see Figure 13–9):

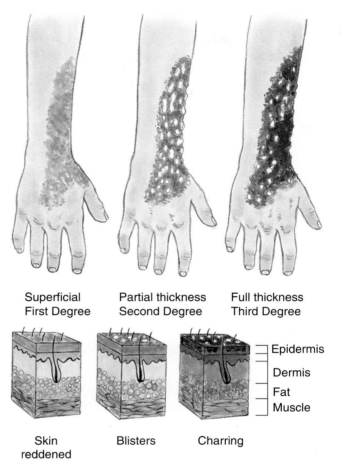

FIGURE 13–9.
Severity of burns.

Superficial
First Degree

Partial thickness
Second Degree

Full thickness
Third Degree

Epidermis
Dermis
Fat
Muscle

Skin
reddened

Blisters

Charring

■ Superficial or *first-degree burns* are surface burns.

■ Partial thickness or *second-degree burns* are deeper or just below the surface, and blistering occurs.

■ Full thickness or *third-degree burns* are even deeper, destroying both surface and underlying tissue.

Burns around the mouth or nose may indicate that the airway is burned. This can cause swelling that may obstruct the airway. If breathing stops, follow the procedure for rescue breathing as discussed at the beginning of this unit. Blistering and swelling may not appear until later. A full thickness burn destroys nerve endings, so a burn victim may not feel pain in that area, but surrounding areas may be painful. The absence of pain *does not* indicate a mild burn. Do the following for a burn victim:

■ Relieve pain
■ Minimize the chance of infection
■ Prevent shock (page 287)

Procedure

Treating Burns

ALERT: Follow Standard Precautions.

First-Degree Burn

1. Put on disposable gloves.
2. Apply cool water to burn area, or submerge burn site in cool water; this will reduce pain.
3. Large surface burns may be dried with sterile dressing. Apply a cold pack over dressing to reduce discomfort. Partial thickness or deeper burns (full thickness) require the following procedure.

Second- and Third-Degree Burns

1. Put on disposable gloves.
2. Stop the burning process by smothering or dousing with water and removing smoldering or hot clothing.
3. Cover burned area with dry sterile dressing. Do not pull away clothing that is stuck to burn site.
4. Place a dry cold pack over dressing if not too heavy.
5. Follow procedure to prevent shock.
6. Call or send for advanced medical assistance as soon as possible.

■ NON-LIFE-THREATENING SITUATIONS

The bone fractures described below are examples of non-life-threatening conditions. Such conditions require first aid or medical care but not urgent care.

Bone Fractures

There are two main types of fractures: closed and open.

■ A *closed fracture* is difficult to determine. The following are signs and symptoms of closed fractures to look for:

• Swelling • Pain • Change in the color of the skin • Deformity

■ An *open fracture* is present when the skin over the fracture site is broken or open and/or the broken bone protrudes through the skin.

Call or send for advanced medical help if you believe a fracture is present. If medical help is not available or the victim must be taken to a medical facility, splint the fracture (see Figure 13–10).

A fracture of the arm usually requires a sling. Apply a triangle sling so that the victim's hand and forearm are slightly higher than the elbow. This helps to minimize the swelling. A sling is a triangular bandage used to support the arm. Once the patient's arm is placed in a sling, a **swathe** can be used to hold the patient's arm against the side of the chest. Commercial slings are available. Roller bandage can be used to form a sling and swathe. Velcro straps can be used to form a swathe. Use whatever materials you have on hand, provided that they will not cut into the patient. Remember: Shirts, ties, and wide belts can be used to make both sling and swathe.

swathe Bandage.

FIGURE 13–10. Long-board splinting for a fractured hip or for any bone in the leg.

Procedure

Applying a Splint

ALERT: Follow Standard Precautions.

1. Put on disposable gloves.
2. Move fractured area as little as possible.

3. Splint area with a firm object, such as newspapers, magazines folded flat, wood, or a commercially made splint.
4. Secure splint in place using roller gauze, wrapping it snugly and overlapping about two-thirds each wrap, or secure splint to extremity with strips of cloth. You can wrap over the fracture site.
5. If it is an open fracture, apply dressing over wound and secure in place with tape or with roller gauze that holds splint in place.

Procedure

Applying a Triangular Sling

ALERT: Follow Standard Precautions.

1. Put on disposable gloves.
2. Make a sling from a piece of cloth, clothing, towel, or sheet; fold or cut this material into shape of a triangle. The ideal sling is about 50 to 60 inches long at its base and 36 to 40 inches long on each side.
3. Position triangular material over top of client's chest opposite the injured arm, as shown in Figure A. Fold patient's arm across chest. If patient cannot hold his or her own arm, have someone assist you, or provide support for client's arm until you are ready to tie sling. Note that one point of triangle should extend beyond patient's elbow on injured side.
4. Take bottom point of triangle and bring this end up over client's arm. When you are finished, this bottom point should be taken over top of patient's shoulder on the side of injured arm. (See Figure B.)

5. Draw up on ends of sling so that patient's hand is about 4 inches above elbow. Tie the two ends of the sling together, making sure that the knot does not press against back of client's neck. Leave patient's fingertips exposed so that you can see any color changes that indicate lack of circulation. Check for radial pulse. If pulse has been lost, take off sling and attempt to reposition arm to regain pulse, then repeat procedure.
6. Take point of material at patient's elbow and fold it forward. Pin it to front of sling. This forms a pocket for client's elbow. If you do not have pin, twist excess material and tie knot in point. This will provide a shallow pocket for patient's elbow. (See Figure C.)
7. Create a swathe by folding a triangular bandage in half and then folding it to a 4″ width. This swathe is tied around chest and injured arm, over sling. Do not place this swathe over patient's arm on uninjured side. (See Figure D.)

A

B

C

D

■ DRESSINGS AND BANDAGES

Dressings prevent infectious bacteria from entering a wound. Dressings also aid when direct pressure is necessary to control bleeding. There are many types of dressings used for various body locations. Bandages hold dressings in place.

Principles of Bandaging

■ Always wear disposable gloves and follow Standard Precautions.

■ Never tie a bandage around the neck; taping a bandage to the neck is safer. Anything that encircles the neck could strangle the victim.

■ The bandage needs to be snug enough to hold the dressing in place but not tight enough to stop the circulation.

■ Leave fingers and toes exposed so that you can watch for discoloration of the skin or swelling.

■ Check the skin temperature. Cold skin may indicate poor circulation. Check the bandage to be certain it is not too tight.

■ Loosen bandages if the patient complains of numbness or a tingling feeling.

■ Do not remove a dressing once it has been applied. If blood soaks through, add another layer of dressings and secure with a bandage.

Procedure

Triangular Bandaging of a Head Wound

ALERT: Follow Standard Precautions.

1. Put on disposable gloves.
2. Fold triangular bandage to make 2-inch hem along base.
3. Apply gauze pad over wound. With folded edge face out, position bandage on client's forehead, just above eyes. Make certain that point of bandage hangs down behind patient's head.

4. Draw ends of bandage behind patient's head and tie them.
5. Next, pull ends to front of client's head and tie them together.
6. Tuck in the tail at back.

Procedure

Circular Bandaging of a Small Leg or Arm Wound

ALERT: Follow Standard Precautions.

1. Put on disposable gloves.
2. Apply dressing to wound and elevate extremity.
3. Place end of gauze roll (1 to 2 inches wide) on dressing. Anchor end of gauze roll over dressing with two initial wraps. Continue to wrap from distal (far) end of extremity to proximal (near the torso) end until entire dressing is covered. Bandage will overlap dressing on both sides. Pull bandage snug as you wrap. Overlap each wrap by about two-thirds. Cut gauze and tape end or tie gauze to secure in place.

Procedure

Spiral Bandaging of a Large Wound

ALERT: Follow Standard Precautions.

1. Put on disposable gloves.
2. Apply dressing to wound.
3. Place end of gauze roll (3 to 6 inches wide) on lower edge of dressing.
4. Anchor end. (Place end of gauze over the dressing. Wrap gauze around the area once. Fold angled corner of gauze back over wrapped gauze.)
5. Wrap gauze around arm or leg at an angle and overlap the edges.
6. If you use up the gauze, continue the wrap with another roll.
7. Secure end by taping or tying off.

Procedure

Bandaging of an Ankle or Foot Wound

ALERT: Follow Standard Precautions.

1. Put on disposable gloves.
2. Apply dressing to wound.
3. Place end of gauze roll (1 to 2 inches wide) on top of foot just above toes, and anchor ends.
4. On second wrap around foot, bring gauze around back of ankle and over top of foot. Bring gauze under foot and over top of foot again. Wrap around ankle and over top of foot, then under foot. Continue these steps until dressing is covered, and secure gauze by tying off or taping.

■ SUMMARY

In this unit, you learned very basic first-aid skills. You have been introduced to the general principles of handling both life-threatening and non-life-threatening situations. You have learned about rescue breathing, obstructed airway, and heart attack. We have discussed the treatment for shock, poisoning, serious wounds, and burns. It is very important for you to become proficient in first aid. To do this, you should attend a class given by a qualified American Red Cross instructor.

Thinking Critically: Check Your Understanding

1. **Communication** During an emergency it is important to communicate the urgency and severity of the situation without causing panic. Imagine that you just received a bomb threat over the telephone. Write an explanation of each step you would take following the call. Clearly indicate how you would prevent patients and co-workers from panicking.

2. **Legal and Ethical** When you stop to help those involved in an accident, do the laws of your state protect you against legal action if something goes wrong? What is the law called? Give an example of a recent case in which the law protected a rescuer or did not protect a rescuer.

3. **Patient Education** Identify ways people are educated about safety precautions—related to hazardous material, radiation, exits, and so on—in a medical facility. Give some examples of the training provided.

4. **Case Study** The facility you work in is being evacuated for the bomb threat described in point 1. When the fire department arrives, they find a patient who was not evacuated from an examination room. The patient panics, starts screaming, and then faints. Later, in the parking lot, the patient complains of chest pain and is transferred to the hospital. A week later, it is determined that the patient suffered a heart attack during the evacuation episode. The patient and family are threatening to sue your employer.

   Can you justify leaving the patient in a room during the evacuation? Can you predict the outcome of the lawsuit?

Portfolio Connection

Reading product labels correctly is a key component of many of our daily projects. We need to know if products will do what we want them to do. We need to know if there is a risk in using a product. In this chapter, we discussed MSDS sheets. You learned that MSDS sheets provide all the primary information needed for any product in the work environment. If you become a home health aide, you work in clients' homes. There will not be an MSDS book to refer to. You will have to read the labels on products for the information you need. Choose three household products from home—for example, toothpaste, a cleaning product, White-Out, a synthetic food product—and create your own MSDS sheet for each of these three products. Use the following headings in your forms.

1. Product Identification
2. Hazardous Ingredients of Mixture
3. Physical Data
4. Fire and Explosion
5. Reactivity Data
6. Health Hazard Data
7. Emergency and First-Aid Procedures
8. Spill or Leak Procedures
9. Protection Information/Control Measures
10. Special Precautions

Completion of this assignment for your portfolio shows your ability to assimilate information and transfer your knowledge into a usable format for your daily use. When you appropriately apply each step of your learning, you show others that you are capable of taking responsibility in a work environment. Place these three forms in the section of your portfolio labeled "Written Reports and Assignments."

EMPLOYABILITY AND LEADERSHIP

14

Steps to success

1. Read this unit.
2. Complete Worksheets 1 through 6 in the Student Workbook as assigned.
3. Ask your instructor to review and comment about your completed portfolio.
4. When you are confident that you can meet each objective for this unit, ask your instructor for the unit evaluation.

Rationale

Before you apply the skills you have learned, you must find a job and be hired as an employee. It is important to learn the skills needed to find a job and to keep a job. This enables you to practice the health care career that you worked so hard to learn.

Objectives

When you have completed this unit, you will be able to do the following:

✓ List seven places to seek employment opportunities and explain the benefits of each.
✓ Explain four ways to contact an employer.
✓ Name three occasions when a cover letter is used.
✓ List eight items required on a résumé.
✓ Identify seven items generally requested on a job application form.
✓ Write a cover letter and a résumé.

✓ Complete a job application.

✓ List five do's and five don'ts of job interviewing.

■ FINDING A JOB

Looking for and finding a job takes planning and requires use of many skills. In this chapter, you learn the steps to follow when you are ready to find a job. These skills give you the tools to be successful in job seeking and save you a lot of time.

■ YOUR VOCATIONAL PORTFOLIO

As time approaches to begin your search for a job, review your portfolio notebook. Obtain a new cover and section dividers so your finished portfolio has a clean, crisp look. Identify the items that best reflect your knowledge level, skills, and personality. When you complete your résumé and other portfolio requirements place them in the appropriate section of your new portfolio.

■ PLACES TO SEEK EMPLOYMENT

■ *Newspaper ads.*   Jobs in health care careers appear in newspaper ads. When you look for a job in the newspaper, turn to the classified ads and look under "Help Wanted." There are different ways of listing jobs. Some papers list all health care positions under "Medical." Others list them under a particular job. See Figure 14–1 for some examples of ads from several newspapers. You also need to become familiar with some of the abbreviations used by newspapers.

Common Abbreviations

appl.	applicant	immed.	immediately
asst.	assistant	incl.	included
cert.	certified	lic.	licensed
exp.	experience	N.A.	nurse aide
FT	full time	PT	part time

FIGURE 14–1. Examples of newspaper advertisements for health care jobs.

■ *Directly to the employer.*   If you are looking for a position in a laboratory, you might apply directly to a medical laboratory. If you want to work in a hospital, you go to the **personnel** department. The Yellow Pages of your phone book offer an excellent resource of possible employers.

■ *Friends and relatives.*   You may know of someone working in the health care field who can suggest a place to apply or who can introduce you to a possible employer.

■ *School counselors.*   Many schools have career counselors and/or work experience counselors. They are a good resource for the types of jobs available in your community.

■ *School bulletin boards.*   If you have a career center or a bulletin board where jobs are listed, be sure to check it daily.

■ *Employment agencies.*   There are both public and private employment agencies. Employers call these agencies to list the job openings that they have. A public agency does not charge a fee; however, a private agency charges either the employer or the person seeking a position. The Yellow Pages list employment agencies, and some of them specialize in health care careers. The public agencies are listed in the white pages under "Government Agencies."

■ *Internet.*   If you have access to a computer that is connected to the Internet, go to Search and type in the words *"job search"* or *"job link."*

personnel People who work in an establishment; a personnel office is where a worker goes to apply for a job.

■ WAYS TO CONTACT AN EMPLOYER

Now that you know where to look for a job, you need to know how to make the contact and how to present yourself.

Telephone

If you have a lead on a possible job, you may choose to call for an appointment. Give your name and the job you are interested in and ask when you may come in to apply.

Cover Letter

You may be asked to send a letter in order to apply for a particular position. You need a cover letter when

■ You are applying for a job that is out of town.
■ You are answering a newspaper advertisement.
■ A potential employer requests a letter.

Your cover letter is a sales letter. You want to sell yourself to the employer in order to get an interview. (A sample cover letter is shown in Figure 14–2.) Your letter should

■ Be neat
■ Have all the words spelled correctly
■ State where you heard about the job opening
■ State what you are applying for and why you are qualified for this specific position
■ Give a brief overview of your education, experience, and qualifications
■ Refer to your portfolio with work samples, skills checkoff lists, and evaluations
■ Request an interview
■ Give your address and phone number

FIGURE 14–2.
Sample cover letter to potential employer.

888 Whitegate Avenue
Los Angeles, CA 90820

January 25, 1999

Mr. E. B. Burns
Director of Nurses
St. Joseph's Hospital
P.O. Box 123
Los Angeles, CA 90880

Dear Mr. Burns:

I am responding to your advertisement in <u>Nurses World</u> on January 14, 1999. I am interested in applying for the position of nurse assistant. I graduated from Medical Technologies High School on December 15, 1998. I studied nursing assisting and am well qualified for this position. My course work included communication, CPR, and a core of courses that prepared me to be employed as a nursing assistant. I also worked in a hospital setting eight hours a week for sixteen weeks. My attendance is excellent, and I am very reliable. My goal is to use my skills as a nursing assistant and to be an exemplary employee.

My résumé is enclosed. Also included is a list of skills I have mastered. I know that I am well qualified for this position. I am looking forward to an opportunity to interview for this position. I will call on Monday, February 3, at 9:00 a.m. and hope to arrange an interview at that time.

If you require additional information, or want to contact me, please call me at (123) 456-7890 after 3:00 p.m.

Sincerely,

Mark Adams, CNA

Résumé

In addition to your cover letter, it is helpful for a potential employer to have more details about you and your qualifications. This is accomplished by preparing a résumé. (See the example in Figure 14–3.) A résumé includes the following:

- Your name, address, phone number, and message number
- Career plans
- Details about your education
- Your past work experience—paid or unpaid
- What honors you have earned
- What activities you like
- Skills, strengths, and abilities
- References (always ask permission to use someone as a reference)

800 N. Euclid
New York, New York 00333

Home: 220-666-8340
Message: 220-620-9180

Mary Jane Rodgers

Career Plans	Complete 2 year Associate of Science Nursing Program
	Short-range: Nursing assistant
	Long-range: Complete a Bachelor of Science Program as a registered nurse

Experience

1998-present   Henry's Hamburger Shop   New York, NY
Sales Clerk

- Food preparation
- Counting inventory
- Customer service
- Operating a cash register and making change
- Maintaining health standards

1994-1998   June Allison   New York, NY
Baby Sitter

- Meal preparation
- Overnight care of two children, 8 and 10 years of age
- Planning recreation

Family Responsibilities

- Prepare dinner 2-3 times a week
- Weekly gardening
- Perform minor household tasks

Experience

Diploma candidate 1999   Hoover High School   New York, NY

Interests

Dancing, classical music, reading, skiing, member of Explorer Scouts Medical Post and Health Occupation Students of America

Skills and Strengths

Fluent in oral and written Spanish communication

Proficient in Windows programs including Word, Word Perfect, Excel, and Lotus applications

FIGURE 14–3. Sample résumé.

Job Application

Most employers require that you fill out an application. When you fill out a job application, you give the employer needed information and also have an opportunity to demonstrate that you are neat and well organized. Use the information in your vocational portfolio to fill out an application. Included should be

- Your complete address with the zip code.
- Your Social Security number.
- Your phone number or a number where you can be reached.
- A list of the schools you have attended, with dates.
- A list of any special training that you have.
- A prepared list of any past jobs, the address of the employer, the dates you worked there, and what your duties were.
- A list of people who can give you a reference. Be certain that you have their addresses and phone numbers. Also be certain that you have asked permission to use them as a reference.

There are also other ways that you can prepare. Be sure that you

- Carry a pen—do not use a pencil.
- Read the application all the way through.
- Print unless you are told to write.
- Spell accurately.
- Answer every question. Put "NA" (not applicable) in the space to show that you did not overlook the question.
- Recheck for errors.

■ INTERVIEW

The interviewer wants to be sure that you are the best fit for the job. She is assessing your skills from the time she receives your résumé. Her focus during the interview is to determine if your explanations and behaviors match the job requirements. This evaluation occurs throughout the interview process, even when conversation is about the weather or hobbies. It is important to make a good first impression. The following guidelines tell you what to do and what not to do during an interview.

Interview Guidelines

Follow these guidelines for a positive interview experience.

- Be well groomed.
- Dress neatly and appropriately (no jeans).
- Be on time.
- Greet the interviewer by name, and smile.
- Shake hands firmly.
- Stand until asked to sit.
- Answer questions truthfully and sincerely.
- Be enthusiastic.
- Do not chew gum.
- Do not criticize former employers or teachers.

- Look at the interviewer when you talk.
- Do not talk about personal problems.
- When the interview is over, thank the interviewer and leave quickly.

Interview Preparation

The interviewer expects you to answer a variety of questions pertinent to the job you are applying for. Be prepared to give at least three examples of your behavior in various situations. Each experience should describe the

- *Situation.* What exactly happened?
- *Behavior.* What did you do?
- *Outcome.* What were the results?

Read the following questions and determine how to answer them.

- Tell me about the most difficult decision you made at school or work in the last few months.
- Tell me how you get along with people at school or work.
- Tell me about the most difficult job or school task you've done. Why was it difficult? How did you get past the difficulties?
- Explain a recent situation that demonstrates your ability to be a team player.
- Describe a situation in which you had to work under pressure. What kind of pressure were you facing? How did you handle the situation? What was the outcome?
- Describe a situation where you had to be very flexible. How did your actions demonstrate your flexibility?

After the Interview

The interviewer will do a reference check to verify that your résumé and application are honest and correct. She will also rate your responses to help her make a decision about which candidate is best for the job. The following is an example of an interview rating form.

	Excellent	**Average**	**Not Acceptable**
Appearance			
Manner			
Qualifications			
Experience			
Job fit			

After the interview, send a letter of thanks to the interviewer. (See the example in Figure 14–4.) This lets the interviewer know that you are interested in the position, and it may increase your chance of getting the job.

Finding a job and then getting a job takes effort on your part. Careful planning is the key to your success, and you will be glad that you took time to prepare yourself.

FIGURE 14–4.
Sample thank-you
letter to interviewer.

888 Whitegate Avenue
Los Angeles, CA 90820

February 10, 1999

Mr. E. B. Burns
Director of Nurses
St. Joseph's Hospital
P.O. Box 123
Los Angeles, CA 90880

Dear Mr. Burns:

Thank you for interviewing me yesterday afternoon. The position interests me very much, and I know that I will do a good job for you. I hope that you will give me an opportunity to work for the nursing department at St. Joseph's.

Sincerely,

Mark Adams, CNA

■ SUMMARY

Finding a job requires effort on your part. When you decide to look for a job, check the newspaper; go to a personnel department; ask friends, relatives, and your school counselor if they know of an opening; check employment agencies and bulletin boards; and search the Internet. After finding a possible opening, contact the employer. Call for an appointment, or send a cover letter with your résumé. You will also have to fill out a job application.

The last step is your interview with the employer. There are some important rules to follow when you go to an interview. After your interview, send a thank-you note to the interviewer.

UNIT 2   Keeping a Job

Steps to success

1. Complete Vocabulary Worksheet 1 in the Student Workbook.
2. Read this unit.
3. Complete Worksheet 2 as assigned.
4. When you are confident that you can meet each objective for this unit, ask your instructor for the unit evaluation.

Rationale

You spend a lot of time and effort learning the skills for a career in health care. You also spend a lot of time and effort finding a job and then getting the job. Now that you have the job, you want to keep it. Employers have very specific things that they are looking for in an employee. The information in this unit tells what these things are and how you can be a good employee.

Objectives

When you have completed this unit, you will be able to do the following:

✓ Define vocabulary words.
✓ List four employer responsibilities.
✓ List four responsibilities of a good employee.

■ RESPONSIBILITIES

The Good Employer

An employer has responsibilities to you, and you have responsibilities to the employer. The good employer demonstrates

■ *Dignity,* by respecting each employee as an important member of the health care team. Providing a safe, clean working environment is an example of treating employees and patients with dignity.

■ *Excellence,* by encouraging personal and professional development, accountability, teamwork, and a commitment to quality health care. Employers who support routine activities and provide the necessary materials that allow you to do the best possible job show a dedication to excellence.

■ *Service,* by establishing standards and guidelines directing appropriate, caring, compassionate health care to those dependent on the health care services. Providing clear guidelines for employees to follow gives the direction necessary to accomplish the job in a caring, compassionate manner.

■ *Fairness and justice,* by establishing employee salaries and benefits that are fair and reliable. An employer who provides a reasonable salary for agreed-upon work and establishes a standard salary and benefit structure for all employees is striving to be a fair, equitable employer.

The Good Employee

As a good employee, you demonstrate

■ *Dignity* through communication and interpersonal effectiveness, by

• Being open, honest, and respectful • Listening actively and seeking understanding • Providing positive, helpful feedback

■ *Excellence* through teamwork and accountability, by

• Creating an environment of continuous improvement • Trying new ways to improve performance, processes, and service • Seeking growth and development opportunities for you and others • Taking responsibility for individual and team actions, decisions, and results • Adapting to changing needs and learning new skills, knowledge, and behaviors

FIGURE 14–5.
Together everyone
accomplishes more.

■ *Service* through being flexible and customer focused, by

• Responding to the needs of those served and showing concern for meeting those needs • Responding quickly and effectively to problems that arise while providing service

■ *Fairness and justice* by

• Using equipment and supplies in an appropriate manner • Treating and responding to all people in the work environment with the same dignity, excellence, and service standards

Teamwork and team building is essential if you and your fellow workers expect to accomplish your goals (see Figure 14–5). When you follow these guidelines, your job gives you a sense of accomplishment. Being able to keep a job until you are ready to leave builds your references for the future. Remember that each job you have becomes an important part of your professional experience, and you want it to be a positive experience.

■ SUMMARY

Once you acquire a job, you and your employer agree to work together to accomplish the job you are hired to do. Your behavior reflects your attitude and values. Continually evaluate your actions using the Dignity, Excellence, Service, and Fairness/Justice criteria as a measure of your progress in the work environment. Be a team player by respecting your co-workers and encouraging them to do the best job they can do.

UNIT 3   Becoming a Professional Leader

Steps to success

1. Read this unit.
2. Complete Worksheets 1 and 2 in the Student Workbook.
3. When you are confident that you can meet each objective for this unit, ask your instructor for the unit evaluation.
4. Complete "Your Link to Success" at the end of this chapter.

Rationale

Student and professional health care organizations enhance the delivery of compassionate, high-quality care by providing knowledge, skill, and leadership development. Committed students and professionals seek opportunities provided by these organizations to keep current and to provide patients with good-quality care.

Objectives

When you have completed this chapter, you will be able to do the following:

✓ Define vocabulary words.
✓ Name the three main benefits of being a member of a student health vocational organization.
✓ Name six benefits of being a member of a professional organization.
✓ Identify ways to find a professional organization.
✓ Identify steps to becoming a leader.
✓ Define HOSA and VICA.
✓ Summarize why you plan to participate in a student and professional organization.

■ MEMBERSHIP IN AN ORGANIZATION

Membership in your student or professional organization gives you an opportunity to gain occupational knowledge and skills. It also provides opportunities to develop leadership skills. Some of the skills that you learn include the following:

- Professional ethics
- Communication and interpersonal relations
- Leadership skills
- Ability to recognize and initiate change
- How to organize activities and people
- Time management
- Establishing priorities

■ Budgeting
■ Fund raising
■ Current health issues

Health Occupations Students of America (HOSA)

Health Occupations Students of America (HOSA) is the student organization for health occupation students (see Figure 14–6). Among HOSA's primary goals are to

■ Promote high standards in ethics, skills, scholarship, and safety
■ **Foster** respect for the dignity of work
■ Provide recognition and **prestige** that will foster physical, mental, and social well-being
■ Develop leadership abilities through various activities
■ Promote involvement in current health care issues

foster To develop; to promote; to stimulate.

prestige Influence obtained through success, wealth, or some other source.

Benefits of Membership

Benefits available to HOSA members include the following:

■ Introduction to various health careers
■ Development of a responsible attitude through service to the community
■ Available guidance that develops knowledge, skills, and characteristics necessary in preparing to be a health care worker
■ Help for students to gain self-confidence through the development of leadership skills
■ Occasional offers of scholarships

Skills Competitions

Membership in HOSA provides an opportunity to travel and compete in skills competition. Competitions are at three levels: The first level is local competition; those who win go on to the second level. The second level is state competition; those who win go on to the third level. The third level is national competition.

Competitive event categories include:

FIGURE 14–6.
Emblem of HOSA.
(Reprinted by permission of Health Occupations Students of America.)

■ Category I: Health occupations related

• Medical math • Medical spelling • Medical terminology • Dental spelling
• Dental terminology

■ Category II: Health occupations skills

• Medical assisting—clerical • Medical assisting—clinical • Dental assisting
• Nursing assisting • Practical/vocational nursing • CPR/first aid

■ Category III: Individual leadership

• **Extemporaneous** speaking • Extemporaneous health display • Extemporaneous writing • Job-seeking skills • Prepared speaking

extemporaneous
Completed with little
preparation.

■ Category IV: Team leadership

• Community awareness • HOSA Bowl

■ Category V: Recognition

• Outstanding HOSA chapter • National recognition program

Competition requirements include the following:

■ Student must be an active HOSA member.
■ Student must be identified as either a secondary student (currently enrolled in
a high school) or a postsecondary student (graduate from high school or over 18
years of age).

Students attending HOSA functions follow a strict code of conduct and official
HOSA uniform and competitive event dress codes. Experiencing the challenges,
structure, and competition in HOSA teaches students how to reach for and achieve
their highest potential.

Vocational Industrial Clubs of America (VICA)

Vocational Industrial Clubs of America (VICA) is the organization serving high
school students and students enrolled in training programs in technical, skilled,
and service occupations, including health occupations (see Figure 14–7). Effective
July 1999, VICA will change its name to SkillsUSA-VICA. The new name reflects
VICA's expanded role in preparing students for the workplace. The information in
the next two sections is excerpted from VICA's fact sheet, which is published at the
following Web address: http:///www.vica.org/facts.html.

FIGURE 14–7.
Emblem of VICA.

Purpose Statement

"VICA prepares America's high performance workers. It provides quality education experiences for students in leadership, teamwork, citizenship and character development. It builds and reinforces self-confidence, work attitudes and communications skills. It emphasizes total quality at work, high ethical standards, superior work skills, life-long education and pride in the dignity of work. VICA also promotes understanding of the free enterprise system and involvement in community service activities."

VICA Programs

"VICA programs include local, state and national competitions in which students demonstrate occupational and leadership skills. . . . VICA programs also help to establish industry standards for job skill training in the classroom.

"*The VICA Total Quality Curriculum* enhances VICA's Quality at Work movement by preparing students for the world of work starting in the classroom. The curriculum emphasizes the competencies and essential workplace basic skills identified by employers and the U.S. Secretary of Labor's Commission on Achieving Necessary Skills (SCANS).

"*The Professional Development Program* is a self-paced curriculum for secondary and college students. It teaches skills such as effective communication and management, teamwork, networking, workplace ethics, job interviewing and more. The curriculum involves local industry and academics and can be used in day-trades, apprenticeship training, cooperative education."

■ PROFESSIONAL ORGANIZATIONS

Professional organizations help professionals keep current in the latest technology and trends. Being aware of the advantages offered through involvement in such organizations motivates health care workers to become active in the professional group for their chosen occupation.

There are numerous professional organizations for the health care worker. Most organizations have a local chapter, state chapter, and national chapter. Each supports the other, and all work toward common goals. Belonging to a professional organization provides the following benefits:

■ Updates on new technological advances
■ Communication with other geographical areas
■ Shared resources
■ Resources for employment opportunities
■ Current legislative issues
■ Interaction with other health professionals
■ Pooled money to accomplish changes for the good of the occupation/ profession
■ Power as a united group to encourage positive change
■ Development of new ideas that support growth

When you classes are complete, find your professional organization by

■ Referring to Chapter 2 of this book
■ Asking fellow employees

■ Reading the bulletin boards at work
■ Reading your professional journals
■ Reading brochures
■ Attending occupationally related inservice programs
■ Checking the *Occupational Outlook Handbook*

■ LEADERSHIP

Becoming a leader in your occupational area takes time and patience. To become a leader you must take several important steps. These include the following:

■ Developing a superior skill level
■ Becoming a decision maker
■ Being a good communicator
■ Developing a balanced focus on tasks and people

Tom Peters, author of *A Passion for Excellence,* says:

"A leader is a . . .	A leader is not a . . .
cheerleader	cop
enthusiast	referee
nurturer	devil's advocate
coach	naysayer
facilitator	pronouncer"

A true leader unites people and works toward positive outcomes.

■ SUMMARY

Participation in HOSA or VICA is an important part of your career development and professionalism. As a member, you are introduced to various health careers, develop a responsible attitude toward your community, develop knowledge and skills for the work world, and gain self-confidence.

Membership prepares you to be a leader in your chosen occupation; it also helps you prepare to become a valuable member of your professional organization when you join the workforce.

To become a leader you must develop superior skill levels, become a decision maker, be a good communicator, and develop a balanced focus on tasks and people.

For more information, write

National HOSA	VICA
6021 Morriss Road	Vocational Industrial Clubs of America
Suite 111	P.O. Box 3000
Flower Mound, TX 75028	Leesburg, VA 20177-0300
(800) 321-4672	(703) 777-8810
FAX (972) 874-0063	FAX (703) 777-8999
Web site: http://www.hosa.org	Web site: http://www.vica.org
e-mail: info@hosa.org	e-mail: anyinfo@vica.org

Thinking Critically: Check Your Understanding

1. **Communication** Preparing for an interview requires time and practice. To prepare adequately for an interview,

■ Write answers to the questions on page 305.
■ Think through how you want to use your tone of voice to emphasize certain points.
■ Practice saying your answers to questions in front of the mirror.
■ Ask another person (a professional who interviews in his or her work setting is best) to ask you these questions and to hear your responses.
■ Ask the questioner to evaluate you and make recommendations.

2. **Computers** Search the Internet for job opportunities.

■ List ways that you can use a computer to apply for a position.
■ List available opportunities in your chosen occupations and within a reasonable vicinity.

3. **Medical Math** Concepts in medical math apply in calculating values pertinent to choosing a job. You make the best job choice when you take all of the benefits of a job into consideration. Some jobs pay less but have excellent benefits. Other jobs pay a high salary and provide only minimum benefits. Calculate the full value of three different jobs by determining the dollar value of health insurance, paid vacation time, stock or retirement benefits, and life insurance benefits. Compare your findings and evaluate which job is best for you.

Portfolio Connection

The cover letter, résumé, and thank-you letter are the primary tools for acquiring a job. There are ways to make your application packet stand out from others. Here are some of them:

■ Prepare each item perfectly so that it presents you as the best possible candidate.
■ Include a job objective at the top of your résumé—use key phrases that indicate your special talents and desires. *Example:* "I am seeking the position of a Clinical Medical Assistant in the ambulatory care setting. I am qualified for this position because it provides an opportunity to use my skills and training as a Clinical Medical Assistant."
■ Add a statement to your cover letter that tells about your values concerning client-centered care and about teamwork. *Example:* "My school and work experience reflects a dedication to excellence through teamwork and responsibly carrying out assignments. My grades demonstrate an ability to focus on learning and to apply the learning in a clinical area.
■ Add a statement to your thank-you letter that indicates your confidence in being capable of doing the job and your interest in the position. *Example:* "I am

confident that my skill level as a Medical Assistant is appropriate for your office and that our common goals to serve patients and families through providing responsible health care will make me an asset to your team."

Rewrite your cover letter, résumé, and thank-you letter samples with these additional elements. Place them in your portfolio behind their tabs. When you complete training in a specific occupation, refer back to these documents and adapt them to focus specifically on the job you are applying for.

15 NURSE ASSISTANT/PATIENT CAREGIVER

Steps to success

1. Complete Vocabulary Worksheet 1 in the Student Workbook.
2. Read this unit.
3. Complete Worksheets 2 and 3 as assigned.
4. When you are confident that you can meet each objective for this unit, ask your instructor for the unit evaluation.

Objectives

When you have completed this unit, you will be able to do the following:

✓ Complete all objectives in Part One of this book.
✓ Match vocabulary words with their correct meanings.
✓ Identify the following:
  • Responsibilities of the nurse assistant
  • Personal care equipment used by residents
  • Four skin conditions requiring special attention
  • Areas on the body where pressure sores usually develop
  • Antipressure aids
  • Occupied bed, closed bed, and open bed
  • Causes and symptoms of **dehydration**
  • Common types of specimens collected for analysis
  • Six common prosthetic devices
✓ List the following:
  • Four types of bathing

dehydration Severe loss of fluid from tissue and cells.

316

- Two body areas requiring special attention during the bathing process
- Four changes in the skin that may indicate the beginning of a pressure sore
- Four techniques for positioning residents
- Seven reasons why **ambulation** is important
- Signs of diabetic coma and **insulin shock**
- Nine steps to preparing a resident for a meal
- Six ways to prevent pressure sores
- Causes and symptoms of edema
- Ways to help residents who have a colostomy, ileostomy, or ureterostomy
- Symptoms that indicate a resident is about to faint, and precautions that prevent injury
- Five conditions that may develop when using **postural supports**
- Five things you must do when using postural supports
- Five rules for oxygen safety.

✓ Explain the following:
- Four important reasons to give mouth care
- Six important reasons for routine bathing
- Nine conditions poor body **alignment** causes
- Why residents with diabetes must have their toenails cut by a podiatrist
- Why a urinary drainage bag is not raised above the level of insertion
- Six causes of incontinence
- Procedures for bowel and/or bladder training
- Important observations about urine
- Important observations about stool

✓ Define the following terms:
- *AM* and *PM care*
- *Good body alignment*
- **Seizure**
- **Syncope**
- *Soft postural supports*
- *Guarding technique* and *guarding belt* from Chapter 19

✓ Match range-of-motion vocabulary words with their meanings.

✓ **Calculate** in cc's and record fluid intake properly.

✓ Evaluate and determine appropriate action for a given situation.

✓ Demonstrate each procedure in this chapter.

✓ Demonstrate the following in
- Chapter 19: Ambulating with a walking belt
   Walking with crutches
   Walking with a walker

ambulation Walking.

insulin shock Condition caused by too much insulin.

postural supports Soft restraints used to protect resident.

alignment Keeping a resident in proper position.

seizure Involuntary muscle contraction and relaxation.

syncope Fainting.

calculate Figure out.

■ RESPONSIBILITIES OF A LONG-TERM CARE NURSE ASSISTANT

Nurse assistants are important members of the health care team. They are responsible for giving personal care to the resident. They spend more time with the resident than the other members of the team. This gives them an opportunity to give extra support and understanding to the resident. They may work in an acute care hospital or in long-term care. Long-term care nurse assistants are required to complete training that meets the OBRA 1987 guidelines. They must also pass a test and receive a nursing assistant certification. (See pages xxiii–xxv.) Many long-term care nurse assistants choose to learn additional skills and work in the long-term care/ rehabilitation sub-acute care area. These additional skills are described in Unit 2 of this chapter. The acute care and assistive personnel care skills are in your teacher's Instructors Guide. If you are interested in these areas, talk to your instructor about your interest (see Figure 15–1).

As a long-term nurse assistant you will

admit To let someone in, take in.

impaction Being tightly wedged into a part (e.g., fecal material wedged into the bowel that requires mechanical means to remove).

enemas Solution introduced into the rectum.

perineal Region between the vulva and anus in a female, or between the scrotum and anus in a male.

- **Admit,** discharge, and transfer residents.
- Provide AM and PM care.
- Provide oral hygiene.
- Offer the bedpan and urinal.
- Understand the seriousness of **impaction.**
- Understand the use of **enemas.**
- Assist with dressing and/undressing.
- Bathe residents.
- Give **perineal** care.
- Give good skin care.
- Follow the patient care plan (see Figure 15–2).
- Perform range of motion.
- Provide body alignment and positioning.
- Care for hair and nails.
- Shave the resident.
- Apply hot and cold applications.

FIGURE 15–1. The interdisciplinary team is made up of professionals and nonprofessionals from many healthcare fields.

FIGURE 15–2.
Components of the patient care plan.

- Make the bed.
- Assist residents to move and ambulate.
- Apply prosthetic devices and supports.
- Assist with feeding the resident.
- Record intake and output.
- Care for the **incontinent** resident.
- Understand tubes and **catheters.**
- Collect specimens.
- Measure height and weight.
- Take seizure precautions.
- Give **stoma** care.
- Do **postmortem** care.

incontinent Unable to control the bowel or bladder.

catheters Tubes inserted into body opening or cavity.

stoma Opening, e.g., opening in abdomen in an ostomy.

postmortem After death.

FIGURE 15-3.
Admitting a resident.

■ ADMISSION

You are one of the first people the resident and family see (see Figure 15–3). Be pleasant and try to put everyone at ease. The facility where you work has a procedure for you to follow when you admit the resident. Do not rush the resident. Give the person time to adjust to the new environment. When a resident is admitted to the hospital, there are some basic procedures that are followed. (See Figure 15–4 for a sample of an admission checklist.) These include the following:

■ Making a clothing list
■ Making a list of personal items

FIGURE 15-4.
Sample admission checklist.

A SAMPLE ADMISSION CHECK LIST
(Fill in every statement and check every appropriate item)

Resident's name _____   Room number _____

Time of admission _____ a.m./p.m.   Date of admission _____
Unit ready to receive resident? Yes☐No☐ Equipment ready? Yes☐No☐
Admitted by stretcher _____ wheelchair _____ walking _____
Check identification bracelet? Yes☐No☐ Bed tag in place? Yes☐No☐
Did the resident need help to get undressed? Yes☐No☐
Is the resident in bed at this time? Yes☐No☐ Time _____ a.m./p.m.
Siderails up? Yes☐No☐
Bruises, marks, rashes, or broken skin noted? Yes☐No☐
    If yes, describe_____
Weight _____ Height _____ Scale Used? Yes☐No☐
Temperature_____ Pulse _____ Respirations _____ Blood Pressure _____
Admission urine specimen collected? Yes☐No☐ Sent to lab? Yes☐No☐
Unusual behavior noted? Yes☐No☐ Unusual appearance noted? Yes☐No☐
    If yes, describe_____
Does the resident have any difficulty with the English language? Yes☐No☐
Is the resident allergic to food? Yes☐No☐ Allergic to drugs? Yes☐No☐
Reason for admission _____
Complaints_____
Dentures? Yes☐No☐ Partial? Yes☐No☐ Full? Yes☐No☐ Denture cup? Yes☐No☐
Vision problems? Yes☐No☐ Does the resident wear glasses? Yes☐No☐ Contact lenses? ☐
Valuables: Money? Yes☐No☐ Describe_____
    Jewelry? Yes☐No☐ Describe _____
Is the resident hard of hearing? Yes☐No☐ Hearing aid? Yes☐No☐ Contact lenses? Yes☐No☐
    Artificial limb? Yes☐No☐ Brace? Yes☐No☐
Is the resident calm? Yes☐No☐ Is the resident very anxious? Yes☐No☐
    Angry? Yes☐No☐ Is the resident agitated or very excited? Yes☐No☐
Has the resident been admitted to this hospital before? Yes☐No☐
Is the clothing list completed? Yes☐No☐ Signed by _____
Is the signal cord attached to the bed? Yes☐No☐
Have drugs brought into the hospital by the resident been given to the charge nurse? Yes☐No☐
Name of the nurse drugs were given to _____
Additional comments _____
Admitted by _____

■ Requesting that the family take home valuables or see that they are put in a safe place

■ Taking vital signs

■ Weighing the resident

■ Explaining the call light and routine

■ Collecting urine specimens if required

Procedure

Admitting a Resident

ALERT: Follow Standard Precautions.

1. Wash hands.
2. Assemble equipment.
   a. Admission checklist
   b. Admission pack (may be all disposable depending on facility)
      (1) Bedpan
      (2) Urinal
      (3) Emesis basin
      (4) Wash basin
      (5) Tissues
   c. Gown or pajamas
   d. Portable scale
   e. Thermometer
   f. Blood pressure cuff
   g. Stethoscope
   h. Clothing list
   i. Envelope for valuables
3. Fan-fold bed covers to foot of bed. (See the procedure "Making an Open Bed.")
4. Put resident's equipment away.
5. Put gown or pajamas on foot of bed.
6. Greet resident and introduce yourself.
7. Identify resident by looking at arm band and asking name. (See Figure A.)
8. Introduce resident to roommates.
9. Explain
   a. How call signal works
   b. How bed controls work (see Figure B)
   c. Hospital regulations
   d. What you will be doing to admit him or her
10. Provide privacy by pulling privacy curtains.
11. Ask resident to put on gown or pajamas.
12. Check weight and height.

13. Help to bed if ordered. (Check with nurse.)
14. Put side rails up if required.
15. If resident has valuables:
    a. Make a list of jewelry, money, wallet, etc.
    b. Have resident sign list
    c. Have relative sign list
    d. Either have relative take valuables home or send to cashier's office in valuables envelope.

A

B

Procedure box continued

16. Take and record the following:
    a. Temperature, pulse, respiration
    b. Blood pressure
    c. Urine specimen, if required
17. Complete admission checklist.
    a. Allergies
    b. Medications being taken
    c. Food preferences and dislikes

    d. Any prosthesis
    e. Skin condition
    f. Handicaps (e.g., deafness, sight, movement)
18. Orient resident to meal times, visiting hours, etc.
19. Record information according to your facility's policy.
20. Wash hands.

■ HEIGHT AND WEIGHT

Residents are weighed and measured for height when they are admitted. These measurements provide a baseline during the resident's stay. Measurements must be accurate, as they are important to the well-being of the resident. The resident's weight is important because it indicates

■ Nutritional status
■ Any change (weight loss or gain) in condition

There are several different types of scales. Each is designed for ease in weighing residents with varying problems. The three types of scales are the

■ Standing scale
■ Scale with mechanical lift
■ Wheelchair scale (Figure 15–5)

FIGURE 15–5.
Chair scale.

Residents who are wheelchair-bound can be left in the wheelchair and weighed. Allowance is made for the weight of the wheelchair and platform by subtracting a certain amount from the weight or by having the scale adjusted to allow for the extra weight. You can also use a mechanical lift that has a scale. It is operated by using a hydraulic pump to raise and lower the resident. This makes weighing a bedfast resident much easier.

Height is used as an indicator of the ideal weight of the resident. You may have to measure the resident with a measuring tape if the person is unable to stand. If the resident can stand, use the measure on the standing scale.

Procedure

Measuring Weight on Standing Balance Scale

ALERT: Follow Standard Precautions.

1. Wash hands.
2. Assemble equipment.
   a. Portable balance scale
   b. Paper towel
   c. Paper and pencil/pen
3. Identify resident.
4. Explain what you are going to do.
5. Take resident to scale or bring scale to resident's room.
6. Place paper towel on platform of scale (with standing scale).
7. Put both weights to the very left on zero.
8. Balance beam pointer must stay steady in middle of balance area. (If pointer does not center, turn balance screw until it remains centered.)
9. Have resident remove shoes and stand on scale.

Note: The balance bar raises to top of bar guide and pointer is not centered.

10. Move large weight to estimated weight of resident.
11. Move small weight to right until balance bar hangs free halfway between upper and lower bar guide.
12. The largest (lower) weight is marked in increments of 50 pounds; the smaller (upper weight) is marked in single pounds. The even-numbered pounds are marked with numbers (e.g., 2, 4, 6). The uneven pounds are unmarked long lines and the short line is one-fourth of a pound.
13. Write weight down on a notepad.
14. Help resident with shoes and make him or her comfortable.
15. Replace scale.
16. Wash hands.
17. Chart weight. Report any unusual increases or decreases in weight.

Procedure

Measuring Weight on a Chair Scale

ALERT: Follow Standard Precautions.

1. Place wheelchair on scale or transfer resident to chair on scale.
2. Follow the directions in the procedure "Measuring Weight on a Standing Balance Scale."
3. Write down weight on notepad.
4. Make resident comfortable.
5. Wash hands.
6. Chart weight.

Wheelchair scale

Procedure

Measuring Weight on a Mechanical Lift

ALERT: Follow Standard Precautions.

1. Wash hands.
2. Assemble equipment.
   a. Mechanical lift
   b. Sling
   c. Clean sheet
3. Identify resident.
4. Explain what you are going to do.
5. Pull privacy curtain.
6. Lower side rail on side you are working on.
7. Cover sling with clean sheet.
8. Help resident roll on side and place sling with top at shoulders and bottom at knees.
9. Fan-fold remaining sling.
10. Help resident roll to other side onto one half of sling and pull other half of sling through.

Scale with mechanical lift

Procedure box continued

11. Broaden base of lift.
12. Wheel lift to side of bed with base beneath bed.
13. Position lift over resident.
14. Attach sling using chains and hooks provided. *(Keep open end of hook away from resident to avoid injury.)*
15. Use hand crank or pump handle to raise resident from bed. Make certain that buttocks are not touching bed.
16. Check to be certain that resident is in center of sling and is safely suspended.
17. To weigh resident:
    a. Swing feet and legs over edge of bed; move lift away from bed so that no body part contacts bed.

    b. If bed is low enough, raise resident above bed so that no body part contacts bed.
18. Adjust weights until scale is balanced. (See the procedure "Measuring Weight on a Standing Balance Scale.")
19. Return resident to bed by reversing steps.
20. Replace mechanical lift.
21. Wash hands.
22. Note weight and write on pad.

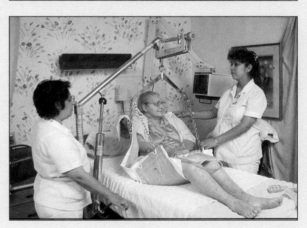

Procedure

Measuring Height

ALERT: Follow Standard Precautions.

1. Wash hands.
2. Assemble equipment.
   a. Balance scale with height rod
   b. Paper towels
3. Identify resident.
4. Explain what you are going to do.
5. Have resident remove shoes.
6. Raise measuring rod above head.
7. Have resident stand with back against measuring rod.
8. Instruct resident to stand straight, with heels touching measuring rod.
9. Lower measuring rod to rest on resident's head.
10. Check number of inches indicated on rod. This number is found where the sliding rod enters the hollow post.
11. Record in inches, centimeters, or feet and inches according to hospital policy.
12. Help resident with shoes.
13. Chart height.

Height measuring rod

■ TRANSFER

When you assist in transferring the resident to another area, the resident may be unhappy about the move. Be calm and pleasant, and explain that you will make the move as easy as possible. Be certain that all of the resident's belongings are transferred to the new area and that the nurse assistant who is responsible for the resident knows that the resident has arrived. Follow the policies and procedures of your facility for transferring residents.

■ DISCHARGE

A resident cannot be discharged without an order from his or her physician. If your resident plans to leave when it has not been ordered, report it to the head nurse immediately. Each facility has a policy and procedure for discharging the resident. Know what you are expected to do if you are asked to assist in discharging the resident. Be sure that you check to see that the resident has all his or her personal belongings. If the resident has valuables that were put away for safekeeping, remind the person to take them home. This is usually a happy time for the resident.

Procedure

Moving Resident and Belongings to Another Room

ALERT: Follow Standard Precautions.

1. Wash hands.
2. Assemble equipment.
   a. Resident's chart   b. Nursing care plan
   c. Medications   d. Paper bag
3. Identify resident.
4. Explain what you are going to do.
5. Determine location to which resident is being transferred.
6. Gather resident belongings. (Check admission list.)
7. Determine how resident is to be transported.
   a. Wheelchair   b. Stretcher
   c. Entire bed   d. Ambulation
8. Transport resident to new unit.
9. Introduce to staff on new unit.
10. Introduce to new roommate.
11. Make resident comfortable.
12. Put away belongings.
13. Wash hands.
14. Give transferred medications, care plan, and chart to nurse.
15. Before leaving unit, record the following:
    a. Date and time of transfer
    b. How transported (e.g., wheelchair)
    c. How transfer was tolerated by resident
16. Return to original unit and report completion of transfer.

Procedure

Discharging a Resident

ALERT: Follow Standard Precautions.

1. Check chart for discharge order.
2. Wash hands.
3. Identify resident.
4. Explain what you are going to do.
5. Provide privacy by pulling the privacy curtain.
6. Help resident dress.
7. Collect resident's belongings.
8. Check belongings against admission list.
9. Secure and return valuables.
   a. Verify with resident that all valuables are there.
   b. Have resident sign for them.
10. Check to see if resident has medications to take home.
11. Check to see if any equipment is to be taken home.
12. Help resident into wheelchair.
13. Help resident into car.
14. Return to unit.
    a. Remove all items left in unit (e.g., basins, disposable items).
    b. Clean unit according to your facility's policy.
15. Wash hands.
16. Record discharge.
    a. Date and time
    b. Method of transport
    c. Who resident left with

■ STANDARD PRECAUTIONS

Always follow Standard Precautions when caring for a resident. You must evaluate the situation before you start a procedure to determine when you must wear protective gear. The following procedures indicate when to put on gloves and when to discard them. However, you are responsible for determining when to wear gloves.

There are times when you need gloves to protect yourself from body fluids that may not be addressed in a procedure. Carefully think through the care you are giving and protect yourself and others.

■ MORNING AND EVENING CARE (AM AND PM CARE)

The beginning of the day is very important. How you care for the resident when he or she first awakens sets the tone for the entire day. This care is called AM care and is given before breakfast. Awaken the resident quietly; never be loud or abrupt. Do not shake the person by the shoulder. Touch him or her on the arm and say the person's name. After the person is awake, there are several steps in the care you give. Follow the AM care procedures.

Procedure

AM Care

1. Wash hands.
2. Gently awaken resident.
3. Assemble equipment.
   a. Washcloth and towel
   b. Toothbrush and toothpaste
   c. Emesis basin
   d. Glass of water
   e. Denture cup if needed
   f. Clean gown if necessary
   g. Clean linen if necessary
   h. Comb and brush
   i. Disposable gloves (two pair)
4. Explain what you plan to do.
5. Provide privacy by pulling privacy curtain.
ALERT: Follow Standard Precautions.
6. Elevate head of the bed if allowed.
7. Put on disposable gloves.
8. Provide a bedpan or urinal if needed, or escort resident to bathroom.

9. Empty bedpan or urinal, rinse it, and dispose of gloves.
10. Put bedpan or urinal out of sight.
11. Allow resident to wash hands and face.
12. Put on disposable gloves.
13. Provide oral hygiene.
14. Provide a clean gown if necessary.
15. Smooth sheets if resident remains in bed.
16. Transfer to a chair if resident is allowed out of bed.
17. Allow resident to comb hair; assist if necessary.
18. Prepare the overbed table.
    a. Clear tabletop.
    b. Wipe off.
19. Position overbed table if resident is to remain in the room, or transport resident to dining room.
20. Remove and discard gloves.
21. Wash hands.

The PM care given to residents just before sleep is also important. Use this time to make residents comfortable for the night. Unhurried care allows the residents to feel relaxed, and they sleep better. If you take care of all their needs before you leave the room, it gives you time to finish your other duties. If you do not make them comfortable (e.g., see if they need to go to the bathroom), you have to return frequently to their rooms. Follow the PM care procedures.

Procedure

PM Care

1. Wash hands.
2. Tell resident what you are going to do.
3. Provide privacy.
4. Assemble equipment.
   a. Washcloth and towel
   b. Toothpaste and toothbrush
   c. Glass of water
   d. Emesis basin
   e. Denture cup, if necessary
   f. Night clothes
   g. Lotion
   h. Linen as needed
   i. Disposable gloves
5. Encourage resident to do his or her own care if capable.

ALERT: Follow Standard Precautions.

6. Assist if unable to do his or her own care.
7. Put on disposable gloves.
8. Provide bedpan or urinal if necessary, or escort to bathroom.

9. Empty bedpan or urinal.
10. Rinse and place in a convenient place for nighttime use.
11. Remove and dispose of gloves.
12. Wash resident's hands and face.
13. Put on gloves.
14. Provide for oral hygiene.
15. Change resident into night clothes.

16. Transfer resident from chair or wheelchair into bed, if out of bed.
17. Give back rub with lotion.
18. Observe skin for irritations or breakdown.
19. Smooth the sheets.
20. Change draw sheets if necessary.
21. Provide extra blankets if necessary.
22. Position side rails as ordered after resident is in bed.
23. Remove and discard gloves.
24. Wash hands.
25. Provide fresh drinking water.
26. Place bedside table within resident's reach.
27. Secure call light within resident's reach.
28. Chart procedure.

■ SKIN MANAGEMENT

Skin is the first defense against infection. When you bathe your residents, you have an opportunity to observe their skin. You should look for

■ Dryness
■ Bruising

■ Any unusual condition
■ Broken area (pressure sore/decubitus)

Pressure sores/*decubiti* are very serious. Residents must be moved to help remove pressure on the skin, or pressure sores develop. This pressure can occur when residents are in bed or when they are sitting. They must be moved at least every 2 hours. The following areas are very sensitive to pressure:

■ Shoulders   ■ Heels
■ Elbows   ■ Ankles
■ Hips   ■ Ears
■ Sacrum   ■ Toes

Watch these areas carefully (see Figures 15–6 and 15–7). The bones press against the skin and stop circulation of blood. This causes the skin and tissue to break down. Pressure sores/decubiti are very painful and very difficult to heal. They can become very deep and require a surgical procedure to help them heal. They can be prevented! Report any changes, such as redness, heat, tenderness, or broken skin, to the charge nurse.

To help prevent pressure sores/decubiti:

■ Change the resident's position at least every 2 hours.
■ Keep skin clean.
■ Massage reddened areas over sharp, bony areas to increase circulation.
■ Provide back rubs to increase circulation and relax the resident.
■ Keep linen dry and free of wrinkles.
■ Use foam padding, fiber-filled overlay, gel-filled pads, or sheepskin.
■ Use a foot cradle to keep linen off feet.

Residents who are stationary for long periods of time can be protected by using special cushions on beds. For example:

■ An egg-crate cushion made of foam rubber can be placed on a bed or cut to fit a chair.

Places to Check for Signs of Bedsores

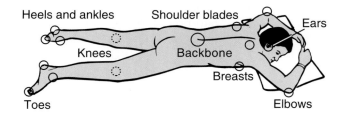

FIGURE 15–6. Places to check for signs of pressure sores.

FIGURE 15–7. Pressure from the ischial bones and sacrum with the resident in the sitting position.

Procedure

Giving a Back Rub

1. Wash hands.
2. Assemble equipment.
   a. Lotion
   b. Powder
   c. Towel
   d. Washcloth
   e. Soap
   f. Water (105°F)
   g. Disposable gloves
3. Tell resident what you are going to do.

ALERT: Follow Standard Precautions.

4. Provide privacy by pulling privacy curtains.
5. Place lotion container in warm water to help warm it.
6. Raise bed to a comfortable working height.
7. Lower side rail on the side you are working on.
8. Put on disposable gloves.
9. Position resident on side or in prone position.
10. Place a towel along back to protect linen if resident is in a side-lying position.
11. Wash back thoroughly.
12. Rub a small amount of lotion into your hands.
13. Begin at base of spine and apply lotion over entire back.
14. Use firm, long strokes, beginning at buttocks and moving upward to neck and shoulders.

15. Use firm pressure as you stroke upward, and light circular strokes returning to buttocks.

Note: Pay special attention to bony prominences.

16. Use a circular motion over each area (shoulder blades, backbone).
17. Observe skin for irritation or breakdown.

Note: Do not rub or apply lotion to any open area on the skin.

18. Repeat several times (3 to 5 minutes).
19. Dry back.
20. Adjust gown for comfort.
21. Remove towel.
22. Position resident comfortably.
23. Return bed to lowest height.
24. Put side rail up if required.
25. Secure call light in reach of resident.
26. Remove and discard gloves.
27. Wash hands.
28. Record procedure and any observations (e.g., redness, broken areas, dry skin).

■ Rotating air mattresses circulate air through canals. The circulating air allows pressure from mattress to alternate. This alternating pressure allows blood circulation to keep skin healthy.

■ Turning beds are used when a resident cannot move freely or easily. There are a variety of types of beds that allow a resident to be sandwiched between two mattresses. The bed is then turned and the top mattress is removed until the resident is repositioned.

■ Water mattresses conform to the body weight and shape. The water redistributes with movement to prevent pressure.

■ ORAL HYGIENE

Good mouth care should be provided at least three times a day: before breakfast when you give AM care, after lunch, and after dinner. It is important because it

■ Reduces odor
■ Helps prevent tooth decay
■ Is refreshing
■ Relieves dry lips and mouth, especially if the resident has an elevated temperature or breathes through the mouth

dentures False teeth.   Some residents may have **dentures.** Often residents are sensitive about removing their dentures. Provide privacy and encouragement for oral care. Learn the correct method of handling dentures so that you do not break them.

Procedure

Self-Care Oral Hygiene

ALERT: Follow Standard Precautions.

1. Wash hands.
2. Assemble equipment.
   a. Toothbrush
   b. Toothpaste
   c. Mouthwash
   d. Cup of water with straw, if needed
   e. Emesis basin
   f. Bath towel
   g. Tissues
3. Identify resident and explain what you are going to do.
4. Screen resident by pulling privacy curtain around bed.
5. Raise head of the bed if resident is allowed to sit up.
6. Place towel over blanket and resident's gown.
7. Place toothbrush, toothpaste, mouthwash, emesis basin, and glass of water on overbed table.
8. Remove overbed table when resident has completed brushing.

9. Put towel away and make resident comfortable.
10. Put side rails up if required.
11. Secure call bell within resident's reach.
12. Put all equipment away and tidy unit.
13. Wash hands.
14. Chart procedure.

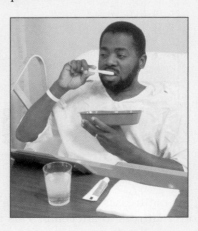

Procedure

Brushing the Resident's Teeth

1. Wash hands.
2. Assemble equipment.
    a. Toothbrush
    b. Toothpaste
    c. Mouthwash
    d. Cup of water with straw, if needed
    e. Emesis basin
    f. Bath towel
    g. Tissues
    h. Disposable nonsterile gloves

ALERT: Follow Standard Precautions.

3. Identify resident and explain what you are going to do.
4. Screen resident by pulling privacy curtain around bed.
5. Raise head of bed if resident is allowed to sit up.
6. Place a towel over blanket and resident's gown.
7. Put on gloves.
8. Pour water over toothbrush; put toothpaste on brush.
9. Insert brush into the mouth carefully.

10. Place brush at an angle on upper teeth and brush in an up-and-down motion starting at rear of mouth.
11. Repeat on lower teeth.
12. Give resident water to rinse mouth. If necessary, use a straw.
13. Hold emesis basin under chin. Have resident expectorate (spit) water into the basin.
14. Offer tissues to resident to wipe mouth and chin. Discard tissues.
15. Provide mouthwash if available. Use emesis basin and tissues as above.
16. Return all equipment.
17. Remove gloves and put in hazardous waste.
18. Wash hands.
19. Tidy up unit.
20. Put side rails up if required.
21. Secure call bell within resident's reach.
22. Make resident comfortable before leaving the room.
23. Chart procedure and how resident tolerated it.

Procedure

Oral Hygiene: Ambulatory Resident

ALERT: Follow Standard Precautions.

1. Wash hands.
2. Tell resident what you are going to do.
3. Set up equipment at sink.
    a. Toothbrush
    b. Toothpaste
    c. Tablets or powder to soak dentures in
    d. Towel
    e. Glass
4. Rinse equipment and put away.
5. Wash hands.

Procedure

Denture Care

1. Wash hands.
2. Assemble equipment.
   a. Tissues
   b. Paper towel or gauze squares
   c. Mouthwash
   d. Disposable denture cup
   e. Toothbrush or denture brush
   f. Denture paste or toothpowder
   g. Towel
   h. Disposable nonsterile gloves

ALERT: Follow Standard Precautions.

3. Identify resident.
4. Explain what you are going to do.
5. Pull privacy curtain.
6. Lower side rails.
7. Raise head of bed if allowed.
8. Place towel across resident's chest.
9. Prepare emesis basin by placing tissue or paper towel in bottom of basin.
10. Put on gloves.
11. Have resident remove his or her dentures.
12. Remove dentures if resident cannot.

Upper Denture

   a. Explain what you are going to do.
   b. Use a gauze square to grip upper denture.
   c. Place your index finger between top ridge of denture and cheek.
   d. Gently pull on denture to release suction.
   e. Remove upper denture.

Lower Denture

   a. Use a gauze square to grip lower denture.
   b. Place your index finger between lower ridge and cheek.
   c. Gently pull on denture to release suction.
   d. Remove lower denture.

13. Place dentures in lined emesis basin and take to sink or utility room.
14. Hold dentures firmly in palm of hand.
15. Put toothpowder or toothpaste on toothbrush.
16. Hold dentures under cold running water and brush dentures until clean.

17. Rinse dentures under cold running water.

18. Place in denture cup.
19. Place a solution of mouthwash and cool water in cup.
20. Help resident rinse mouth with mouthwash; if food particles are between cheek and gumline, gently swab away with gauze.
21. Have resident replace dentures.
22. Place dentures in labeled denture cup next to bed, if dentures are to be left out.
23. Rinse equipment and put away.
24. Remove gloves; dispose of in hazardous waste.
25. Wash hands.
26. Position resident.
27. Raise side rails if required.
28. Secure call bell within resident's reach.
29. Chart procedure and how it was tolerated.

Note: The resident may want to soak dentures overnight after PM care has been given. Place dentures in a solution in a denture cup and store in a safe place.

Procedure

Oral Hygiene for the Unconscious Resident

1. Wash hands.
2. Tell resident what you are going to do. When resident is unconscious he or she may hear even if he or she cannot respond.
3. Provide privacy.
4. Assemble equipment.
   a. Emesis basin
   b. Towel
   c. Lemon glycerin swabs
   d. Tongue blades
   e. 4 × 4 gauze
   f. Lip moisturizer
   g. Disposable nonsterile gloves

   ALERT: Follow Standard Precautions.
5. Position bed at a comfortable working height.
6. Put on gloves.
7. Position resident's head to side and place towel on bed under resident's cheek and chin.
8. Secure emesis basin under resident's chin.
9. Wrap a tongue blade with 4 × 4 gauze and slightly moisten. Swab mouth being certain to clean gums, teeth, tongue, and roof of mouth.

10. Apply lip moisturizer to lips and swab mouth with lemon and glycerin if available.
11. Remove towel and reposition resident.
12. Discard disposable equipment in hazardous waste.
13. Clean basin and put away.
14. Remove gloves and put in hazardous waste.
15. Wash hands.
16. Report and document resident's tolerance of procedure.

■ OFFERING THE URINAL AND/OR BEDPAN

Eliminating waste products from the body is necessary for good health. When residents are confined to bed, they must use a bedpan or urinal. Male residents use urinals to empty the bladder. Women use the bedpan for both urine and the elimination of solid waste (bowel movement). Men also use a bedpan for the elimination of solid waste. Solid waste is called *feces* or *stool*. When residents eliminate liquid waste, we call it *urinating* or *voiding*.

If your resident does not eliminate liquid waste from the bladder, he or she may develop a urinary tract infection. This is very painful and serious. Small amounts of liquid elimination may indicate infection, dehydration, or fluid retention in the body. If solid waste is not eliminated, large amounts of stool may cause an impaction. When a large amount of stool stays in the bowel it causes discomfort, and the resident experiences nausea and sometimes vomiting. This can be prevented by carefully recording bowel movements and letting the charge nurse know if a resident has not had a bowel movement. The charge nurse will give the resident a **laxative, suppository,** or enema (see Figure 15–8), which is discussed later in this chapter.

laxative Liquid or pill that causes evacuation of the bowel.

suppository Bullet shaped mass inserted into rectum to stimulate bowel movement.

FIGURE 15–8.
Cleansing enema.

Procedure

Offering the Bedpan

1. Wash hands.
2. Assemble equipment.
   a. Bedpan with cover
   b. Toilet tissue
   c. Soap and water
   d. Towel
   e. Disposable nonsterile gloves (two pairs)

ALERT: Follow Standard Precautions.

3. Ask visitors to wait outside room.
4. Provide privacy for resident.
5. Remove bedpan from storage space.
6. Warm metal bedpans by running warm water over them and drying.
7. Lower head of bed if it is elevated.
8. Put on gloves.
9. Fold top covers back enough to see where to place the pan. Do not expose resident.
10. Ask resident to raise hips off bed. Help support resident by placing your hand at resident's mid-back.
    a. Roll the resident onto his or her side if the resident is unable to lift the hips.
    b. Place bedpan on buttocks.
    c. Hold in place with one hand and help resident roll back onto bedpan.
11. Slide bedpan into place.

Procedure box continued

12. Cover resident again.
13. Raise head of bed for comfort.

14. Remove gloves.
15. Wash your hands.
16. Leave call light with resident.

17. Leave room to provide privacy.
18. Watch for call light to signal resident's readiness to be removed from bedpan.
19. Put on gloves.
20. Assist resident as necessary to ensure cleanliness.
21. Remove bedpan and empty.
22. Measure urine if on I & O.
23. Remove gloves.
24. Wash hands.
25. Provide washcloth, water, and soap for resident to wash hands.
26. Provide comfort measures for resident.
27. Secure call light in resident's reach.
28. Open privacy curtain.
29. Chart the following:
    a. Bowel movement amount, color, consistency
    b. Amount voided if on I & O

Procedure

Offering the Urinal

1. Wash hands.
2. Assemble equipment.
    a. Urinal with cover
    b. Soap and water
    c. Towel
    d. Disposable nonsterile gloves
ALERT: Follow Standard Precautions.
3. Ask visitors to wait outside room.
4. Provide privacy for resident.
5. Hand urinal to resident.
    a. Place call light at resident's side.
    b. Wash your hands.
    c. Leave room until resident signals with the call light.
    (If the resident is unable to place urinal, place penis in urinal. If necessary, stand and hold urinal until resident has finished voiding.) Wear gloves for this step.
6. Return to room when resident has finished voiding.

7. Put on gloves.
8. Place cover over urinal and carry it into bathroom.
9. Check to see if resident is on I & O or if a urine specimen is needed. (See I & O and specimen collection in this chapter.)
10. Observe urine color, consistency, and odor.
11. Empty into toilet.
12. Rinse urinal with cold water.
13. Cover and place in a convenient location for the resident.
14. Remove gloves.
15. Wash hands.
16. Secure call light in reach of resident.
17. Report and document unusual color, odor, or consistency of urine.
18. Record amount if on I & O.

Procedure

Bedside Commode

1. Wash hands.
2. Assemble equipment.
   a. Bedside commode
   b. Toilet tissue
   c. Washcloth
   d. Warm water
   e. Soap
   f. Towel
   g. Disposable nonsterile gloves

ALERT: Follow Standard Precautions.

3. Identify resident.
4. Explain what you are going to do.
5. Place commode chair next to bed facing head of bed. *Lock wheels!*
6. Check to see if receptacle is in place under seat.
7. Provide privacy by pulling privacy curtains.
8. Lower bed to lowest position.
9. Lower side rail.
10. Help resident to sitting position.
11. Help resident swing legs over side of bed.
12. Put resident's slippers on and assist to stand.
13. Have resident place hands on your shoulders.
14. Support under resident's arms, pivot resident to right, and lower to commode. (See the procedure "Pivot Transfer from Bed to Wheelchair.")
15. Place call bell within reach.
16. Place toilet tissue in reach.
17. Remain nearby if resident seems weak.
18. Return immediately when resident signals.
19. Put on gloves.
20. Assist resident to stand.
21. Clean anus or perineum if resident is unable to help self.
22. Remove gloves and put in hazardous waste.
23. Help resident wash hands.
24. Assist back to bed and position comfortably.
25. Put side rail up if required.
26. Put on gloves.
27. Put cover on commode chair down and remove receptacle.
28. Empty contents, measuring if on I & O.
29. Empty and clean per hospital policy.
30. Remove gloves and put in hazardous waste.
31. Wash hands.
32. Replace equipment and tidy unit.
33. Record the following:
    a. Bowel movement
       (1) Amount
       (2) Consistency
       (3) Color
    b. Any unusual observations, such as
       (1) Weakness
       (2) Discomfort

■ MOVEMENT AND AMBULATION OF THE RESIDENT

You are responsible for moving your resident in many different ways:

- ■ Into a chair or wheelchair
- ■ Into bed from a chair or wheelchair
- ■ From bed to gurney
- ■ From gurney to bed

■ Transferring into a wheelchair
■ Transporting by gurney
■ Using a mechanical lift (see Figure 15–9)

Be careful not to injure the residents or yourself when you move them. Review the unit on body mechanics in Chapter 13. Always remember to evaluate whether you need help before you start to move the resident, and do not hesitate to ask someone to give you a hand.

When residents first try to get out of bed, they may feel dizzy. Help them sit on the side of the bed. Encourage the resident to swing his or her legs slightly back and forth until you determine that he or she is strong enough to stand and walk.

When your residents are able to walk, encourage them to do as much as they are capable of. They may seem slow, and it may take you a little extra time, but it is important for them. Walking (ambulating)

■ Helps maintain stamina
■ Increases joint mobility
■ Improves muscle tone
■ Helps prevent lung congestion
■ Improves circulation
■ Helps maintain independence
■ Provides a sense of accomplishment

Your residents may need a device such as a cane, crutches, or walker. They may need a wheelchair much of the time but still be able to ambulate in a limited way. Learn the procedures for ambulation in Chapter 19.

Before residents are moved, check to see if there are tubes or catheters in place. You must be careful not to pull them out, crimp them, or put a strain on them. If residents have drainage equipment (e.g., Foley bag [urine drainage bag]), do not raise the tubing above the level of insertion into the body. If they have an IV, do not allow the tubing to drop below the bed level. Never let any tubing touch the floor. If you have any question about moving residents, *ask your instructor or the charge nurse before moving them.*

Boom

Pump

Sling

Mast

Base

FIGURE 15–9.
Mechanical lift.

Procedure

Pivot Transfer from Bed to Wheelchair

ALERT: Follow Standard Precautions.

1. Wash hands.
2. *Lock* wheels on chair.
3. Lift foot rests or swing leg supports out of way.
4. Position wheelchair along side of bed. (See instructor for directions in working with stroke residents.) Lock wheels.
5. Move resident to edge of bed, with legs over side.

7. Support him or her at midriff and ask resident to stand, if resident is not dizzy.
8. Once standing, have resident pivot (turn) and hold onto armrest of wheelchair with both arms or one strong arm.

6. Have resident dangle legs for a few minutes. Encourage some slow deep breaths and observe for dizziness. (See the section on syncope in this chapter.)

9. Gently ease resident into a sitting position.
10. Position yourself at back of wheelchair. Ask resident to push on the floor with feet as you lift gently under each arm to ease resident into a comfortable position against backrest.
11. Return foot rests to normal position and place feet and legs in a comfortable position on rests.

Procedure box continued

12. Do not leave a resident who requires a postural support until it is in place.

13. Reverse above procedure to return resident to bed.
14. Wash hands.

Procedure

Sliding from Bed to Wheelchair and Back

ALERT: Follow Standard Precautions.

1. Wash hands.
2. Assemble equipment: wheelchair with removable arms.
3. Position wheelchair at bedside with back parallel to head of bed. *Lock* wheels.
4. Remove wheelchair arm nearest to bedside.
5. Place bed level to chair seat height if possible. *Lock* bed wheels.

6. Raise head of bed so that resident is in sitting position.
7. Position yourself beside wheelchair and carefully assist resident to slide from bed to wheelchair.
8. Position resident for comfort and apply postural supports PRN.
9. Wash hands.

Procedure

Two-Person Lift from Bed to Chair and Back

ALERT: Follow Standard Precautions.

1. Wash hands.
2. Assemble equipment: chair.
3. Ask one other person to help.
4. Tell resident what you are going to do.
5. Position chair next to bed with back of chair parallel with head of bed. *Lock* wheels.
6. Position resident near edge of bed.
7. Position co-worker on side of bed near feet.
8. Position yourself behind chair at head of bed.

9. Place your arms under resident's axillae and clasp your hands together at resident's mid-chest.
10. Co-worker places hands under resident's upper legs.
11. Count to three. On the count of three, lift resident into chair.

12. Position for comfort and secure postural supports PRN.
13. Wash hands.

Procedure

Sliding from Bed to Gurney and Back

ALERT: Follow Standard Precautions.

1. Wash hands.
2. Assemble equipment.
   a. Gurney   b. Cover sheet
3. Ask a co-worker to help.
4. Explain what you are going to do and *lock* wheels on bed.
5. Cover resident with sheet and remove bed covers.
6. Raise bed to gurney height: lower side rail and move resident to side of bed.
7. Loosen draw sheet on both sides so it can be used as a pull sheet.

8. Position gurney next to bed and *lock* wheels on gurney.

Procedure box continued

9. Position yourself on outside of gurney—one at the head, the other at the hips. Co-worker is on other side of bed.
10. Reach across gurney and securely hold edge of draw sheet. Pull resident onto gurney and cover. (If resident is large, a third person on the opposite side of bed may be necessary.)

11. Position resident for comfort.
12. Secure with safety straps or raise side rails.
13. Wash hands.

Procedure

Lifting with a Mechanical Lift

ALERT: Follow Standard Precautions.

1. Wash hands.
2. Gather equipment.
   a. Mechanical lift
   b. Sheet or blanket for resident comfort
   c. Sling
3. Check all equipment to be sure it is in good working order and that the sling is not damaged or torn.
4. Ask one other person to help.
5. Prepare resident's destination.
   a. Chair
   b. Gurney
   c. Bathtub
   d. Shower
6. *Lock* wheels on bed and explain what you are going to do.
7. Roll resident toward you.
8. Place sling on bed behind resident.
   a. Position top of sling at shoulders.
   b. Position bottom of sling under buttocks.
   c. Leave enough of sling to support body when the body is rolled back. Fan-fold remaining sling next to body. It will be pulled through when resident is rolled back.
9. Roll resident to other side of bed and pull fan-folded portion of sling flat. Remove all wrinkles and allow resident to lie flat on back.
10. Position lift over resident, being sure to broaden base of lift. This stabilizes the lift while raising resident.
11. Raise head of bed to a semi-Fowler's position.

12. Attach straps on lift to sling loops. Shorter straps must be attached to shoulder loops. Longer straps are attached to loops at hips. *(Important! If you reverse the strap attachment, the resident's head will be lower than his or her hips.)*
13. Reassure resident. Let resident know you will keep him or her from falling. Gently raise resident from bed with hand crank or pump handle.
14. Keep resident centered over base of lift as you move lift and resident to his or her destination. (It is helpful to have a helper stand by and steady resident while moving so that resident doesn't swing.)
15. Position resident over chair, commode, bathtub, shower chair, etc. Ask a co-worker to steady chair.
16. Slowly lower resident into chair using foot-pedal positioning.
17. Unhook sling from lift straps and carefully move lift away from resident.
18. Provide all comfort measures for resident.
19. Secure postural supports if necessary.
20. Return lift to storage area.
21. Wash hands.
22. Reverse procedure when returning resident to bed.

Note: The mechanical lift is an expensive item. Depending on the size of the facility you are in, there may be a limited number available. Always return the lift to its storage area so that it will be available for others to use.

Procedure

Moving a Resident on a Gurney

ALERT: Follow Standard Precautions.

1. Position bed to gurney height.
2. *Lock* all the brakes on gurney and bed.
3. Follow the procedure for transferring to and from a gurney.
4. Stand at the resident's head and push the gurney with resident's feet moving first down the hallway.
5. Slow down when turning a corner. Always check the intersection mirrors for traffic.
6. Enter an elevator by standing at resident's head and pulling gurney into elevator. The feet will be the last to enter elevator.
7. Leave elevator by carefully pushing the gurney out of elevator into corridor.
8. Position yourself at resident's feet, and back a resident on a gurney down a hill.
9. Never leave a resident unattended on a gurney.
10. Raise side rails and secure a safety strap.

Procedure

Moving a Resident in a Wheelchair

ALERT: Follow Standard Precautions.

1. Position wheelchair.
2. *Lock* all brakes on wheelchair and bed.
3. Follow procedure for transferring resident to and from a wheelchair.
4. Push wheelchair carefully into hallway, watching for others who may be near doorway.
5. Move cautiously down hallway, being especially careful at intersections.
6. Always back a resident in a wheelchair over bumps, doorways, and into or out of elevators.
7. Always back a resident in a wheelchair down a hill.
8. Check resident for comfort measures before leaving.
9. Always notify appropriate person resident has arrived.

Procedure box continued

■ POSITIONING AND BODY ALIGNMENT

Always position your residents with the head in a straight line with the spine and the body in a comfortable, normal alignment. If a resident is bent in an unnatural position (slumped forward, rolled in a ball) the resident may experience

- Breathing problems
- Added pressure to the bony areas, causing skin breakdown (decubiti)
- Strain on the lumbar spine
- Contractures
- Decreased circulation
- Discomfort and pain
- Edema
- Foot drop

When the resident is confined to bed, the side-lying position is best. This allows for drainage of mucus from the nose and mouth and reduces the areas of pressure on the skin. If a resident must be on his or her back, check frequently for reddened areas, and be certain that antipressure aids are under them (egg-crate mattress, flotation mattress, sheepskin). Some of the techniques you can use are

- Pillow support at back for side lying
- Pillow support from the knee to ankle to support upper leg
- Trochanter support to prevent outward rotation
- Footboard and padded splints to prevent foot drop

Good body alignment is important at all times. This includes when the resident is lying in bed, sitting in a chair, and sitting in a wheelchair. When your residents are positioned in good body alignment, they look comfortable.

Procedure

Helping the Helpless Resident to Move Up in Bed

ALERT: Follow Standard Precautions.

1. Wash hands.
2. Ask a co-worker to help move resident. (Co-worker will work on opposite side of bed.)
3. Identify resident and explain what you are going to do. (Even if the resident seems unresponsive, he or she may be able to hear.)
4. Lock wheels of bed. Raise bed to comfortable working position, and lower side rails.
5. Remove pillow and place it at head of bed or on a chair.
6. Loosen both sides of draw sheet.
7. Roll edges toward side of resident's body.
8. Face head of bed and grasp rolled sheet edge with hand closest to resident.
9. Place your feet 12 inches apart with foot farthest from the edge of bed in a forward position.
10. Place your free hand and arm under resident's neck and shoulders, supporting head.
11. Bend your hips slightly.
12. On the count of three, you and your co-worker will raise resident's hips and back with draw sheet, supporting head and shoulders, and move resident smoothly to head of bed.

13. Replace pillow under resident's head and check for good body alignment.
14. Tighten and tuck in draw sheet and smooth bedding.
15. Raise side rails and lower bed.
16. Wash hands.

Procedure

Assisting Resident to Sit Up in Bed

ALERT: Follow Standard Precautions.

1. Wash hands.
2. Identify resident and explain what you are going to do.
3. Lock bed and lower all the way down.
4. Face head of bed, keeping your outer leg forward.
5. Turn your head away from resident's face.
6. Lock your arm nearest resident with resident's arm. To lock arms, place your arm between resident's arm and body, and hold upper arm near shoulder. Have resident hold back of your upper arm.
7. Support resident's head and shoulder with your other arm.
8. Raise resident to sitting position. Adjust head of bed and pillows.
9. Wash hands.

Procedure

Logrolling

ALERT: Follow Standard Precautions.

1. Wash hands.
2. Identify resident and explain what you are going to do.
3. Provide privacy by pulling privacy curtain.
4. Lock wheels of bed. Raise bed to a comfortable working position.
5. Lower side rail on side you are working on.
6. Be certain that side rail on opposite side of bed is in up position.
7. Leave pillow under head.
8. Place a pillow lengthwise between resident's legs.
9. Fold resident's arms across chest.
10. Roll resident onto his or her side like a log, turning body as a whole unit, without bending joints.
11. Check for good body alignment.
12. Tighten and tuck in draw sheet and smooth bedding.
13. Tuck pillow behind back for support.
14. Raise side rails and lower bed.
15. Secure call light in resident's reach.
16. Wash hands.
17. Chart position of resident and how procedure was tolerated.

Procedure

Turning Resident Away from You

ALERT: Follow Standard Precautions.

1. Wash hands.
2. Identify resident and explain what you are going to do.
3. Lock bed and elevate to a comfortable working height.
4. Lower side rail on side you are working from.
5. Have resident bend knees. Cross arms on chest.
6. Place arm nearest head of bed under resident's shoulders and head. Place other hand and forearm under small of the resident's back. Bend your body at hips and knees, keeping your back straight. Pull resident toward you.
7. Place forearms under resident's hips and pull resident toward you.
8. Place one hand under ankles and one hand under knees and move ankles and knees toward you.

As a safety measure, this procedure must be done before turning a patient onto his side. It ensures that the patient, when turned, is located in the center of the mattress.

Procedure box continued

9. Cross resident's leg closest to you over other leg at ankles.

10. Roll resident away from you by placing one hand under hips and one hand under shoulders.

11. Place one hand under resident's shoulders and one hand under resident's head. Draw resident back toward center of bed.

12. Place both hands under resident's hips and move hips toward center of bed.

13. Put a pillow behind resident's back to give support and keep resident from falling onto his or her back.

14. Be certain resident is in good alignment.

15. Place upper leg on a pillow for support.

16. Replace side rail on near side of bed and return bed to lowest height.

17. You may place a turning sheet under a helpless or heavy resident to help with turning. Use a folded large sheet or half sheet and place it so that it extends just above shoulders and below hips.

18. Wash hands.

A Bend the resident's farthest arm next to her head and place the other arm across her chest. Cross her near leg over the other leg.

B Place one hand on the resident's shoulder and the other on her hip. Turn her away from you onto her side.

C Place pillows under her upper arm and leg for support.

Procedure

Turning Resident Toward You

ALERT: Follow Standard Precautions.

1. Wash hands.

2. Identify resident and explain what you are going to do.

3. Lock bed and elevate to a comfortable working height.

4. Lower side rail on side you are working from.

5. Cross resident's far leg over leg that is closest to you.

6. Place one hand on resident's far shoulder. Place your other hand on the hip.

7. Brace yourself against side of bed. Roll resident toward you in a slow, gentle, smooth movement.

8. Help resident bring upper leg toward you and bend comfortably (Sims position).

Procedure box continued

9. Put up side rail. Be certain it is secure.
10. Go to other side of bed and lower side rail.
11. Place hands under resident's shoulders and hips. Pull toward center of bed. This helps maintain side-lying position.
12. Be certain to align resident's body properly.
13. Use pillows to position and support legs if resident is unable to move self.
14. *Check tubing to make certain that it is not caught between legs or pulling in any way if resident has an indwelling catheter.*
15. Tuck a pillow behind resident's back. This forms a roll and prevents resident from rolling backward onto back.
16. Return bed to low position.
17. Secure call light in resident's reach.
18. Wash hands.

■ RANGE OF MOTION

Range-of-motion (ROM) exercises are very important for the resident who has limited movement. ROM exercises are given to

- Stimulate circulation
- Encourage **flexibility** and mobility of the joints
- Prevent contractures (permanent **contraction** of the muscle)

Residents are encouraged to move each joint to the best of their ability. This is active ROM. When you do passive ROM for your residents, you move the joints for them.

range of motion (ROM) Moving all joints of the body, can be active or passive.

flexibility Ability to bend easily.

contraction Drawing up.

Procedure

Range of Motion

Note: The use of passive and active range of motion (ROM) is related to resident's ability level.

■ Active ROM.   Resident is able to perform all movements without assistance.

■ Passive ROM.   Health care worker moves body parts for resident.

1. Wash hands.
2. Assemble equipment.
   a. Sheet or bath blanket
   b. Treatment table or bed
   c. Good lighting
3. Identify resident.
4. Explain what you are going to do.
5. Ask visitors to wait outside, and provide privacy.

Procedure box continued

ALERT: Follow Standard Precautions.

6. Place resident in a supine position on bed or treatment table and cover with sheet or bath blanket. *Instruct resident to do the following movements at least five times each or to tolerance.*

Head Flexion and Extension

7. Bend head until chin touches chest (flexion) then gently bend backward (extension).

Right/Left Rotation

8. Turn head to right (right rotation), then turn head to left (left rotation).

Right/Left Lateral Flexion

9. Move head so that right ear moves toward right shoulder (right lateral flexion), then move head to central position and continue moving head so that left ear moves toward left shoulder (left lateral flexion).

Shoulder Flexion and Extension

10. Raise one arm overhead keeping elbow straight. Return to side position. Repeat with other arm.

Shoulder Abduction and Adduction

11. Raise arm overhead, then lower, keep arm out to side. Repeat with other arm.

Elbow Flexion and Extension

12. Bend one hand and forearm toward shoulder (flexion) and straighten (extension). Repeat with other arm.

Procedure box continued

Forearm Pronation and Supination

13. Bend arm at elbow and rotate hand toward body (pronation), then rotate away from body (supination). Repeat with other arm.

Wrist Flexion and Extension

14. Bend hand at wrist toward shoulder (flex), then gently force backward past a level position with arm (extension) to below arm level (hyperextension). Repeat with other hand.

Ulnar and Radial Deviation

15. Holding hand straight, move toward thumb (radial deviation), then move hand toward little finger (ulnar deviation). Repeat with other hand.

Finger Flexion and Extension

16. Bend thumb and fingers into hand making a fist or (flexion), then open hand by straightening fingers and thumb (extension). Repeat with other hand.

17. Move thumb away from hand (abduct) then toward hand (adduct). Repeat with other hand.

Finger/Thumb Opposition

18. Move thumb toward little finger, touch tips. Touch tip of thumb to each finger. Open hand each time. Repeat with other hand.

Finger Adduction and Abduction

19. Keeping fingers straight, separate them (abduction), then bring them together (adduction). Repeat with other hand.

Procedure box continued

Hip/Knee Flexion and Extension

20. Raise leg, bend knee, then return to bed straightening knee. Repeat with other leg.

Straight Leg Raising

21. Keep knee straight. Slowly raise and lower leg. Repeat with other leg.

Hip Abduction and Adduction

22. Separate legs (abduction) then bring back together (adduction). Then turn both legs so knees face outward. Turn legs so knees face inward.

23. Rotate one foot toward other foot (internal rotation), then rotate away from other foot (external rotation). Repeat with other foot.

Ankle Dorsiflexion and Plantar Flexion

24. Move foot so that toes move toward knee (dorsal flexion), then move foot so that toes point away from head (plantar flexion). Repeat with other foot.

Toe Flexion and Extension

25. Spread toes apart (abduction) on one foot, then bring toes together (adduction). Repeat on other foot.

26. Turn resident in a prone position.

Arm Abduction and Adduction

27. Move arm toward ceiling; do not bend elbows (hyperextension), then return to bed. Repeat with other arm.

Leg Flexion and Extension

28. Bend leg so that foot moves toward resident's back (flexion), then straighten leg (extension). Repeat with other leg.

29. Position resident for comfort.

30. Place bath blanket or sheet in laundry basket.

31. Wash your hands.

32. Report and document resident's tolerance of procedure.

■ BATHING THE RESIDENT

Providing for your residents' cleanliness is an important responsibility. Bathing is important because it

- ■ Removes perspiration and dirt
- ■ Removes odor
- ■ Increases circulation
- ■ Allows for some exercise
- ■ Gives you an opportunity to observe the residents' skin
- ■ Provides relaxation

You may be asked to give several different types of baths. This depends on the resident's condition. Always check the chart to see what type of bath is ordered. The following are types of baths:

- ■ Bed bath
- ■ Tub bath
- ■ Whirlpool bath
- ■ Shower

Residents may not have a complete bath every day. Sometimes they are bathed only twice a week. This is especially true of elderly residents, who have drier skin, less subcutaneous fat, and more fragile tissues. Always wash the perineum (pericare) and the underarms every day. These areas tend to develop an odor because they have more bacteria and are not open to the air. Good pericare is especially important when there is a urinary catheter in place. Good pericare helps prevent infection.

Procedure

Giving a Bed Bath

1. Wash hands.
2. Assemble equipment.
   a. Soap and soap dish
   b. Face towel
   c. Bath towel
   d. Washcloth
   e. Hospital gown or resident's sleepwear
   f. Lotion or powder
   g. Nailbrush and emery board
   h. Comb and brush
   i. Bedpan or urinal and cover
   j. Bed linen
   k. Bath blanket
   l. Bath basin, water at 105°F
   m. Disposable nonsterile gloves

ALERT: Follow Standard Precautions.

3. Place linens on chair in order of use and place towels on overbed table.
4. Identify resident.
5. Explain what you are going to do.

Procedure box continued

6. Provide for privacy by pulling the privacy screen.

7. Raise bed to a comfortable working height.

8. Offer bedpan or urinal. *Empty and rinse* before starting bath. *Wash your hands.* (Remember to wear gloves when handling urine.)

9. Lower headrest and knee gatch (raised knee area/bed) so that bed is flat.

10. Lower the side rail only on side where you are working.

11. Put on gloves.

12. Loosen top sheet, blanket, and bedspread. Remove and fold blanket and bedspread, and place over back of chair.

13. Cover resident with a bath blanket.

14. Ask resident to hold bath blanket in place. Remove top sheet by *sliding* it to foot of bed. *Do not expose resident.* (Place soiled linen in laundry container.)

15. Leave a pillow under resident's head for comfort.

16. Remove resident's gown and place in laundry container. If nightwear belongs to resident, follow hospital policy (i.e., send home with family or to hospital laundry).

17. To remove gown when the resident has an IV:
    a. Loosen gown from neck.
    b. Slip gown from free arm.
    c. Be certain that resident is covered with a bath blanket.
    d. Slip gown away from body toward arm with IV.
    e. Gather gown at arm and slip downward over arm and tubing. *Be careful not to pull on tubing.*
    f. Gather material of gown in one hand and slowly draw gown over tip of fingers.
    g. Lift IV free of standard with free hand and slip gown over bottle.
    h. *Do not lower bottle! Raise gown.*

18. Fill bath basin two-thirds full with warm water.

19. Help resident move to side of bed nearest you.

20. Fold face towel over upper edge of bath blanket. This will keep it dry.

21. Form a mitten by folding washcloth around your hand.

Procedure box continued

22. Wash resident's eyes from nose to outside of face. Use different corners of washcloth.

23. Ask resident if he or she wants soap used on the face. Gently wash and rinse face, ears, and neck. Be careful not to get soap in eyes.

24. To wash resident's arms, shoulders, axilla:
    a. Uncover resident's far arm (one farthest from you).

    b. Protect bed from becoming wet with a bath towel placed under arm. Wash with long, firm, circular strokes, rinse, and dry.
    c. Wash and dry armpits (axillae). Apply deodorant and powder.

25. To wash hand:
    a. Place basin of water on towel.
    b. Put resident's hand into basin.
    c. Wash, rinse, and dry and push back cuticle gently.

26. Repeat on other arm.

27. To wash chest:
    a. Place towel across resident's chest.
    b. Fold bath blanket down to resident's abdomen.
    c. Wash chest. Be especially careful to dry skin under female breasts to prevent irritation. Dry area thoroughly.

28. To wash abdomen:
    a. Fold bath blanket down to pubic area.
    b. Wash, rinse, and dry abdomen.

    c. Pull bath blanket up to keep resident warm.
    d. Slide towel out from under bath blanket.

29. To wash thigh, leg, and foot:
    a. Ask resident to flex knee if possible.
    b. Fold bath blanket to uncover thigh, leg, and foot of leg farthest from you.
    c. Place bath towel under leg to keep bed from getting wet.
    d. Place basin on towel and put foot into basin.
    e. Wash and rinse thigh, leg, and foot.

    f. Dry well between toes. Be careful to support the leg when lifting it.

30. Follow same procedure for leg nearest you.

31. Change water. You may need to change water before this time if it is dirty or cold.

32. Raise side rail on opposite side if it is down.

Procedure box continued

33. To wash back and buttocks:
    a. Help resident turn on side away from you.
    b. Have resident move toward center of bed.
    c. Place a bath towel lengthwise on bed, under resident's back.
    d. Wash, rinse, and dry neck, back, and buttocks.

    e. Give resident a back rub. Massage back for at least a minute and a half, giving special attention to shoulder blades, hip bones, and spine. *Observe for reddened areas.* (See the procedure "Giving a Back Rub.")
34. To wash genital area:
    a. Offer resident a clean, soapy washcloth to wash genital area.
    b. Give the person a clean wet washcloth to rinse with and a dry towel to dry with.
35. Clean the genital area thoroughly if resident is unable to help. To clean the genital area:
    a. When washing a female resident always wipe from front to back.
    b. When washing a male resident, be sure to wash and dry penis, scrotum, and groin area carefully.
    c. Remove gloves and put in hazardous waste.
36. If range of motion is ordered, complete at this time. (See the procedure "Range of Motion.")
37. Put a clean gown on resident.
38. If resident has an IV:
    a. Gather the sleeve on IV side in one hand.
    b. Lift bottle free of stand. *Do not lower bottle.*

    c. Slip bottle through sleeve from inside and rehang.
    d. Guide gown along the IV tubing to bed.
    e. Slip gown over the resident's hand. Be careful not to pull or crimp tubing.
    f. Put gown on arm with IV, then on opposite arm.
39. Comb or brush hair.

40. Follow hospital policy for towels and washcloths. (Some have you hang them for later use, others have you place them in the laundry containers immediately.)

41. Leave resident in a comfortable position and in good body alignment.
42. Place call bell within reach. Replace furniture and tidy unit.
43. Wash hands.
44. Chart procedure and how resident tolerated it. Note any unusual skin changes or resident complaints.

Procedure

Giving a Partial Bath (Face, Hands, Axillae, Buttocks, and Genitals)

1. Wash hands.
2. Assemble equipment.
   a. Soap and soap dish
   b. Face towel
   c. Bath towel
   d. Washcloth
   e. Hospital gown or resident's sleepwear
   f. Lotion or powder
   g. Nail brush and emery board
   h. Comb and brush
   i. Bedpan or urinal and cover
   j. Bath blanket
   k. Bath basin, water at 105°F
   l. Clean linen, as needed
   m. Disposable gloves

ALERT: Follow Standard Precautions.

3. Identify resident.
4. Explain what you are going to do.
5. Provide privacy by pulling privacy screen.
6. Offer bedpan or urinal. Empty and rinse before starting bath. (Wear gloves if handling body fluid.)
7. Raise headrest to a comfortable position, if permitted.
8. Lower side rails if permitted. If they are to remain up, lower only side rail on side where you are working.
9. Put on gloves.
10. Loosen top sheet, blanket, and bedspread. Remove and fold blanket and bedspread and place over back of chair.
11. Cover resident with a bath blanket.
12. Ask resident to hold bath blanket in place. Remove top sheet by sliding it to the foot of bed: *Do not expose resident.* (Place soiled linen in laundry container.)
13. Leave a pillow under the resident's head for comfort.
14. Remove resident's gown and place in laundry container. If nightwear belongs to resident, follow hospital policy (i.e., send home with family or to hospital laundry).
15. To remove gown when resident has an IV, see the procedure "Giving a Bed Bath."
16. Fill bath basin two-thirds full with warm water and place on overbed table.
17. Put overbed table where resident can reach it comfortably.

18. Place towel, washcloth, and soap on overbed table.
19. Ask resident to wash as much as he or she is able to and tell the person that you will return to complete bath.
20. Place call bell where resident can reach it easily. Ask resident to signal when ready.
21. Remove gloves, wash your hands, and leave unit.
22. When resident signals, return to unit, wash your hands, and put on gloves.
23. Change water. Complete bathing areas the resident was unable to reach. Make sure that face, hands, axillae, genitals, and buttocks are dry. To wash the genital area:
   a. Offer the resident a clean, soapy washcloth to wash genital area. Provide a clean wet washcloth to rinse with and a dry towel to dry with. If resident is unable to help, you will need to clean the genital area thoroughly.
   b. When washing a female resident, always wipe from front to back.
   c. When washing a male resident, be sure to wash and dry penis, scrotum, and groin area carefully.
   d. Remove gloves and put in hazardous waste. If range of motion is ordered, complete it at this time. (See the procedure "Range of Motion.")
24. Give a back rub. (See the procedure "Giving a Back Rub.")
25. Put a clean gown on resident.
26. If resident has an IV, see the procedure "Giving a Bed Bath."
27. Assist resident in applying deodorant and putting on a clean gown.
28. Change bed according to hospital policy. Not all facilities change linen every day.
29. Put side rails up if required.
30. Leave resident in a comfortable position and in good body alignment.
31. Remove and discard gloves.
32. Wash hands.
33. Place call bell within reach. Replace furniture and tidy unit.
34. Chart procedure and how it was tolerated.

Procedure

Tub/Shower Bath

1. Wash hands.
2. Assemble equipment on a chair near the tub. Be certain the tub is clean.
   a. Bath towels
   b. Washcloths
   c. Soap
   d. Bath thermometer
   e. Wash basin
   f. Clean gown
   g. Bathmat
   h. Disinfectant solution
   i. Shower chair if necessary

ALERT: Follow Standard Precautions.

3. Identify resident and explain what you are going to do.
4. Provide privacy by pulling privacy curtain.
5. Help resident out of bed.
6. Help with robe and slippers.
7. Check with head nurse to see if the resident can ambulate or if a wheelchair or shower chair is needed. If a shower chair is used, always do the following:

a. Undress resident in room so that shower is not tied up for long periods of time while residents are dressing or undressing.
b. Cover resident with a bath blanket or sheet so that resident is not exposed in any way.
c. Before leaving room with resident, step back and walk around resident to see if he or she is exposed from any view.

8. Take resident to shower or tub room.
9. For tub bath, place a towel in bottom of tub to help prevent falling.

10. Fill tub with water or adjust shower flow (95–105°F).
11. Help resident undress. Give a male resident a towel to wrap around his midriff.
12. Assist resident into tub or shower. If shower, leave weak resident in shower chair.
13. Wash resident's back. Observe carefully for reddened areas or breaks in skin.
14. Resident may be left alone to complete genitalia area if feeling strong.

Note: If resident shows signs of weakness, remove plug from tub and drain water, or turn off shower. Allow resident to rest until feeling better.

15. Assist resident from tub or shower.
16. Wrap bath towel around resident to prevent chilling.

Procedure box continued

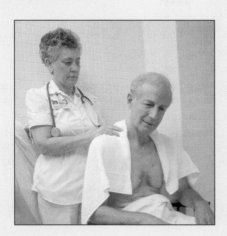

17. Assist in drying and dressing.
18. Return to unit and make comfortable.
19. Put equipment away.

20. Clean bathtub with disinfectant solution.

21. Wash hands.
22. Chart procedure and how resident tolerated it.
Use gloves if you are in contact with body fluids.

Procedure

Resident Gown Change

1. Wash hands.
2. Assemble equipment: clean resident gown.
3. Tell resident what you are going to do.
4. Provide privacy by pulling privacy curtain.

ALERT: Follow Standard Precautions.

5. Untie strings of gown at neck and midback. (It may be necessary to assist resident onto side.)
6. Pull soiled gown out from sides of resident.
7. Unfold clean gown and position over resident.
8. Remove soiled gown one sleeve at a time.
9. Leave soiled gown laying over resident's chest; insert one arm into sleeve of clean gown.
10. Fold soiled gown to one side as clean gown is placed over resident's chest.

11. Insert other arm in empty sleeve of gown.
12. Tie neck string on side of neck.
13. Tie midback tie if resident desires.
14. Remove soiled gown to linen hamper.
15. Slip gown under covers, being careful not to expose resident.
16. Position resident for comfort.
17. Raise side rails when necessary.
18. Place bedside stand and call light in resident's reach.

Use gloves if you are in contact with body fluids.

Perineal Care

1. Wash hands.
2. Assemble equipment.
   a. Bath blanket
   b. Bedpan and cover
   c. Graduate pitcher
   d. Solution, water, or other if ordered
   e. Cotton balls
   f. Waterproof protector for bed
   g. Disposable gloves
   h. Perineal pad and belt if needed
   i. Bag to dispose of cotton balls

ALERT: Follow Standard Precautions.

3. Identify resident.
4. Explain what you are going to do.
5. Provide privacy by pulling privacy curtain.
6. Put warm water in graduate pitcher (about 100°F).
7. Raise bed to a comfortable working height.
8. Lower side rail.
9. Put on disposable gloves.
10. Remove spread and blanket.
11. Cover resident with bath blanket.
12. Have resident hold top of bath blanket, and fold top sheet to bottom of bed.
13. Place waterproof protector under resident's buttocks.

14. Pull bath blanket up to expose perineal area.
15. Provide male and female pericare.
    a. Circumcized male:
       (1) Wipe away from urinary meatus as you wash with soap and water, rinse, and dry.
    b. Uncircumcized male:
       (1) Gently move foreskin back away from tip of penis. Wash as directed in step a. After drying, gently move foreskin back over tip of penis.
    c. Female:
       (1) Instruct resident to bend knees with feet flat on bed.
       (2) Separate resident's knees.
       (3) Separate the labia and wipe from front to back away from the urethra as you wash with soap and water, rinse, and dry.
16. Remove waterproof protector from bed and dispose of gloves.
17. Cover resident with sheet and remove bath blanket.
18. Return top covers.
19. Return bed to lowest position and put side rails up if required.
20. Secure call bell within resident's reach.
21. Put gloves on.
22. Clean equipment; dispose of disposable material according to hospital policy.
23. Discard gloves and wash hands.

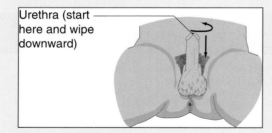

Urethra (start here and wipe downward)

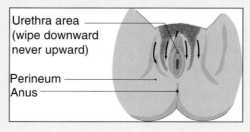

Urethra area (wipe downward never upward)

Perineum

Anus

Vaginal Douche

The doctor may order a vaginal douche for your patient. A vaginal douche is given by flowing a solution into the vagina and letting it flow back out. A douche is given only when the doctor orders it. Douching often removes the normal, protective (good) secretions and can cause increased inflammation or infection. A vaginal douche is used to cleanse the vagina or before an examination

- To remove excessive discharge.
- To reduce inflammation caused by infection.

Procedure

Vaginal Douche

1. Wash your hands.
2. Assemble equipment.
   a. Disposable douche kit
      (1) Tubing clamp
      (2) Douche nozzle
      (3) Irrigating container
   b. Cleansing solution
   c. Cotton balls
   d. Bedpan and cover
   e. Waterproof bed protector
   f. Disposable gloves
   ALERT: Follow Standard Precautions.
3. Identify patient.
4. Explain what you are going to do.
5. Provide privacy by pulling privacy curtains.
6. Put gloves on and offer bedpan; empty after use.
7. Remove and discard gloves; wash hands.
8. Raise bed to comfortable working height.
9. Place waterproof protector under patient's buttocks.
10. Open douche kit.
11. Clamp tubing and pour solution into douche container.
12. Put on gloves.
13. Place bedpan under patient.
14. Pour cleansing solution over cotton balls.
15. Cleanse vulva with cotton balls by spreading lips (labia) and wiping one side from front to back.
16. Discard cotton balls into bedpan. Wipe other side and discard cotton ball.
17. Open clamp to expel air from tubing.
18. Allow solution to flow over vulva. Do not touch vulva with nozzle.
19. Insert douche nozzle into vagina as solution is flowing. Insert about 2 inches with an upward, then downward, and backward gentle movement.
20. Allow solution to flow into vagina while holding douche container no more than 18 inches above mattress.
21. Rotate nozzle until all solution has been used.
22. Clamp tubing and remove nozzle gently.
23. Place nozzle and tubing in douche container for disposal.
24. Assist patient to upright position on bedpan to help drain solution from vagina.
25. Help patient dry perineal area.
26. Remove bedpan.
27. Remove waterproof protector.
28. Empty bedpan; rinse, and put away.
29. Remove gloves and discard according to facility policy.
30. Wash hands.
31. Lower bed to lowest position.
32. Position patient comfortably.
33. Put side rails up if required.
34. Secure call bell within patient's reach.
35. Wash hands.
36. Record procedure.

■ CARE OF HAIR AND NAILS

Hair and nail care helps residents feel good about themselves. Good grooming adds to a feeling of well-being. Hair is always kept clean and neatly arranged. Style hair appropriately for the age of the client. For example, ponytails are not a hairstyle that an elderly person would normally select. If residents can have a tub bath or shower, shampoo their hair at bath time. If they are on bedrest, shampoo their hair while they are in bed.

Procedure

Shampooing the Hair in Bed

ALERT: Follow Standard Precautions.

1. Wash hands.
2. Assemble equipment.
   a. Chair
   b. Basin of water (105°F)
   c. Pitcher of water (115°F)
   d. Paper or Styrofoam cup
   e. Large basin
   f. Shampoo tray or plastic sheet
   g. Waterproof bed protector
   h. Pillow with waterproof cover
   i. Bath towels
   j. Small towel
   k. Cotton balls
3. Identify resident.
4. Explain what you are going to do.
5. Provide privacy by pulling privacy curtain.
6. Raise bed to a comfortable working position.
7. Place a chair at side of bed near resident's head.
8. Place small towel on chair.
9. Place large basin on chair to catch water.
10. Put cotton in resident's ears to keep water out of ears.
11. Have resident move to side of bed with head close to where you are standing.
12. Remove pillow from under head. Cover pillow with waterproof case.
13. Place pillow under resident's back so that when he or she lies down the head will be tilted back.
14. Place bath blanket on bed.
15. Have resident hold top of bath blanket, and pull top covers to foot.
16. Place waterproof protector under head.
17. Put shampoo tray under resident's head (i.e., plastic bag with both ends open).
18. Place end of plastic in large basin.
19. Have resident hold washcloth over eyes.
20. Put basin of water on bedside table with paper cup. Have pitcher of water for extra water.
21. Brush resident's hair thoroughly.
22. Fill cup with water from basin.
23. Pour water over hair; repeat until completely wet.
24. Apply small amount of shampoo; use both hands to massage the resident's scalp with your fingertips. Be careful not to scratch the scalp with your fingernails.
25. Rinse soap off hair by pouring water from cup over hair. Have resident turn head from side to side. Repeat until completely rinsed.
26. Dry resident's forehead and ears.
27. Remove cotton from ears.
28. Lift resident's head gently and wrap with bath towel.
29. Remove equipment from bed.
30. Change resident's gown and be certain resident is dry.
31. Gently dry resident's hair with towel. (Use a hair dryer if allowed by your facility.)
32. Comb or brush hair and arrange neatly.
33. Remove bath blanket and cover resident with top covers.
34. Make resident comfortable.
35. Lower bed to its lowest position.
36. Put side rail up if required.
37. Return equipment.
38. Tidy unit.
39. Wash hands.
40. Record procedure.

Procedure

Shampooing in Shower or Tub

ALERT: Follow Standard Precautions.

1. Assemble equipment.
   a. Shampoo
   b. Washcloth
   c. Towel
   d. Cream rinse, if desired
2. Explain what you are going to do.
3. Instruct resident to tip head back.
4. Wet hair with water, being careful not to get eyes wet.
5. Give resident a washcloth to wipe his or her face as needed.
6. Apply a moderate amount of shampoo to hair. Massage head and hair until a lather develops. (Be careful not to use fingernails.)
7. Rinse hair with clean, clear water until shampoo has disappeared.
8. Repeat shampooing procedure a second time. When rinsing, be sure to remove all shampoo.
9. If a cream rinse is used, apply a small amount to hair, paying special attention to ends of hair.
10. Allow rinse to remain on hair for a few seconds before rinsing.
11. Rinse thoroughly with clean, clear water.
12. Towel dry.
13. Gently comb or brush hair to remove tangles.
14. Use a hair dryer to dry hair.
15. Arrange in an appropriate hairstyle for the resident's age and manner. (Remember that ponytails, pigtails, etc., are not appropriate for a 70-year-old resident.)

Procedure

Arranging the Hair

ALERT: Follow Standard Precautions.

1. Wash hands.
2. Assemble equipment.
   a. Comb and/or brush
   b. Towel
3. Identify resident.
4. Explain what you are going to do.
5. Provide privacy by pulling privacy curtain.
6. Raise bed to a comfortable working height.
7. Assist as needed.
8. If total assistance is needed:
   a. Section the hair, starting at one side, working around to other side.
   b. Comb or brush hair thoroughly, being careful not to pull it.
   c. Arrange hair neatly.
9. Lower bed to lowest position.
10. Put side rail up if required.
11. Secure call light in resident's reach.
12. Clean and replace all equipment.
13. Wash hands.
14. Report procedure and observations (e.g., dry scalp, reddened areas).

Keep nails trimmed and clean. Long nails may scratch the resident or someone else. They break more easily and are more difficult to clean when they are not kept short. Toenails may become very thick and hard. Often it is necessary to have a podiatrist (foot doctor) cut them. If the resident has diabetes, *do not cut the nails*. Diabetic residents tend to have poor circulation and do not heal well. This results in severe **ulcerations** if their skin is knicked or broken. Whenever you cut fingernails or toenails, check first with the charge nurse.

ulcerations Open areas, or sores.

Procedure

Nail Care

ALERT: Follow Standard Precautions.

1. Wash hands.
2. Assemble equipment.
   a. Warm water
   b. Orange sticks
   c. Emery board
   d. Nail clippers
   Do not clip a diabetic resident's nails.
3. Identify resident.
4. Cleanse nails by soaking in water.
5. Use slanted edge of orange stick to clean dirt out from under nails.
6. File nails with emery board to shorten. (Clip if permitted by your facility.)
7. Use smooth edge of emery board to smooth.
8. Apply lotion to help condition cuticle.
9. Massage hands and feet with lotion.
10. Make resident comfortable.

11. Raise side rail if required.
12. Return equipment.
13. Wash hands.
14. Record procedure and any unusual conditions (e.g., hangnails, broken nails).

■ SHAVING THE RESIDENT

Men usually shave every day when they are able to care for themselves. Encourage them to shave themselves when possible. They will feel much better, and their day will be better. If they are unable to shave themselves, take time to shave them. Women tend to have facial hair when they age. This can be very distressing to the resident. Follow the procedures that your facility has to remove the facial hair. In some facilities it is plucked; in others it is shaved. Be certain to look in the procedure book.

Procedure

Shaving the Resident

1. Wash hands.
2. Assemble equipment.
   a. Electric shaver or safety razor
   b. Shaving lather or an electric preshave lotion
   c. Basin of warm water
   d. Face towel
   e. Mirror
   f. Aftershave
   g. Disposable gloves

ALERT: Follow Standard Precautions.

3. Identify resident and explain what you are going to do.
4. Provide privacy by pulling privacy curtains.
5. Raise head of bed if permitted.
6. Place equipment on overbed table.
7. Place a towel over resident's chest.
8. Adjust light so that it shines on resident's face.
9. Shave resident.
   a. If you are using a safety razor:
      (1) Put on gloves.
      (2) Moisten face and apply lather.
      (3) Start in front of ear; hold skin taut and bring razor down over cheek toward chin. Use short firm strokes. Repeat until lather on cheek is removed and skin is smooth.
      (4) Repeat on other cheek.
      (5) Wash face and neck. Dry thoroughly.
      (6) Apply aftershave lotion or powder if desired.
      (7) Discard gloves according to facility policy.

   b. If you are using an electric shaver:
      (1) Put on gloves.
      (2) Apply preshave lotion.
      (3) Gently shave until beard is removed.
      (4) Wash face and neck. Dry thoroughly.
      (5) Apply aftershave lotion or powder if desired.
      (6) Remove gloves.
10. Wash hands.
11. Chart procedure and how procedure was tolerated.

■ DRESSING AND UNDRESSING THE RESIDENT

It is very important for the resident to be up and dressed. Residents must not remain in bed unless the doctor orders bedrest. Being up and dressed gives a feeling of well-being. When the resident is up and dressed, it creates an attitude of wellness. Staying in bedclothes presents an attitude of "being sick." Be certain that residents are dressed nicely and that their clothes are in good repair. Match the clothing rather than just throwing on "anything that's handy."

For residents who have a handicap, take special care in how you put their clothes on. This is also true of residents who have an IV. The following are some rules to follow:

limb Arm, leg.

■ Always dress the weak or most involved side first. A **limb** that does not function well slides into a sleeve or pant leg if you start on that side.

■ Always undress the weak or most involved side last.

■ If the resident has an IV, be very careful not to disturb or dislodge it. Ask your instructor how to do this.

■ PROSTHETIC DEVICES

A prosthesis or prosthetic device replaces or aids a body part that is injured, lost, or not working correctly. These include

■ Dentures
■ Glasses/contact lenses
■ Hearing aids
■ Artificial limbs
■ Artificial eyes
■ Artificial breasts (after mastectomy)
■ Pacemaker

These devices are very important to the well-being of the resident and are treated carefully. You need to learn the correct way to put them on. Your resident is an excellent source of information on how they fit. Always put them in the same place when the resident is not using them so that they are not lost and the resident can find them.

■ BEDMAKING

When bedding is wrinkled or wet it causes irritation to the skin and is very uncomfortable. Keeping the bed smooth and dry prevents decubitus, a severe breakdown of the skin (see the section "Skin Management"). The number of times that you change the bed depends on whether or not the resident is continent. When the resident is in bed, check to be sure that the wrinkles are smoothed out and that the bed is dry.

The hospital bed has a small sheet, called a draw sheet, that is placed in the midsection of the bed between the resident's knees and shoulders. This provides protection to the bottom sheet and can be changed easily without having to change the entire bottom sheet. Often, a plastic cover is placed over the bottom sheet and under the draw sheet to prevent soiling. Be certain that the plastic sheet is always smooth.

There are several ways that hospital beds are made. If the resident is up and around, you make a closed bed. If the resident must remain in bed, you have to make an occupied bed. When the resident is in and out of bed during the day you make an open bed.

Procedure

Making a Closed Bed

ALERT: Follow Standard Precautions.

1. Wash hands.
2. Assemble equipment.
   a. Mattress pad and cover
   b. Plastic or rubber draw sheet (if used in your facility)
   c. Two large sheets or fitted bottom sheet and one large sheet
   d. Draw sheet or half-sheet
   e. Blankets as needed
   f. Spread
   g. Pillow
   h. Pillowcase

A

3. Raise bed to a comfortable working height. Lock wheels on bed.
4. Place a chair at the side of bed.
5. Put linen on chair in the order in which you will use it. (First things you will use go on top.)
6. Position mattress at head of bed until it is against head board.
7. Place mattress cover even with top of mattress and smooth it out.
8. Work on one side of bed until that side is completed. Then go to other side of bed. This saves you time and energy.
9. Bottom sheet is folded lengthwise. Place it on bed with center fold in center of mattress from head to foot. Place large hem to head of bed and narrow hem even with foot of mattress.

10. Open sheet. Check to see that it hangs the same distance over each side of bed.
11. Leave about 18 inches of sheet to tuck under head of mattress.
12. To make a mitered corner:
    a. Pick up edge of sheet at side of bed approximately 12 inches from head of bed.
    b. Place folded corner (triangle) on top of mattress.
    c. Tuck hanging portion of sheet under the mattress.
    d. While you hold the fold at the edge of mattress, bring folded section down over side of mattress.
    e. Tuck sheet under mattress from head to foot. Start at head and pull toward foot of bed as you tuck.

B Grasp the edge of the sheet 10-12 inches from the top of the bed and fold it onto the mattress.

C Tuck the part of the sheet that is hanging down under the mattress.

Procedure box continued

D Bring the folded part down over the mattress.

E Tuck the entire side of the sheet under the mattress.

13. Fold draw sheet in half and place about 14 inches down from top of mattress. Tuck it in. Check to be sure that each piece of linen is straight and even as you tuck it in.

F

14. Top sheet is folded lengthwise. Place on bed.
    a. Place the center fold at center of bed from head to foot.

b. Put large hem at head of bed, even with top of mattress.
    c. Open the sheet. Be certain rough edge of hem is facing up.
    d. Tightly tuck the sheet under at foot of bed.
    e. Make a mitered corner at foot of bed.
    f. Do not tuck sheet in at side of bed.

G

15. Blanket is folded lengthwise. Place it on bed.
    a. Place center fold of blanket on center of bed from head to foot.
    b. Place upper hem 6 inches from top of mattress.
    c. Open blanket and tuck it under foot tightly.
    d. Make a mitered corner at foot of bed.
    e. Do not tuck in at sides of bed.
16. Bedspread is folded lengthwise. Place it on bed.
    a. Place center fold in center of bed from head to foot.
    b. Place upper hem even with upper edge of mattress.
    c. Have rough edge down.
    d. Open spread and tuck it under at foot of bed.
    e. Make a mitered corner.
    f. Do not tuck in at sides.
17. Go to other side of bed. Start with bottom sheet.
    a. Pull sheet tight and smooth out all wrinkles.
    b. Make a mitered corner at top of bed.
    c. Pull draw sheet tight and tuck it in.
    d. Straighten out top sheet. Make a mitered corner at foot of bed.
    e. Miter foot corners of blanket and bedspread.

Procedure box continued

18. Fold top hem of spread over top hem of blanket.

19. Fold top hem of sheet back over edge of spread and blanket to form cuff. The hem should be on the underside so that a rough surface does not come in contact with resident's skin and cause irritation.

20. Put pillowcase on pillow.

    a. Hold pillowcase at center of end seam.

    b. With your other hand turn pillowcase back over hand holding end seam.

    c. Grasp pillow through case at center of end of pillow.

J Grasp the pillow at the center of one end with the hand that is inside the pillowcase.

    d. Bring case down over pillow and fit pillow into corners of case.

    e. Fold extra material over open end of pillow and place it on bed with open end away from door.

H With one hand, hold the pillowcase at the center of the seamed end.

K Pull the pillowcase down over the pillow with your free hand.

I Turn the pillowcase back over that hand with your free hand.

L Straighten the pillowcase.

21. Put bed in lowest position.
22. Wash hands.

Procedure

Making an Occupied Bed

ALERT: Follow Standard Precautions.

1. Wash hands.
2. Assemble equipment.
   a. Draw sheet
   b. Two large sheets or fitted bottom sheet and one large sheet
   c. Two pillowcases
   d. Blankets as needed
   e. Bedspread (if clean one is needed)
   f. Pillow
   g. Disposable gloves if needed
3. Identify resident and explain what you are going to do.
4. Raise bed to comfortable working height. Lock wheels on bed.
5. Place chair at side of bed.
6. Put linen on chair in the order in which you will use it. (First things you will use go on top.)
7. Provide for privacy by pulling privacy curtain.
8. Lower headrest and kneerest until bed is flat, if allowed.
9. Loosen linens on all sides by lifting edge of mattress with one hand and pulling bedclothes out with the other. *Never shake linen: This spreads microorganisms.*
10. Push mattress to top of bed. Ask for assistance if you need it.
11. Remove bedspread and blanket by folding them to the bottom, one at a time. Lift them from center and place over back of chair.
12. Place bath blanket or plain sheet over top sheet. Ask resident to hold top edge of clean cover if he or she is able to do so. If resident cannot hold the sheet, tuck it under resident's shoulders.
13. Slide soiled sheet from top to bottom and put in dirty linen container. Be careful not to expose resident.
14. Ask resident to turn toward the opposite side of bed. Have resident hold onto the side rail. Assist resident if he or she needs help. Resident should now be on far side of bed from you.
15. Adjust pillow for resident to make him or her comfortable.
16. Fan-fold soiled draw sheet and bottom sheet close to resident and tuck against resident's back. This leaves mattress stripped of linen.

17. Work on one side of bed until that side is completed. Then go to other side of bed. This saves you time and energy.
18. Take large clean sheet and fold it lengthwise. Be careful not to let it touch floor.
19. Place sheet on bed, still folded, with fold on middle of mattress. Small hem should be even with foot of mattress.
20. Fold top half of sheet toward resident. Tuck folds against resident's back.
21. Miter corner at head of mattress. Tuck clean sheet on your side from head to foot of mattress.
22. Place clean bottom draw sheet that has been folded in half with fold along middle of mattress. Fold top half of sheet toward resident. Tuck folds against resident's back.
23. Raise side rail and lock in place.
24. Lower side rail on opposite side.
25. Ask resident to roll away from you to other side of bed and onto clean linen. Tell resident that there will be a bump in the middle. (Be careful not to let resident become wrapped up in bath blanket.)
26. Remove old bottom sheet and draw sheet from bed and put into laundry container.
27. Pull fresh linen toward edge of mattress. Tuck it under mattress at head of bed and make mitered corner.
28. Tuck bottom sheet under mattress from head to foot of mattress. Pull firmly to remove wrinkles.
29. Pull draw sheet very tight and tuck under mattress.
30. Have resident roll on back, or turn resident yourself. Loosen bath blanket as resident turns.
31. Change pillowcase.
    a. Hold pillowcase at center of end seam.
    b. With your other hand turn pillowcase back over hand, holding end seam.
    c. Grasp pillow through case at center of end of pillow.
    d. Bring case down over pillow and fit pillow into corners of case.
    e. Fold extra material over open end of pillow and place pillow under resident's head.
32. Spread clean top sheet over bath blanket with wide hem at the top. Middle of sheet should

Procedure box continued

run along middle of bed with wide hem even with top edge of mattress. Ask resident to hold hem of clean sheet. Remove bath blanket by moving it toward foot of bed. Be careful not to expose resident.

33. Tuck clean top sheet under mattress at foot of bed. Make toepleat in top sheet so that resident's feet can move freely. To make a toepleat, make 3-inch fold toward foot of bed in topsheet before tucking in sheet. Tuck in and miter corner.

34. Place blanket over resident, being sure that it covers the shoulders.

35. Place bedspread on bed in same way. Tuck blanket and bedspread under bottom of mattress and miter corners.

36. Make cuff.
    a. Fold top hem edge of spread over blanket.
    b. Fold top hem of top sheet back over edge of bedspread and blanket, being certain that rough hem is turned down.

37. Position resident and make comfortable.

38. Put bed in lowest position.

39. Open privacy curtains.

40. Raise side rails, if required.

41. Place call light where resident can reach it.

42. Tidy unit.

43. Wash hands.

44. Chart linen change and how the resident tolerated procedure.

Procedure

Making an Open Bed

1. Wash hands.
2. Grasp cuff of bedding in both hands and pull to foot of bed.

Fan fold to foot of bed

3. Fold bedding back on itself toward head of bed. The edge of cuff must meet fold. (This is called fan-folding.)

Fold sheet back toward head of bed

4. Smooth the hanging sheets on each side into folds.
5. Wash hands.

■ FEEDING THE RESIDENT

Mealtime is a pleasant time for residents. It is often the most pleasurable event of the day. This should be an unhurried, enjoyable experience. Be certain that the resident is prepared for meals before the food arrives. The preparation for the meal includes the following:

emesis Vomit.

■ Assisting residents or reminding them to wash their hands
■ Removing any unpleasant items from the area, such as **emesis** basins and bedpans
■ Offering the opportunity to use the bedpan or the bathroom
■ Providing for the resident's comfort:

• Raise the head of the bed. • Position the resident in a chair. • Transport the resident to the dining area.

■ Checking to be certain that you have the right tray for the resident and that it is the correct diet
■ Always placing the food within reach
■ Checking the tray to be certain that everything is there
■ Preparing any item that the resident cannot manage
■ Tell the resident where each item is according to the face of a clock if the resident is blind

Procedure

Preparing the Resident to Eat

ALERT: Follow Standard Precautions.

1. Wash hands.
2. Assemble equipment.
   a. Bedpan or urinal
   b. Toilet tissue
   c. Washcloth
   d. Hand towel
3. Assist resident as needed to empty bladder and wash hands and face.
4. Explain that you are getting ready to give resident a meal.
5. Clear bedside table.
6. Position resident for comfort and a convenient eating position.
7. Wash your hands.
8. Identify resident and check name on food tray to ensure that you are delivering the correct diet to resident.
9. Place tray in a convenient position in front of resident.

10. Open containers if resident cannot.
11. If resident is unable to prepare food, do it for resident.
    a. Butter the bread
    b. Cut meat
    c. Season food as necessary
12. Follow the procedure for feeding a resident if resident needs to be fed.
13. Wash hands.

Procedure

Feeding the Resident in the Dining Room

ALERT: Follow Standard Precautions.

1. Wash hands.
2. Help resident take care of toileting needs.
3. Assist with handwashing.
4. Take resident to dining room.
5. Position resident in wheelchair at table that is proper height for wheelchair.
6. Be certain resident is sitting in a comfortable position in wheelchair.
7. Provide adaptive feeding equipment if needed.
8. Bring resident tray.
9. Identify resident.
10. Serve tray and remove plate covers.
11. Provide assistance as needed (e.g., cut meat, butter bread, open containers).
12. Remove tray when finished, noting what resident ate.

13. Assist with handwashing and take resident to area of choice.
14. Wash hands.
15. Record what resident ate.
16. Record I & O if necessary. (See the section "Measuring Intake and Output" later in the unit.)

Procedure

Assisting the Resident with Meals

ALERT: Follow Standard Precautions.

1. Wash hands.
2. Check resident's ID band with name on food tray to ensure that you will be feeding correct diet to resident.
3. Tell resident what food is being served.
4. Ask resident how he or she prefers food to be prepared (e.g., salt, pepper, cream or sugar in coffee).
5. Position resident in a sitting position, as allowed by physician. If ordered to lie flat, turn resident on side.
6. Position yourself in a comfortable manner so that you won't be rushing resident because you are uncomfortable. (Do not sit on bed.)
7. Cut food into small bite-size pieces.

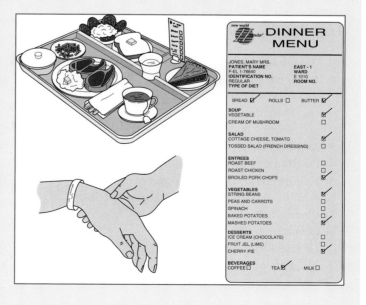

Procedure box continued

8. Place a napkin or small hand towel under resident's chin.

9. Put a flex straw in cold drinks. Hot drinks tend to burn mouth if taken through a straw.

10. Use a spoon to feed resident small to average-size bites of food. (Encourage resident to help self as much as possible.)

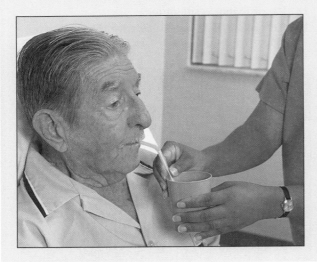

11. Always feed resident at a slow pace. It may take more time for him or her to chew and swallow than you think is necessary.

12. Always be sure that one bite has been swallowed before you give another spoonful to resident.

13. Tell resident what is being served and ask which item he or she prefers first, if resident cannot see food.

14. Encourage resident to finish eating, but do not force.

15. Assist resident in wiping face when resident is finished eating.

16. Observe amount of food eaten.

17. Remove tray from room.

18. Position resident for comfort and safety.

19. Place call light in a convenient place.

20. Wash hands.

21. Record amount of food eaten (half, three-fourths, one-fourth, etc.) on chart, and indicate if food was tolerated well or not well.

Procedure

Feeding the Bed Resident (Self-Help)

ALERT: Follow Standard Precautions

1. Wash hands.

2. Assemble equipment.
   a. Food tray with diet card
   b. Flex straws
   c. Towel

3. Assist resident with bedpan or urinal.

4. Position in a sitting position if possible.

5. Help resident wash hands and face.

6. Remove unsightly or odor-causing articles.

7. Clean overbed table.

8. Check tray with diet card for
   a. Resident's name
   b. Type of diet

   c. Correct foods according to diet (e.g., diabetic, puréed, chopped, regular)

9. Set up tray and help with foods if needed (e.g., cut meat, butter bread, open containers). *Do not add foods to the tray until you check on diet.*

10. Encourage resident to eat all foods on tray.

11. Remove tray when finished and note what resident ate.

12. Help resident wash hands and face.

13. Position resident comfortably.

14. Remove tray.

15. Be certain that water is within reach.

16. Wash hands.

17. Record I & O if required.

18. Record amount eaten.

Procedure

Feeding the Helpless Resident

ALERT: Follow Standard Precautions.

1. Wash hands.
2. Bring resident's tray.
3. Check name on card with resident ID band.
4. Explain to resident what you are going to do.
5. Tuck a napkin under resident's chin.
6. Season food the way resident likes it.
7. Use a spoon and fill only half full.
8. Give food from tip, not side of spoon.
9. Name each food as you offer it if resident cannot see food.
10. Describe position of food on plate (e.g., hot liquids in right corner, peas at the position of 3 o'clock on a clock) if resident cannot see but can feed self.
11. Tell resident if you are offering something that is hot or cold.
12. Use a straw for giving liquids.

13. Feed resident slowly and allow time to chew and swallow.
14. Note amount eaten and remove tray when finished.
15. Help with washing hands and face.
16. Position resident comfortably.
17. Wash hands.
18. Record amount eaten and I & O if required. See following pages for directions on recording I & O.

INTAKE AND OUTPUT SHEET

Hospital #_____   Patient Name _____

Date _____   Room #_____

Time 7-3	INTAKE			OUTPUT			
	BY MOUTH	TUBE	PARENTERAL	URINE		GASTRIC	
				VOIDED	CATHETER	EMESIS	SUCTION
TOTAL							
Time 3-11							
TOTAL							
Time 11-7							
TOTAL							
24 HOUR TOTAL							
24 Hour Grand Total • Intake				24 Hour Grand Total • Output			

Procedure

Serving Nourishments

ALERT: Follow Standard Precautions.

1. Wash hands.
2. Assemble equipment.
   a. Nourishment
   b. Cup, dish, straw, spoon
   c. Napkin
3. Identify resident.

4. Take nourishment to resident.
5. Help if needed.
6. After resident is finished, collect dirty utensils.
7. Return utensils to dietary cart or kitchen.
8. Record intake on I & O sheet if required.
9. Wash hands.
10. Record nourishment taken.

You may have a resident with a nasogastric (N/G) tube. The nasogastric tube is used when the resident has difficulty swallowing or has no swallow reflex. It is a soft, plastic tube that is inserted in the nostril and goes down the back of the throat through the esophagus to the stomach. The tube is taped to the resident's nose. Fluids such as liquid food and medication are put into the tube. Another type of tube is the gastric tube. This tube enters the stomach through the abdominal wall. It is left in place and capped after each feeding. Be very careful not to pull these tubes out.

■ MEASURING INTAKE AND OUTPUT

One of your most important responsibilities is helping the resident with fluid balance. Normally, our bodies maintain this balance without our thinking about it. We take in fluids in our foods and liquids. About the same amount is eliminated by the kidneys (urine), respiration, and perspiration. However, in some residents, fluid balance becomes a very serious problem (see Figure 15–10). Fluid imbalance occurs when fluid stays in the tissues, causing edema, or when there is excessive loss of fluid (dehydration).

Dehydration is caused by

- Diarrhea
- Vomiting
- Bleeding
- Excessive perspiration (diaphoresis)
- Poor fluid intake

If you notice any of the following symptoms of dehydration, report them immediately:

- Fever is present.
- There is a decrease in urine.
- Urine is concentrated.
- Weight loss occurs.
- Membranes are dry, and patient has difficulty swallowing.

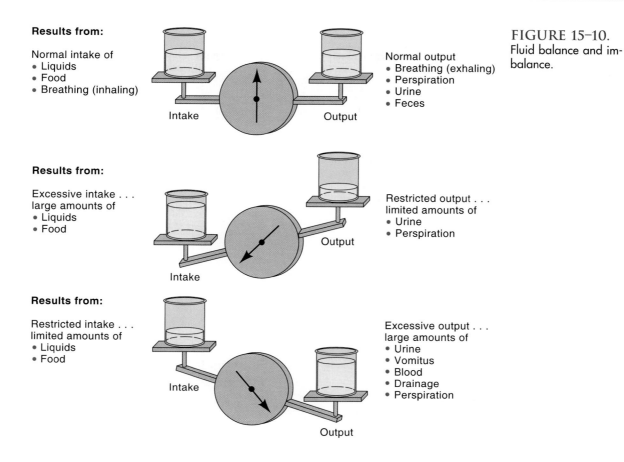

Results from:

Normal intake of
• Liquids
• Food
• Breathing (inhaling)

Intake   Output

Normal output
• Breathing (exhaling)
• Perspiration
• Urine
• Feces

Results from:

Excessive intake . . .
large amounts of
• Liquids
• Food

Output

Intake

Restricted output . . .
limited amounts of
• Urine
• Perspiration

Results from:

Restricted intake . . .
limited amounts of
• Liquids
• Food

Intake

Output

Excessive output . . .
large amounts of
• Urine
• Vomitus
• Blood
• Drainage
• Perspiration

FIGURE 15–10.
Fluid balance and imbalance.

■ Tongue is coated and thickened.
■ Skin becomes hard and cracks and is dry and warm.

Edema is serious; it is caused by

■ High salt intake
■ Infections
■ Injuries or burns
■ Certain kidney diseases
■ Certain heart diseases or heart inefficiencies
■ Sitting too long in one position
■ Infiltration of IV fluid

If you notice any of the symptoms of edema, report them immediately:

■ Decrease in urine output
■ Gain in weight
■ Puffiness or swelling
■ Sometimes shortness of breath

When any of these situations occur, the doctor writes an order to record intake and output (I & O). You record any fluid taken in and any fluid that is eliminated. To measure intake, record the amount of fluid consumed by mouth (see Figure 15–11). Be sure to include the following:

FIGURE 15–11.
Fluid intake.

■ All liquid taken by mouth
■ Any food item that turns to liquid at room temperature (e.g., gelatin, ice cream)
■ All fluid taken by IV or tube feeding

Your facility has a charting method for you to use. Record the amount of liquid taken at the time it is taken. This way, you do not forget this important task. You are probably most familiar with measuring liquid in ounces. When you record liquid intake, you record it in cubic centimeters (cc). This is a metric measure and is used in medical facilities. Most facilities have a chart that helps you determine how many cubic centimeters are in a serving (see Table 15–1). If you need to change ounces to cubic centimeters, use the formula on page 379.

TABLE 15–1 Customary Liquid Measures and Their Equivalents*

1cc/1mL	15 drops
1cc/1mL	1/4 teaspoon
5cc/mL	1 teaspoon
15cc/mL	1 tablespoon
30cc/mL	1 oz
60cc/mL	2 oz
120cc/mL	4 oz
180cc/mL	6 oz
240cc/mL	8 oz (1 cup)
500cc/mL	16 oz (1 pint)
1,000cc/mL	32 oz (1 quart)
4,000cc/mL	64 oz (1 gallon)

*cc, cubic centimeter; mL, milliliter; oz, ounce.

FIGURE 15–12.
Nasogastric suction.

$$30 \times (\text{number of ounces}) = \text{number of cc}$$

For example:

$$30 \times 8 \text{ ounces} = 240 \text{ cc}$$

To measure resident output, measure all

- Urine
- Emesis (vomit)
- Suctioned secretion
- Drainage
- Excessive perspiration

Suctioned secretion (see Figure 15–12) and perspiration are estimated. It is a good idea to have an experienced person help you determine the amount. When you have measured input and output, record them on the chart provided. You may be asked to empty a urinary bag and measure the urine at the end of your shift. The totals are taken each 24 hours. If you notice any unusual recordings, be absolutely certain that you report it.

Procedure

Measuring Urinary Output

1. Wash hands.
2. Assemble equipment.
   a. Bedpan, urinal, or special container
   b. Graduate or measuring cup
   c. Disposable nonsterile gloves
   ALERT: Follow Standard Precautions.
3. Put on gloves.
4. Pour urine into measuring graduate.
5. Place graduate on flat surface and read amount of urine.
6. Observe urine for
   a. Unusual color

   b. Blood
   c. Dark color
   d. Large amounts of mucus
   e. Sediment

7. Save the specimen and report to nurse immediately if you notice any unusual appearance.
8. Discard if urine is normal.
9. Rinse graduate or pitcher and put away.
10. Remove gloves and discard according to facility policy.
11. Wash hands.
12. Record amount of urine in cc on I & O sheet.

■ SPECIAL PROCEDURES

Enemas

You may have the responsibility of giving the resident an enema. Fluid is run into the rectum to remove feces and gas from the bowel. The solution in the bowel causes the resident to feel uncomfortable and want to force the fluid out. Encourage him or her to retain the fluid as long as possible. This gives better results. An enema is given only when there is a doctor's order. There are several different kinds of enemas. These include tap water, soap suds, saline, and prepackaged enemas. An oil retention enema is held in the bowel longer than the cleansing enema. Encourage the resident to retain the oil solution for 20 to 30 minutes. See pages 380–384 for enema procedures.

Procedure

Oil Retention Enema

1. Wash your hands.
2. Assemble equipment.
   a. Prepackaged oil retention enema
   b. Bedpan and cover
   c. Waterproof bed protector
   d. Toilet tissue
   e. Towel, basin of water, and soap
   f. Disposable gloves

ALERT: Follow Standard Precautions.

3. Identify patient.
4. Ask visitors to leave the room.
5. Explain what you are going to do.
6. Put on gloves.
7. Cover patient with a bath blanket, and fan-fold linen to foot of bed.
8. Put bedpan on foot of bed.
9. Place bed protector under buttocks.
10. Help patient into the Sims position.
11. Tell patient to retain enema as long as possible.
12. Open a prepackaged oil retention enema.
13. Lift patient's upper buttock and expose anus.
14. Tell patient when you are going to insert prelubricated tip into anus. (Instruct patient to take deep breaths and try to relax.)
15. Squeeze container until all solution has entered rectum.
16. Remove container; place in original package to be disposed of in contaminated waste according to facility policy and procedure.

17. Instruct patient to remain on side.
18. Remove gloves and discard according to facility policy.
19. Check patient every 5 minutes until fluid has been retained for at least 20 minutes.
20. Position patient on bedpan or assist to bathroom. Instruct patient not to flush toilet.
21. Raise head of bed if permitted if using a bedpan.
22. Place toilet tissue and call bell within easy reach.
23. Stay nearby if patient is in bathroom.
24. Put on gloves.
25. Remove bedpan or assist patient to return to bed. Observe contents of toilet or bedpan for
    a. Color, consistency, unusual materials, odor
    b. Amount of return
26. Cover bedpan and dispose of contents.
27. Remove gloves and discard.
28. Replace top sheet and remove bath blanket and plastic bed protector.
29. Give patient soap, water, and towel for hands and face.
30. Wash your hands.
31. Chart the following:
    a. Type of enema given
    b. Consistency and amount of bowel movement
    c. How the procedure was tolerated

Prepackaged Enemas

1. Wash your hands.
2. Assemble equipment.
   a. Prepackaged enema
   b. Bedpan and cover
   c. Waterproof bed protector
   d. Toilet tissue
   e. Towel, basin of water, and soap
   f. Disposable gloves

ALERT: Follow Standard Precautions.

3. Identify patient.
4. Ask visitors to leave room.
5. Explain what you are going to do.
6. Cover patient with a bath blanket, and fan-fold linen to foot of bed.
7. Put on gloves.
8. Place bed protector under buttocks.
9. Put bedpan on foot of bed.
10. Help patient into the Sims position.

11. Tell patient to retain enema as long as possible.
12. Open a prepackaged enema.
13. Lift patient's upper buttock and expose anus.

14. Tell patient when you are going to insert prelubricated tip into anus. (Have patient take deep breaths and try to relax.)
15. Squeeze container until all the solution has entered the rectum.
16. Remove container; place in original package to be disposed of according to facility policy.
17. Remove gloves.
18. Instruct patient to remain on side and to hold solution as long as possible.

19. Put on gloves.
20. Position patient on bedpan or assist to bathroom. Instruct patient not to flush toilet.
21. Raise head of bed if permitted if patient is using a bedpan.
22. Place toilet tissue and call bell within easy reach.
23. Stay nearby if patient is in bathroom.
24. Remove bedpan or assist patient to return to bed.
25. Observe contents of toilet or bedpan for
   a. Color, consistency, unusual materials, odor
   b. Amount of return
26. Cover bedpan and dispose of contents.
27. Remove gloves and dispose of according to facility policy.
28. Replace top sheet and remove bath blanket and plastic bed protector.
29. Give the patient soap, water, and towel for hands and face.
30. Wash hands.
31. Chart the following:
   a. Type of enema given
   b. Consistency and amount of bowel movement
   c. How the procedure was tolerated

When removing a bedpan, always cover it.

Procedure

Tap Water, Soap Suds, Saline Enemas

1. Wash your hands.
2. Assemble equipment.
   a. Disposable gloves
   b. Disposable enema equipment
      (1) Plastic container
      (2) Tubing
      (3) Clamp
      (4) Lubricant
   c. Enema solution as instructed by the head nurse, e.g.:
      (1) Tap water, 700–1,000 cc water (105°F)
      (2) Soap suds, 700–1,000 cc (105°F), one package enema soap
      (3) Saline, 700–1,000 cc water (105°F), 2 teaspoons salt
   d. Bedpan and cover
   e. Urinal, if necessary
   f. Toilet tissue
   g. Waterproof disposable bed protector
   h. Paper towel
   i. Bath blanket

ALERT: Follow Standard Precautions.

3. Identify patient.
4. Ask visitors to leave room.
5. Tell patient what you are going to do.
6. Attach tubing to irrigation container. Adjust clamp to a position where you can easily open and close it. Close clamp.

7. Fill container with warm water (105°F).
   a. Add one package enema soap for soap suds enema.
   b. Add 2 teaspoons salt for saline enema.
   c. For tap water enema, do not add anything.
8. Provide privacy by pulling privacy curtain.
9. Cover patient with a bath blanket. Remove upper sheet by fan-folding to foot of bed. *Be careful not to expose patient.*
10. Put on gloves.
11. Put waterproof protector under patient's buttocks.
12. Place bedpan on foot of bed.
13. Place patient in the Sims position.
14. Open clamp on enema tubing and let a small amount of solution run into bedpan. (This eliminates air in tubing and warms tube.) Close clamp.
15. Put a small amount of lubricating jelly on tissue. Lubricate enema tip. Check to be certain that the opening is not plugged.
16. Expose buttocks by folding back bath blanket.
17. Lift the upper buttock to expose anus.
18. Tell patient when you are going to insert lubricated tip into anus.
19. Hold rectal tube about 5 inches from tip and insert slowly into rectum.

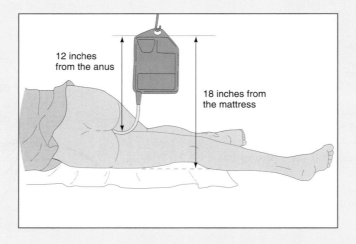

Procedure box continued

20. Tell patient to breathe deeply through mouth and to try to relax.
21. Raise container 12 to 18 inches above patient's hip.
22. Open clamp and let solution run in slowly. If patient complains of cramps, clamp tubing for a minute and lower can slightly.
23. When most of solution has flowed into rectum, close clamp. Gently withdraw rectal tube. Wrap tubing with paper towel and place into enema can.
24. Ask patient to hold solution as long as possible.
25. Help patient onto bedpan and raise head of bed if permitted.
26. Assist patient to bathroom and stay nearby if patient can go to bathroom. Ask patient not to flush toilet.
27. Place call light within reach and check patient every few minutes.
28. Dispose of enema equipment while you are waiting for patient to expel enema. *Follow hospital policy.*

29. Remove bedpan or assist patient back to bed.
30. Observe contents for
    a. Color, consistency, unusual materials
    b. Note amount (i.e., large or small)
31. Cover bedpan and remove bed protector.
32. Remove gloves and dispose of according to facility policy. Wash hands.
33. Replace top sheet and remove bath blanket.
34. Give patient soap, water, and a towel to wash hands.
35. Secure call light in patient's reach.
36. Clean and replace all equipment used and wash your hands.
37. Chart the following:
    a. Date and time
    b. Type of enema given
    c. Results (amount, color, consistency) of bowel movement
    d. How the procedure was tolerated

Harris Flush

Excess gas in the bowel causes **distension** and is very painful. To relieve the excess gas, a Harris flush may be ordered by the doctor. A small amount of water is introduced into the rectum and allowed to flow out. When the irrigation can is lowered, the water runs out of the bowel and gas is removed. This can be repeated several times until the patient is more comfortable and the distension is relieved.

distension Stretched out; bloated.

Procedure

Harris Flush

1. Wash your hands.
2. Assemble equipment.
   a. Disposable gloves
   b. Disposable enema equipment
      (1) Plastic container
      (2) Tubing
      (3) Clamp
      (4) Lubricant
   c. 500 mL of tap water (105°F)
   d. Toilet tissue

Rectal tube

Flatus bag

Tip

Procedure box continued

e. Waterproof disposable bed protector

f. Bath blanket

ALERT: Follow Standard Precautions.

3. Identify patient.

4. Ask visitors to leave room.

5. Tell patient what you are going to do.

6. Attach tubing to irrigation container. Adjust clamp to a position where you can easily open and close it. Close clamp.

7. Fill container with warm water (105°F).

8. Provide for privacy by pulling privacy curtain.

9. Cover patient with a bath blanket. Remove upper sheet by fan-folding to foot of bed. *Be careful not to expose patient.*

10. Put on gloves.

11. Put waterproof protector under patient's buttocks.

12. Place patient in a left Sims position.

13. Place bedpan on foot of bed.

14. Open clamp on enema tubing and let a small amount of solution run into bedpan. (This eliminates air in tubing and warms tube.) Close clamp.

15. Put a small amount of lubricating jelly on tissue. Lubricate enema tubing tip. Check to make certain that opening is not plugged.

16. Expose buttocks by folding back bath blanket.

17. Lift upper buttock to expose anus.

18. Tell patient when you are going to insert lubricated tip into anus.

19. Hold rectal tube about 5 inches from tip and insert slowly into rectum.

20. Tell patient to breathe deeply through mouth and to try to relax.

21. Raise container 12 to 18 inches above patient's hip.

22. Open clamp and let 200 mL of solution run in slowly.

23. Lower irrigating can about 12 inches below level of bed and allow fluid to flow out of rectum into can.

24. Continue process until gas is expelled. When all fluid has returned, clamp tube, and gently withdraw rectal tube. Wrap tubing with paper towel and place in enema can.

25. Position patient for comfort.

26. Dispose of equipment according to facility policy.

27. Remove gloves and dispose according to facility policy.

28. Replace top sheet and remove bath blanket. Straighten bed and make patient comfortable.

29. Put side rails up if required.

30. Secure call bell within patient's reach.

31. Wash your hands.

32. Chart the following:

a. Date and time

b. Type of procedure (Harris flush)

c. Amount of flatus expelled

d. How procedure was tolerated by patient

Procedure

Inserting a Rectal Suppository

1. Wash your hands.

2. Assemble equipment.

a. Ordered suppository

b. Lubricant

c. Disposable gloves

d. Toilet tissue

e. Bedpan with cover

ALERT: Follow Standard Precautions.

3. Identify patient.

4. Ask visitors to leave the room.

5. Explain what you are going to do.

6. Provide privacy by pulling privacy curtain.

7. Raise bed to comfortable working position.

8. Position patient on left side with one knee bent toward chest (left Sims position).

9. Put on gloves.

10. Lift sheet and expose buttocks.

11. Apply lubricant to gloved finger.

12. Apply lubricant around anus.

Procedure box continued

13. Hold suppository between thumb and index finger. Insert gently into anus as far as lubricated index finger will reach.
14. Remove finger and hold toilet tissue against anus for short time.
15. Remove gloves by turning inside out, and discard in hazardous waste.
16. Reposition patient and ask him or her to hold suppository as long as possible.
17. When patient signals for assistance, lower bed and assist to bathroom. Ask patient not to flush toilet.
18. Put on gloves.
19. Provide privacy and assist patient onto bedpan.
20. Raise head of bed to a comfortable position.
21. Provide toilet tissue and place call bell within patient's reach.
22. Remove gloves and discard according to facility policy.
23. Wash hands.
24. Return every few minutes until patient has expelled suppository or had a bowel movement.
25. Put gloves on to help patient clean self.
26. Dispose of waste.
27. Clean bedpan, cover and place in storage area.
28. Remove gloves and discard, and wash hands.
29. Reposition bed to lowest position (if bed patient).
30. Put side rail up if required.
31. Secure call bell within patient's reach.
32. Wash your hands.
33. Record time suppository given and results.

Rectal Suppositories

A rectal suppository is ordered to

- Help relieve constipation
- Soften the feces
- Help regulate the bowel
- Give medications

Ostomy

A patient may require an ostomy (Figure 15–13). When the bowel is diseased or injured, it may be necessary to operate and create a new passage for feces. A part of the bowel is brought through the abdominal wall. Sometimes this is permanent. Sometimes the bowel can be reconnected after it has healed. The new opening is called a *stoma,* and fecal material is expelled through it. This can cause irritation and an unpleasant odor. Patients often feel depressed and may have difficulty accepting the new ostomy. Be careful not to show any reaction that might make them feel worse about themselves. The registered nurse cares for a new ostomy. However, you may be asked to care for one that is not new. The patient needs an ostomy bag to collect the drainage. Skin care around the stoma is very important, and proper placement of the bag requires careful attention. Check the hospital policy before you care for an ostomy.

Some illnesses, injuries, and diseases may require surgery that leaves an opening in the wall of the digestive or urinary tract (see Figure 15–14), such as:

- Into the colon: colostomy
- Into the ileum: ileostomy
- Into the ureter: ureterostomy

FIGURE 15–13.
Common ostomies.

Ileostomy

Descending
colostomy

These openings may be temporary or permanent. Be aware that the resident suffers a change in self-image, which can be very difficult for him or her. Give help by

■ Being a good listener
■ Giving support
■ Keeping the ostomy (opening) clean and dry
■ Being alert for odor that is unpleasant
■ Observing the skin for irritation or breakdown
■ Notifying the charge nurse about any change, pain, or discomfort

FIGURE 15–14
Ostomy appliance in place over the stoma.

Place the wafer over the stoma and attach
a clean bag.

Procedure

Changing an Ostomy Bag

1. Wash your hands.
2. Assemble equipment.
   a. Bedpan
   b. Waterproof bed protector
   c. Disposable gloves
   d. Basin of water and soap
   e. Washcloth
   f. Towel
   g. Skin protector (ordered by doctor)
   h. Biohazard waste bag

ALERT: Follow Standard Precautions.

3. Identify patient.
4. Ask visitors to leave room.
5. Explain what you are going to do.
6. Raise bed to comfortable working height.
7. Position patient on back with head elevated, if allowed.
8. Put waterproof protector on bed next to stoma (opening to ostomy).
9. Fill basin with water (105°).
10. Put on gloves.
11. Place bedpan where you can reach it easily.
12. Expose abdomen; keep genital area covered.
13. Carefully open ostomy belt.
14. Remove soiled or full ostomy bag by gently peeling away from skin. (Use toilet tissue to protect skin from feces.)
15. Put soiled ostomy bag in bedpan.
16. Check contents of ostomy bag for undigested food, blood, or any change in consistency of feces.
17. Remove belt if soiled.
18. Apply lubricant, skin protector, or skin cream around stoma.
19. Carefully observe surrounding area for redness, tenderness, or sores.
20. Place a clean bag over stoma.
21. Remove gloves and discard according to facility policy.
22. Wash hands. Position patient comfortably.
23. Put a clean belt around patient.
24. Lower bed to lowest position.
25. Put side rail up, if required.
26. Secure call bell within patient's reach.
27. Put on gloves.
28. Dispose of bag according to your facility's policy.
29. Wash bedpan and return to storage.
30. Remove gloves and dispose of according to facility procedure.
31. Wash your hands.
32. Document procedure.
33. Report any unusual observations.

■ INCONTINENT RESIDENT

When a resident is incontinent, he or she loses the ability to control the bowel or bladder or both. This is embarrassing to most residents. They are often irritable and depressed. You can help them by having a positive attitude and by being patient and kind. Some of the causes of incontinence are

- ■ Infections
- ■ Surgical problems, e.g., prostate surgery
- ■ Spinal cord injuries
- ■ Loss of sphincter control (muscle control)
- ■ Some diseases, such as multiple sclerosis and central nervous system damage
- ■ Disorientation

Bladder training is one method that is used to help relieve incontinence. This requires the cooperation of the health care workers and the resident. Your part in helping with the retraining of the bladder is to follow instructions carefully. They include the following:

- ■ Keeping a careful intake and output record
- ■ Giving fluids at very specific times
- ■ Taking the resident to void at specific intervals
- ■ Watching for symptoms of bladder distension:

  • Restlessness • Dribbling • Distended lower abdomen • Sensation of pressure • **Residual** urine

residual Left over.

Staying on a schedule is the only way that bladder training can be successful. Everyone who cares for the resident must cooperate.

When bladder training is not successful and urinary incontinence continues, the doctor may order an indwelling catheter (see Figure 15–15). This is a sterile tube that is inserted into the bladder and drains the urine into a bag. Use of the catheter helps keep the resident dry and prevents skin irritation. However, careful technique is absolutely essential, because the catheter also increases the chances of infection. When you are caring for the resident, notice the urine that is in the bag. It should be

- ■ Clear, not cloudy
- ■ Straw-colored, pale yellow (not deep in color)
- ■ 1,200 to 1,500 cc per day; if less than 30 cc per hour, notify the charge nurse

If you notice anything unusual about the urine, report it immediately. This includes blood, mucus, or deep color.

NOTE Never allow the urinary drainage bag to be higher than the hips of the resident. Keeping the bag lower provides drainage away from the urinary bladder. If the drainage bag were higher, urine could flow back into the bladder and cause an infection.

How to Loosely Tape Tubing in Place
(b)

(a)

FIGURE 15–15. Urinary catheter.

Procedure

Disconnecting an Indwelling Catheter

1. Wash hands.
2. Assemble equipment.
   a. Disinfectant
   b. Sterile gauze sponges
   c. Sterile cap or plug
   d. Disposable gloves

ALERT: Follow Standard Precautions.

3. Identify resident.
4. Explain what you are going to do.
5. Put on gloves.
6. Disinfect connection between catheter and drainage tubing where it is to be disconnected by applying disinfectant with cotton or gauze.
7. Disconnect catheter and drainage tubing. *Do not allow catheter ends to touch anything!*

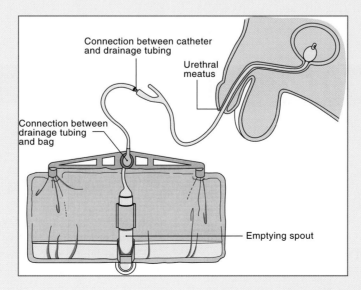

Procedure box continued

8. Insert a sterile plug in end of catheter. Place sterile cap over exposed end of drainage tube.
9. Carefully secure drainage tube to bed.
10. Remove gloves and discard according to facility policy.

11. Wash hands.
12. Record procedure. *Reverse procedure to reconnect.*

Procedure

Giving Indwelling Catheter Care

1. Wash hands.
2. Assemble equipment.
   a. Antiseptic solution
   b. Waterproof bed protector
   c. Disposable nonsterile gloves

ALERT: Follow Standard Precautions.

3. Identify resident.
4. Explain what you are going to do.
5. Provide privacy by pulling the privacy curtains.
6. Put on gloves.
7. Put waterproof protector on bed.
8. Carefully clean perineum.
9. Observe around catheter for sores, leakage, bleeding, or crusting. Report any unusual observation to nurse.
10. For females, separate labia with forefinger and thumb. Apply antiseptic solution around area where catheter enters the urethra.

11. For males, pull back foreskin on uncircumcised resident and apply antiseptic to entire area.
12. Apply antiseptic ointment (if allowed in your facility).
13. Position resident so catheter does not have kinks and is not pulling. *Be sure the tubing is free of kinks and is draining!*
14. Remove waterproof protector.
15. Cover resident.
16. Dispose of supplies according to facility policy.
17. Remove gloves.
18. Position resident comfortably.
19. Secure call light within resident's reach.
20. Wash hands.
21. Record procedure.

Procedure

Urinary Catheter Condom

1. Wash hands.
2. Assemble equipment.
   a. Basin warm water
   b. Washcloth
   c. Towel
   d. Waterproof bed protector
   e. Gloves
   f. Plastic bag

   g. Tincture of benzoin
   h. Condom with drainage tip
   i. Paper towels

ALERT: Follow Standard Precautions.

3. Identify resident.
4. Explain what you are going to do.
5. Provide privacy by pulling privacy curtain.
6. Raise bed to comfortable working height.

Procedure box continued

7. Cover resident with bath blanket. Have resident hold top of blanket, and fold cover to bottom of bed.

8. Put on gloves.

9. Place waterproof protector under resident's buttocks.

10. Pull up bath blanket to expose genitals only.

11. Remove condom by rolling gently toward tip of penis.

12. Wash and dry penis.

13. Observe for irritation, open areas, bleeding.

14. Report any unusual observations.

15. Check condom for "ready stick" surface. If there is none, apply a thin spray of tincture of benzoin. *Do not spray on head of penis.*

16. Apply new condom and drainage tip to penis by rolling toward base of penis.

17. Reconnect drainage system.

18. Remove and dispose of gloves.

19. Pull up top bedding and remove bath blanket.

20. Replace equipment.

21. Lower bed to lowest position.

22. Put side rail up if required.

23. Secure call light within resident's reach.

24. Tidy unit.

25. Wash hands.

26. Record procedure.

Tubing from resident

- Check tubing for kinks.
- Be sure patient is not lying on tubing.
- If level remains the same or increases rapidly, report to your head nurse or team leader.
- Hang plastic urine container on bed frame below level of the patient's urinary bladder.

CC
– 2000
– 1800
– 1600
– 1400
– 1200
– 1000
– 800
– 600
– 400

100
50

Drain for emptying the container

Procedure

Emptying the Urinary Drainage Bag

1. Wash hands.

2. Assemble equipment.
   a. Graduate or measuring cup
   b. Disposable gloves

ALERT: Follow Standard Precautions.

3. Put on disposable gloves.

4. Carefully open drain outlet on urinary bag. *Do not allow container outlet to touch floor!* This will introduce microorganisms into bag and can cause infection.

5. Drain bag into graduate and reattach drainage outlet securely.

6. Observe urine for
   a. Dark color
   b. Blood
   c. Unusual odor
   d. Large amount of mucus
   e. Sediment

7. Report any unusual observations to nurse immediately (do not discard urine).

8. Hold graduate at eye level and read amount of urine on measuring scale.

9. Discard urine if normal.

Procedure box continued

10. Rinse graduate and put away.
11. Remove gloves and discard in hazardous waste.
12. Wash hands.
13. Record amount of urine in cc on the I & O record.

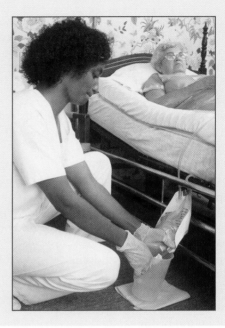

Bowel Incontinence

The resident may be incontinent of stool. This can be more embarrassing for the resident and more unpleasant for you than bladder incontinence. The same principles apply to bowel training as to bladder training:

■ Everyone must participate.
■ A specific time to evacuate the bowel is identified.
■ Avoid between-meal snacks.
■ Give 2,000 cc of fluid intake per day.

There are additional aids for stimulating the bowel and helping to time evacuation. The nurse is responsible for giving these aids, but she relies on the reports of everyone caring for the resident. Mechanical aids used include the following:

■ Suppositories (medication)
■ Laxatives (medication)
■ Enemas

Observe the stool for

■ *Color:* brown, light or dark (may be black from certain medications)—this is reported because black stool can also indicate bleeding.

■ ***Consistency:*** usually soft and formed (report dry, hard stool and stool that is watery, runny, frequent, or has mucus in it).

■ *Odor.*

consistency
Thickness.

Always report a bowel movement and/or any unusual changes.

■ SPECIMEN COLLECTION

Specimens that you collect from your residents are sent to the laboratory and tested. These tests give the physician information that helps him or her treat the resident. It is important that specimens be collected carefully and properly. They must also be labeled correctly.

Urine specimens are collected in different ways. The following are five common urine specimen collection procedures:

■ Routine urine specimen
■ Clean-catch urine specimen
■ Fresh fractional urine
■ 24-hour urine specimen
■ Strained urine

When obtaining urine specimens, always observe and record

■ *Color:* may range from light straw color to dark amber
■ *Clearness, cloudiness,* or *particles*
■ *Odor:* normal, strong, or unusual

Use the urine specimen collection procedures to guide you in the correct way to collect useful specimens.

Other specimens commonly collected for testing include stool and sputum (see Figure 15–16). The stool samples are examined for occult (hidden) blood and for microorganisms. Sputum samples help the physician determine what is causing an illness of the respiratory system.

When obtaining these specimens always observe and record

■ Color
■ Consistency
■ Odor

Use the correct specimen collection procedures to guide you when obtaining these specimens.

FIGURE 15–16.
(a) Collecting the sputum specimen; (b) collecting a stool specimen; (c) straining the urine; (d) collecting a 24-hour specimen

(a)

(b)

(c)

(d)

Procedure

Routine Urine Specimen

1. Wash hands.
2. Assemble equipment.
   a. Graduate (pitcher)
   b. Bedpan or urinal
   c. Urine specimen container
   d. Label
   e. Paper bag
   f. Disposable nonsterile gloves

ALERT: Follow Standard Precautions.

3. Identify resident.
4. Explain what you are going to do.
5. Label specimen carefully:

   a. Resident's name
   b. Date
   c. Time
   d. Room number
6. Provide privacy by pulling privacy curtain.
7. Put on gloves.
8. Have resident void (urinate) into clean bedpan or urinal.
9. Ask resident to put toilet tissue into paper bag.
10. Pour specimen into graduate.
11. Pour from graduate into specimen container until about three-quarters full.

Procedure box continued

12. Place lid on container.
13. Discard leftover urine.
14. Clean and rinse graduate, bedpan, or urinal, and put away.
15. Remove gloves.
16. Position resident comfortably.
17. Assist resident to wash hands.

18. Wash hands.
19. Store specimen according to direction for lab pickup.
20. Report and record procedure and observation of specimen.

Procedure

Midstream Clean-Catch Urine, Female

1. Wash hands.
2. Assemble equipment.
   a. Antiseptic solution or soap and water or towelettes
   b. Sterile specimen container
   c. Tissues
   d. Nonsterile gloves

ALERT: Follow Standard Precautions.

3. Identify resident.
4. Explain what you are going to do.
5. Label specimen:
   a. Resident's name   c. Time obtained
   b. Date
6. If resident is on bedrest:
   a. Put on gloves.
   b. Lower side rail.
   c. Position bedpan under resident.
7. Have resident carefully clean perineal area if able; if not, you will be responsible for cleaning perineum:
   a. Wipe with towelette or gauze with antiseptic solution from front to back.
   b. Wipe one side and throw away wipe.
   c. Use a clean wipe for other side.
   d. Use another wipe down center.
   e. Then proceed with collecting midstream urine.
8. Explain procedure if resident is able to obtain own specimen.
   a. Have resident start to urinate into bedpan or toilet.
   b. Allow stream to begin.

   c. Stop stream and place specimen container to collect midstream.
   d. Remove container before bladder is empty.
9. Wipe perineum, if on bedpan.
10. Remove bedpan.
11. Rinse bedpan and put away.
12. Remove gloves and discard according to facility policy and procedure.
13. Raise side rail.
14. Secure call light in resident's reach.
15. Dispose of equipment. Never handle contaminated equipment without gloves.
16. Wash hands.
17. Record specimen collection.
18. Report any unusual
    a. Color   c. Consistency
    b. Odor

Procedure

Midstream Clean-Catch Urine, Male

1. Wash hands.
2. Assemble equipment.
   a. Antiseptic solution or soap and water or towelettes
   b. Sterile specimen container
   c. Tissues
   d. Disposable gloves

ALERT: Follow Standard Precautions.

3. Identify resident.
4. Label specimen:
   a. Resident's name
   b. Date
   c. Time obtained
5. Explain procedure (if possible allow resident to obtain his own specimen).
   a. Put on gloves.
   b. Cleanse head of penis in a circular motion with towelette or gauze and antiseptic. (If resident is uncircumcised, have him pull back foreskin before cleaning.)
   c. Have resident start to urinate into bedpan, urinal, or toilet. (If he is uncircumcised, have resident pull back foreskin before urinating.)
   d. Allow stream to begin.
   e. Stop stream and place specimen container to collect midstream.
   f. Remove container before bladder is empty.
6. Dispose of equipment according to facility policy.
7. Remove and discard gloves according to facility policy and procedure.
8. Wash hands.
9. Record specimen collection.

Procedure

HemaCombistix

1. Wash hands.
2. Assemble equipment.
   a. Bottle of HemaCombistix
   b. Nonsterile gloves

ALERT: Follow Standard Precautions.

3. Identify resident.
4. Explain what you are going to do.
5. Put on gloves.
6. Secure fresh urine sample from resident.
7. Take urine and reagent to bathroom.
8. Remove cap and place on flat surface. Be sure top side of cap is down.
9. Remove strip from bottle by shaking bottle gently. *Do not touch areas of strip with fingers.*
10. Dip reagent stick in urine. Remove immediately.
11. Tap edge of strip on container to remove excess urine.
12. Compare reagent side of test areas with color chart on bottle. Use time intervals that are given on bottle.

Note: Do not touch reagent strip to bottle.

13. Remove gloves and discard according to facility policy and procedure.
14. Replace equipment.
15. Wash hands.
16. Record results.
    a. Date and time
    b. Name of procedure used
    c. Results

Procedure

Straining the Urine

1. Wash hands.
2. Assemble equipment.
   a. Paper strainers or gauze
   b. Specimen container and label
   c. Bedpan or urinal and cover
   d. Laboratory request for analysis of specimen
   e. Sign for resident's room or bathroom explaining that all urine must be strained
   f. Nonsterile gloves

ALERT: Follow Standard Precautions.

3. Identify resident.
4. Tell the resident to urinate into a urinal or bedpan and that the nurse assistant must be called to filter each specimen. Tell resident not to put paper in specimen.
5. Put on gloves.
6. Pour voided specimen through a paper strainer or gauze into a measuring container.
7. Place paper or gauze strainer into a dry specimen container if stones or particles are present after pouring urine through.

Note: Do not attempt to remove the particles from strainer.

8. Measure the amount voided and record on intake and output record.
9. Discard urine and container according to facility policy and procedure.
10. Clean urinal or bedpan and put away.
11. Remove gloves and discard according to facility policy and procedure.

12. Wash hands.
13. Label specimen:
    a. Resident's name
    b. Date
    c. Room number
    d. Time
14. Return resident to comfortable position.
15. Place call button within reach of resident.
16. Provide for resident safety by raising side rails when indicated or using postural supports as ordered.
17. Wash hands.
18. Report collection of specimen to supervisor immediately.
19. Record specimen collection.

Procedure

24-Hour Urine Collection

1. Wash hands.
2. Assemble equipment.
    a. One-gallon plastic disposable container
    b. Funnel
    c. Graduate (pitcher)
    d. Bedpan, urinal, or specipan (may be called *hat*)
    e. Tag to place over or on bed and in resident's bathroom to indicate that a 24-hour specimen is being collected
    f. Disposable nonsterile gloves
    g. Paper bag

ALERT: Follow Standard Precautions.

3. Identify resident.
4. Explain what you are going to do.
5. Fill in tag with
    a. Resident's name
    b. Date
    c. Time of first collection
6. Fill a large bucket/basin with ice.
7. Place tag over or on resident's bed. This alerts all staff that collection is being taken so that urine is not discarded.
8. When resident/client is on bedrest do the following:
    a. Provide for privacy by pulling privacy curtains
    b. Put gloves on
    c. Offer bedpan/urinal
    d. Ask resident/client to void and put toilet tissue in paper bag
    e. Discard gloves
    f. Wash hands

    When resident/client is out of bed do the following:
    a. Place specipan/hat in toilet
    b. Instruct resident to void into the specipan and to discard toilet tissue into the toilet avoiding the specipan and to turn on call light for attendant to handle specimen
9. Put on gloves.
10. Start the 24-hour collection by discarding the first specimen. Place all additional urine voided into the 24-hour iced container.

11. Remove and discard gloves.
12. Wash hands.
13. Instruct resident to void the final specimen at the end of the 24-hour collection.
14. Put gloves on.
15. Measure specimen and place it in the iced specimen container.
16. Discard ice and process graduate for cleaning.
17. Remove gloves.
18. Wash hands.
19. Record the following:
    a. Amount of the last specimen on I & O sheet
    b. Completion of 24-hour collection in medical record and I & O sheet
20. Notify your supervisor that 24-hour urine collection is complete.
21. Process 24-hour specimen according to facility policy and procedure.
22. Wash hands.

Procedure

Stool Specimen Collection

1. Wash hands.
2. Assemble equipment.
   a. Stool specimen container with label
   b. Wooden tongue depressor
   c. Disposable gloves
   d. Bedpan and cover

ALERT: Follow Standard Precautions.

3. Identify resident.
4. Explain what you are going to do.
5. Be certain container is properly labeled with
   a. Resident's name   c. Time
   b. Date   d. Room number
6. Provide privacy by pulling privacy curtains.
7. Put on gloves.
8. Take bedpan into bathroom after resident has had bowel movement.
9. Use tongue depressor to remove about 1 to 2 tablespoons of feces from bedpan.
10. Place specimen in specimen container.
11. Cover container immediately.
12. Wrap tongue depressor in paper towel and discard.
13. Remove gloves and dispose of according to facility policy.
14. Wash hands.
15. Follow instruction for storage of specimen for collection by lab.
16. Position resident comfortably.
17. Report and record procedure.

Procedure

Occult Blood Hematest

1. Wash hands.
2. Assemble equipment.
   a. Hematest Reagent filter paper
   b. Hematest Reagent tablet
   c. Distilled water
   d. Tongue blade
   e. Disposable gloves

ALERT: Follow Standard Precautions.

3. Identify resident.
4. Explain what you are going to do.
5. Put on gloves.
6. Secure stool specimen from resident.
7. Place filter paper on glass or porcelain plate.
8. Use tongue blade to smear a thin streak of fecal material on filter paper.
9. Place Hematest Reagent tablet on smear.
10. Place 1 drop distilled water on tablet.
11. Allow 5 to 10 seconds for water to penetrate tablet.
12. Add second drop, allowing water to run down side of tablet onto filter paper and specimen.
13. Gently tap side of plate to knock water droplets from top of tablet.
14. Observe filter paper for color change (2 minutes). Positive is indicated by blue halo on paper.
15. Dispose of specimen and equipment according to your facility's policy.
16. Remove gloves and dispose of according to your facility's policy.
17. Wash hands.
18. Report and record results (e.g., date, time, procedure, and results).

Procedure

Sputum Specimen Collection

1. Wash hands.
2. Assemble equipment.
   a. Sputum container
   b. Disposable nonsterile gloves

ALERT: Follow Standard Precautions.

3. Identify resident.
4. Explain what you are going to do.
5. Label container:
   a. Resident's name
   b. Date
   c. Time taken
   d. Room number
6. Put on gloves.
7. Help resident rinse mouth if he or she has just eaten.

8. Ask resident to take three deep breaths. On the third breath tell resident to cough deep from lungs and try to bring up thick sputum. (Saliva is not adequate for this test.)
9. Have resident try several times until you get a good specimen. (You need 1 to 2 tablespoons.)
10. Cover container immediately.
11. Remove gloves and discard according to facility policy.
12. Wash hands.
13. Report to nurse that specimen has been collected. (It needs to go to lab immediately.)
14. Record that specimen has been taken and record color, amount, odor, and consistency.

■ DIABETES MELLITUS

Diabetes mellitus is an endocrine problem. This disease is caused when the islets (islands) of Langerhans in the pancreas do not produce enough insulin. When there is an insulin imbalance, you must watch the resident carefully for signs of diabetic coma or insulin shock. Diabetic coma occurs when the diabetic resident does not have enough insulin, when there is an infection, or if there is increased stress. The following are symptoms of diabetic coma:

- Loss of appetite
- Abdominal discomfort or pain
- Dry skin
- Flushed skin
- Sweet or fruity odor of the breath
- Soft eyeballs
- Generalized aches
- Increased urination
- Air hunger, increased respiration, labored breathing
- Nausea and/or vomiting
- Dulled senses
- Weakness
- Excessive thirst

Insulin shock occurs when the resident receives too much insulin, misses a meal, or exercises too much. *Remember to report a missed meal to the head nurse.* The following are symptoms of insulin shock:

- Excessive sweating, perspiration
- Hunger
- Numbness of tongue and lips
- Faintness, weakness, dizziness
- Headache
- Irritability, personality change, nervousness
- Inability to awaken, stupor, unconsciousness, coma
- Tremors, trembling
- Blurred or impaired vision

Your responsibility in caring for the diabetic resident includes securing a fresh urine sample to test for sugar and acetone. These tests are usually done ½ hour before meals and again at bedtime. A reagent stick test is dipped into the fresh urine to measure glucose, acetone, and protein in the blood. Follow the procedure in Chapter 18, "Using Reagent Sticks to Test Urine." Report any reading on the dipstick above negative to your supervisor. The most common test for glucose levels is the blood test. This test is performed with a glucose meter. The procedure for glucose monitoring with a meter is in Chapter 18, "Monitoring Glucose." These tests are essential for the health of the resident. Errors in testing can result in diabetic coma or insulin shock.

▉ THERAPIES

Oxygen Therapy

Some residents require oxygen to help them breathe. Concentrated oxygen helps these residents breathe more easily. The following are common ways to give oxygen therapy:

- ■ *Nasal cannula:* A two-pronged tube that fits into the nostrils and is secured with an elastic strap that stretches around the back of the head
- ■ *Nasal catheter:* A small tube that fits into a nostril and is secured with tape on the nose and side of the face
- ■ *Mask:* A plastic see-through mask that fits over the nose and mouth and is secured with an elastic strap that stretches around the back of the head

You have specific responsibilities when you care for a resident on oxygen therapy, including the following:

- ■ Ensuring that all oxygen safety rules are followed. Review Chapter 13, Unit 3.
- ■ Checking the elastic strap for chafing and a firm fit.
- ■ Cleaning the cannula, catheter, or mask and checking the skin for irritation.
- ■ Providing oral hygiene by moistening the lips and mouth frequently. Encourage fluid intake if allowed.
- ■ Keeping tubing free of kinks or blockage.
- ■ Checking flow rate and oxygen humidifier frequently.
- ■ Immediately reporting to supervisor any changes or problems, e.g., cyanosis, dyspnea, shortness of breath.

Hot and Cold Applications

You may give hot or cold applications. Be certain that this is allowed by your facility and by state law. These applications help provide healing but must be done correctly. Read the information in Chapter 19 of this text on thermotherapy and cryotherapy and be certain that you have demonstrated competency before giving any treatments.

▉ SPECIAL PRECAUTIONS

Seizure Precautions

Seizures are caused by

- ■ Strokes
- ■ Poisoning
- ■ Infection with high temperature
- ■ **Epilepsy**

epilepsy Chronic disease of the nervous system.

A seizure is serious; the resident can be hurt. A seizure is an involuntary contraction and relaxation of the muscles. There are two common types:

- ■ *Grand mal:* The entire body becomes stiff, followed by the muscles jerking. This lasts several minutes.
- ■ *Petit mal:* The eyes roll back and the muscles may quiver. The resident seems to be daydreaming. This lasts about 30 seconds.

Procedure

Seizure Precautions

ALERT: Follow Standard Precautions as needed.
   If you are with a resident who has a seizure:

1. Use call signal or shout to get help. *Do not leave resident.*
2. Assist resident to lie down to prevent falling.
3. Protect head with pillow or soft cushion.
4. Move furniture to prevent limbs from bumping into it.
5. Turn resident on side to allow secretions to drain from mouth.
6. Observe resident for
   a. Length of time of seizure
   b. Part of body where seizure began
   c. Incontinence
   d. Injury (where and severity)
   e. Severity of convulsions
7. Help resident to bed when seizure is over.
8. Make resident comfortable.
9. Put side rails up.
10. Wrap side rails with blanket, sheet, or soft material to pad them.
11. Wash hands.
12. Chart seizure and observations.
13. Report seizure to charge nurse.

You cannot stop the seizure, but you can follow seizure precautions to help protect the resident from injury. The dangers to the resident include

- Physical injury to limbs and body parts
- Aspiration
- Biting cheeks and tongue if the jaws clamp closed

Syncope

Syncope is another term for fainting. It is caused when the brain does not have an adequate supply of blood. Symptoms of syncope include the following:

- Feeling of uneasiness
- Lightheadedness
- Pale, cool, **clammy** skin
- Dilated pupils

clammy Moist, cold skin.

Several different things can cause this:

- Fear of pain
- Sight of blood or needles
- Emotional disturbance
- Pain
- Long periods of time without movement, causing poor blood circulation
- Dehydration
- Standing up too fast may cause dizziness

If a resident complains of any of these symptoms, take proper precautions to prevent an accident or injury to the resident or to yourself. You should

■ Have the resident put his or her head between the knees, with arms hanging loose at his or her sides. Place your hands on the back of the resident's head. Instruct resident to apply upward pressure with the head.

■ Break open a spirits of ammonia ampule and place under the resident's nose.

■ Have the resident lie down, with the head lower than the legs, if possible.

■ Place a cold towel on the forehead.

■ Loosen any tight clothing.

■ Have resident remain quiet until you are sure he or she has adjusted and is not dizzy.

■ SPECIAL CARE DEVICES

Antiembolism Hose

Antiembolism hose are used to prevent blood from pooling in the legs. This reduces the possibility of developing phlebitis and blood clots. Elasticized hose are called TEDS or antiembolism hose. Sometimes elastic bandages are used. These extend from the ankle or foot to calf or midthigh. They are applied after surgery and when there is danger of a clot forming and causing thrombophlebitis. They must be ap-

Procedure

Elastic Hose (Antiembolism Hose)

ALERT: Follow Standard Precautions as needed.

1. Wash hands.
2. Select elastic hose. Check to be sure that they are the correct size and length.

3. Identify resident.
4. Have resident lie down; expose one leg at a time.

Procedure box continued

5. Hold the hose with both hands at top and roll toward toe end.
6. Place hose over toes, positioning opening at base of toes unless toes are to be covered. The raised seams should be on outside.
7. Check to be sure that the stocking is applied evenly and smoothly. There must be no wrinkles.

8. Repeat on opposite leg.
9. Record the following in the medical record
   a. Date and time applied
   b. Any skin changes, temperature change, or swelling
10. Remove and reapply at least once every 8 hours, or more often if necessary.

plied so that they are smooth and even and do not cut off the circulation. Be certain to remove them and reapply them at least once every 8 hours.

Postural Supports

Soft postural supports (soft cloth ties used on arms and legs, or vests are used to protect elderly or disoriented residents from hurting themselves or someone else (see Figure 15–17). It is much better if you do not have to use them. They can be used only if they are ordered by the doctor. Precautions must be taken when they are used as they may create the following conditions:

■ Increased agitation
■ Immobilized resident
■ Increased risk of pneumonia
■ Skin breakdown
■ Decreased circulation

When postural supports are used, you must

■ Anticipate elimination needs.
■ Check for swelling above, below, and at the site of supports.
■ Release the supports periodically.
■ Provide for hydration by offering fluids.
■ Change position frequently.

There are times when postural support must be used:

■ To prevent resident from pulling out tubes and catheters
■ To prevent resident from scratching or injuring self and others
■ To keep resident from falling out of bed or chair

However, there must be a valid reason for using the supports. Do not use them just because you are annoyed that the resident takes too much of your time.

FIGURE 15–17
Soft protective devices:
(a) limb, (b) vest, (c)
body, (d) mitten

Procedure

How to Tie Postural Supports

ALERT: Follow Standard Precautions.

1. Wash hands.
2. Assemble equipment: a postural support that has been ordered.
3. Tie a half-bow knot or quick release knot. Tie the same way you tie a bow on a shoe. Once bow is in place, grasp one loop and pull end of tie through knot.

4. Knot can be easily released pulling end of loop.

Note: Half bow knot/quick release knot is always used when a restraint is attached to wheelchair or mattress support. This allows quick release if it is necessary to move resident in a hurry.

Procedure

Postural Supports: Limb

ALERT: Follow Standard Precautions.

1. Wash hands.
2. Assemble equipment: a limb support.
3. Identify resident.
4. Explain what you are going to do.
5. Place soft side of limb support against skin.
6. Wrap around limb and put one tie through opening on other end of support (see Figure 15–17a).
7. Gently pull until it fits snugly around limb.
8. Buckle or tie in place so that support stays on limb.
9. Tie out of resident's reach. (See the procedure "How to Tie Postural Supports.")
   a. Tie to bed frame *(not side rails)*.
   b. Tie to wheelchair *(do not tie to stationary chair)*.
10. Check for proper alignment and comfort of resident.
11. Check to be certain that knots or wrinkles are not causing pressure.
12. Check to be certain that support is snug but does not bind. *(You should be able to put two fingers under edges.)*
13. Place call light where it can be easily reached.
14. Check resident frequently and move at least every 2 hours.
15. Chart the following:
    a. Reason for use of support
    b. Type of support used
    c. When it was applied
    d. When it was released
    e. Times of repositioning
    f. How resident tolerated it

Procedure

Postural Supports: Mitten

ALERT: Follow Standard Precautions.

1. Wash hands.
2. Assemble equipment: a soft cloth mitten.
3. Identify resident.
4. Explain what you are going to do.
5. Slip mitten on hand with padded side against palm and net on top of hand.
6. Lace mitten (see Figure 15–17d).
7. Gently pull until it fits snugly around wrist.
8. Tie with a double bow knot so that support stays on hand.

Note: Double bow knot helps secure the restraint to the resident. Use only a half bow/quick release knot to tie a postural support to a bed, wheelchair, or other furniture.

9. Check for proper alignment and comfort of resident.
10. Check to be certain knots or wrinkles are not causing pressure.
11. Check to be certain support is snug but does not bind. *(You should be able to put two fingers under edges.)*
12. Place call light where it can be easily reached.
13. Check resident frequently and move at least every 2 hours.
14. Chart the following:
    a. Reason for use of support
    b. Type of support used
    c. When it was applied
    d. When it was released
    e. Times of repositioning
    f. How resident tolerated it

Procedure

Postural Supports: Vest

1. Wash hands.
2. Assemble equipment: a vest support.
3. Identify resident.
4. Explain what you are going to do.
5. Put arms through armholes of vest with opening to back (see Figure 15–17b).
6. Cross back panels by bringing tie on left side over to right and right tie to left.
7. Carefully smooth material so that there are no wrinkles.
8. Tie where resident cannot reach. (See the procedure "How to Tie Postural Supports.")
   a. Tie to bed frame *(not side rails)*.
   b. Tie to wheelchair *(not stationary chair)*.
9. Check for proper alignment and comfort of resident.
10. Check to be certain that knots or wrinkles are not causing pressure.
11. Check to be certain that support is snug but does not bind. *(You should be able to put two fingers under edges.)*
12. Place call light where it can be easily reached.
13. Check resident frequently and move at least every 2 hours.
14. Chart the following:
    a. Reason for use of support
    b. Type of support used
    c. When it was applied
    d. When it was released
    e. Times of repositioning
    f. How resident tolerated it

■ TERMINAL AND POSTMORTEM CARE

You may be called upon to provide care for someone who is dying. Refer to Chapter 9, Unit Four, "Psychological Stages in the Terminally Ill." This helps you understand the stages the resident goes through. Always be gentle and respectful both before and after death. Before death occurs, gently wash away discharges that have accumulated. As death approaches, the muscles lose their tone and the body openings drain. Gently straighten the limbs and make the resident as comfortable as possible. After death occurs, you may be asked to prepare the body. Check the procedures of the facility you work in and follow the steps your facility provides.

Procedure

Postmortem Care

1. Wash hands.
2. Assemble equipment.
   a. Wash basin with warm water
   b. Washcloth and towel
   c. Shroud/postmortem set:
      (1) Sheet or plastic container
      (2) Strap to tie chin (to keep mouth closed)
      (3) Identification tags
      (4) Large container for personal belongings
      (5) Plastic pad
   d. Gurney or morgue cart
   e. Nonsterile disposable gloves
   ALERT: Follow Standard Precautions.
3. Close privacy curtains.
4. Put on gloves.
5. Position body in good alignment in supine position.
6. Keep one pillow under head.
7. Straighten arms and legs.

Procedure box continued

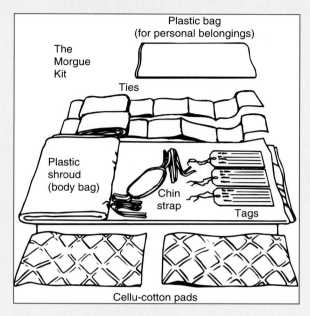

The Morgue Kit

Plastic bag (for personal belongings)

Ties

Plastic shroud (body bag)

Chin strap

Tags

Cellu-cotton pads

8. Gently close each eye. Do not apply pressure to eyelids.

9. Put dentures in mouth or in a denture cup. If placed in a denture cup, put cup inside shroud so that mortician can find.

10. Secure chin with a chin strap. Use pads under straps along side of face to prevent marking.

11. Remove all soiled dressings or clothing.

12. Bathe body thoroughly.

13. Apply clean dressings where needed.

14. Tie wrists loosely together over abdomen. Use pads under ties to prevent marking.

15. Tie ankles loosely together. Use pads under ties to prevent marking.

16. Attach identification tags to wrists and ankles. Fill in tags with
    a. Name
    b. Sex
    c. Hospital ID number
    d. Age

17. Place body in a shroud, sheet, or other appropriate container. Do this in the following way:
    a. Ask for assistance from a co-worker.
    b. Logroll body to one side. Place shroud behind body leaving enough material to support body when rolled back. Fan-fold remaining shroud next to body.
    c. Place a plastic protection pad under buttocks.
    d. Roll body on its back and then to the other side.
    e. Pull fan-folded portion of shroud until flat.
    f. Roll body on its back.
    g. Cover entire body with shroud.
    h. Tuck all loose edges of cover in.
    i. Position a tie above elbows and below knees and secure around body.
    j. Attach ID tag to tie just above elbows.

18. Remove gloves and discard according to facility policy and procedure.

19. Wash hands.

20. Place all personal belongings in a large container. Label container with
    a. Resident's name
    b. Age
    c. Room number

21. Place list of belongings in container and on resident's chart.

22. Follow your facility's procedure for transporting body and belongings through hallways.

23. Remove all linen and other supplies from room.

24. Wash hands.

25. Report procedure completed to charge nurse.

UNIT 2 Advanced Roles/Sub-Acute Care

Steps to success

1. Complete Vocabulary Worksheet 1 in the Student Workbook.
2. Read this unit.
3. Complete Worksheets 2 through 4 as assigned.
4. When you are confident that you can meet each objective for this unit, ask your instructor for the unit evaluation.
5. Complete "Your Link to Success" at the end of this chapter.

Objectives

When you have completed this unit, you will be able to do the following:

✓ List types of services in the sub-acute area.
✓ Explain transitional care.
✓ Describe the nurse assistant's role in the sub-acute area.
✓ List 11 observations for the postoperative patient.
✓ Explain why proper body alignment is important.
✓ List five devices used to align the body and explain how they work.

■ SUB-ACUTE CARE

Patients are often well enough to leave the acute care hospital but not well enough to return to their homes. Many long-term care facilities have a sub-acute area where these patients receive the care and rehabilitation they require. The goal in these units is to provide transitional care at a lower cost than acute care. The lower cost allows care to be provided with less time restraint, allowing the patient to progress according to their level of ability. The goal of transitional care is to help the patient regain physical and living skills through physical therapy and occupational therapy, allowing a return to an independent lifestyle when possible. The nurse assistant is an important part of the interdisciplinary rehabilitation team. The sub-acute area also provides residents in long-term care with additional services when needed. Patients in this specialized care area usually require treatment or services for

■ Postoperative care
■ Complex wound care
■ Intravenous infusions
■ Tracheostomy care
■ Ventilator/respiratory care
■ Multiple trauma and head injuries
■ Stroke care
■ Physical, occupational, and speech therapy

■ RESPONSIBILITIES OF A SUB-ACUTE NURSE ASSISTANT

Nurse assistants in the sub-acute area use all of their CNA skills. They must also learn some additional specialized skills:

- Organize patient care so that it does not interfere with treatment.
- Observe, recognize, and report vital signs, symptoms, and complications.
- Perform neurological checks.
- Protect intravenous lines or Port-a-caths from pulling or dislodging.
- Prevent infection at insertion sites.
- Recognize problems related to intravenous infusions.
- Observe wounds and recognize symptoms of infection.
- Clean the area around tracheostomies.
- Participate on rehabilitation team.
- Observe, recognize, and report problems related to intravenous infusions.
- Observe, recognize, and report problems related to tracheostomy care.
- Observe, recognize, and report changes in patients with head and brain injuries.

NOTE You may use additional or expanded skills. Chapter 25 in the Instructor's Guide provides these skills.

■ POSTOPERATIVE CARE

Patients are in the sub-acute area for monitoring of vital signs and neurological status, pain management, infection control, and rehabilitation. The nurse assistant's role is to monitor the patient carefully and report any changes to the charge nurse. Use Table 15–3 on page 415 as a checklist for monitoring the postoperative patient.

Supportive Devices and Equipment

Fractures and joint replacement are two major areas in sub-acute postoperative care. Keeping the patient in good alignment is very important. Poor alignment can cause a new hip joint to move out of the socket and cause improper healing of fractures. The following are some of the common supportive devices:

- *Trochanter roll:* A towel or small blanket is rolled and put next to the greater trochanter (femur). It keeps the hip from rotating outward and prevents permanent disability or difficulties with walking.
- *Abduction splint:* This is a device that keeps the thighs apart and keeps the hip joints in proper alignment.
- *Abductor wedge:* A wedge-shaped, spongy material is placed between the legs. The wedge is used to keep the hip that has been replaced or fractured away from the center of the body. This prevents excessive strain on the hip and prevents a dislocation of the repair.
- *Footboard:* A padded board is placed at the feet when the patient is in a prone or supine position. The feet naturally extend when lying in this position. If the feet are not aligned correctly, contractures occur and cause problems with walking.
- *Pillows:* Pillows of different sizes and shapes are placed to support joints and provide support for proper body alignment.

Ambulatory Devices

There are many different ambulatory devices, such as walkers, crutches, and canes. These are discussed in Chapter 19.

■ WOUND CARE AND OBSERVATION

Patients who have suffered a trauma or surgery have very specific needs. Their wounds may be life threatening and must be cared for properly. As a nurse assistant, your primary responsibility in caring for wounds includes careful, specific observations and reporting.

You must understand wounds in order to make good observations and reports. Always observe and report the location, size, appearance, and odor of the wound; the condition of the surrounding skin; and the type and amount of drainage. Wounds often have drainage, and there are other complications to watch for. Refer to Table 15–3 for help with observation and charting.

Types of Wounds

Wounds are described as being either *open* or *closed*.

■ *Closed wounds:* Tissue is injured, but the skin is not broken. These wounds can be caused by bruising, sprains, and twists.

■ *Open wounds:* The skin or mucous membrane is broken. These wounds can be caused by bites, cuts, and incisions. Whenever there is an open wound there is a chance of infection.

Open wounds can be either partial thickness or full thickness wounds.

■ *Partial thickness wounds:* The dermis and epidermis are broken.

■ *Full thickness wounds:* The dermis, epidermis, and subcutaneous tissue are penetrated. Muscle and bone may be involved.

The following are some common types of wounds.

■ *Abrasion:* partial thickness wound caused by scraping the skin away

■ *Contusion:* closed wound caused by a blow to the body

■ *Incision:* intentional wound made with a scalpel

■ *Laceration:* open wound with jagged edges and torn tissue

■ *Penetrating wound:* open wound caused by piercing the underlying tissues of the skin

■ *Puncture wound:* open wound caused by a sharp object entering the skin and underlying tissues

■ HOW WOUNDS HEAL

Types of Healing

Wounds are allowed to heal in different ways.

■ *Primary (first) intention:* The wound is pulled together by suturing, stapling, taping, clipping, or gluing. This is a clean wound that usually heals quickly.

■ *Secondary (second) intention:* The wound edges are not brought together. The wound is cleaned, and dead tissue is removed. This method is often used in infected and contaminated wounds.

■ *Third intention:* The wound is left open and may be closed at a later time. Poor circulation and infection are common reasons for using this method.

Medical Emergencies in Wound Healing

Wound healing is dependent on many factors, including the type of wound and the patient's age, nutrition, and lifestyle. The patient's medical history is also very important. Poor circulation, diabetes, some medications, and a weakened immune system can cause complications. The following are major complications:

■ *Dehiscence:* The skin layer and/or the underlying tissues separate, reopening the wound. Stress to the wound from coughing, vomiting, and abdominal distension is usually the cause of dehiscence. This is a surgical emergency. Notify your supervisor immediately.

■ *Evisceration:* The skin layer is separated by the **protrusion** of an internal organ through the wound. The causes are the same as in dehiscence. This is also a surgical emergency. Notify your supervisor immediately.

protrusion Pushing through.

■ *Hemorrhage:* Excessive bleeding that is life threatening. *Hemorrhage is a medical emergency and must be reported to your supervisor immediately.* The patient is in immediate danger.

• *External hemorrhage* is easily seen. Dressings soak with blood and blood may flow under the body. Always check under the patient for pooling blood when you see saturated dressings. • *Internal hemorrhage* cannot be seen. The bleeding is in the tissue of the body and in the body cavities. Signs of internal bleeding include the patient's vomiting blood or coughing up blood, shock, and loss of consciousness. A hematoma may form (i.e., blood collects under the skin, causing swelling and discoloration).

Types of Drainage

Wound drainage occurs during the inflammatory stage of healing when healing fluid and cells escape from the surrounding tissues. The overlying skin heals, but the underlying tissue does not. Drainage that is trapped in the wound and underlying tissue causes swelling and pain and may cause infection. The doctor puts in a drainage tube when large amounts of drainage are expected.

There are several different types of drainage, including the following:

■ *Purulent drainage:* thick green, yellow, or brown drainage.

■ *Sanguineous drainage:* bloody drainage. Large amounts may indicate hemorrhage.

■ *Serous drainage:* watery, clear drainage.

■ *Serosanguineous drainage:* thin, watery, blood-tinged drainage.

Remember always to follow Standard Precautions when in contact with any type of drainage.

■ INTRAVENOUS THERAPY

When a needle or catheter is inserted into a vein it is called intravenous (IV) therapy. IV therapy is ordered to provide fluids when the patient is not allowed to drink or eat; to replace needed vitamins and minerals lost in injury or illness; to administer medications and blood; and to replace sugar for energy.

The following equipment is used for IV therapy:

■ *IV pole:* May be attached to the bed or stand alone. It is used to hang the IV solution.

■ *Solution container:* Plastic bags are most common. You may also see a glass bottle. The containers come in different sizes from 50 to 1,000mL.

■ *Infusion pump:* This is a device that controls the rate of infusion.

■ *Catheters and needles:* These come in different sizes and are inserted into the vein to allow the solution to circulate through the body. A catheter may be implanted in the upper chest area when repeated use is necessary. This is called a peripherally inserted central catheter (PICC line) or Port-a-cath.

■ TRACHEOSTOMY CARE

Tracheostomies may be permanent or temporary. They are permanent when the patient's airway structure is removed due to disease or injury. They are temporary when the patient requires only temporary ventilation. The tracheostomy tube is inserted through an incision in the trachea. Normally, foreign bodies are filtered as they pass through the nose. The patient with a tracheostomy, or "trache," does not have this protection, and foreign bodies such as bacteria enter directly into the lungs. This causes mucus and secretions that make it difficult for the patient to breathe. These secretions must be removed by suction through the tracheostomy. A licensed nurse does suctioning. The patient may be on mechanical ventilation, which means that a machine is moving the air in and out of the lungs to maintain the oxygen supply to the body.

As a nurse assistant, you are responsible for making good observations and reporting them. Use Table 15–3 as a guideline for observing the patient with a tracheostomy.

■ MULTIPLE TRAUMA AND HEAD INJURIES

cerebrovascular accidents (CVA) Complete or partial loss of blood flow to brain tissue caused by blood vessel spasms, intracranial bleeding, and/or obstruction of the blood vessels in the brain.
irreversible Cannot be changed; condition will remain the same.
intracranial Inside the skull.

Accidents and sports injuries cause head and brain injuries. Brain tumors and **cerebrovascular accidents (CVA)** also cause brain trauma. They happen at any age and can cause paralysis, seizures, **irreversible** coma, loss of bowel and bladder control, and mental retardation. Most nerve pathways cross inside the brain. This means that signs and symptoms will appear on the opposite side of the body. The type of impairment depends on which side of the brain is injured and on the severity of the damage (see Table 15–2). Recovery may be very slow, and the patient often has to relearn how to speak, to perform simple tasks, and to function as normally as possible.

A major problem with head and brain injuries is increased **intracranial** pressure caused by bleeding and cerebrospinal fluid. The increased pressure can cause permanent brain injury and brain death. As a nurse assistant, you are responsible for making good observations and reporting them. Use Table 15–3 as a guideline for observing the patient with a head or brain injury.

TABLE 15–2   Possible Results of Left and Right Brain Injuries

Left Brain Injury	Right Brain Injury
Causes partial or complete paralysis of the right side of body, with loss of feeling (e.g., touch, temperature, and pain).	Causes partial or complete paralysis of the left side of body, with loss of feeling (e.g., touch, temperature, and pain).
Affects speech and communication centers; causes aphasia, an inability to communicate verbally.	Affects thought processes, memory, written computation, ability to tell time, judgment of movement, size, and distance.
Patient may act cautiously and slowly.	Patient may act impulsively and unsafely.

TABLE 15-3   Guidelines for the Nurse Assistant in Sub-Acute Care

Postoperative Observations	Loose dressing or dressing with drainage showing through. IV fluid that is not flowing and tubing that is crimped. IV that is beginning to run out. Skin where the needle is placed is swelling, red, or wet. Drainage tubes or catheters that are bent or plugged, or that have unusual-looking drainage. Pulse rate over 100 or below 60. Respirations that are labored, shallow, above 30, or below 14. Changes in blood pressure. Nausea or vomiting. Cyanosis of the skin, lips, or nailbeds. Bleeding. Complaints of pain, or moaning.
Wound Care	Location (e.g., lower-left abdominal quadrant). Size: Measure in centimeters. Measure side to side. Appearance: Is wound red, swollen, discolored, warm to touch? Wound edge parted or closed? Odor: Is it foul or unusual? Surrounding skin: Is it swollen, discolored, intact? Drainage: Observe type and amount.
Intravenous Care	Alarm ringing on infusion pump. Changes in flow rate. Empty or near-empty bottle or bag. Bleeding at site. Puffiness, redness, and swelling at site. Changes in skin temperature, blood pressure. Pulse change (e.g., tachycardia, bradycardia, arrhythemia). Respiration change (e.g., rapid or shallow breathing, shortness of breath, or dyspnea). Confusion or mental changes. Pain (e.g., headache, chest pain). Skin color (e.g., paleness or cyanosis).
Tracheostomy Care	Dislodged tracheostomy tube. Bleeding at site. Bubbling of mucus at site. Respiratory change: rapid, slow, labored. Changes in skin, nailbed color (e.g., cyanosis or grayness). Alarm ringing on mechanical respirator. Any equipment that is loose or kinked.
Head and Brain Injuries	Complaints of headache, blurred or double vision, dizziness. Vomiting. Loss of sensation. Change in ability to move (weakness, paralysis). Changes in vital signs. Slurred or changed speech pattern. Change in alertness. Disorientation and/or confusion. Pupils not equal in size. Pupils do not react to light (i.e., pupil does not become smaller when flashlight is directed at eye). Convulsions.

Thinking Critically:
Check Your Understanding

1. **Communication** Mr. Ramsey doesn't want to get out of bed or to dress. He likes to stay in bed. He sometimes asks to have his breakfast tray brought to him. Then he asks to stay in bed and read. You know that he wants to stay in bed all the time. Explain how you can convince Mr. Ramsey that it is very important for him to get up and to attend activities.

2. **Medical Terminology** Mrs. Sherman experienced a stroke four months ago. Using appropriate medical terms, describe each passive range-of-motion exercise performed on her weak side and what you will say to instruct Mrs. Sherman in how to do active range of motion on her stronger side.

3. **Legal and Ethical** Putting side rails up for patients who are in bed in a long-term care facility is an important part of keeping patients/clients safe. Explain the legal issues of concern related to leaving a bedside rail down with approval.

4. **Patient Education** You are assigned to a new patient who just arrived for admission to the facility. Write a list of things you will explain about safety, daily routine, and meeting the patient's needs. Describe how you will educate the patient and family about each of these items.

5. **Medical Math** Calculate how many cc of fluid Miss White ate during her lunch. She ate the following: turkey sandwich with lettuce and tomato, 8 ounces of cream of mushroom soup, 6 ounces of tea, two chocolate chip cookies, and 4 ounces of sherbet.

Portfolio Connection

Write a description of two patient care events with which you feel you really helped the patient or the patient's family during your training. Include details about how staff and/or instructors were involved in the event.

Write a paper describing your doubts and realizations and the barriers that you were able to overcome during your nurse assistant experience. For example, were you afraid that you couldn't learn to use the equipment? Describe the ways you plan to use the skills, information, and insights that you gained about people and about this job. This assignment must be in standard report format.

HOME HEALTH AIDE

16

Steps to success

1. Complete Vocabulary Worksheet 1 in the Student Workbook.
2. Read this chapter.
3. Complete Worksheets 2 through 5 as assigned.
4. Practice and demonstrate all procedures.
5. When you are confident that you can meet each objective for this chapter, ask your instructor for the chapter evaluation.
6. Complete "Your Link to Success" at the end of this chapter.

Objectives

When you have completed this chapter, you will be able to do the following:

✓ Complete all objectives in Part One of this book.
✓ Complete all objectives in Chapter 15.
✓ Define vocabulary words.
✓ List the following:
  • Five causes of mental impairment
  • Items included when charting
  • Six rights to check when assisting a client with medication
  • Seven basic rules to follow when using household cleaners
  • Ten safety concerns specific to the client's home
  • Eight elements to remember when planning food/menus

✓ Explain the following:
  • Why correct charting is important
  • Proper care of a sterile and nonsterile dressing
  • The basic guidelines to follow when storing medications
  • Why deep breathing is important for bedridden clients
  • The elements of an escape plan to use in case of fire
  • The basic guidelines for food storage
  • The definition of *sterile*
  • The home health aide's responsibilities when there are children in the home
✓ Develop an action plan to use when caring for
  • Children
  • The aged
  • The dying
✓ Demonstrate all procedures in this chapter.
✓ Demonstrate all procedures in Chapter 15.
✓ Complete the following objectives in Chapter 20:
  • List three methods of packaging items.
  • Demonstrate envelope wrap and square wrap.
✓ Apply medical terminology when charting and discussing the patient's/client's condition.
✓ Demonstrate putting on a nonsterile dressing.

■ RESPONSIBILITIES OF A HOME HEALTH AIDE

Home health aides are the members of the health care team who provide personal care for clients at home. They perform a variety of tasks under the supervision of a registered nurse.

As a home health aide, you perform the following skills:

■ Transfer clients from place to place.
■ Assist with bathing.
■ Help clients with walking and prescribed exercise.
■ Help with braces or artificial limbs.
■ Check and record temperature, pulse, and respiration.
■ Check and record blood pressure.
■ Change surgical dressings.
■ Change bed linens.
■ Provide emotional support.
■ Do laundry.
■ Clean clients' living quarters.
■ Plan and prepare meals.
■ Shop for clients' food.
■ Report findings and observations to supervisors.
■ Document daily activities and observations.

■ HOME HEALTH CARE AGENCIES

Home health care agencies are the major employers of home health aides. The goal of most home health care agencies is to promote the highest level of function for their clients. As a home health aide, you are the major personal care provider for your client. A registered nurse will instruct you about the procedures to follow and decide the best plan to follow for the client's care. The home care team includes the following caregivers:

- Physicians
- Therapists
- Social worker
- Nutritionist/dietician
- Registered nurse
- Licensed vocational/licensed practical nurse
- Home health aide
- Homemaker
- Housekeeper
- Sitter/companion

■ WORKING WITH CLIENTS IN THE HOME

Mentally Impaired

Review Unit 2, "Understanding Human Needs," in Chapter 4. When we understand basic needs and the reasons that people react to situations in different ways, we understand some occasional unacceptable behavior in people. In some cases, people who behave in socially unacceptable ways may have some type of mental impairment. Some of these behaviors can be changed through **psychotherapy.** Usually, psychotherapy helps clients who are reacting to their environment, stress, or a lack of problem-solving abilities. Other types of mental impairments may be caused by

- **Heredity**
- Extreme high body temperature
- Impaired circulation
- Drugs
- Venereal disease

Your role in providing care is focused on basic personal care needs and protecting clients from harming themselves and others.

psychotherapy Method of treatment using mental applications, such as hypnotherapy.

heredity Characteristics passed from parent to child.

Ill and Disabled

To fully understand the implications of illness and disability, review Unit 3, "Disabilities and Role Changes," in Chapter 9. An ill or recently disabled person in the home may cause many disruptions. The family unit has longstanding methods for **coping** with all kinds of situations. Do not try to change the coping devices that each family member is using to survive during a difficult situation. As a health care provider, you may observe behaviors and attitudes that create tension and stress. Report these observations to your supervisor. Be a good listener, and use your best health care techniques. This provides a sense of caring and trust. When you establish trust, you help ease unnecessary worry about your ability to give the client or the family proper care.

coping Handling difficult situations.

Children

Review Unit 1, "Development and Behavior," in Chapter 9. Ask your instructor for a copy of *The Pediatric Patient*. As a home health aide, you interact with children of the clients you are caring for. You also interact with children who are assigned to you as clients. Your responsibility in each of these situations differs from household to household. Always discuss with your supervisor your primary responsibility to all family members. When a child is present in the home of a client, always be sensitive to the implications of the client's condition and the environment the child is exposed to. Noise and activity may be restricted for a child. A few positive comments about how much their cooperation is appreciated are helpful. When it is possible, answer children's questions truthfully and openly. If you are uncomfortable discussing questions children ask, *do not ignore them* but refer them to your supervisor or another adult in the household. Remember, children usually like to be helpful, so, when appropriate, include them in teaching about the client's care or condition.

If the child is the client, he or she will be most interested in his or her own care. Do not talk behind his or her back or just outside his or her room. Fears may develop when the child feels that secrets are being kept from him or her. Always remember that you are in a client's home. Do not overstep your bounds with children by disciplining them before you discuss it with the client or other adult in the home.

The Aged

Review Unit 2, "Aging and Role Change," in Chapter 9. It provides information on attitudes and physical changes of the aged. It is important when you are working in clients' homes to respect their wishes about when and how you perform each task. Try to make arrangements that are acceptable to both of you. However, these arrangements should not affect the treatment. Your overall attitude about the aged affects the way you interact with geriatric patients. It is important to evaluate your thinking about older people in general. Consider the following:

- How do you picture an old person?
- What is old?
- When does a person stop being of value?
- Does the amount of money a person has make a difference in deciding that person's value?
- When does a person stop wanting to have fun?
- Is there a time when a person would not be worth your giving of time and energy?

Answer these questions honestly, and then discuss your answers with others. When you discuss the various responses to the same questions, you become more aware of your attitude toward aging.

The Dying

Many people are choosing to die at home rather than in the hospital. They are comfortable in their own environment and feel that they have more control at home. Remember to review the five stages of dying discussed in Chapter 9. These help you understand your clients' many needs and desires. Try to provide a sense of normalcy by keeping the routine standard. Encourage activity as tolerated. Remember, humor and laughter can be the best medicine.

Continued relationships with others are an important part of each day. These relationships provide a sense of being cared about and feeling worthwhile. Take time just to be there for patients (e.g., sit quietly with them, listen to them, have a conversation with them). When you perform your duties in a professional manner and with confidence, your clients and their families maintain a sense of security knowing that all that can be done is being done.

As the moment of death draws near, a spiritual leader may be requested. At this time, ensuring privacy and quiet may be the most important task you perform. Remember that you do not have to agree with the spiritual belief of the household to provide good care at this time. The time of death may be difficult for you as the caregiver, especially if you have provided care for the same client and family for a long period of time. It is all right to express your own sadness, but do not become an extra burden. When providing personal care for the client, always be respectful both before and after death. As death approaches, the muscles lose their tone and the body openings may drain. Before death occurs, gently wash away discharges that have accumulated around the orifices of the body. Gently straighten the limbs and make the patient as comfortable as possible.

When death occurs, the physician must be notified. Before the body is moved to a funeral home, the physician must establish that the client has died. If the cause of death is not certain, an **autopsy** may be required. The agency you work for will have specific procedures to guide you at this time. Usually, you will need to bathe the body and change the bed. This is especially important if family or friends will be viewing the body before it is taken from the home. Always notify your supervisor as soon as possible when a client dies.

autopsy Medical procedure after death to determine the cause of death.

Recording Observations

Insurance companies and other third-party payers **reimburse** for care you provide only when appropriate documentation is prepared in a timely manner. It is essential that you document each procedure you provide for the patient's needs. You must keep your records accurate and up to date. Each agency has specific terms and phrases that it requires for reimbursement purposes. Be sure you use your agency's guidelines when recording observations and procedures. Do not hesitate to ask your supervisor for assistance. Review "Charting and Observation" in Unit 2 of Chapter 5.

reimburse To pay back for something given or spent.

When charting about care given in the home, include the following:

- Caregiver's name, title, and Social Security number
- Client's name and case number
- Date and times care was provided
- Reason for the visit
- Statements describing the client's condition when you arrived
- Statements describing the time, treatment, or activity done and the patient's tolerance of the activity or procedure
- Description of teaching completed
- Your signature
- The client's signature, which is often required

It is important to remember that no matter how efficient you are as a home health aide, if your records are not properly prepared, you may be fired.

Patient/Client Movement and Ambulation in the Home

See the discussion on ambulation in Chapter 19 for ambulation procedures and precautions. In the home, it is important to keep the floor free of clutter. The walking space should be adequate and allow freedom of movement. Throw rugs and carpet edges are hazards and can cause serious falls. Place wide masking tape over carpet edges to prevent tripping. Throw rugs must be secured or picked up. Electrical cords, children's toys, shoes, socks, and any loose items on the floor must be removed to ensure safe ambulation. Clients who have been in bed for a long period of time may be weak. When they are allowed to be out of bed, it helps to have another health care worker assist you until the client shows adequate strength. Ask your supervisor to help you make the appropriate decisions.

Special Procedures

Nonsterile Dressings

Dressings are used to protect an open area on the skin from infection, to absorb drainage, or to keep medicines that aid healing on the open area. The licensed nurse changes sterile dressings (dressings that are free of all living microorganisms). If your patient has a sterile dressing in place and drainage is showing through, tape a sterile dressing over the wet dressing. Make absolutely certain that

Procedure

Dressings: Clean, Nonsterile

1. Wash hands.
2. Assemble equipment.
   a. Clean dressings
   b. Tape
   c. Cleansing solution
   d. Paper or plastic bag
   e. Medication to be applied by patient
   f. Disposable nonsterile gloves
   ALERT: Follow Standard Precautions.
3. Identify patient/client.
4. Explain what you are going to do.
5. Position patient comfortably.
6. Open paper bag.
7. Open clean dressings. *Do not touch center of bandage.*
8. Put on gloves.
9. Remove old dressing and
   a. Check amount of drainage.
   b. Check color, consistency, odor.
   c. Check skin around wound.
   d. Note size of wound.
10. To cleanse wound:
   a. Use circular motions.
   b. Clean from center of wound to skin.

11. Assist client with application of medication, if ordered.
12. Apply clean dressing.
   a. Hold dressing by corner.
   b. Tape bandage securely in place.
13. Discard bandages according to agency procedures.
   a. Close bag with soiled bandages inside.
   b. Tape bag closed.
   c. Discard in covered container.
14. Remove gloves and discard according to agency procedures.
15. Clean equipment and put away.
16. Wash hands.
17. Chart the following:
   a. Time and date
   b. Any observation made:
      (1) Drainage (amount, color, odor)
      (2) Size of wound
      (3) Surrounding skin condition
   c. Type of bandage applied
   d. How procedure was tolerated

you do not touch the area of the dressing that contacts the wet dressing. Notify your supervisor as soon as possible. You may be asked to replace a dressing that is clean (but not sterile).

Assisting with Medication

Each state has guidelines that outline who can and cannot give medications. As a home health aide (including certified home health aide), you are *not* licensed to give medications. If you choose to give medications to a client, you may be fined or held liable for your actions. The agency you work for is also liable for your actions. It is important that you remember this when assisting with medications. There is a legal difference between administration and assisting. The licensed nurse coordinator tells you what medication your client needs and the time it should be taken.

When assisting your client with medications, always check the six "rights."

The Rights of Medication

- The right client — Is the medication order for the correct person?
- The right medication — Is this the correct medication?
- The right time — Is this the prescribed time to take it?
- The right route — How to take it? By mouth, apply to the skin, swallow it, suck on it?
- The right amount — Is this the prescribed quantity?
- Document the right way — Are rights documented in the patient record?

Procedure

Assisting with Medication in the Home

Always follow the six rights of medication.

1. Wash hands.
2. Assemble supplies.
   a. Glass of water or juice
   b. Appropriate medication
   c. Spoon or measuring device, if needed
3. Remind patient when it is time to take medication.
4. Read label on medication.
5. Read physician's order for medication.
6. Read label on medication again.
7. Steady or guide client's hand if necessary.
8. Assist with pouring correct amount of medication into a container. (Pills are to be counted and placed in a container; liquids are measured.)
9. Close medicine container and read label again.
10. Assist patient in taking medication.
11. Record on patient care notes: time, type, route, amount of medication taken.
12. Wipe up spills and replace soiled linen or client's clothing, if necessary.
13. Replace medication in proper storage place.
14. Wash hands.

Medication Guidelines

There are some basic guidelines to follow when assisting with medications:

disoriented Being confused about time, place, and identity of persons and objects.

- Always throw old medications in the toilet where they cannot be taken by others. Old medication loses its strength and does not produce the effect it was prescribed for. It can also become toxic and cause illness. Many medications are dated. Do not use after the expiration date.
- Never allow a client to take medication from an unlabeled container.
- Keep medications out of reach of children and **disoriented** clients.
- Always discuss the placement of medications. Clients may take medication by its placement on a shelf rather than by reading the directions (especially when the client is vision-impaired).

Deep-Breathing Exercises

Deep breathing is an important procedure to remember when working with clients. We normally take a deep breath every few minutes during the day. This deep breath is called a sigh. When we are sleeping or inactive, we do not sigh or deep breathe. Without the sigh, mucus and fluid begin to develop in the lowest part of the lungs. This extra fluid may cause the client to feel short of breath and cause pneumonia. Pneumonia is still a leading complication in most illnesses. You can help prevent this from occurring by encouraging your clients to take a few slow deep breaths every hour. This simple procedure helps remove mucus and fluid from the lungs. Another way to encourage clients to take a deep breath is to have them cough. The cough helps to force fluid and mucus up the bronchial tree and out of the lungs. This keeps the lungs clear.

Sitting the Patient/Client on the Bedside

When getting a client out of bed, it is a good idea to take a few minutes and have the client sit on the side of the bed (dangling his or her legs) and take a few slow, deep breaths. By allowing the client this time and encouraging slow, deep breaths, your client takes oxygen into the lungs, and the blood pressure is able to equalize. (Have you ever felt dizzy after standing up too fast? If so, this probably happened because it took a few seconds for the blood to reach your brain. You do not want this to happen with your client.) Review the discussion on syncope in Chapter 15.

■ STERILIZATION IN THE HOME

It may be necessary to use sterilized articles in the process of caring for your client. Remember that sterilization means that all living microorganisms are dead. Just being clean does not mean that an item is sterile. Many agencies purchase disposable items that are used once and then discarded. It is important to remember that sterile disposable supplies are contaminated when they have been used. Do not try to save money by reusing supplies that are used or opened. Microorganisms are too small to see, so even though an article looks clean, it may be contaminated. You may find it necessary to sterilize items in the home. This can be done in two different ways. The method you use depends on the item to be sterilized. Articles that can tolerate moisture and high heat are sterilized by using wet heat (Figure 16–1). Articles that cannot tolerate moisture are sterilized in a dry heat process (Figure 16–2). When working with clients, always remember the aseptic techniques you learned in Chapter 12. It is essential to practice good technique at

FIGURE 16–1. Wet heat sterilization.

FIGURE 16–2. Dry heat sterilization.

all times. This protects your client, the family, and yourself! Follow the procedure your agency recommends for sterilizing.

■ MAINTAINING A CLEAN ENVIRONMENT

As a home health aide, you may be expected to do some basic cleaning, cooking, and shopping for the client. Your supervisor will establish the jobs that are required to promote the client's progress toward improved health. Your primary responsibility is to the client's health needs. If the environment is not clean, the client may be in jeopardy. The bathroom and kitchen require frequent cleaning to help prevent the spread of microorganisms. You will be expected to keep the bathroom and kitchen clean. It is important for you to understand the client's values concerning cleanliness. Dust on the furniture may be tolerable to the client, but messy cabinets may be intolerable. Things that you are not concerned about may concern the client. To establish a good working relationship, try to discover these details early in your assignment. It usually works best to involve all family members in a plan to maintain a clean environment. A good plan can be organized by deciding what jobs need to be completed each week. Then determine which tasks have to be completed on certain days. Balance the week by assigning tasks to all days so that one day is not extremely busy and another light. When you or your supervisor can encourage the family members to volunteer for some of the tasks, the plan becomes a working agreement.

Housecleaning Method

Try to use the products that are available in the home. If new items are needed, discuss your preferred items, but be flexible and adjust to the products the client prefers. There are a few basic rules to remember when using cleaning products.

■ Never mix cleaning products. They may cause a harmful reaction to occur (e.g., fumes that irritates eyes or lungs, a corrosive effect on the surface being cleaned).

■ Never use cleansers or **abrasive** agents (cleaners with a gritty feel) until you have checked with the client or family. Some newer finishes can easily be scratched.

■ Always read instructions thoroughly and follow them exactly.

■ When using a tub or container of cleaning solution, change the solution before it becomes dirty. Trying to clean with a dirty solution is impossible.

■ Never store cleaning products or tools near food.

■ Discard any bottles that are not labeled.

■ Remember that most cleaners are toxic, so keep them away from children and disoriented clients.

abrasive Compound used to rub away or scrape away another substance.

Procedure

Establishing a Work Plan

1. Evaluate the need for basic household duties to be performed.
2. Make a list of the duties you decide must be routinely completed.
3. Ask the family to make a list of duties they feel must be routinely completed.
4. Plan a meeting with family members to discuss routine duties to be completed.
5. Discuss and agree upon the basic duties that will be done by each member of the family.
6. See sample work plan and use it or develop your own.

Sample Work Plan

Day	Duty	Responsible Person
Monday		
Tuesday		
Wednesday		
Thursday		
Friday		
Saturday		
Sunday		

Remember that bacteria cannot move from place to place on their own. They can move only when carried. The most common carriers of bacteria are dust, insects, pests, and people. Proper cleaning reduces dust and discourages insects and pests. People can reduce the chance of spreading bacteria by remembering the importance of washing their hands after going to the bathroom and before handling food for themselves or others.

■ SAFETY IN THE HOME

The units on safety in Chapter 13 are appropriate for safety in the home. There are additional concerns in the home environment, however, that you need to be aware of.

■ Proper lighting must be available at all times.

■ Floors and walking areas must be free from clutter, and adequate walking space must be available.

■ Stairways need to be blocked by doors or railings to prevent falls.

■ Throw rugs are a hazard and may cause clients to fall. Pick them up to provide a safe walkway.

■ Use wide masking tape on loose carpet edges.

■ Stay with clients while they are smoking, especially if they are sleepy or disoriented.

■ Keep ashtrays clean and free of litter so they do not create a fire hazard.

■ Be alert about how your client and visitors extinguish cigarettes. Watch furniture for smoke or smoldering.

■ The use of extension cords or multiple-socket adapters can create a fire hazard. It is always better to unplug something rather than to overload the electrical system.

■ See that a nonskid pad or decals are placed in showers and tubs to prevent slipping.

■ Safety rails or bars can be installed around the tub and toilet, if necessary, to provide support for an unstable client.

■ Keep all poisons away from food and locked in a cabinet whose use is only for poisons.

■ Be sure that all combustible items are kept away from heat and stored in a cool place.

■ Remember: *No smoking* must be enforced if the client is using oxygen. A No Smoking sign should be displayed.

■ Turn oxygen off before putting a plug in the wall or removing a plug from the wall. The spark that occurs at this time could cause an explosion.

■ A client with portable oxygen must not go into an area where there is an open flame (e.g., gas stove with pilot, water heater with pilot).

The kitchen can be especially hazardous. Keep in mind the following precautions when the client and others are in the kitchen.

■ A fire extinguisher should be available.

■ Keep all handles turned toward the center of the stove when cooking so that they are less likely to be knocked off and so that children cannot pull them off.

■ Do not use towels or aprons to lift hot items. The edges can easily catch fire. Use only potholders that provide adequate protection.

■ Never reach over an open flame. Turn off the flame before reaching.

■ Clients with pacemakers must be kept away from a microwave oven.

■ Check the water heater and house heater area for proper circulation of air. These areas should not be used to store other things. If they are cluttered, they are a fire hazard.

Fire is always unexpected. Taking the proper fire precautions will save lives. Take the time to make an escape plan with the family. Only well-thought-out plans can be implemented with assured success. Don't be caught unprepared. Your plan should include the following:

■ An operational smoke detector, properly mounted in an appropriate location

■ Various routes of escape

■ Properly placed equipment (e.g., drop ladder for a second story or a slide)

■ Method to remove the client in a safe manner

■ An assigned meeting place outside the house

REMINDER Escape is most important, not valuables. Valuables can be replaced. Family members cannot.

■ SHOPPING AND PLANNING FOR MEALS

Review Chapter 10 on nutrition. As a home health aide, you may be responsible for planning, shopping, and preparing meals for your client. It is very important for you to follow the diet ordered by the physician. If the client is on a regular diet, it is important for you to discuss the menus with the client. You also want to know the client's preference for between-meal snacks. When planning menus, keep in mind that the meals should be well balanced over a 24-hour period. Each of the food groups should be included in the proper proportions. For some clients, mealtime is the best time of day. For others, meals are unenjoyable. Every person needs healthy, well-balanced meals to maintain or regain good health. The following are things to keep in mind when planning meals:

■ Prepare nutritionally balanced meals.
■ Do not serve foods that are the same texture.
■ Always plan for a variety of foods.
■ Serve meals in an attractive manner (e.g., a variety of colors present, not all the same color).
■ Keep the cost moderate or within the family budget. Once the menu is decided upon, develop a grocery list.
■ Check the household grocery supply for amounts of food on hand.
■ Be certain that there are enough of the foods used daily.
■ Check other household supplies, such as toilet paper, paper towels, toothpaste, and laundry soap. It saves time if you plan a week's shopping. This keeps you or others from having to return to the store.

specifications Exact way something should be done.

When purchasing food, always check the labels of packaged foods. The ingredients are important for people on special diets. The ingredients are listed according to the amount of each item in the package (see Table 16–1). If your client is on a restricted diet, you must carefully select food that meets the diet's **specifications.** If you are unsure, do not buy it. Check with the doctor or your supervisor first.

Storing Food

Proper storage of food is essential. If food is not properly stored, nutrients are lost, and foods may spoil before they are used. Proper storage also prevents the growth of bacteria. Only use foods that are fresh. Discard the following:

■ All food with an expired date
■ Foods that have a strange smell
■ Foods that are moldy

TABLE 16–1   Hot Cocoa Mix Ingredients
sugar
sweet dairy whey
cocoa
corn syrup
solids
nonfat dry milk
hydrogenated vegetable oil
vanilla flavoring

Sugar is the largest amount. Vanilla flavoring is the smallest amount. You might not realize how much sugar is in cocoa mix unless you read the ingredients.

The following are basic guidelines for food storage:

■ Use meat within 48 hours of placing in the refrigerator.

■ Defrost frozen meat in the refrigerator, not on a counter in the kitchen.

■ Fish spoils rapidly. Prepare it as soon as possible after purchase.

■ Fruits and vegetables remain fresh longer if they are kept in the refrigerator. Fruits that are not ripe will ripen faster if placed at room temperature.

■ Breads can be frozen if wrapped carefully or kept in an airtight container. In humid climates, bread will develop mold faster than it will in dry climates.

■ Milk should be refrigerated. Nonfat milk will last longer than whole milk or lowfat milk because there is no fat to sour.

■ Canned foods should be stored in a cool, dark place.

■ Frozen foods can be stored for long periods as long as they remain frozen. Once they have started to thaw, they should be cooked, and then they can be re-frozen. A cookbook will provide guidelines for the safe freezing periods of most foods.

Preparing Food

Food preparation varies from person to person. Discuss with clients their food preferences. Try to please them by preparing foods as close to their desires as possible. If they express a desire to try a special food, or if they especially like the way you prepare food, feel free to use your imagination. Your main restrictions are the ordered diet the client must follow.

Your link to success

Thinking Critically:
Check Your Understanding

1. **Communication** Mr. Vanderlong had a stroke six months ago. He is gradually recovering his speech and mobility. He is still very slow about moving from place to place. He prefers using his walker to the using the wheelchair. When you have a lot to do, it is easier to move him in the wheelchair. What should you do and say, and why?

2. **Legal and Ethical** Mr. Dimas is very ill. He asks you to arrange for his priest to visit. You belong to a different religion and do not approve of his. You wonder if it is a good idea to call your minister to see him. What should you do, and why?

3. **Patient Education** Write down instructions you would give to a patient or the patient's family explaining what to do when a sterile dressing becomes saturated with drainage.

4. **Medical Math** In the home where you are working, all containers are marked in ounces, pints, and quarts. The agency you work for requires that you chart all intake in cubic centimeters (cc). Choose three examples of containers marked in ounces and convert the measurements to cc.

5. **Case Study** Johnny is a 4-year-old you have taken care of for about five months. He has leukemia, and it cannot be cured. You are very attached to him because he is such a loving child. Everyone around him feels very sad that he is going to die soon. What do you think you will feel when he dies, and how will you react to this situation?

Portfolio Connection

Once you attain competence as a home health aide, ask for permission to copy your documentation. (Remove all patient identifiers.) Place this copy in your portfolio as evidence of your skills. Place a copy of your on-site trainer's evaluation in your portfolio.

Write a paper describing your doubts and realizations and the barriers that you were able to overcome during the home health aide experience. For example, were you afraid that you couldn't learn to use the equipment? Describe the ways you plan to use the skills, information, and insights that you gained about people and about this job. This assignment must be in standard report format.

ELECTROCARDIOGRAM TECHNICIAN

17

Steps to success

1. Read this chapter.
2. Complete Worksheets 1 and 2 in the Student Workbook as assigned.
3. Practice and demonstrate all procedures.
4. When you are confident that you can meet each objective for this chapter, ask your instructor for the chapter evaluation.
5. Complete "Your Link to Success" at the end of this chapter.

Objectives

When you have completed this chapter, you will be able to do the following:

EKG/ECG Graphic record of the electrical currents produced by the heart.

✓ Complete all objectives in Part One of this book.
✓ Match vocabulary words with their correct meanings.
✓ List two reasons why the doctor orders an **EKG/ECG.***
✓ List four conditions that are determined by an EKG/ECG.
✓ Label a diagram of an EKG/ECG machine and describe the function of each part.
✓ Label a normal EKG/ECG complex.
✓ List three waves recorded on the EKG/ECG cycle, and relate them to the activity of the heart.
✓ List the 12 leads recorded on an EKG/ECG.
✓ Identify the leads according to color and correct placement.
✓ List three common sources of artifacts.

*EKG/ECG are both used to indicate an electrocardiogram. Either is correct.

✓ Identify eight common causes of artifacts and their remedies.

✓ Perform an EKG.

✓ Mount EKG/ECG readings.

✓ Compare and contrast normal EKG/ECG readings with abnormal readings.

✓ Attach a Holter monitor to a patient and give clear instructions to the patient.

✓ Explain what a Holter monitor records and why it is used for diagnostic purposes.

✓ Demonstrate the following skills:
- From Chapter 15: Pivot transfer from bed to wheelchair and back
  Sliding from bed to gurney and back
  Moving a patient/client in a wheelchair
  Moving a patient/client on a gurney
- From Chapter 22: List five filing systems.
  Demonstrate alpha and numeric filing.

■ RESPONSIBILITIES OF AN EKG/ECG TECHNICIAN

irregularities Different than normal.

An ECG technician works in a general hospital or clinic, or for a physician in private practice. ECG technicians operate equipment that makes a record of the electrical changes that occur during a heartbeat. These recordings help physicians diagnose **irregularities** or changes in the patient's/client's heart. These tests are done routinely after a client reaches a certain age, before surgery, and as a diagnostic tool to detect heart disease and dysfunctions, such as

■ Previous heart attack

■ **Heart block**

heart block Interference with the conduction of the electrical impulses of the heart that is either partial or complete.

■ Enlarged heart muscle

■ Rhythm disturbances

As an EKG technician, you are required to do the following tasks:

■ Prepare patients/clients for testing.

■ Operate the EKG machine and record 12-lead EKG rhythm strips.

■ Mount EKG strips.

■ File paperwork.

■ Maintain equipment and order supplies.

■ Prepare copies of EKGs.

■ Notify your supervisor immediately of deviations from normal on EKG strips.

■ Transport patient/client.

■ ELECTROCARDIOGRAPH

electrocardiograph Instrument that records electric currents produced by the heart.

An EKG/ECG is taken with an **electrocardiograph.** An ECG shows the path of the electrical stimulation to the heart.

ECG Functions

See Figure 17–1.

■ *Electrodes* are small pieces of metal that pick up the electrical activity of the heart.

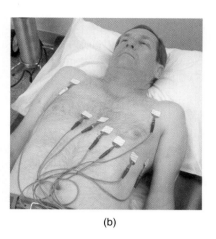

(b)

(a)

FIGURE 17–1.
ECG technician performing an ECG on a client.

■ *Leads* are wires carrying impulses from the electrodes on the patient's skin to the machine.

■ *Lead indicator switches* (on old machines) tell the machine which lead to read.

■ The *stylus* records the heart's electrical activity on graph paper.

■ *Amplifiers* **magnify** the electrical signal the heart generates so that it can be recorded.

■ *Speed switches* regulate the speed at which the graph paper runs through the machine.

■ *Standardization buttons* (on old machines) are like a ruler. They are a guide to the physician reading the ECG. If you forget to use the standardization button, the ECG may be read incorrectly (see Figure 17–2 for a strip standardization indicator).

■ The *sensitivity switch* changes the height of the standard measurement.

■ EKG/ECG machines record single leads (Figure 17–3 on page 434) or multi-channel lead strips (Figure 17–4 on page 434).

magnify Enlarge.

ECG/EKG Paper

The ECG/EKG paper is graph paper with small squares that measure the time it takes for each heartbeat (see Figure 17–5 on page 434). ECG paper is heat and pressure sensitive. The stylus makes an imprint as it moves over the paper. It is important to handle the paper carefully, as it marks easily.

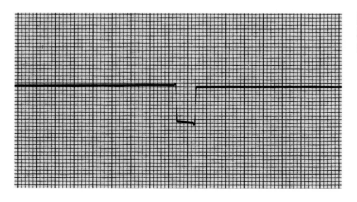

FIGURE 17–2.
Standardization markings.

FIGURE 17–3.
Single-channel paper prints one lead at a time.

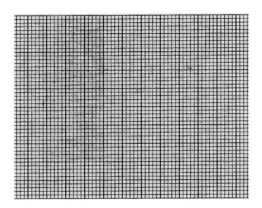

FIGURE 17–4.
Multichannel paper allows all twelve leads to be printed on a full sheet of paper (reduced 20%).

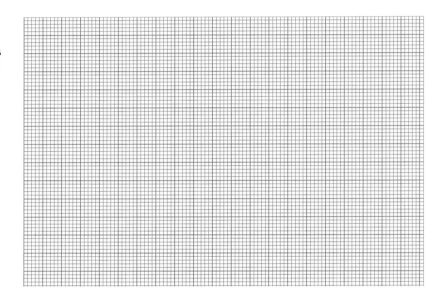

FIGURE 17–5.
ECG graph paper measures electrical° activity of the heart and the time it takes to complete each part of that activity.

FIGURE 17–6.
ECG rhythm strip.

In a healthy heart, each cardiac cycle would
be expected to correlate with the patient's
individual pulse beats.

The marks made during an ECG are labeled "PQRST" waves. Each letter identifies an activity in the heart (see Figure 17–6). Each PQRST equals one heartbeat.

EKG/ECG Leads

The standard 12-lead electrocardiogram records electrical activity from 12 different angles of the heart. Recognizing a normal recording from each lead is important. Each angle is identified by a lead name or number (see Figures 17–7 to 17–18). The last six leads are the chest leads. Chest leads (see Figure 17–19) read

LEADS 1 THRU 3

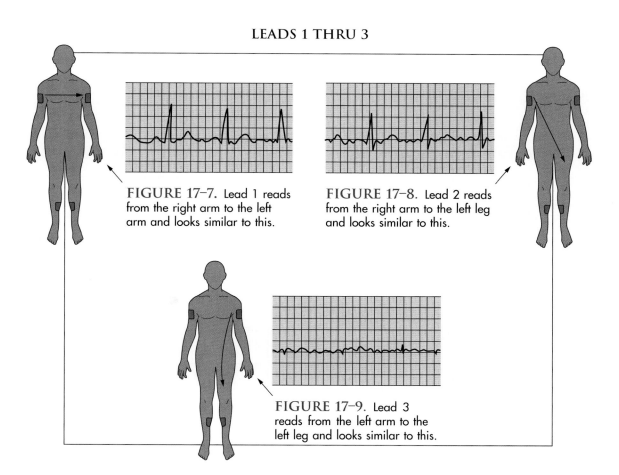

FIGURE 17–7. Lead 1 reads from the right arm to the left arm and looks similar to this.

FIGURE 17–8. Lead 2 reads from the right arm to the left leg and looks similar to this.

FIGURE 17–9. Lead 3 reads from the left arm to the left leg and looks similar to this.

AUGMENTED VOLTAGE (LEADS)

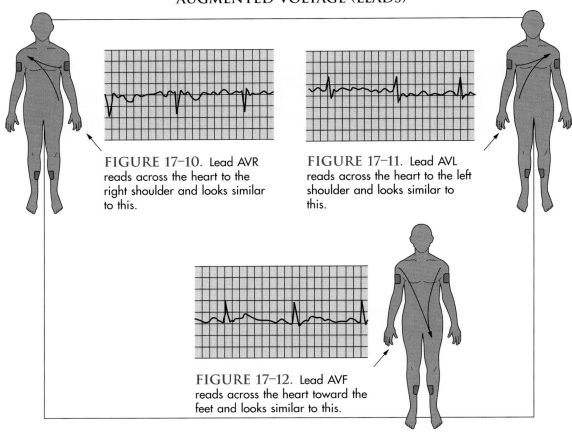

FIGURE 17–10. Lead AVR reads across the heart to the right shoulder and looks similar to this.

FIGURE 17–11. Lead AVL reads across the heart to the left shoulder and looks similar to this.

FIGURE 17–12. Lead AVF reads across the heart toward the feet and looks similar to this.

augmented Increased (e.g., augmented voltage leads show an increase in graph size).

FIGURE 17–13. Lead V1.

FIGURE 17–14. Lead V2.

FIGURE 17–15. Lead V3.

FIGURE 17–16. Lead V4.

FIGURE 17–17. Lead V5.

FIGURE 17–18. Lead V6.

FIGURE 17–19.
Chest or V-lead placement.

from the ventral to the dorsal surface (see Figures 17–13 to 17–18). They are called V leads and are placed in very exact places on the chest. To obtain correct readings, EKG technicians must place all leads correctly. Technicians are responsible for reporting abnormal recordings immediately.

■ PERFORMING AN EKG/ECG

Placing the Leads on the Patient/Client

Always explain to the patient/client that there is no pain or discomfort during an EKG/ECG. Reassure patients that their privacy is respected and that they are kept covered as much as possible. Tell them the test takes only a few minutes. Reassure patients that there is nothing wrong with them if you have to adjust leads because **artifacts** appear on the strip. Explain that the machine is very sensitive and that it is necessary to hold very still. Talk with patients as you put the leads in place to help them relax and feel more at ease.

Correct lead placement is important (see Figures 17–7 through 17–12 and 17–19). The blue squares on Figures 17–7 through 17–12 are placement sites for limb leads. Figure 17–19 shows placement sites for chest or V leads.

artifacts Unwanted marks on an electrocardiogram.

EKG/ECG Machines

There are many types of ECG machines. The basic procedure for operating each type of machine may be slightly different. The most common machines are the 12-lead manual EKG machine and the three-channel computerized machine. There is also a single-channel EKG machine. A very high tech machine can interpret the reading and mount the strips automatically. Some patients use a device at home that sends their EKG **impulses** over the telephone for interpretation.

impulses Measures of electrical activity to the heart tissue recorded on a graph.

Machine Controls

It is important to set each control on the machine so that a correct reading is recorded. Follow all procedures carefully to ensure that you will have an accurate reading.

Procedure

Using a Multilead Electrocardiograph (Placing Leads on the Patient/Client, Setting Machine Controls)

ALERT: Follow Standard Precautions.

Placing Leads on Patient/Client

1. Wash hands.
2. Assemble equipment.
   a. EKG machine with electrodes
   b. Electrode pads
   c. Alcohol wipes or skin cleansing agent
   d. Bath blanket/sheet
   e. Patient gown
3. Identify patient/client.
4. Explain what you are doing and reassure patient that this procedure is painless.
5. Help client change into a patient gown if necessary.
6. Position patient on bed or treatment table in a supine position with arms relaxed beside body.
7. Cover patient with a blanket, leaving arms and legs exposed.
8. Position machine at the side of client.
9. Identify correct location for leg, arm, and chest leads. (Avoid bony areas.)
10. Wipe skin with a cleansing agent to remove oils, scaly skin, or perspiration.
11. Apply electrode patches.
12. Attach leads to snap-on electrode patches. Each lead is color coded to ensure proper placement.
    a. White lead to right arm
    b. Black lead to left arm
    c. Green lead to right leg
    d. Red lead to left leg
    e. Brown leads are chest leads—place each one as indicated:
       (1) V1: fourth intercostal space just to the right of sternum
       (2) V2: fourth intercostal space just to the left of sternum

       (3) V3: midway between position of the fourth and fifth intercostal spaces
       (4) V4: fifth intercostal space
       (5) V5: same level as V4 and just anterior of midaxillary line
       (6) V6: same level as V4 and V5 at midaxillary line

Setting Machine Controls

13. Set machine controls.
    a. Set speed switch to run 25 mm per second. (If there is a severe tachycardia, it may be necessary to set at 50 mm per second.)
    b. Position stylus in center of paper.
    c. Set sensitivity at 1 for normal complexes. If complexes are too small to recognize each wave, set at 2. If complexes are so large that they will not fit on the graph paper, set the sensitivity at ½.
    d. Standardize each lead as instructed by your teacher.
14. Turn on machine.
15. Turn run button on. (Most multichannel EKG machines automatically standardize and record each lead when run button is pushed. See manufacturer's instructions to operate your machine properly.)
16. Turn machine off when all leads are recorded.
17. Remove all leads and electrode patches.
18. Clean remaining gel or paste left from patches.
19. Assist patient in dressing if necessary.
20. Label EKG with patient's name and physician's name.
21. Clean machine so that it is ready for next procedure.
22. Mount EKG and deliver as instructed for interpretation. (See the procedure "Mounting EKGs.")

*P*rocedure

Using a Single-Lead Electrocardiograph (Placing Leads on the Patient/Client, Setting Machine Controls, Performing an EKG)

ALERT: Follow Standard Precautions.

Placing Leads on Patient/Client

1. Wash hands.
2. Assemble equipment.
   a. EKG machine with electrodes
   b. Conductive gel
   c. Alcohol wipes or skin cleansing agent
   d. Gauze
   e. Rubber electrode straps
   f. Bath blanket/sheet
   g. Patient gown
3. Identify patient/client.
4. Explain what you are doing and reassure client that this procedure is painless.
5. Help patient change into patient gown if necessary.
6. Position patient on bed or treatment table in supine position with arms relaxed beside the body.
7. Cover client, leaving arms and legs exposed.
8. Position machine at the side of patient.
9. Identify correct location for arm and leg leads on fleshy areas. (Avoid bony areas.)
10. Wipe skin with a cleansing agent to remove oils, scaly skin, or perspiration.
11. Apply conductive gel or paste and electrodes. Secure with rubber straps.
12. Connect leads to electrodes. Each lead is color coded to ensure proper placement.
    a. White lead to right arm
    b. Black lead to left arm
    c. Green lead to right leg
    d. Red lead to left leg
    e. Brown lead not attached at this time

Setting Machine Controls

13. Set machine controls. Now that leads are in the proper place, it is important that you set each control on the machine in order to have a correct reading.
    a. Be certain to set speed switch to run 25 mm per second. (If there is a severe tachycardia, it may be necessary to set at 50 mm per second.)
    b. Position stylus in center of paper.
    c. Set sensitivity at 1 for normal complexes. If complexes are too small to recognize each wave, set at 2. If complexes are so large that they will not fit on graph paper, set the sensitivity at $\frac{1}{2}$.
    d. Standardize each lead as instructed by your teacher.
    e. Record 8 to 10 inches for each lead.
14. Turn on machine. A light will come on if the machine is on.
15. Turn lead selector switch to standardization position and quickly press standardization button.
16. Turn lead selector to an off position.
17. Check standardization mark on EKG paper. If machine is operating correctly, this mark will be 10 small blocks high, or two large blocks high. Press standardization button as you run each lead.
18. Label each lead automatically if the machine does not.
19. Turn lead selector to lead I and run an 8- to 10-inch strip.
20. Repeat step 19 for leads II and III.
21. Repeat step 19 for AVL, AVR, and AVF, but run only 4- to 6-inch strips.
22. Place brown chest leads in the following locations on the chest wall. After each placement, standardize and run a 4- to 6-inch strip.
    a. V1: fourth intercostal space just to the right of the sternum
    b. V2: fourth intercostal space just to the left of the sternum
    c. V3: midway between position of the fourth and fifth intercostal spaces
    d. V4: fifth intercostal space
    e. V5: same level as V4 and just anterior of midaxillary line
    f. V6: same level as V4 and V5 at midaxillary line
23. Turn machine off.
24. Remove all leads and electrodes.
25. Clean remaining gel or paste from skin.
26. Assist client in dressing if necessary.
27. Label EKG with patient's name and physician's name.
28. Clean electrodes thoroughly so that machine is ready for the next procedure.
29. Mount EKG and deliver as instructed for interpretation. (See the procedure "Mounting EKGs.")

■ ARTIFACTS

Artifacts are unwanted marks on the electrocardiogram. These marks are caused not by heart activity but by another source of electrical activity. These unwanted marks make it difficult to read the EKG. There are three common causes:

1. *Alternating-current (AC) interference* occurs when there is an electrical leak from equipment nearby (see Figure 17–20).

Common Causes	Remedies
Improper grounding	Check to be certain that equipment is grounded.
Other equipment leaking electricity	Turn off nearby equipment and unplug.
Lead wires crossed and not pointed toward the hands and feet	Adjust the position of the lead wire.
Corroded or dirty electrodes	Clean the electrodes.

2. *Somatic (body) tremors* can be recognized by a "quivering" baseline (Figure 17–21).

Common Causes	Remedies
Shivering or tense muscles	Warm the patient if cold; reassure if frightened.
Moving or talking	Refrain from moving and talking.
Nervous disorders	Place the patient's hands under the hips to help control tremors.

3. A *wandering baseline* can be recognized because it drifts away from the center of the graph paper (Figure 17–22).

FIGURE 17–20. AC (60-cycle) interference.

FIGURE 17–21. Somatic/muscle tremors.

FIGURE 17–22. Wandering baseline.

Common Causes	**Remedies**
Old conductive solution or too little solution	Use fresh solution and apply an adequate amount.
Improperly applied electrodes	Be certain that the electrodes are not too loose or too tight.
Corroded or dirty electrodes	Keep the electrodes clean.
Lead wires that are pulling on electrodes	Remove tension from the lead wire.
Creams or lotions on the skin under the electrodes	Clean the skin properly.

■ MOUNTING THE EKG/ECG

Mounting the EKG/ECG strips and submitting them to the physician for interpretation is the final step of the ECG procedures.

Procedure

Mounting EKGs

There are a variety of standard mount forms used in medicine. Mount the EKG records according to the physician's preference or the standard form used in your facility. Regardless of the form used, there are a few important steps you must follow in mounting every EKG.

1. Neatly trim strips to fit in space provided.
2. Include any unusual-looking complexes in the mounted strip.
3. Fill in the appropriate blanks on the form portion of mount.
4. Sign your name and deliver the completed EKG to the appropriate person for interpretation.

■ HOLTER MONITORING

Patients who experience occasional chest pain or discomfort without EKG/ECG changes are often tested with a Holter monitor. A Holter monitor is small and easy to carry. The wires are bulky but painless. A small recording device is carried on a strap around the waist or in a shoulder strap (Figure 17–23). Five electrodes are placed on the chest (Figure 17–24). The Holter records all heart activity during the time it is attached to the patient. The patient is instructed to follow routine activities. Instruct the patient that if pain, discomfort, or any symptoms occur, he or she should

1. Push the event button on the monitor.
2. Document in the diary the time of the event and the length of time that the symptoms last.

FIGURE 17–23. The medical assistant shows the client the diary and gives instructions regarding the Holter monitor before securing it around the patient's waist.

FIGURE 17–24. Anatomical placement of chest electrodes for Holter monitoring.

The physician determines when the client returns to have the monitor and electrodes removed. The recording cassette is removed and placed in a computerized analyzer, where a printout is made from the recording. The printout is analyzed by the physician, who determines treatment or need for additional testing. See the Holter monitor procedure for step-by-step directions in applying the monitor and electrodes.

Procedure

Using the Holter Monitor

ALERT: Follow Standard Precautions.

1. Wash hands.
2. Assemble equipment.
   a. Prejelled adhesive electrodes
   b. Holter monitor with lead wires
   c. Alcohol wipes
   d. Monitor belt
   e. Razor and shaving cream
   f. Cassette and batteries
   g. Diary for patient records
   h. Nonallergic tape to secure electrodes if needed
   i. Patient's medical record
   j. Pen
   k. Patient gown for women
3. Explain what you are going to do, and show monitor and leads to patient.
4. Ask client to remove clothes from the waist up. Provide a gown for women, instructing them to place the opening in front.
5. Test monitor for proper operation and insert new batteries each time you apply monitor.
6. Shave chest at electrode placement sites if necessary.
7. Rub electrode sites with gauze to prepare skin for good contact.
8. Place electrodes as indicated in Figure 17–24. Follow manufacturer's instructions for details.
9. Place monitor belt with monitor in place around patient's waist or over the shoulder.
10. Instruct client in care of monitor according to manufacturer's instructions.

11. Give patient the diary and instruct him or her to follow a normal routine. If pain, discomfort, or any symptoms should occur, the patient is to
    a. Push event button on monitor.
    b. Document in diary time of event and length of time that symptoms last.
12. Assist client in dressing.
13. Wash hands.
14. Record the following in patient medical record:
    a. Date and time monitor was applied
    b. What instructions were given to patient; initial
15. Schedule client for a return visit.

To Remove Monitor:

16. Wash hands.
17. Assist client in removing clothes from the waist up.
18. Remove monitor strap, electrodes, and wires.
19. Clean skin at electrode sites.
20. Assist patient in dressing if necessary.
21. Collect diary from patient.
22. Instruct client according to physician's orders.
23. Wash hands.
24. Place diary in patient's medical record and record time monitor was returned; initial.
25. Place cassette in analyzer for reading.
26. When printout is received from analyzer, attach to medical record, initial, and send or give to physician.

Being an EKG/ECG technician is an important job on the health care team. You must follow the steps carefully, or the strip that you run will not be accurate and could cause the physician to make a mistake in the diagnosis and treatment. Learn all the steps, and practice until they are very familiar to you. Follow the instructions in the ECG/EKG procedure.

■ JOBS AND PROFESSIONS

- ■ Assistive personnel
- ■ Nurse assistant
- ■ Clinical medical assistant
- ■ Licensed vocational/practical nurse
- ■ Registered nurse
- ■ Cardiology technician
- ■ Paramedic

Your link to success

Thinking Critically: Check Your Understanding

1. **Medical Terminology** Use information in Part One of this text and a medical dictionary to list ten medical symptoms and conditions of the heart. Use these ten medical terms to write a scenario about a patient with a heart condition.

2. **Cultural Competency** Identify cultures that may object to a male technician performing an ECG/EKG on a female. Explain ways to prevent or eliminate alarm or conflict.

3. **Patient Education** Identify patient information describing what a patient wearing a Holter monitor or similar monitor can and cannot do. Explain how to instruct the patient in the use of the monitor and to confirm the patient's level of understanding.

4. **Medical Math** ECG/EKG graph paper can be run through the EKG machine at different speeds. The standard speed is 25 mm per second. Use Figures 17–5 and 17–6 to determine how fast the pulse rate is in Figure 17–6.

5. **Case Study** Mrs. Marcolis refuses to allow you to place the electrodes on her chest. She is sure that those "new-fangled machines" will electrocute her. She has been having a lot of chest pain, and the doctor wants to determine if there are changes to her EKG that indicate heart damage. She tells you that this is exactly why she hasn't been to a doctor in fifty years: "The doctors always want to do all these silly tests." You have explained everything about the test very carefully. What can you do to ensure that she allows you to complete the test?

Portfolio Connection

Once you attain competence as an ECG/EKG technician, ask for permission to copy an electrocardiogram that is mounted and ready for the medical record. (Remove all patient identifiers.) Place this copy in your portfolio as evidence of your skills. Place a copy of your on-site trainer's evaluation in your portfolio.

Write a paper describing your doubts and realizations and the barriers that you were able to overcome during the electrocardiography experience. For example, were you afraid that you couldn't learn to use the equipment? Describe the ways you plan to use the skills, information, and insights that you gained about people and this job. This assignment must be in standard report format.

18 LABORATORY ASSISTANT/ MEDICAL ASSISTANT LABORATORY SKILLS; PHLEBOTOMIST

UNIT 1 **Laboratory Skills**

Steps to success

1. Complete Vocabulary Worksheet 1 in the Student Workbook.
2. Read this unit.
3. Complete Worksheets 2 through 7 as assigned.
4. Practice and demonstrate procedures.
5. When you are confident that you can meet each objective for this unit, ask your instructor for the unit evaluation.

Objectives

When you have completed this unit, you will be able to do the following:

✓ Complete all objectives in Part One of this book.
✓ Match vocabulary words with their correct meanings.
✓ Follow twelve general laboratory guidelines.
✓ Practice laboratory safety.
✓ Practice aseptic technique.
✓ Demonstrate loading and operating an autoclave.
✓ Dispose of hazardous materials according to facility policy.
✓ List six ways that laboratory tests help the physician.
✓ Identify information required on all laboratory slips.
✓ Discuss the importance of advance preparation for laboratory tests.
✓ List eight types of specimen studies.
✓ Identify general rules for testing specimens.
✓ List three methods for testing specimens.

✓ Discuss quality control in the laboratory.

✓ Label a diagram of a microscope.

✓ List five ways to prevent loss of your specimen in a centrifuge.

✓ Identify steps to acquire a midstream clean-catch urine specimen for male and female.

✓ Define *urinary sediment*.

✓ List three infectious diseases that can be diagnosed with a sputum test.

✓ Explain the reason for testing stool specimens for occult blood.

✓ Demonstrate the following:

- Obtaining a throat culture
- Preparing a direct smear
- Streaking an agar plate
- Preparing a slide from culture grown in an agar plate
- Gram staining a slide

✓ Identify seven items learned from a CBC.

✓ Explain why a hematocrit and hemoglobin test are important.

✓ Explain the reason for blood glucose testing.

✓ Explain the importance of counting WBCs and RBCs.

✓ State reasons for doing a WBC differential.

✓ List the four blood types.

✓ Explain agglutination.

✓ Explain an erythrocyte sedimentation rate.

✓ Identify the tests done in blood chemistries.

✓ Demonstrate the following:

- Finger stick
- Hematocrit test
- Blood glucose test with a glucose meter
- Diluting blood cells with an Unopette
- Preparing a blood smear slide
- Completing a differential white cell count
- Typing your blood
- Determining the erythrocyte sedimentation rate

■ RESPONSIBILITIES OF A LABORATORY ASSISTANT/MEDICAL ASSISTANT

Laboratory assistants/medical assistants perform a variety of tests. Some of the tests are highly technical: laboratory assistants/medical assistants run tests that assist in diagnosing an illness or disease. Their duties include the following:

■ Cleaning laboratory equipment

■ Preparing cleaning solutions

■ Drying glassware and instruments using a cloth, hot air dryer, or acetone bath

■ Examining clean equipment for cracks or chips

■ Operating an autoclave to sterilize equipment

■ Preparing stains, solutions, and culture media

■ Counting blood cells

- Separating plasma from whole blood using a centrifuge
- Incubating cultures
- Using computerized test equipment to test blood specimens
- Performing venipuncture with a Vacutainer™ and/or a needle and syringe
- Monitoring control tests
- Performing laboratory tests on stool, urine, blood, and sputum
- Preparing specimens for processing
- Giving patients instructions for specimen collection or self-testing

Importance of Laboratory Tests

Laboratory tests are important because they are

- A valuable diagnostic tool
- Used to monitor the amount of medication a patient has in his or her system (therapeutic drug level)
- A measure of the body's chemical balance that compares blood and urine samples with normal test values
- A way to use blood and urine tests to diagnose a certain disease or condition

CLIA (see below) periodically sends tests to labs for reading. Tests are returned to CLIA to confirm the laboratory's readings. This is CLIA's quality control on laboratories.

■ LABORATORY STANDARDS

Medical laboratories and medical offices that perform lab tests on human specimens are regulated by a federal amendment called the Clinical Laboratory Improvement Amendment of 1988 (or CLIA). CLIA sets standards and regulates all laboratories, physician's offices, and other labs that use human specimens to diagnose, prevent, or treat disease.

As a laboratory assistant/medical assistant you can perform simple tests allowed by CLIA. The lab or medical office must have a CLIA waiver certificate before you perform these tests. The tests include the following:

- Dipstick or tablet reagent urinalysis for bilirubin, glucose, hemoglobin, ketone, leukocytes, nitrite, pH, protein, urobilinogen, specific gravity
- Ovulation tests: visual color test to tell if human luteinizing hormone is present
- Urine pregnancy tests: visual color comparison test
- Erythrocyte sedimentation rate (nonautomated)
- Hemoglobin copper sulfate (nonautomated)
- Fecal occult blood
- Spun microhematocrit
- Blood glucose by glucose monitoring devices cleared by the Food and Drug Administration for home use

Do not perform these tests unless you know that there is a waiver certificate and you have been trained properly.

uniformity A state of being all the same; does not vary.

Operating a laboratory with **uniformity** and maintaining standards of measure quality are important. People who work in the laboratory must follow the same guidelines that all laboratory workers follow. These guidelines are as follows:

■ Clean and cover microscope daily according to manufacturer guidelines.
■ Maintain all infection control logs.
■ Report all defective equipment immediately to your supervisor.
■ Maintain and observe quality control logs.
■ Follow all directions to ensure accurate results from each test.

• Refrigerate promptly. • Transport specimens in racks. • Follow instructions when watching for serum separation. • Instruct patients in proper collection of all specimens. • Use appropriate technique with all specimen collections.

■ Check temperatures of appliances daily.
■ Learn new techniques for testing new material or equipment changes.
■ Check expiration dates of all reagents and testing kits weekly.
■ Do quality control checks on all testing materials and equipment following manufacturer's directions and CLIA standards.
■ Ask the supervisor for help when in doubt regarding any procedure or result.
■ Recognize the importance of correct and accurate test results for doctors.
■ Report all "stats" immediately.

The medical laboratory is an environment with hazards. The laboratory assistant/medical assistant or anyone working with laboratory tests must be aware of possible dangers. In the laboratory, you work with patient specimens that must be treated as **hazardous** materials. You also work with various chemicals that can react when mixed together. Some of these chemicals are harmful to the skin, eyes, and/or the respiratory system. To be safe in the laboratory:

hazardous Dangerous.

■ Learn safety measures and follow them carefully.
■ Always follow Standard Precautions (review in Chapter 12).

General Safety Practice Guidelines

Personal Safety

The protective equipment you wear includes the following:

■ A nonpermeable lab coat to protect your clothes
■ Safety eye goggles/glasses to guard your eyes from splashes
■ Gloves to keep you from being contaminated by infectious material
■ A rubber apron to protect you from **acids** that can spill or splash
■ Metal tongs when working with hot objects

acids Substances that cause the urine to have an acid pH.

Other safety considerations are as follows:

■ Never use your mouth to pipette.
■ Do not eat, drink, or apply makeup in the laboratory area.
■ Flush eyes first, then report eye contamination immediately to supervisor for eye treatment.
■ Dispose of all broken glass, needles, or other sharp objects in a sharps container.
■ Do not bend, break, or recap needles.
■ Follow Standard Precautions and consider all specimens as highly infectious.
■ Disinfect counters, surfaces, and equipment daily.

Fire Prevention

■ Locate the fire extinguisher.
■ Participate in fire drills.
■ Report all potential electrical hazards to the supervisor immediately.
■ Use grounded plugs for equipment.

Additional Safety Practice Guidelines

reagents Chemical substances that react to the presence of other substances in the blood and urine.

■ Clearly label and date all **reagents.**
■ Label all waste containers with a biohazard symbol.
■ Complete incident reports:

• Incident or injury to patients or self • Chemical spills • Electrical or fire hazards

■ Keep trash from building up in any area.
■ Keep all posters and decorations away from lights and vents.
■ Inspect areas where heating elements are used for possible fire hazards.
■ Keep spills wiped up and use a disinfectant when necessary.
■ Discard any rag with a flammable substance on it in a metal container with a self-closing lid.

Sterilization

You must sterilize all items in the laboratory that have contact with body tissue or fluids. The most effective way to sterilize equipment is in an autoclave (see Figure 18–1 and Chapter 20). The autoclave produces steam under pressure. The high heat of the steam kills organisms that cause disease. Keep items that you are sterilizing in the autoclave for the specified length of time to ensure that all microorganisms are killed. The autoclave is a heavy piece of equipment with a chamber that withstands high degrees of temperature and a great deal of pressure. Steam under pressure can burn skin, hair, and eyes. Always follow these basic rules when operating an autoclave:

1. Read the directions for the autoclave you are using.
2. Use protective gloves when placing articles in an autoclave or taking them out.

FIGURE 18–1.
Autoclave.

3. Protect yourself if the autoclave is hot from recent use.

4. Do not overload. If you pack material into the autoclave too tightly, the steam cannot circulate and the items will not be sterilized.

5. Allow the temperature and pressure to return to normal before opening the autoclave when sterilization is complete.

6. Clean the autoclave according to the manufacturer's directions. (See Chapter 20 for additional information on sterilization.)

Items that you cannot reuse are not sterilized. Never put body tissue, body fluid, or any article that has been in contact with blood, body fluids, or tissues in the regular trash. Dispose of them in a biohazard container following your facility's policies. All health care workers have the responsibility to protect themselves and others.

The increased concerns over hazardous and/or toxic materials in all areas of work create the need for strict guidelines to protect people. The federal Occupational Safety and Health Administration (OSHA) provides guidelines to help ensure safety. Your laboratory supervisor has these guidelines in a notebook with material safety data sheets (MSDS; see Figure 13–1). The MSDS sheets follow OSHA guidelines by explaining how to dispose of and handle hazardous materials safely. The sheets also describe possible physical symptoms of overexposure and proper first-aid treatment if exposed. Ingredients of the hazardous product are also identified on MSDS forms. It is important to follow the general guidelines above and check the MSDS for specific information on each substance.

Contaminated/Hazardous Material

Specimens being analyzed in the laboratory come from patients. The physician often does not know what is causing a client's illness, so you must treat every specimen as though it is contaminated and potentially hazardous. *Always follow Standard Precautions.* When you work in a laboratory or medical office, you must practice good aseptic technique at all times. The most important steps include washing your hands before and after each procedure. Always wear gloves when working with specimens.

Biohazardous Waste Containers

In the medical setting, you must dispose of all contaminated biohazardous materials in biohazardous waste containers. The laboratory containers are lined with red plastic. Put all discarded contaminated/biohazardous materials in the red-lined containers marked "Biohazardous." Empty all containers at the end of each shift or when full. Carefully tie the bag and be certain that it will stay closed. Mark the tied bag "Biohazardous." Reline the container with a new red bag. Place the marked bag in a red sealed container for pickup. Handle all contaminated/hazardous materials according to OSHA guidelines. Never mix them with ordinary trash.

■ LABORATORY TESTS

Laboratory workers are responsible for testing specimens. The most common specimens include urine, blood, sputum, and stool. The results of these tests provide information about the patient's health. This information helps

- Diagnose the illness
- Determine the cause of the illness

■ Confirm a diagnosis
■ Evaluate progress
■ Regulate treatment
■ Establish a baseline for future tests

Guidelines for Laboratory Tests

When you receive a laboratory request, check it for all information. This information includes

■ Client's name and address
■ Client's age and sex
■ Name of test requested
■ Time and date of collection
■ Physician's name and address
■ Method of collection
■ Possible diagnosis
■ Type and source of specimen
■ Medications the patient is taking
■ Stat or routine tests

Preparation of Patients/Clients

There are many different kinds of laboratory tests. Some of the tests require very specific preparation. The results of some tests are affected by medication, food, time of day, and type of activity. Know the advance preparation for each test. If you are not certain about preparation, look it up in the procedures manual. Instruct the patient to follow the preparation orders exactly. Advance preparation may include

■ *Fasting.* Eating before some tests changes the results of the test (e.g., fasting blood sugar [FBS], glucose tolerance test [GTT], SMA-12 profile). During fasting, patients must not eat or drink fluid (except water). They usually fast for 12 to 14 hours before the test.

■ *Medication restriction.* Many medications can change the chemical and physical qualities of the specimen. The patient needs special instruction if taking medications that can change test results. Medication affects urine specimens more than it affects blood. If the patient can be off the medication without causing injury, the medication is stopped 48 to 72 hours before the tests. The physician makes this decision.

Analyzing Specimens

There are many different studies that help identify and diagnose physical problems.

■ *Urinalysis.*   Examines urine chemically, physically, and microscopically
■ *Hematology.*   Examines blood for disease conditions
■ *Microbiology.*   Identifies pathogens in the body
■ *Histology.*   Microscopic study of body tissues to detect diseased tissues

■ *Cytology.* Microscopic examination to discover abnormal cells
■ *Clinical chemistry.* Examines substances in body fluids, feces, tissues
■ *Serology and blood banking.* Study of antigen-antibody reactions to discover presence of foreign substance or disease
■ *Parasitology.* Determines parasite that is causing illness

General Rules for Testing the Specimen

There are basic steps to follow for testing all specimens.

1. Measure the amount of specimen required for the test very carefully. This is very specific.
2. Combine the correct chemical reagent for the test with the specimen.
3. Process the specimen correctly (e.g., centrifuge, heat in a water bath, incubate, heat fix, etc.).
4. Assess the sample by manual or automatic method.
5. Calculate results by hand or machine.
6. Record all the information on the lab report sheet, including
   a. Patient's name b. Age and sex c. Time and date d. Source of specimen
   e. Name of test completed f. Results of test g. Name of classification

Always follow the approved procedure in your facility.

Methods of Testing Specimens

The *manual method* requires carefully following a series of steps. Some small labs and physicians' offices use manual methods for simple tests (e.g., urinalysis).

Semiautomated analysis is a combination of manual and automated testing (e.g., glucose monitor). To perform a glucose test, you stick the finger to get blood. The glucose monitor measures the glucose in the blood. *Automatic analyzers* can do more than one specimen at a time. These analyzers measure the specimen, add reagent, process the specimen, and give the results.

Quality Control for Specimen Testing

There must be a method for quality control when performing laboratory tests. Performing these test controls tells you that the test is accurate. Quality control helps ensure that the test result is a true picture of the patient's condition. Some tests have the control built in. When the information is reliable, the physician can make a diagnosis. Quality control methods include

■ Discarding outdated reagents
■ Following the procedure for exact testing
■ Routinely verifying that laboratory equipment is reading specimens accurately
■ Maintaining equipment by having it serviced routinely

Quality control includes keeping accurate logs. The log includes important information about the test (e.g., expiration date, lot number, date tested, and pass/fail of control). You must initial each test in the log.

■ LABORATORY EQUIPMENT

There are many kinds of laboratory equipment. The simple microscope and centrifuge are found in all laboratories. Some equipment is more complicated than others, for example, very advanced computers and analyzers.

Microscope

The microscope is an important tool that magnifies and enlarges objects (see Figure 18–2). You use it to see microorganisms and other components that are too small to see without magnification. The ability to see these components helps find the cause of illnesses. Learning to use the microscope is necessary for laboratory workers.

How to Use a Microscope

There are different types of microscopes. Some microscopes have one eyepiece. These are **monocular** microscopes. Microscopes with two eyepieces are **biocular.**

monocular Having one eyepiece.

biocular Having two eyepieces.

Basic Parts of the Microscope

■ *Base.*   Supports the microscope. It keeps the microscope from falling over.

■ *Arm.*   Supports the eyepiece and is used to carry the microscope.

■ *Stage.*   Holds slides that are put on the stage after you prepare them.

■ *Slide clips.*   Hold the prepared slide in place.

■ *Iris diaphragm.*   Adjusts the amount of light that enters the microscope through the opening in the stage.

■ *Mirror or illumination light.*   Provides light so that you can see the object on the slide. You control the amount of light with the iris diaphragm. When you use a mirror, you turn the mirror to pick up a light source and *reflect* it into the microscope.

■ *Eyepiece.*   Lets you see the object on the slide. Some microscopes have eyepieces that magnify to ten times (10×), others to twenty times (20×).

FIGURE 18–2.
Microscope.

Stereo type lens set

Microscope body

Coarse & fine adjustments (2)

Magnification control

Stage

Illuminator

Base

■ *Objectives.* Magnify what you have on the slide. Most microscopes have three objectives. The most common objectives are

• High-power objectives that magnify the objects forty times (40×). • Medium-power objectives that magnify the object ten times (10×). • Low-power objectives that magnify four times (4×). • Oil immersion: the oil immersion objective magnifies 95× to 100×. You put a drop of oil on a specimen that is dark and hard to see. The oil concentrates the light and makes the specimen easier to see.

■ *Body tube.* Connects the eyepiece to the objectives, which are on the revolving nosepiece.

■ *Revolving nosepiece.* The objectives are attached to the revolving nosepiece. You turn it to place the objective over the specimen.

How tpo Determine Total Magnification of the Specimen

Specimens are very small samples. It is important to know how many times the specimen is magnified. To determine how many times the specimen is magnified, multiply the power of the eyepiece by the power of the objective. For example:

Power of eyepiece　10×
Power of objective　4×
10 × 4 = 40

This means that the specimen is enlarged 40 times its actual size.

Procedure

Using a Microscope

ALERT: Follow Standard Precautions.

1. Assemble equipment.
   a. Microscope
   b. Lens paper
   c. Slides and slide cover
   d. Specimen
   e. Oil if using oil immersion
2. Wash hands.
3. Place specimen (e.g., hair, scraping from under nails, scraping from tooth) on clean slide (one drop only if liquid specimen).
4. Add required solution.
5. Drop clean slide cover over specimen.
6. Clean eyepiece with lens paper.
7. Clean objectives with lens paper.
8. Turn on illuminating light.
9. Open iris diaphragm.
10. Turn revolving nosepiece to low-power objective.
11. Place slide on stage under slide clips.
12. Turn coarse adjustment knob to move objective close to slide.
13. Look into eyepiece and turn coarse adjustment to move tube upward until you focus specimen.
14. Turn fine-adjustment knob until specimen is clear and focused.
15. Continue steps 11 through 14 using higher objectives until you have best possible focus for specimen.
16. Observe specimen. If setup is for technician or physician, tell that person that slide is ready.
17. Remove slide after it is read.
18. Discard slide according to procedure in your facility.
19. Clean lens and objective with lens paper.
20. Turn off illuminating light.
21. Fill out lab slips according to your facility's policies.

There are both a coarse adjustment and a fine adjustment on the microscope:

■ *Coarse adjustment.*   Upper knob on the arm, which moves the objectives up and down. This helps you put the specimen in rough focus.
■ *Fine adjustment.*   Lower, smaller knob, which moves the objective more slowly. This helps you have a clear image of the specimen (see Figure 18–2).

The microscope must be taken care of. Remember to

■ Use special lens paper to clean the eyepiece, or you will scratch the lens.
■ Watch the objectives when you move them up and down. This prevents damaging the objectives or breaking the slide.
■ Cover the microscope when you are not using it. This keeps dust out.
■ Keep the microscope in a safe place where it cannot be knocked to the floor (see the procedure "Using a Microscope").

Centrifuge

The centrifuge is a device that spins at high speed. As the centrifuge spins, it separates heavy or solid components from liquid. The heavy or solid components move to the lower part of the container. This separation allows you to study all components of the specimen. There is one type of centrifuge to process urine and blood in a test tube (Figure 18–3) and another type to process blood in a capillary tube.

Guidelines for Using a Centrifuge

■ Counterbalance the tube by placing another tube directly opposite it. This tube must contain a liquid of equal weight. You can usually use water.
■ Do not use cracked or scratched tubes. If the tube breaks, the specimen will spill out.
■ Turn off centrifuge immediately if a tube breaks.
■ Put on rubber gloves and clean the centrifuge.
■ Follow the instruction in each procedure for using the centrifuge.

FIGURE 18–3.
Examples of a centrifuge used for blood and for urine.

■ URINALYSIS

A routine urinalysis provides information about the patient. The urinalysis gives the physician information about the physical, chemical, and microscopic characteristics of the urine. This information tells many different things about the patient's health.

Urine Collection

Proper urine collection is important. The way you collect the urine affects the test. The following are some general guidelines for urine collection:

■ Use a clean, dry container.

■ A specimen over 32 hours old may give inaccurate test results.

■ Refrigerate it and write the collection time on the label if it is necessary to keep a specimen over 2 hours.

■ If possible, collect on-site for immediate testing.

Reagent Strips

Your facility may use reagent strips and or other individual tests. Always follow the procedures of your facility.

Reagent strips have small pads that react to a specific substance. When you dip the strip in a fresh urine sample, there is a chemical reaction. Carefully match the reagent strip with the color chart on the container label. The procedure for using all reagent strips is similar.

Guidelines for Using Reagent Strips

■ Check the bottle for an expiration date.

■ Keep the bottle in a cool dry area with the top tightly closed. (Do not refrigerate.)

■ Check the strips for a change in color. A tan-to-brown color change indicates deterioration. Do not use the strips.

■ Keep the specimen container clean.

■ Use freshly voided urine. Urine over 2 hours old gives poor results. Refrigerate if it stands more than 2 hours.

■ A clean-catch urine is best for determining leukocytes.

■ First urine in the morning is best for determining nitrates.

■ Match colors on strips to the color chart on the label. Follow the times on the label carefully.

■ Write the type of strips used when recording the type of test.

Microscopic Examination of the Urine

Urinary sediment contains the solid materials in the urine. There are many components in the sediment that help the **provider** confirm or determine a diagnosis. The sediment may contain renal or kidney cells, casts, crystals, bacteria, parasites, mucus, or other substances. The sediment settles to the bottom of a centrifuged urine specimen. A small sample of the sediment is placed on a slide for the provider to look at. The provider looks for a cause of illness (e.g., bacteria causing a bladder infection, renal cells indicating renal damage, or red blood cells from irritation). Spinning urine (centrifuging) will be one of your duties.

provider Physician, physician assistant, nurse practitioner.

Procedure

Using Reagent Strips to Test Urine

1. Wash hands.
2. Assemble equipment.
   a. Reagent strips and bottle
   b. Laboratory report slip
   c. Watch
   d. Urine specimen
   e. Disposable nonsterile gloves
   ALERT: Follow Standard Precautions.
3. Complete laboratory slip.
   a. Name   d. Physician
   b. Sex   e. Date
   c. Age   f. Type of test
4. Put on gloves.
5. Hold specimen to light and observe:
   a. Color (colorless, yellow, light yellow, brown, orange, etc.)
   b. Clarity (clear, hazy, cloudy)
6. Write color and clarity on lab slip.
7. Open reagent jar and remove one strip.
   a. Note expiration date. *Do not use if expired.*
   b. Replace jar cover immediately.

8. Hold strip by clear end and immerse in urine.
9. Remove strip immediately by pulling gently over lip of tube to remove excess urine.
10. Hold strip in horizontal position to prevent mixing of chemicals.
11. Hold strip close to color blocks on bottle label and match carefully.
12. Read strip at time indicated and record results.

13. Discard reagent strip in biohazard waste.
14. Clean and replace equipment.
15. Remove gloves.
16. Wash hands.
17. Record required information.
    a. Date
    b. Time
    c. Results
    d. Signature and classification
18. Report any abnormal results to supervisor immediately.

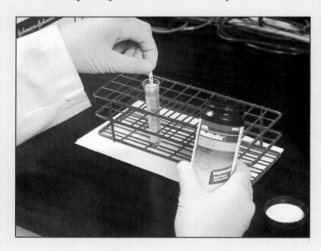

Special Urine Tests
Measuring Specific Gravity

You can measure specific gravity on a reagent stick. The urinometer is another simple way to check specific gravity. Specific gravity gives the dilution of urine. For example, urine is heavier when the patient is dehydrated.

Procedure

Measuring Specific Gravity with Urinometer

1. Wash hands.
2. Assemble equipment.
   a. Disposable gloves
   b. Glass cylinder (5 inches high)
   c. Urinometer
   d. Fresh urine specimen

ALERT: Follow Standard Precautions.

3. Put on gloves.
4. Pour urine into cylinder to ¾ mark.
5. Place urinometer in urine.
6. Spin urinometer gently.
7. Place cylinder with lower line of meniscus at eye level.
8. Read specific gravity:
   a. Look at point where lowest part of meniscus crosses urinometer scale.
   b. Read gauge on nearest line.
9. Record reading to enter in computer or on lab slip.
10. Discard urine according to facility's contaminated waste policy.
11. Rinse urinometer with water and dry.
12. Rinse cylinder with water and dry.
13. Remove gloves and discard in contaminated waste.
14. Wash hands.
15. Record specific gravity in computer or on lab list.

Pregnancy Tests

The physician may request a pregnancy test for several reasons, including the following:

■ To begin prenatal care early in pregnancy
■ To make certain that medication that causes fetal damage is not given
■ To prevent the use of procedures that may cause injury to the fetus

A common test for determining pregnancy is a simple urine test. The test is performed on a concentrated urine specimen. The urine is tested for a hormone called human chorionic gonadotropin (HCG). This hormone is produced by the developing fertilized egg. Some of the hormone is secreted into the urine and blood. It is very important to read the manufacturer's instructions carefully before completing a pregnancy test.

To perform an accurate pregnancy test, follow these guidelines:

■ Use clean urine containers to collect urine.
■ Use the first voided morning specimen for the highest accumulation of HCG.
■ Check the specific gravity. If it is less than 1.010, the urine is too dilute.
■ Have the urine specimen at room temperature.
■ Follow the manufacturer's instructions for storing the reagents.
■ Do not use reagents after the expiration date.
■ Do not contaminate the specimen.

Procedure

Centrifuging a Urine Specimen

1. Wash hands.
2. Assemble equipment.
   a. Centrifuge
   b. Two centrifuge tubes
   c. Microscope slide (number slide)
   d. Coverslip
   e. Pipette
   f. Disposable nonsterile gloves
   g. Urine specimen

ALERT: Follow Standard Precautions.

3. Fill in lab slip:
   a. Name
   b. Date
   c. Time
4. Put on gloves.
5. Mix urine to suspend sediment.
6. Pour 10 mL of urine into centrifuge tube.
7. Put tube with urine into centrifuge.
8. Pour 10 mL with water into second centrifuge tube.
9. Place in centrifuge opposite the tube with urine.
10. Secure centrifuge lid.
11. Set centrifuge timer for 4 to 5 minutes. (Allow it to stop on its own.)

12. Remove tube with urine.
13. Carefully invert urine centrifuge tube quickly over sink to pour 9 mL of urine into sink.
14. Turn tube right side up immediately. (About 1.0 cc will remain in tube.)
15. Mix sediment by snapping end of centrifuge tube with finger.
16. Pipette 1 drop of urine on numbered slide.
17. Put on coverslip. (Redo if air bubbles appear under coverslip.)
18. Put slide on microscope stage.
19. Use 10× objective with coarse adjustment to focus on slide.
20. Adjust light source.
21. Follow your facility's policy for reading slide. (If setup is for technician, tell him or her that slide is ready.)
22. Remove slide after it is read.
23. Discard slide according to facility procedure.
24. Clean lens and objective with lens paper.
25. Clean equipment and replace equipment.
26. Remove gloves, and dispose of according to facility policy.
27. Wash hands.
28. Record results if you read the specimen.

Testing Urine for Drugs

The collection of urine to determine drug use is becoming more and more common. Some reasons for drug testing:

■ Employer requests a preemployment test.
■ Department of Transportation requires testing of pilots, truck drivers, and others.
■ Employer requests test for employee suspected of using drugs.

There are many strict rules that you *must* adhere to when you collect urine for drug testing. Follow the instructions and proceed step by step. *Be very exact.*

Procedure

Abbott Test Pack Plus Pregnancy Test

1. Wash hands.
2. Assemble equipment.
   a. Abbott Test Pack Plus HCG-Urine
   b. Transfer pipettes
   c. Disposable nonsterile gloves
   d. Specimen container for clean-catch urine
   e. Watch or timer
3. Put on gloves.

ALERT: *Follow Standard Precautions.*

4. Remove Abbott Test Pack Plus HCG-Urine reaction disk from pouch.

5. Place on flat, dry surface.
6. Transfer 3 drops of urine into the sample well with pipette.
7. Read test results immediately after appearance of a red color in end of assay window (approximately 5 minutes).

8. A positive (+) sign or negative (−) sign will appear in result window (see figures).
9. *Retest specimen* if a positive (+) or negative (−) sign *fails* to appear in result window.
10. Discard urine cup and pipette in hazardous waste container.
11. Pour urine in sink and rinse sink.
12. Remove gloves and dispose of according to facility procedures.
13. Wash hands.
14. Document on chart:
    a. Procedure (name of test used)
    b. Time
    c. Date
    d. Results
    e. Signature and classification

Clean-Catch Collection

Clean-catch midstream urine collection has a specific procedure. The physician may order a clean-catch urine when he or she suspects that a urinary infection is present or for any urine test. The clean-catch method reduces possible contamination of the specimen. Clean the area around the meatus carefully to remove microorganisms. Collect the urine in a sterile cup using medical aseptic techniques. Pour off part of the specimen for the dipstick test and for spinning down when you collect a clean-catch urine. This leaves the urine in the specimen container uncontaminated. If necessary, you can use it for culture and sensitivity testing.

There are other urine specimen tests that may be ordered. Your facility has a procedure manual with instructions for each test that your lab performs. Follow the instructions for collection carefully.

Procedure

Midstream Clean-Catch Urine, Female

1. Wash hands.
2. Assemble equipment.
    a. Sterile urine container for clean catch
    b. Label
    c. Disposable antiseptic towelettes
    d. Disposable nonsterile gloves: wear if you handle cup with specimen.

ALERT: Follow Standard Precautions.

3. Label container.
4. Instruct client to
    a. Wash hands.
    b. Remove container lid and place on counter with inside of lid facing up.
    c. Separate labia to expose meatus.
    d. Take towelette and wipe on side of urinary meatus from front to back.
    e. Dispose of towelette.
    f. Repeat with new towelette on other side.
    g. Wipe directly over meatus with new towelette.
    h. Continue to hold labia open.
    i. Urinate small amount into toilet.
    j. Stop stream.
    k. Place sterile container under meatus and void into container (60 cc).
    l. Stop stream.
    m. Remove container carefully.
    n. Empty bladder.
    o. Carefully replace lid.
    p. Wipe outside of container with paper towel.
    q. Put in designated area.
5. Put on gloves.
6. Finish testing as ordered (e.g., dipstick, set up microscopic exam, drug test).
7. Document procedure.

Procedure

Midstream Clean-Catch Urine, Male

1. Wash hands.
2. Assemble equipment.
    a. Sterile container for clean catch
    b. Label
    c. Disposable antiseptic towelettes
    d. Disposable nonsterile gloves: wear if handling container with specimen

ALERT: Follow Standard Precautions.

3. Label container.
4. Instruct patient to
    a. Wash hands.
    b. Remove container lid and place on counter with inside of lid facing up.
    c. Cleanse head of penis in a circular motion with towelette. (If uncircumsised, pull back foreskin before cleaning.)
    d. Urinate into toilet. (If uncircumsised, pull back foreskin while urinating.)
    e. Allow stream to begin.
    f. Stop stream and place specimen container to collect midstream.
    g. Remove container before bladder is empty.
    h. Empty bladder into toilet.
    i. Carefully replace lid.
    j. Wipe outside of container with paper towel.
    k. Put in designated area.
5. Put on gloves.
6. Finish testing as ordered (e.g., dip stick, set up microscopic exam, drug test).
7. Document procedure.

Procedure

Collecting Urine from an Infant

1. Wash hands.
2. Assemble equipment.
   a. Specimen container
   b. Disposable urine collector (small plastic bag with opening and sticky area)
   c. Disposable nonsterile gloves

ALERT: Follow Standard Precautions.

3. Identify patient.
4. Explain to parents what you are going to do.
5. Tell child what you are going to do even if you think that he or she is too young to understand. Children often understand.
6. Put on gloves.
7. Remove diaper.
8. Make certain that skin is clean and dry in genital area.
9. Remove outside cover that is around opening of bag. This has a sticky area that is applied to vulva or around penis. Place over vulva or penis (see figures).
10. Replace diaper.
11. Remove gloves and dispose of according to facility procedure.
12. Check every half hour to see if bag has urine in it.
13. Remove bag when specimen is collected.
14. Rinse, clean, and dry genital area.
15. Replace diaper.
16. Put specimen in specimen container for lab.
17. Label with:
    a. Patient's name   c. Time of collection
    b. Date   d. Room number
18. Record collection of specimen.

■ SPUTUM COLLECTION

Sputum is a secretion from the trachea, bronchi, and lungs. It is forced up and out through the mouth by deep coughing. When you collect sputum, make sure that it is not saliva or postnasal drip. Saliva and postnasal drip contaminate a sputum sample. When you collect a sputum sample you must instruct the patient carefully. The doctor orders a sputum specimen to help determine the cause of the illness and whether the patient has an infectious disease. Some of these diseases are

- Tuberculosis
- Pneumonia
- Candidiasis
- Other fungal infections

Procedure

Sputum Specimen Collection

1. Wash hands.
2. Assemble equipment.
   a. Sputum container
   b. Disposable nonsterile gloves
   ALERT: Follow Standard Precautions.
3. Identify client.
4. Explain what you are going to do.
5. Label container with
   a. Client's name
   b. Date
   c. Time taken
   d. Room number
6. Put on gloves.
7. Help patient rinse mouth if he or she has just eaten.
8. Ask client to take three deep breaths. On the third breath tell resident to cough deep from lungs and try to bring up thick sputum. (Saliva is not adequate for this test.)
9. The patient may have to try several times to get a good specimen. (You need 1 to 2 tablespoons.)
10. Cover container immediately.
11. Remove gloves and discard according to facility procedure.
12. Wash hands.
13. Record color, amount, odor, and consistency.

Another test is the Papanicolaou stain. This tests for the presence of cancer cells. Collect the sputum for this test in a 95 percent alcohol solution for a period of 72 hours. Read the procedure for your facility.

■ STOOL COLLECTION

The patient/client may need to collect a stool specimen. The tests on the stool specimen give the physician information about the patient's digestive system (e.g., blood, bacteria, ova, and parasites in stool). The patient needs to collect the specimen at home. Proper instructions are very important. The following are guidelines for collection of a stool specimen:

■ Feces must not be contaminated with urine.
■ Patient must *not* take a laxative unless instructed to do so.

occult Hidden, unseen.

There are several tests performed on stool samples (see Table 18–1), the most common tests are those for **occult** blood. Screening tests to detect bleeding in the intestinal tract are done routinely. Occult blood may indicate

■ Cancer
■ Polyps
■ Lesions in the colon or rectum
■ Gastrointestinal bleeding

Testing for occult blood is a simple technique that you can do in the office or at home. It consists of three slides. The patient must smear a small amount of stool on slide 1, then slides 2 and 3 for the next three bowel movements. Tell the patient/client that it is important to follow the instructions carefully. When you receive slides from the patient, be sure they are properly labeled.

TABLE 18–1   Tests Performed on Stool Specimens

Reason for Test	Type of Specimen
Intestinal amoeba flagellates	Specimen must be at body temperature and checked within 30 minutes.
Ova cystic forms of parasites	Well-formed stool can be taken to lab within a few hours.
Tapeworm	May be examined for ova. If liquid stool, must bring in entire amount. Lab must examine for tapeworm head.

Procedure

Occult Blood Test on Stool Specimen

1. Wash hands.
2. Assemble equipment.
   a. Three occult blood slides
   b. Developer per slide manufacturer
   c. Disposable nonsterile gloves
3. Open the back flap of specimen slide.

ALERT: Follow Standard Precautions.

4. Use the type of liquid developer that coordinates with the type of slide used (i.e., Hemacult developer for Hemacult slides, Serracult developer for Serracult slides).
5. Develop the slides for test results according to manufacturer's directions.
6. Dispose of slides and gloves according to facility's policy.

7. Document the following:
   a. Patient's name
   b. Account number
   c. Date
   d. Time
   e. Physician's name
   f. Type of test
   g. Number of tests
   h. Results
   i. Client's diet
   j. Your initials

(1)   (2)   (3)

■ LABORATORY CULTURES

Physicians need a culture of the microorganism that is causing an illness. Knowing what organism is causing the problem helps with the diagnosis and the treatment. Microorganisms that cause strep throat, staph infections, and other illnesses can be treated when they are identified. You need to know how to

■ Obtain a specimen.
■ Place the specimen on the medium, where it can grow and reproduce.
■ Stain a sample of the culture.

Take a specimen for the culture from the affected body sites. These sites include any skin lesion, such as an open, draining sore. Cultures are also taken from any body opening, such as eyes, ears, nose, throat, and vagina. You must be careful when you take a specimen for culturing. Poor technique causes a false test result. You must use a sterile swab to secure the specimen and be careful not to contaminate the sample.

Procedure

Obtaining a Specimen for Cultures

1. Wash hands.
2. Assemble equipment.
   a. Sterile swab
   b. Culture medium
   c. Kit for culture
   d. Disposable nonsterile gloves
   ALERT: Follow Standard Precautions.

3. Identify patient/client.
4. Put on gloves.
5. Explain what you are going to do.
6. Label culture container from kit.

   a. Patient's name
   b. Date
   c. Physician's name
7. Determine site you are culturing.
8. Remove sterile swab from package.
9. Touch tip of swab to area. *Do not touch anything except area you are culturing.*
10. Rotate tip to cover with specimen.
11. Remove swab from site.
12. Put swab into a sterile container or on culture medium.
13. Be sure that tip is in medium.
14. Prepare as ordered.
15. Dispose of gloves according to contaminated waste policy.
16. Wash hands.
17. Record the following:
    a. Time
    b. Date
    c. Culture site
    d. Where culture is being sent
    e. Signature and classification

A specimen may be placed on a slide immediately. This is a direct smear. When the technician or doctor reads the smear, he or she can identify the organism. Prepare a direct smear slide following the procedure for using a microscope.

The physician may also request that the microorganism be grown on an *agar plate*. The agar in the plate provides food and moisture. The organisms grow and multiply when you place the agar plate in a warm incubator, at 36 to 37° Celsius (97 to 99° Fahrenheit) for 24 to 36 hours.

Procedure

Throat Cultures

1. Wash hands.
2. Assemble equipment.
    a. Culturette, strep test kit, and so on
    b. Nonsterile disposable gloves
    c. Tongue blade
    d. Pen light

ALERT: Follow Standard Precautions

3. Explain procedure to patient/client.
4. Explain that the swab may cause gagging.
5. Have patient in seated position.

6. Put on gloves.
7. Remove applicator from culture tube.

Note: Do not contaminate by touching any surface.

8. Ask client to tilt head back.
9. Depress tongue with a tongue blade and illuminate throat with a penlight.

10. Observe for inflamed or purulent area. (Withdraw the tongue blade and tell patient to breathe deeply if patient starts to gag.)
11. Reinsert tongue blade but not as deeply as before.
12. Swab tonsillar area from side to side, including any inflamed or purulent areas. *(Do not touch the tongue, cheeks, or teeth with the swab.)*

13. Withdraw the swab and tongue blade.
14. Place swab into medium. Do not touch sides.
15. Complete test according to order (e.g., direct smear, manufacturer's test kit, culture, and sensitivity).
16. Label specimen.
17. Clean and replace equipment.
18. Remove gloves and dispose of according to facility policy.
19. Wash hands.

Procedure

Preparing a Direct Smear for Staining

1. Wash hands.
2. Assemble equipment.
   a. Bunsen burner
   b. Saline solution
   c. Clean glass slides
   d. Rubber-tipped slide holder
   e. Wax pencil
   f. Disposable nonsterile gloves
   g. Specimen

ALERT: Follow Standard Precautions.

3. Put on gloves.
4. Label slide.
5. Light Bunsen burner.
6. Roll swab on slide touching all sides of swab.

7. Allow smear to air dry.
8. Hold slide with smear face up.
9. Attach rubber-tipped slide holder.
10. Pass slide over bunsen burner flame quickly (slide is warm, not hot).

11. Cool slide.
12. Process according to orders.
13. Clean equipment and put away.
14. Remove gloves and dispose of according to facility policy.
15. Wash hands.

Procedure

Streaking Agar (Media) Plate for Cultures

1. Wash hands.
2. Assemble equipment.
   a. Agar plate with media
   b. Specimen of a direct smear
   c. Pen or marker
   d. Incubator
   e. Disposable nonsterile gloves

ALERT: Follow Standard Precautions.

3. Label agar plate.
   a. Name of patient
   b. Time
   c. Date
   d. Physician's name
   e. Site of specimen
4. Put on gloves and take swab with specimen from culture tube.
5. Remove lid from agar plate.
6. Place lid on table with inside facing up.
7. Hold plate with agar firmly.
8. Hold swab lightly against agar at top of plate.
9. Roll swab so that all sides touch agar following a side-to-side pattern (see figure).

Procedure box continued

10. Continue halfway down agar, being careful not to break into agar.

Note: Do not go over areas that are already streaked.

11. Roll swab in top-to-bottom pattern in right-hand quarter.

12. Roll swab side to side in left-hand quarter.

Note: See examples of other patterns. Follow your facility's procedure.

13. Discard swab following facility's contaminated waste policy.

14. Replace cover on plate. Do not touch inside of lid.

15. Place plate with specimen in incubator upside down (agar on top).

Note: Temperature is 36 to 37° Celsius.

16. Discard gloves according to policy.

17. Wash hands and record the following:
    a. Patient name
    b. Physician's name
    c. Type of culture (e.g., wound, throat)
    d. Date

18. Clean and replace equipment.

19. Remove gloves and dispose of according to facility policy.

20. Wash hands.

Label lid:
J. White #11333
Wound 1/12/93

A common test is called a culture and sensitivity test. This test identifies the antibiotic that kills the organism. It also identifies the antibiotics to which the organisms are **resistant.** This information helps the physician decide which medication to prescribe. To do a culture and sensitivity test, place paper disks coated with antibiotic on an agar plate streaked with a specimen. If the organism is resistant to the antibiotic, it continues to grow around the disk. If the specimen is sensitive to the antibiotic, the colony around the disk dies. The physician then knows which antibiotic to prescribe for the patient.

resident Able to protect itself.

Gram Stain

Gram staining is a process that dyes and fixes microorganisms. The stain helps make the organism more visible in the microscope. It also helps in identifying the microorganism. The slide can be kept and reviewed if necessary. To prepare a slide from colonies grown in an agar plate for staining, a small colony of organisms is taken from the agar plate. These organisms are placed on a slide and stained.

Procedure

Preparing a Culture Smear from a Growth Medium

1. Wash hands.
2. Assemble equipment.
   a. Culture medium with growth
   b. Slide
   c. Saline solution
   d. Inoculating loop
   e. Disposable nonsterile gloves

ALERT: Follow Standard Precautions.

3. Put on gloves.
4. Light Bunsen burner.
5. Hold inoculating loop in flame until red hot. (This sterilizes the loop.)
6. Air-cool loop for several minutes. *Do not contaminate.*
7. Remove lid from agar plate.
8. Place lid on table with inside facing up.
9. Carefully touch cool loop to colony.
10. Gently move loop over organisms.
11. Replace lid on plate to prevent contaminating culture.
12. Put small drop of normal saline on slide.
13. Mix specimen on loop with saline on slide.
14. Follow policy in your facility for slide preparation.
15. Allow slide to air dry.
16. Hold loop in flame to destroy microorganisms.
17. Heat-fix smear.
    a. Attach rubber-tipped clamps to slide.
    b. Hold slide with smear face up.
    c. Pass slide over bunsen burner flame quickly.

18. Label slide.
    a. Name
    b. Date
    c. Physician's name
19. Clean equipment and put away.
20. Remove gloves and dispose of according to facility policy.
21. Wash hands.

Slide may be prepared:

Placed thinly in circles   Loop

M. Kehli Wound 1/2/93

or

Spread thinly on slide   Loop

D. Collins Throat 2-6-93

Staining a Smear with Gram Stain

1. Wash hands.
2. Assemble equipment.
   a. Staining rack
   b. Crystal violet
   c. Gram's iodine
   d. 95 percent ethyl alcohol
   e. Safranin
   f. Wash bottle with distilled water
   g. Slide with fixed smear
   h. Timer or watch
   i. Absorbent paper
   j. Disposable nonsterile gloves
   k. Face shield (check your facility's policy)
   l. Nonpermeable gown (check your facility's policy)

ALERT: Follow Standard Precautions

3. Put on
   a. Gloves   b. Face shield   c. Gown
4. Put slide face up on staining rack. Do not touch specimen.
5. Flood slide with crystal violet. Time for 30 seconds to 1 minute.

6. Wash dye off with stream from water wash.

7. Use forceps to tip slide to remove water.
8. Replace slide on stain rack.
9. Flood slide with Gram's iodine and tip to allow runoff.
10. Flood slide again with Gram's iodine. Time for 1 to 2 minutes.

11. Wash dye off with stream from water wash.

12. Use forceps to tip slide to remove water.
13. Wash slide with 95 percent ethyl alcohol for 30 to 60 seconds until smear no longer gives off dye.

Procedure box continued

Note: This step removes stain from gram-negative organisms, which helps identify organism on smear.

14. Replace on rack and rinse with distilled water.

15. Flood slide with Safranin. Time for 30 to 60 seconds.

Note: This will stain red everything that decolorized.

16. Wash slide with distilled water.

17. Wipe underside of slide (away from smear) with alcohol to remove any stain.
18. Blot slide dry with absorbent paper.

19. Clean work area.
20. Discard gloves according to facility's contaminated waste policy.
21. Remove face shield and gown.
22. Wash hands.

■ BLOOD, BLOOD COMPOSITION, AND BLOOD TESTING

Components of Blood

Whole blood has many formed elements that are suspended in a clear yellow liquid called *plasma*. Plasma makes up 55 percent of the whole blood. The other 45 percent has the formed elements. These elements are

- *Erythrocytes.* RBC (carry O_2 to cells, carry away CO_2)
- *Leukocytes.* WBC (protect against infection and disease)
- *Thrombocytes.* Platelets (start the clotting process)

The average adult has 6 to 8 quarts of blood.

Blood Tests

Physicians order blood tests for routine checkups and to help diagnose an illness. There are many blood tests available. This chapter covers the blood tests that the physician orders frequently. (See Table 18–2, which gives you the important reasons for the tests you are doing.) Refer back to the table before you practice a blood test procedure.

The laboratory most often uses capillary/peripheral blood and venous blood. You usually obtain capillary blood from the finger and sometimes from the earlobe. You use a heel stick for infants. The amount of blood is limited to a few drops. This is enough blood to do the following:

■ Complete blood count (CBC)
■ Hematocrit/microhematocrit
■ Some bleeding and coagulation times
■ Some chemical and **agglutination** tests

agglutination
Clumping together (e.g., red blood cells clump together).

When you need a larger amount of blood, you draw venous blood from the veins with a Vacutainer™ or syringe and needle. Some states and schools do not allow students to perform blood tests. Your teacher will tell you what you can do. *Never practice these tests without training.*

Complete Blood Count

The laboratory worker performs many different types of blood tests. The most frequently ordered test is a complete blood count. The complete blood count (CBC) gives a lot of information about the patient's condition. It includes the following:

■ RBC (red blood cell) count
■ WBC (white blood cell) count
■ Hemoglobin determination
■ Hematocrit determination
■ Differential white blood cell count
■ Estimate of the number of platelets
■ RBC morphology (size and shape)

Hematocrit/Microhematocrit

A hematocrit measures the volume of packed red blood cells in the blood. When you do this test you separate cell elements from the plasma. You perform this test with a few drops of capillary blood. Collect the blood in a **heparinized** capillary tube from a finger or earlobe stick for adults. In infants collect the blood from a heel stick. Centrifuge the blood to pack the cells. Low hematocrit readings tell the physician that there is a problem (e.g., anemia). High hematocrit readings provide important information (e.g., **polycythemia**) (see Table 18–2).

heparinized Containing heparin, an anticoagulant.

polycythemia Condition of having too much blood.

Hemoglobin

Hemoglobin (HGB) tests measure the oxygen-carrying capacity of the blood. Hemoglobin has the *heme*, which carries iron, and *globin*, which is the protein in the red blood cell. Hemoglobin picks up oxygen in the lungs and transports it to the cells. It also helps carry waste product, CO_2, from the body cells back to the lungs. One way to measure hemoglobin is with a hemoglobinometer.

TABLE 18–2   Common Blood Tests

Test	Abbreviation	Normal Range	Examples of Possible Diagnosis	
			Increase	Decrease
White blood cell count	WBC	5000–10,000 mm^3	Acute infection, leukemia, mononucleosis	Viral infections, bone marrow depression
Red blood cell count	RBC	Female: 4–5 million/mm^3 Male: 5–6 million/mm^3	Polycythemia, poisoning, pulmonary fibrosis	Anemia, multiple myeloma, lupus erythemia
Differential white blood cell count	Diff	Neutrophils 50–70%	*Neutrophilia:* acute bacterial infections, parasitic infections, liver disease	*Neutropenia:* acute viral infections, blood diseases, hormone diseases
		Eosinophils 1–4%	*Eosinophilia:* allergic conditions, parasitic infections, lung and bone cancer	*Eosinopenia:* infectious mononucleosis, congestive heart failure, aplastic and pernicious anemia
		Basophils 0–1%	*Basophilia:* Leukemia, hemolytic anemia, Hodgkin's disease	*Basopenia:* acute allergic reactions, hyperthyroidism, steroid therapy
		Lymphocytes 20–35%	*Lymphocytosis:* acute and chronic infections, carcinoma, hyperthyroidism	*Lymphopenia:* cardiac failure, Cushing's disease, Hodgkin's disease
		Monocytes 3–8%	*Monocytosis:* viral infections, bacterial and parasitic infections, collagen diseases, cirrhosis	*Monocytopenia:* prednisolone treatment, hairy cell leukemia
Hemoglobin	Hgb	Female: 12–16 g/100 mL Male: 14–18 g/100 mL	Congestive heart failure, (CCHF) chronic obstructive pulmonary disease (COPD), severe burn	Hodgkin's disease, hyperthyroidism, cirrhosis
Hematocrit/ microhematocrit	Hct, HCT	Female: 40–54% Male: 37–47%	Shock, dehydration, burns	Anemia, leukemia, acute blood loss
Prothrombin time	PT	11–16 sec	Anticoagulant therapy, liver disease, biliary obstruction	Diuretics, pulmonary embolism, multiple myeloma
Erythrocyte sedimentation rate	ESR	(According to method used)	Collagen disease, inflammatory disease, rheumatoid arthritis	Sickle cell anemia, CHF, polycythemia
Platelet count		200,000– 400,000/mm^3	Cancer, leukemia, splenectomy	Bone-marrow-depressant drug, pneumonia infection

Finger Stick with Regular Lancet

A regular lancet is used for the puncture if there is no spring-loaded instrument or if the patient has very tough skin (older patients, manual laborers, diabetics).

1. Wash hands.
2. Assemble equipment.
   a. Test supplies
   b. Cotton sponge
   c. Alcohol sponge
   d. Lancet
   e. Small bandage (e.g., Band-Aid)
   f. Disposable nonsterile gloves and face shield

ALERT: Follow Standard Precautions.

3. Explain procedure to patient/client.
4. Wash hands.
5. Put on gloves and face shield.
6. Select finger for stick: third or fourth finger on nondominant hand.

Note: Do not use finger with sores, scars, thickened skin.

7. Wipe finger with alcohol sponge.
8. Remove lancet from package and hold it between thumb and index finger.
9. Hold patient's finger firmly with your thumb and forefinger.
10. Make a quick, firm, deep puncture.
11. Wipe away first drop of blood with dry cotton sponge.
12. Collect specimen.
13. Give client a dry cotton sponge to apply pressure to wound.
14. Put small bandage on site.
15. Discard lancet into sharps container.
16. Discard all materials according to facility policy.
17. Remove gloves and discard according to facility's contaminated waste policy.
18. Wash hands.

Finger Stick with Spring-Loaded Puncture Instrument

1. Wash hands.
2. Assemble equipment.
   a. Test supplies
   b. Cotton sponges
   c. Alcohol sponge
   d. Spring-loaded puncture instrument
   e. Small bandage (e.g., Band-Aid)
   f. Disposable nonsterile gloves and face shield

ALERT: Follow Standard Precautions.

3. Explain procedure to patient/client.
4. Wash hands.
5. Put on gloves and face shield.
6. Insert lancet into spring-loaded device and set spring for use. (Follow manufacturer's instructions.)
7. Select the finger.
   a. Small children: use thumb.
   b. Adults/older children: use fourth finger on nondominant hand.

Procedure box continued

8. Ask patient to relax hand and dangle it down across the blood-drawing chair or exam table.
9. Wipe finger site with alcohol sponge, allow to dry.
10. Massage finger starting at base of finger and moving to tip of finger.
11. Exert some pressure on fingertip by holding it between your thumb and index finger—"pumping" or "milking" it.
12. Place spring-loaded device against side of fingertip between center pad and outside rim of nail (not dead center) and release according to manufacturer's instructions.
13. Release your hold from finger and wait a few seconds for a drop of blood to begin to form.
14. Wipe away first drop of blood with dry cotton sponge.
15. Collect the following:

    a. Platelet count specimen first
    b. Blood for peripheral smear
    c. Blood for any other test

Note: Always wipe away any blood that accumulates between collection of specimens for different tests.

16. Give client a cotton sponge to apply pressure to wound.
17. Apply small bandage.
18. Remove used lancet and place in contaminated sharps container.
19. Discard all materials according to facility policy.
20. Remove gloves and discard in contaminated waste according to facility's policy.
21. Remove face shield.
22. Wash hands.

Procedure

Heel Puncture

1. Assemble equipment.
    a. Disposable nonsterile gloves and face shield
    b. Alcohol sponge/iodine wipe
    c. Sterile gauze, 3 × 3
    d. Sterile regular lancet (2.4 mm)
    e. Test supplies
    f. Small bandage (e.g., Band-Aid)
2. Explain procedure to patient's caregiver.
3. Wash hands.
4. Instruct caregiver to remove baby's lower torso clothing to expose legs and feet. If there is another adult who can hold infant, drape the person's lap with a nonpermeable towel to protect clothing from dropped blood. Infant should be held so that the feet are free and hanging down. If there is no one to hold child, lay the child down on his or her stomach on center of exam table.

5. Put on gloves and face shield.

ALERT: Follow Standard Precautions.

6. Examine infant's feet and select heel site.

Note: Heel sticks should be performed only on lateral and medial curves of heel (etched areas in figure).

7. Clean bottom of heel with alcohol sponge or iodine wipe. Allow to dry.
8. Take sterile 3 × 3 gauze and wipe area to dry and to increase blood flow to skin.

Procedure box continued

Note: Do not contaminate gauze before using.

9. Open a blue, regular-sized (2.4 mm), sterile lance package.
10. Hold foot tightly and quickly stab site at heel.
11. Withdraw lancet and immediately make a *second* stab perpendicular to first stab, producing T-shaped wound.
12. Release foot for a few seconds.
13. Wipe away first drop of blood with sterile gauze.
14. Hold foot firmly, *avoiding* excessive squeezing to collect blood. If a capillary tube is used, hold it so that blood flows down.

15. Hold sterile gauze over puncture site until bleeding stops after collection is complete.
16. Put small bandage over site.
17. Discard lancet into sharps container.
18. Discard contaminated material according to facility policy.
19. Remove and discard gloves in contaminated waste.
20. Remove face shield.
21. Wash hands.

Procedure

Microhematocrit

1. Assemble equipment.
   a. Two heparinized microhematocrit tubes
   b. Disposable nonsterile gloves
   c. Face shield
   d. Nonpermeable gown
   e. Lancet
   f. Hematocrit tube clay sealant
   g. Microhematocrit reader card (if not on machine)
   h. Microhematocrit centrifuge
   i. Miscellaneous requisition
   j. Alcohol swab
   k. Dry sponge
   l. Small bandage (e.g., Band-Aid)

ALERT: Follow Standard Precautions.

2. Explain procedure to patient/client.
3. Wash hands.
4. Select specimen site.
   a. Adult: use fourth finger of nondominant hand.
   b. Child over 3 months: use finger (see the procedures "Finger Stick with Regular Lancet" and "Finger Stick with Spring-Loaded Puncture Instrument").
   c. Young children who are likely to pull away: use thumb.
   d. Infants to 3 months: use heel (see the procedure "Heel Puncture").
5. Put on gloves and face shield.
6. Wipe site with alcohol sponge, allow to dry.
7. Puncture site with lancet.
8. Do not squeeze finger excessively (causes hemolysis and inaccurate results).
9. Gently milk finger.

Procedure box continued

10. Wipe away first drop of blood with a gauze pad. Use second drop of blood.

11. Hold capillary tube to puncture site with marked end away from collection site, tilting in downward direction (allows tube to fill faster). Hold end to puncture site (avoids air bubbles, which cause inaccurate results).

12. Place a finger over end of tube to prevent loss of blood.

13. Fill opposite end of capillary tube with clay sealant. *Do not pack sealant into both ends of tube.*

14. Fill second capillary tube.

15. Put clean gauze over site.

16. Have patient hold firmly.

17. Place both capillary tubes (sealed end to outside) in centrifuge across from each other.

18. Record centrifuge slot numbers on requisition to avoid confusing specimens.

19. Place cover on centrifuge and lock.

20. Close lid and lock.

21. Spin 3 minutes at 10,000 rpm.

22. Apply bandage over puncture site if needed.

23. Wait until centrifuge stops, turning before opening lid. Do not try to stop spinning.

24. Remove capillary tubes and read within 5 minutes.

25. Place tube at right edge of hematocrit scale (top of plasma line at 100 percent mark).

26. Slide tube left until top of clay sealant is at bottom line, "0."

27. Record point at which top of red cell column crosses line of hematocrit scale. That line is microhematocrit value on the hematocrit scale.

28. Read second tube. Results should agree within 2 percentage points (2 percent). If more than 3 points, repeat entire process.

29. Note color of plasma.
    a. Clear or normal
    b. Yellow (may indicate elevated bilirubin; report to the physician)
    c. Pink or red (suggests either hemoglobinemia or poor collection)

30. Discard hematocrit tubes into sharps container.

31. Discard contaminated materials according to facility policy.

32. Remove gloves, place with contaminated waste.

33. Remove face shield.

34. Wash hands.

35. Document on lab slip:
    a. Patient's name
    b. Account number
    c. Date
    d. Site
    e. Results
    f. Physician's name

36. See reference hematocrit values:

Reference Microhematocrit Values

	Average Normal (%)	**Minimal Normal (%)**
Children		
At birth	56.6	51.0
First day	56.1	50.5
End of first week	52.7	47.5
End of second week	49.6	44.7
End of third week	46.6	42.0
End of fourth week	44.6	40.0

Procedure box continued

	Average Normal (%)	**Minimal Normal (%)**
Children *continued*		
End of second month	38.9	35.1
End of fourth month	36.5	32.9
End of sixth month	36.2	32.6
End of eighth month	35.8	32.3
End of tenth month	35.5	32.0
End of first year	35.2	31.7
End of second year	35.5	32.0
End of fourth year	37.1	33.4
End of sixth year	37.9	34.2
End of eighth year	38.9	35.1
End of twelfth year	39.6	35.7
Men		
End of fourteenth year	44	39.6
End of eighteenth year	47	42.3
18–50 years	47	42.3
50–60 years	45	40.5
60–70 years	43	38.7
70–80 years	40	36.0
Nonpregnant women		
14–50 years	42	36
50–80 years	40	36
Pregnant women		
End of fourth month	42	30
End of fifth month	40	30
End of sixth month	37	30
End of seventh month	37	30
End of eighth month	39	30
End of ninth month	40	30

Source: J. B. Miale, *Laboratory Medicine: Hematology.* St. Louis, Mo.: C. V. Mosby, 1977, p. 426. Reprinted with permission.

Procedure

Using a Hemoglobinometer

1. Wash hands.
2. Assemble equipment.
   a. Sterile lancet or spring-loaded lance device
   b. Alcohol swab
   c. Cotton balls
   d. Hemoglobinometer
   e. Hemolysis applicator stick
   f. Blood chamber
   g. Lens paper
   h. Small bandage (e.g., Band-Aid)
   i. Disposable nonsterile gloves and face shield

ALERT: Follow Standard Precautions.

3. Identify patient/client.
4. Explain what you are going to do.
5. Put on gloves and face shield.
6. Clean blood chamber with lens paper.
7. Do finger stick (see the procedure "Finger Stick with Regular Lancet" or "Finger Stick with Spring-Loaded Puncture Instrument").
8. Wipe off first drop of blood with cotton ball.
9. Use second drop of blood to place on clean chamber.
10. Have client hold cotton ball over stick to stop bleeding.

11. Roll hemolysis applicator stick in blood. (This hemalyzes the blood.)

Note: Blood looks red and cloudy at start. It becomes clear or transparent when it hemolyzes.

12. Cover chamber with coverglass.
13. Push chamber and cover into clip.
14. Look into hemoglobinometer.
15. Slide slide button until the two halves of field are equally light and colors match.
16. Read scale through eyepiece (e.g., 12, 12.5, 13; normal values 12 to 18).
17. Record reading.
    a. Hgb 13 g (example)
    b. Patient's name
    c. Date
    d. Physician's name
18. Place small bandage on patient's finger.
19. Clean and replace equipment according to facility's policy.
20. Remove gloves and face shield.
21. Wash hands.

Blood Glucose Testing

Diabetic Patient/Client

Diabetes is a disease that affects many people. The diabetic patient does not produce enough insulin. This causes glucose to remain in the blood. Too much glucose in the blood can cause

- Circulatory problems
- Poor healing of lesions on legs and feet
- Changes in the retina (which can lead to blindness)
- Nerve disorders

Some patients with diabetes can successfully control sugar levels in the blood with diet and exercise. Others need medication to control their sugar levels.

The diabetic client controls the disease with diet, exercise, and medication. A clinical study conducted between 1983 and 1993 called the DCCT showed that controlling glucose levels reduces the risk of eye, kidney, nerve, and cardiovascular disease. A laboratory test called Glycosolated Hemoglobin (HbA$_1$C) provides indications of glucose control. Each number above 7 grams HbA_1C means an increase in the risk of disease for patients with diabetes. Patients who need insulin must check the level of glucose in their blood. The level of glucose tells them how much insulin they need. Patients use a glucose meter to measure the sugar level in their blood before taking insulin.

General Guidelines for Testing Blood for Glucose

1. Read all instructions on the reagents and glucose meter carefully.
2. Store reagent strips according to instructions.
3. Keep the lid on the reagent bottle tightly closed.
4. *Do not touch* the pad on the reagent strip.
5. Use careful technique in obtaining blood specimen.

There are many different glucose meters. Each one is a little different from the others. Learn the steps for the meter that is used in your facility.

Counting Blood Cells

Counting blood cells gives the doctor information about a patient's health. To count blood cells, you must dilute the blood. You use blood diluting pipettes and diluting fluids for this procedure. You count the cells using the diluted blood, a counting chamber called a hemacytometer, a hemacytometer coverslip, and a microscope.

Blood-cell diluting pipettes have three basic parts (see Figure 18–4):

■ The calibrated stem is where you aspirate the blood and diluting fluid.
■ The bulb is where you mix the contents.
■ The short stem is where you attach rubber tubing.

The red-cell diluting pipette mixes RBCs and diluent 1:200. The white-cell diluting pipette is similar except that the dilution is 1:20. The diluent for WBCs destroys RBCs, leaving only WBCs.

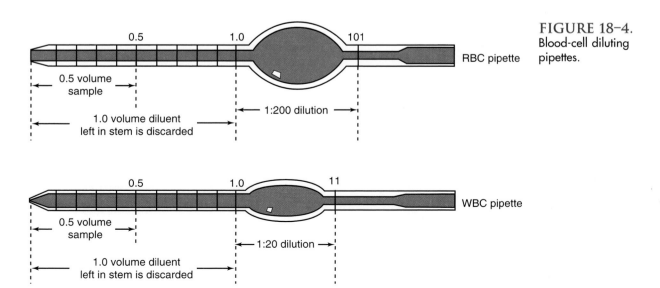

FIGURE 18–4. Blood-cell diluting pipettes.

An Unopette (Becton-Dickinson) is a disposable blood dilutor. It has a prefilled reservoir, capillary pipette, and a pipette shield. There are Unopettes to dilute WBCs, RBCs, and platelets. Follow the directions for using the Unopette carefully. When you use it correctly, it is more accurate than pipettes that require measuring diluents.

You use a hemacytometer to count cells. This is a glass slide. It has two raised areas. There are depressions on three sides. The raised surfaces are marked to help with counting (see Figure 18–5).

Automated Cell Counters

complex Having two or more related parts.

Blood cell counts are often hand counted. There are also many different types of automated equipment that can count cells. The equipment can be simple or very **complex.**

automated Method of lab testing that uses equipment to perform a series of steps, as compared to a manual method.

The **automated** cell counter dilutes the blood first. Then the diluted cells are run through a narrow opening. The cells are counted by a laser in some machines. In other machines the cells are counted by an electrical impulse device. Automated cell counting increases the accuracy of the count. Using automated equipment reduces the risks of exposure of lab workers and medical assistants to bloodborne pathogens such as Hepatitis B virus and HIV virus (AIDS).

Blood Smear

A blood smear allows you to see cells in their most natural state. A blood smear is part of the complete blood count (CBC). When you look at a blood smear through the microscope, you see

- Red blood cells
- Thrombocytes
- White blood cells

biconcave Having a depressed surface on both sides.

There are more red blood cells than white blood cells or thrombocytes. The red blood cells are **biconcave** disks (see Figure 18–6). They do not have a nucleus. When you stain a red blood cell, the hemoglobin turns reddish brown. The red blood cells should all be the same shape and be filled with hemoglobin. You must report any abnormal appearance.

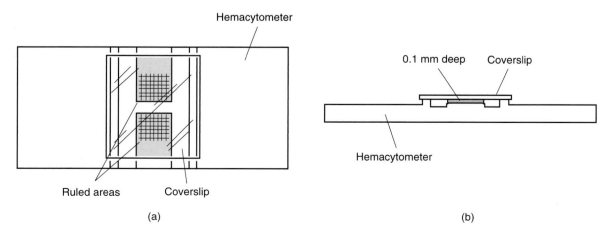

FIGURE 18–5. Hemacytometer: (a) top view; (b) side view.

Procedure

Diluting Blood Cells

1. Wash hands.
2. Assemble equipment.
   a. Red and white blood cell diluting pipettes
   b. EDTA anticoagulant
   c. Diluting fluids
      WBC: 27 acetic acid or 0.1 *N* hydrochloric acid
      RBC: normal saline
   d. Gauze pads
   e. Pipette bulb
   f. Pipette shaker
   g. Test tube rack
   h. Nonsterile gloves and faceshield

   ALERT: Follow Standard Precautions.

3. Put on gloves and face shield.

   Note: Blood may be from vial (mix well) or use finger stick method.

4. Hold pipette horizontal to blood source.
5. Put tip of pipette under surface of blood.
6. Use pipette bulb to fill to 0.5 mark.

   Note: Do not allow air bubbles. Reading is off if there are air bubbles or you are not on 0.5 mark.

7. Wipe outside of pipette with dry gauze pad.
8. Fill diluting fluid container.
9. Put tip of pipette beneath fluid.
10. Hold pipette almost upright.
11. Turn slowly while filling it to 11 mark on WBC pipette or 101 mark on RBC pipette.
12. Put finger over tip of pipette and remove pipette bulb.
13. Rotate pipette to mix sample.
14. Place pipette into tray. (Tray must be labeled with patient's name.)
15. Place pipette on shaker or turn gently to mix.
16. Clean work area.
17. Dispose of materials according to facility's contaminated waste policy.
18. Remove gloves and dispose of according to facility policy.
19. Remove face shield.
20. Wash hands.

FIGURE 18–6.
Components of blood.

Procedure

Counting Red Blood Cells

1. Wash hands.
2. Assemble equipment.
   a. Disposable nonsterile gloves and face shield
   b. Hemacytometer
   c. Counting chamber with coverglass
   d. Microscope
   e. Diluted blood sample
   f. Watch or timer

ALERT: Follow Standard Precautions.

3. Put on gloves and face shield.
4. Discard 3 to 5 drops diluted blood from pipette.
5. Center coverglass on counting chamber.
6. Put 1 drop of diluted blood on chamber platform. Drop must touch edge of coverglass.

Note: Use one drop of blood. If you have air bubbles, repeat steps.

7. Repeat in opposite chamber.
8. Let cells settle for 2 minutes.
9. Put chamber on microscope stage.
10. Use 10× objective to focus on chamber.
11. Bring moat into focus.
12. Move slide to side until indicator arrow appears as a whiter area.
13. Move slide toward you until you see counting area of chamber.
14. Check cells to make sure they are evenly distributed.
15. Find center square of ruled area.
16. Move chamber to center of upper left square of center square.
17. Switch to high power and focus.
18. Count all RBCs in four corner squares.
19. Count all RBCs in center square.
20. Add the five totals together.
21. Multiply by 10,000. This is the RBC count.
22. Repeat on side of chamber. The two counts should be similar.
23. Record number of RBCs.
24. Clean equipment according to facility's procedure.
25. Discard hazardous waste according to policy and remove gloves and face shield.
26. Wash hands.

Thrombocytes (platelets) are the smallest cells. They are round or oval in shape. Thrombocytes do not have a nucleus, and they stain blue (see Figure 18–7). They are small and have irregular shapes.

White blood cells are the largest. There are five different types of white blood cells (see Figure 18–6):

Neutrophils	54–62 percent	
Eosinophil	1–3 percent	
Basophil	0–1 percent	Percentage in blood
Lymphocytes	25–33 percent	
Monocytes	0–9 percent	

A change in the number of white cells tells the physician that something is happening in the body (e.g., allergic reaction, infection). The white blood cell count is very important when making a diagnosis.

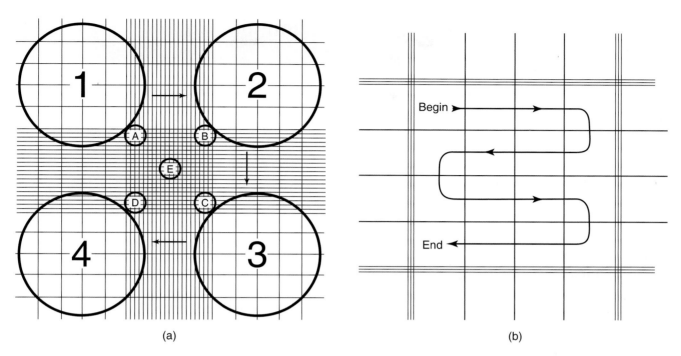

FIGURE 18–7. (a) Hemocytometer. Ruled area is the surface of the counting chamber. Count the white cells in the four large outside corner squares (1, 2, 3, 4). Count the red cells in the five smaller squares in the center (A, B, C, D, E). (b) Pattern for counting cells.

Differential White Cell Count

Use a blood smear slide for a differential count. Choose an area on the slide where red blood cells touch but are not **clumped** together. To do a differential count you count and **classify** 100 **consecutive** white blood cells. You must follow a specific winding pattern. This pattern keeps you from counting the same cell twice (see Figure 18–7). You use a differential cell counter to count the cells.

clumped Stuck together.

classify To put like items together.

consecutive Following one after the other.

Blood Typing: Antigens and Antibodies

Everyone has a blood type. There are four types: A, B, AB, and O. Blood has both antigens and antibodies. The antigens on the surface of your red blood cells determine your blood type. These antigens are inherited through genes and are on the red blood cells in your body (see Figure 18–8).

Type A
A antigen is present
(a)

Type B
B antigen is present
(b)

Type AB
A and B antigens
are present
(c)

Type O
A or B antigens
are not present
(d)

FIGURE 18–8. Blood antigens.

Procedure

Preparing a Blood Smear with Wright Stain

1. Wash hands.
2. Assemble equipment.
   a. Disposable nonsterile gloves and face shield
   b. Clean glass slides
   c. Wright stain
   d. Timer
   e. ECTA anticoagulant blood specimen or capillary blood specimen (wipe off first and use second drop)

ALERT: Follow Standard Precautions.

3. Put on gloves and face shield.
4. Place a small drop of blood on slide.

Note: Center drop on slide about 1/2 inch from end of slide.

5. Hold left side of slide.
6. Put spreader slide in front of drop of blood holding at 30 to 35° angle.
7. Pull spreader slide back into drop of blood.
8. Let blood spread to edges of slide.
9. Push spreader slide forward with a quick smooth motion *(maintain angle).*
10. Air dry.

11. Label slide.
12. Stain slide.
    a. Put smear slide on staining rack.
    b. Cover slide with Wright stain.

Note: Count number of drops used to cover slide. Follow manufacturer's directions.

    c. Time for 1 to 3 minutes.
    d. Add same number of drops of distilled water or buffer to slide.
    e. Blow gently to mix stain and buffer.

Note: Mixture is metallic green.

    f. Rinse thoroughly with distilled water.
    g. Drain water from slide.
    h. Dry back of slide.
    i. Let air dry.
13. Clean work area.
14. Dispose of contaminated waste according to facility's policy and remove gloves and face shield.
15. Wash hands.

Procedure

Performing a White Cell Differential

1. Wash hands.
2. Assemble equipment.
   a. Disposable nonsterile gloves
   b. Immersion oil
   c. Lens tissue
   d. Lens cleaner
   e. Differential cell counter
   f. Stained blood smear

ALERT: Follow Standard Precautions.

3. Clean microscope with lens tissue and put on gloves.

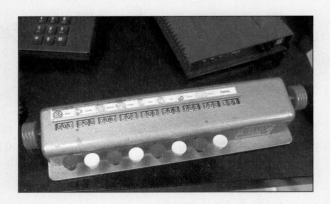

Procedure box continued

4. Put stained blood smear slide in microscope stage. (Use low-power objective.)
5. Find an area on slide where red blood cells barely touch each other.
6. Add drop of oil.
7. Focus with fine-adjustment knob and increased light.
8. Count 100 consecutive white blood cells in winding pattern (see Figure 18–8).
9. Identify each cell (e.g., lymphocyte, eosinophil).
10. Record each cell in differential cell counter.
11. Record variations in red blood cells:

   a. Size (e.g., macrocytosis, microcytosis)
   b. Shape (e.g., sickle cell, target cells)
   c. Content (e.g., hypochromic)

12. Count platelets.

Note: Take an average; multiply average by 15,000. This gives estimate of platelet count. Normal count is 150,000 to 400,000 per column.

13. Clean microscope with lens tissue.
14. Clean work area.
15. Discard contaminated waste according to facility's policy and remove gloves and face shield.
16. Wash hands.

- If you have A antigens, you are type A.
- If you have B antigens, you are type B.
- If you have A and B antigens, you are type AB.
- If you have no antigens, you are type O.

The antibodies are in the blood plasma. An antibody can combine with an antigen. Our bodies never produce antibodies that can combine with their own blood antigens. For example, if the blood has an A antigen, the plasma does not have an A antibody. The B antibody is in the plasma. The B antibody cannot combine with the A antigen. When an A antigen combines with the A antibody, the reaction is life threatening.

- Type A blood, B antibody in plasma
- Type B blood, A antibody in plasma
- Type AB blood, neither A nor B antibody in plasma
- Type O blood, A and B antibody in plasma

Another factor in blood typing is the Rh factor. If the Rh factor is present on the red blood cell, you are Rh+. If it is not present, you are Rh−.

Antigen-Antibody Reactions

When a blood antigen combines with the same type of antibody, *agglutination* occurs. The red blood cells clump together. The clumps of cells cannot pass through the small tubes in the kidney. This can cause kidney failure. The cells also break down and are destroyed (hemolysis). When this happens, oxygen cannot be circulated to the tissues. Carbon dioxide cannot be removed from the tissue, and death results.

Blood Typing and Crossmatching

Blood typing is very important. If the wrong blood is given to a patient, agglutination can occur. To prevent agglutination, you type and crossmatch blood before giving a blood transfusion.

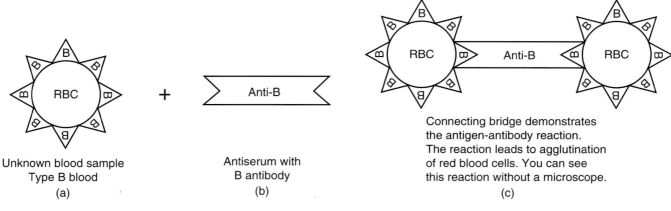

FIGURE 18–9.

To test blood, you use a manufactured antiserum. The antiserum has antibodies in it. If you use an antiserum with B antibodies on blood with B antigen, you will have clumping. If you use an antiserum with B antibodies on A antigen blood, you will not have clumping (see Figure 18–9).

To crossmatch blood before a transfusion, you perform a series of tests on the patient's blood and the donor's blood. The blood you give the patient must match that of the donor.

Erythrocyte Sedimentation Rate (SR, Esr, Sed. Rate)

The sedimentation rate of blood helps in the diagnosis of some diseases. The speed with which red blood cells fall out of plasma is known as the *sedimentation rate*. An increased sedimentation rate can indicate infection, leukemia, or other problems. When the sedimentation rate decreases it can indicate heart disease, liver disease, or polycythemia.

Procedure

Blood Typing

1. Wash hands.
2. Assemble equipment.
   a. Disposable nonsterile gloves and face shield
   b. Anti-A serum at room temperature
   c. Anti-B serum at room temperature
   d. Anti-Rh serum at room temperature
   e. Two clean slides
   f. Wax pencil
   g. Mixing sticks
   h. Blood specimen
   i. Timer

Procedure box continued

ALERT: Follow Standard Precautions.

3. Check expiration date on antiserum.
4. Prepare slides.
   a. Label slides.
   b. Use wax pencil to make two large circles on one slide and one large circle on second slide (see Figure).

Note: Make sure that circle is thick enough to prevent blood from crossing it.

5. Put 1 drop of anti-A serum in A circle.
6. Put 1 drop of anti-B serum in B circle.
7. Put 1 drop of anti-Rh serum in Rh circle.
8. Put on gloves and face shield.
9. Put 1 drop of unknown blood specimen *beside* drop of antiserum in each circle.
10. Mix antiserum with blood specimen in each circle.

Note: Use different mixing stick for each group.

11. Rock slides for 1 minute.

12. Read results before 2 minutes pass.
13. Check slide for agglutination.
14. Record results:

Type of Blood	Anti-A	Anti-B	Anti-Rh or Anti-D
O	Negative	Negative	
A	Positive	Negative	
B	Negative	Positive	
AB	Positive	Positive	
Rh positive			Positive
Rh negative			Negative

15. Clean all equipment.
16. Dispose of contaminated waste according to facility's policy and remove gloves and face shield.
17. Wash hands.

Procedure

Erythrocyte Sedimentation Rate Using Wintrobe Method

1. Wash hands.
2. Assemble equipment.
   a. Disposable nonsterile gloves and face shield
   b. Calibrated ESR tube—Wintrobe method
   c. Sedimentation rate tubes
   d. Transfer pipettes
   e. Tube holder with level
   f. Venous blood with oxalate/anticoagulant
   g. Timer

ALERT: Follow Standard Precautions.

3. Check level indicator on tube holder: *must be level.*
4. Put on gloves and face shield.
5. Put sedimentation tube in sed rack with black line in tube at zero on rack.

16 mm
29 mm

Procedure box continued

6. Take tube of specimen blood with anticoagulant and mix gently.

7. Withdraw blood from specimen tube with pipette.

8. Put pipette on bottom of sed tube and release blood slowly as you withdraw pipette.

9. Fill sed tube to zero line. *Note:* If bubbles occur, start over.

10. Recheck rack. It must be level.

11. Follow your facility's procedure for timing fall of red cells.

12. Read at marked line between cells and plasma.

13. Record readings (e.g., 20 min, 2 mm). Normal readings: male 0–6.5 mm/hr; female 0–15 mm/hr.

14. Clean equipment.

15. Dispose of contaminated waste according to facility's policy and remove gloves and face shield.

16. Wash hands.

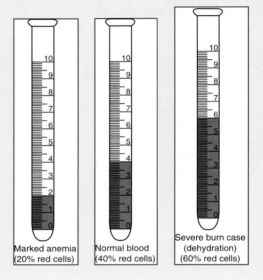

Marked anemia (20% red cells)   Normal blood (40% red cells)   Severe burn case (dehydration) (60% red cells)

Blood Chemistries

The physician uses the results from blood chemistries to help with diagnosis. These chemistries measure chemicals dissolved in the blood. To perform these tests, you need a venous specimen. The phlebotomy unit of this chapter teaches you to draw a venous specimen (see Table 18–3 to familiarize yourself with common blood chemistries). Follow your facility's procedures for tests that you perform.

TABLE 18–3   Most Common Blood Chemistries and Examples of Disorders They Indicate

Test	Abbreviation	Normal Range	Examples of Possible Diagnosis	
			Results Increased	**Results Decreased**
Alkaline phosphate	ALP	30–115 mU/mL	Liver disease, bone disease, mononucleosis	Malnutrition, hypothyroidism, chronic nephritis
Blood urea nitrogen	BUN	8–25 mg/dL	Kidney disease, dehydration, GI bleeding	Liver failure, malnutrition
Calcium	CA	8.5–10.5 mg/dL	Hypercalcemia, bone metastases, Hodgkin's disease	Hypocalcemia, renal failure, pancreatitis
Chloride	Cl	96–11 mEq/L	Dehydration, eclampsia, anemia	Ulcerative colitis, burns, heat exhaustion
Cholesterol	CHOL	120–200 mg/dL	Atherosclerosis, nephrosis, obstructive jaundice	Malabsorption, liver disease, hyperthyroidism
Creatinine	Creat	0.4–1.5 mg/dL	Chronic nephritis, muscle disease, obstruction of urinary tract	Muscular dystrophy
Globulin	Glob	1.0–3.5 g/dL	Brucellosis, rheumatoid arthritis, hepatic carcinoma	Severe burns
Glucose fasting blood sugar	FBS	70–110 mg/100 mL	Diabetes mellitus	Excess insulin
Two-hour postprandial	2-hr PPBS	<140 mg/dL	Cushing syndrome, brain damage	Addison's disease, CA of pancreas
Lactic acid	LDH	100–225 mU/mL	Acute MI, acute leukemia, hepatic disease	
Potassium	K	3.5–5.5 mEq/L	Renal failure, acidosis, cell damage	Malabsorption, severe burn, diarrhea
Serum glutami-coxaloacetic	SGOT	0–41 mU/mL	MI, liver disease, pancreatitis	Uncontrolled diabetes mellitus with acidosis
Serum glutamicpyruvic transaminase	SGPT	0–45 mU/mL	Active cirrhosis, pancreatitis, obstructive jaundice	
Sodium	NA	135–145 mEq/L	Diabetes insipitus, coma, Cushing syndrome	Severe diarrhea, severe nephritis, vomiting
Free thyroxine	T4	1–2.3 mg/dL	Thyroiditis, hyperthyroidism, Graves disease	Goiter, myledema, hypothyroidism
Total bilirubin	TB	0.1–1.2 mg/dL	Liver disease, hemolytic anemia, lupus erythemia	
Triglycerides	TRIG	40–170 mg/dL	Liver disease, atherosclerosis, pancreatitis	Malnutrition
Uric acid	UA	2.2–9.0 mg/dL	Renal failure, gout, leukemia, eclampsia	

UNIT 2   Phlebotomist

S*teps to success*

1. Read this unit.
2. Complete Worksheets 1 through 4 as assigned.
3. When you are confident that you can meet each objective for this unit, ask your instructor for the unit evaluation.
4. Complete "Your Link to Success" at the end of this chapter.

Objectives

When you have completed this unit you will be able to do the following:

✓ Complete all of the objectives in Part One of this book.
✓ List six things the physician can tell from blood samples.
✓ Define vocabulary words.
✓ List three components of blood.
✓ Describe what changes occur in the blood after injury or infection.
✓ List four rules to follow when collecting blood samples.
✓ Match the blood collection tube stopper colors with their content and general use.
✓ Label a diagram of the arm, and identify the veins most often used in **venipuncture.**
✓ State three ways that blood samples are obtained.
✓ Give two reasons why a syringe and needle are used to draw a blood sample.
✓ Discuss why correct disposal of needles, syringes, and contaminated material is important.
✓ List two serious illnesses spread by contaminated needles and materials.
✓ Demonstrate how to use a Vacutainer™ correctly to withdraw blood.
✓ Demonstrate how to use a needle and syringe correctly to withdraw blood.
✓ Demonstrate how to complete a finger stick correctly.
✓ Apply all procedural techniques with confidence.

venipuncture Puncture of a vein.

■ RESPONSIBILITIES OF A PHLEBOTOMIST

Phlebotomists may work in an acute care hospital, private laboratory, physician's office, public health agency, or clinic. They draw blood from the veins of patients for testing by the medical laboratory technician or technologist. The phlebotomist can be a laboratory assistant or medical assistant. Phlebotomy is a job title in some facilities. A phlebotomist may only draw blood and not perform other laboratory or medical assistant tasks. Blood is the primary specimen that laboratory workers use for determining the condition of the patient. The results of these tests give the physician information to help in the diagnosis and treatment of patients. The results of blood tests tell the doctor many things about the patient. Some of these relate to

■ Anemia
■ Infection
■ Organ damage
■ Change in cell structure
■ Liver disease
■ Diabetes

The duties of a phlebotomist include the following:

■ Screen, record, and direct telephone calls.
■ Answer and relay messages.
■ Assist in ordering supplies.
■ Keep work area clean and properly stocked.
■ Keep collection tray clean and stocked.
■ Use sterile techniques.
■ Identify specialized equipment and supplies.
■ Use correct safety precautions.
■ Use equipment and supplies for obtaining blood specimens according to facility policy.
■ Use proper technique in collecting and handling specimens.
■ Obtain blood specimens from patients (must be certified and have a knowledge of correct anticoagulants).
■ Correctly dispose of contaminated materials according to facility policy.

■ ABOUT BLOOD

Blood is the fluid that flows through the arteries and veins. It carries nutrients and oxygen to the cells and carries away waste products. Blood is composed of *red blood cells, white blood cells,* and **plasma.** A specimen of blood tells a doctor many things about a patient. When the body is injured or ill, blood cells rupture and release chemicals that help doctors diagnose conditions. Vital organs also release substances into the blood that indicate normal or abnormal function within the body. Foreign bodies such as bacteria are also detected from blood specimens. Blood counts determine whether an infection is present (increased number of WBCs) and if there are enough red blood cells.

plasma Liquid part of the blood, consisting of water, nutrients, wastes, hormones, antibodies, and enzymes.

Patient Considerations

1. Your patient/client may be afraid of a finger stick or venipuncture. Remain calm and patient. Explain exactly what you are doing.
2. The patient may faint and need you to protect him or her from injury. Review how to treat syncopy in your text.
3. It may be difficult to get into the vein.
   a. Obese patients have fat layers over the vein. **b.** Some patients have small, delicate veins, especially the elderly. **c.** Veins may be injured from past or recent IVs or blood draws. **d.** Veins may roll and be difficult to access.

If you have a problem entering the vein, call your supervisor to help.

Never stick a patient more than two times.

■ PREPARING TO DRAW BLOOD

Venipuncture is an invasive procedure. You break the skin, which is the first line of defense against infection. You must use aseptic technique to protect the patient. Remember to *use Standard Precautions* to protect yourself and your patient.

The following rules help you obtain the specimen you need.

■ Collect enough blood for the test.

hematoma Collection of blood beneath the skin.

■ Obtain the specimen as skillfully and efficiently as possible to prevent a **hematoma** or injury to the patient's vein.

■ Collect the proper specimen.

■ Observe the patient for signs of fainting.

Important Things for You to Know Before You Draw Blood

There are some basic principles that you must learn before you draw blood. Blood is usually tested in two ways:

■ *Uncoagulated.*   Collect the blood in a specimen tube that contains an anticoagulant. This method allows you to test the blood specimen in liquid form with the cells in suspension. The specimen is the same as the blood that circulates through the veins.

■ *Coagulated.*   Collect the blood and let it coagulate (clot). As a clot forms, a clear liquid, called serum, leaves the clotted cells. This serum is used in many tests.

Anticoagulants

Many tests require unclotted blood. Learn which anticoagulant to use for each specific test. Blood with an anticoagulant may be suitable for one test or a group of tests. It may not be suitable for other tests. Collection tubes come prepared with the solutions needed for specific tests. The tubes are color coded for each test. Learn the color codes you use for each test before you draw blood (see Table 18–4).

TABLE 18–4   Selecting the Correct Tube for Venipuncture

Color	Contents	General Use
Red-brown	None	Blood chemistry, multipurpose
Blue	Citrate	Coagulation
Violet	EDTA (anticoagulant)	Hematology
Green	Heparin	Blood gas, pH
Gray	Sodium fluoride	Chemistry (glucose) and alcohol
SST/marble	Coagulant activator and separating jell	Chemistry

■ DRAWING BLOOD

Review the structure of the veins in the arm before you draw blood. This knowledge is essential when you draw blood. Sticking a patient in the wrong place can cause injury. Study Figure 18–10 until you can identify each labeled area and find it on your arm. Review all of the sections in this chapter that are about laboratory safety. Learn the different blood tests and blood chemistries. This helps you understand your job.

Blood can be obtained with a Vacutainer™, syringe and needle, or finger and heel sticks. All three require that you follow the guidelines.

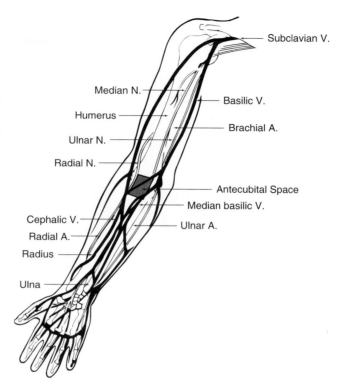

FIGURE 18–10. Diagram of the arm. A, artery; V, vein; N, nerve.

Subclavian V.
Median N.
Basilic V.
Humerus
Brachial A.
Ulnar N.
Radial N.
Antecubital Space
Median basilic V.
Cephalic V.
Ulnar A.
Radial A.
Radius
Ulna

Guidelines for Blood Withdrawal

1. Select the right collection tube (see Table 18–4 for Vacutainers™).
2. Select the site carefully.

   • Never draw blood from an arm with an IV. • Do not use areas that have bruises, a rash, scars, or swelling.

3. Apply a tourniquet above the elbow.
4. Release the tourniquet after 1 minute to prevent bruising and discomfort.
5. Ask the client to open and close the fist to help fill the veins.
6. Cleanse the area for the stick with a sterile swab using a circular motion from the center outward. This removes dirt and bacteria.
7. Hold the skin taut.
8. Use a 15 to 20° angle for entry into the vein.
9. Never press on the vein when removing the needle.
10. *Remember! Do not attempt to draw blood until you are properly instructed in the procedure.*
11. Follow Standard Precautions.

Venipuncture Procedures

Read the following instructions for using a Vacutainer™. Think about each step and why it is important (see Figure 18–11).

Some patients have fragile veins that might be damaged by suction from the Vacutainer™, or have veins that roll. For these patients you can use a syringe and needle. The guidelines are the same as those given in the procedure. The method is different.

FIGURE 18–11. Drawing blood with a Vacutainer™.

g

h

i

j

k

l

FIGURE 18-11. (*continued*)

Procedure

Drawing Blood with a Vacutainer™

1. Wash hands.
2. Assemble equipment.
   a. Alcohol wipes or 70 percent alcohol
   b. Sterile cotton wipes
   c. Sterile compresses
   d. Vacutainer™ system with appropriate tube(s), needle, and holder
   e. Small bandage
   f. Disposable nonsterile gloves
   g. Nonpermeable long-sleeved gown
   h. Face shield

   ALERT: Follow Standard Precautions.

3. If going to client's room, check collection tray for materials required.
   a. Vacutainer™ or syringe
   b. Cotton balls or sterile gauze
   c. Bandages or paper tape
   d. Tourniquet
   e. Tube holders
   f. Packaged alcohol swabs
   g. Needles (various sizes)
   h. Blood culture media
   i. Glass slides
   j. Lancets
   k. Requisitions and marking pen
   l. Disposable nonsterile gloves
4. Identify patient/client.
5. Explain procedure to patient.
6. Attach needle to Vacutainer™ (or syringe).
7. Select correct tube for blood sample you are going to draw.
   a. *Red-brown:* blood chemistry, multipurpose
   b. *Blue:* coagulation
   c. *Violet:* hematology
   d. *Green:* blood gas, pH
   e. *Gray:* chemistry (glucose) and alcohol
8. Insert tube into holder and push tube stopper onto needle.
9. Select site for venipuncture by palpating anticubital space:
   a. Carefully examine both arms.
   b. Select suitable site.
10. Put on gloves and face shield.
11. Apply a tourniquet 3 to 4 inches above patient's elbow.

12. Clean venipuncture site with alcohol wipe. *Do not touch area after cleaning.*
13. Remove needle cover.
14. If you are right-handed, use your left hand to pull skin over puncture site tightly. (If left-handed, use right hand.)
15. Carefully insert needle through skin into vein. (This will take practice to do correctly.)
    a. Bevel tip of needle should be up.
    b. Puncture skin and vein in one motion.
16. Place two fingers at end of holder; with your thumb, push Vacutainer™ onto needle to end of holder. (You may need to use more than one tube.)
17. Release tourniquet as soon as blood begins to enter tube, and obtain as many samples as needed.
18. Remove last Vacutainer™ from holder when enough blood has been obtained.
19. Remove needle from vein when blood stops flowing into tube. Place gauze over puncture site.
20. Apply pressure with sterile compress to puncture site and have patient elevate arm for a few minutes.
21. Discard needle in correct disposal container.
22. If tube contains additives, gently invert 8 to 10 times to mix additives with blood. Do not shake.
23. Apply small bandage to puncture site.
24. Clean area of all used material and discard properly according to facility's contaminated waste policy.
25. Label collection tube:
    a. Patient's name
    b. Date
    c. Time
    d. Technician's initials
26. Remove gloves, face shield, and gown.
27. Check to see that bleeding has stopped.
28. Wash hands.
29. Fill out paperwork or forms that are required.
30. Make certain that blood sample is delivered to proper place for testing.

Procedure

Using a Needle and Syringe to Draw Blood

1. Wash hands.
2. Assemble equipment.
   a. Sterile compresses
   b. Tourniquet
   c. Sterile disposable needle, usually 1½ or 1¼ inches, 21 gauge
   d. Sterile disposable syringe: 5-, 10-, 20-, or 30-cc size
   e. Test tube(s) with or without additives, depending on tests to be done
   f. Disposable nonsterile gloves
   g. Nonpermeable gown with long sleeves
   h. Face shield

   ALERT: Follow Standard Precautions.

3. If you are going to client's room, check collection tray for materials required.
   a. Syringe
   b. Needles (various sizes)
   c. Cotton balls or sterile gauze
   d. Bandages or paper tape
   e. Tourniquet
   f. Tube holders
   g. Packed alcohol swabs
   h. Blood culture media
   i. Glass slides
   j. Lancets
   k. Requisitions and marking pen
   l. Disposable nonsterile gloves
   m. Nonpermeable gown
   n. Face shield
4. Identify patient/client.
5. Explain procedure to patient.
6. Attach needle to syringe. Leave needle cover on.
7. Select correct tube for blood sample you are going to draw.
   a. *Red-brown:* blood chemistry, multipurpose
   b. *Blue:* coagulation
   c. *Violet:* hematology
   d. *Green:* blood gas, pH
   e. *Gray:* chemistry (glucose) and alcohol

8. Select site for venipuncture by palpating anticubital space.
   a. Carefully examine both arms.
   b. Select suitable site.
9. Put on gloves and face shield.
10. Apply tourniquet 3 to 4 inches above patient's elbow.
11. Clean venipuncture site with alcohol wipe. *Do not touch area.*
12. Remove needle cover.
13. If you are right-handed, use your left hand to pull skin over puncture site tightly. (If left-handed, use right hand.)
14. Carefully insert needle through skin into vein. (This will take practice to do correctly.)
    a. Bevel tip of needle should be up.
    b. Puncture skin and vein in one motion.
15. Having entered vein, use your right hand (if you are right-handed) or left hand (if you are left-handed) to pull syringe plunger slowly to withdraw blood. As soon as blood starts to flow into syringe, release tourniquet.
16. When you have drawn required amount of blood, place sterile compress over puncture site and withdraw needle.
17. Apply pressure over puncture site for a few minutes and have patient elevate arm.
18. Remove stopper from Vacutainer™ and fill tube with correct amount of blood.
19. If you are using tubes other than Vacutainers™, cap tubes.
20. Label collection tube with patient's name, date, and time.
21. If tube has an additive, gently invert 8 to 10 times to mix blood and additive. *Do not shake.*
22. Apply small bandage to puncture area.
23. Discard syringe and needle in correct disposal container.
24. Remove gloves, face shield, and gown.
25. Wash hands.

Finger or Heel Stick

You use a finger, heel, or earlobe stick (see procedures in Unit 1 of this chapter) when you need a small amount of blood for a test. You obtain a few drops of blood by this method. This is enough for certain tests (for example, PKU on infants, hematocrit, some coagulation tests, and some chemistry tests).

The Collection Tray

Carry a tray with you when you go to the patient/client. If the patient is coming into the laboratory, you have the equipment that you need at your station. If you carry a tray, you must keep it clean and well stocked. Double-check your tray to be certain that you have all the supplies that you need for the test you are doing. The department that you work in has a list of all the supplies that you should carry. Each lab is slightly different. The following is an example of materials that are in a collection tray.

- Vacutainers™ and syringes
- Cotton balls and/or sterile gauze
- Bandages and or paper tape
- Tube holders
- Packaged alcohol swabs
- Needles (various sizes)
- Blood culture media
- Glass slides
- Lancets
- Requisitions and marking pen
- Disposable gloves

How to Dispose of Used Materials

Carefully dispose of used materials (Figure 18–12). Improper disposal causes injury or illness if someone comes in contact with infected materials. It is especially important to be aware of the dangers of contracting hepatitis and AIDS from accidental needle sticks and/or contact with infected body fluids (see the section "Laboratory Standards" in Unit 1).

FIGURE 18–12.
Sharps container.

Always follow these rules:

■ *Never drop a needle into a wastebasket, where it may injure someone.*

■ Place used needles in a sharps container (see Figure 18–13). Follow the laboratory's procedure for safe disposal of the needles.

■ When drawing blood from a patient who is in isolation, take only the materials that you need into the room. Discard the used needles in the disposal container inside the patient's room. Dispose of them according to the facility's policy for contaminated materials. Follow the rules for the removal of specimens from the isolation room.

■ JOBS AND PROFESSIONS

■ Assistive personnel
■ Clinical medical assistant
■ Laboratory assistant
■ Nurse assistant
■ Licensed vocational/practical nurse
■ Registered nurse
■ Phlebotomist
■ Laboratory technician

Your link to success

Thinking Critically:
Check Your Understanding

1. **Medical Terminology** Use information in Part One of this text and a medical dictionary to list laboratory tests or medical terms used in the laboratory. Use these terms to write a scenario about a patient who had these tests performed.

2. **Legal and Ethical** Control tests are important quality indicators in the laboratory. Explain the legal and ethical reasons for their requirements of accuracy and consistency.

3. **Patient Education** Write the instructions to give a patient for a clean-catch urine specimen. Explain how you can check the patient's understanding of the instructions.

4. **Computers** Identify at least five laboratory tests that are commonly performed by a computerized analyzer. Describe the primary differences (advantages vs. disadvantages) between the computerized test and the manual test that measures the same thing.

5. **Case Study** An 8-year-old girl is in the reception area of the laboratory. Her mother warns you that her daughter is frightened of needles and becomes hysterical every time she gets a shot or has blood drawn. Explain how you will approach the child, what you will communicate to her, and what you are going to do to complete the phlebotomy.

Portfolio Connection

When you are competent in all laboratory assistant and phlebotomy skills, ask for permission to copy the results of tests that you completed. (Remove all patient identifiers.) Place these copies in your portfolio as evidence of your skills. Place a copy of your on-site trainer's evaluation in your portfolio.

Write a paper describing your doubts and realizations and the barriers that you were able to overcome during your laboratory experiences. For example, were you afraid that drawing blood might make you faint? Describe the ways you plan to use the skills, information, and insights that you gained about people and about this job. This assignment must be in standard report format.

PHYSICAL THERAPY AIDE

19

Steps to success

1. Read this chapter.
2. Complete Worksheet 1 as assigned.
3. Practice and demonstrate each procedure.
4. When you are confident that you can meet each objective for this chapter, ask your instructor for the chapter evaluation.
5. Complete "Your Link to Success" at the end of this chapter.

Objectives

When you have completed this chapter, you will be able to do the following:

✓ Complete all objectives in Part One of this book.
✓ Describe the responsibilities of a physical therapy aide.
✓ Name four conditions treated with ultraviolet light.
✓ Describe four conditions treated with diathermy.
✓ Explain the physical therapy aide's main responsibility when setting a patient up for a diathermy treatment.
✓ List three conditions commonly treated by ultrasound.
✓ Document the most important question to ask a patient when preparing for an ultrasound treatment.
✓ Identify two kinds of thermotherapy and the conditions they treat.
✓ Identify two ways to give cryotherapy and conditions they treat.
✓ Define *hydrotherapy* and list the three reasons hydrotherapy is used.
✓ Define *guarding technique* and *guarding belt*.

✓ Explain the purpose of range of motion (Chapter 15).
✓ List five commonly used ambulation devices.
✓ List two transporting devices commonly used (Chapter 15).
✓ Demonstrate the following skills:
  • From Chapter 15: Pivot transfer from bed to wheelchair and back
                    Sliding from bed to gurney and back
                    Moving a patient/client in a wheelchair
                    Moving a patient/client on a gurney
                    Lifting with a mechanical lift
                    Range of motion
  • From Chapter 22: Customer service
✓ Explain the role of physical therapy in the team concept of patient care.
✓ Demonstrate each procedure in this chapter.

■ THE PHYSICAL THERAPY DEPARTMENT

The physical therapy department is made up of a number of trained people who work as a team to assist and direct patients in the rehabilitation process. Their main goal is to reduce pain, prevent deformity, and promote healing. They also attempt to restore function or assist patients/clients by teaching them new ways to adjust to their disabilities. The entry-level job title for this department is "physical therapy aide." Physical therapy workers may be employed in the following facilities and agencies:

■ Acute care facilities
■ Long-term care facilities
■ Rehabilitation centers
■ Schools for the disabled
■ Public health agencies
■ Home health care agencies
■ Sports medicine centers

■ RESPONSIBILITIES OF A PHYSICAL THERAPY AIDE

As a physical therapy aide, you are required to do the following tasks:

■ Prepare equipment (e.g., hydrotherapy pools)
■ Assist patients:

• With walking and gait training • To dress and undress • To position themselves • To remove and replace braces, splints, and slings

■ Change linen on beds and tables
■ Fold linen
■ Clean equipment and work area
■ May inventory materials and supplies

■ PREPARING PATIENTS/CLIENTS FOR THERAPY

As an aide in the physical therapy department, you assist the therapist and prepare

■ The patient   ■ Supplies   ■ Equipment

There are various types of therapy, and each requires a slightly different preparation. Some of the most common types of therapy are discussed below.

Ultraviolet-light therapy is used to treat

■ Acne   ■ Pressure sores   ■ Psoriasis   ■ Wound infections

This treatment can cause severe burning. For this reason, the patient cannot be left unobserved in the room during a treatment.

NOTE Do not turn the light on before the therapist is ready to start the treatment.

Diathermy is a heat-inducing treatment that increases the circulation in the treated area. It is often used to treat

■ Muscle problems   ■ Bursitis
■ Arthritis   ■ Tendonitis

Metal attracts heat during this procedure, so it is your responsibility to

■ Have the patient remove all metal jewelry, belts, hairpins, and so on.
■ Ask the patient if they have any metal implants in joints or in other parts of the body. If they do, report it to the therapist right away.

Ultrasound uses high-frequency sound waves to penetrate deep tissues. It is most commonly used to treat

■ Pain
■ Muscle spasms
■ Problems in circulation

Ultrasound is also used to diagnose. However, physical therapy uses it only in a therapeutic mode. Because ultrasound vibrates tissues, caution has to be taken with patients with joint implants. Always ask patients during the preparation if they have any joint implants. If so, report it to the therapist.

Thermotherapy refers to heat treatments. Heat is used to speed up the healing process. Heat causes the blood vessels to expand (dilate). This allows more blood to circulate to the area and helps the healing process. The blood brings oxygen and food needed for healing. If the area is swollen and/or inflamed, the blood helps absorb and carry away the extra fluid. This type of treatment is used to

■ Relieve pain
■ Promote muscle relaxation
■ Reduce muscle spasms
■ Reduce inflammation
■ Treat skin ulcers

■ Treat perineal lacerations
■ Reduce swelling
■ Promote drainage

There are two kinds of thermotherapy. One type is moist heat. The other type is dry heat. *Moist heat* is applied with

■ Hot soaks
■ Hot compresses
■ Hot packs

Dry heat is applied with

■ Heat lamps   ■ Standard electric bulbs
■ Infrared lights   ■ Heating pads

Procedure

Preparing Moist Hot Soaks

ALERT: Follow Standard Precautions.

1. Wash hands.
2. Assemble equipment.
   a. Hydroculator pad
   b. Towel
3. Identify patient/client.
4. Explain what you will be doing and reassure patient that procedure is painless.
5. Cover warm hydroculator pad with towel.
6. Expose site to be treated.
7. Position patient for comfort.

8. Apply covered warm hydroculator pad to appropriate site.
9. Wash hands.
10. Recheck patient frequently; look for
    a. Severely reddened areas
    b. Irritated areas
    c. Painful areas
11. Remove soaks as ordered.
12. Position client for comfort.
13. Wash hands.
14. Report and record patient's tolerance of treatment and any changes in condition you observed.

You need to prepare hot packs so that they are ready when needed. Always check the skin for signs of extreme redness or burning. If patient complains of discomfort, remove the packs immediately.

Cryotherapy means cold therapy. Cold therapy causes the blood vessels to get smaller (contract). This slows the flow of blood to the area. This reduces the amount of fluid and helps reduce pain. Cold application is used to

■ Relieve pain   ■ Control bleeding   ■ Prevent edema   ■ Reduce body
temperature   ■ Reduce inflammation

Cryotherapy can be given in two ways: dry cold and moist cold. *Dry cold* includes the use of

■ Ice bags   ■ Ice collars

Moist cold includes the use of

■ Cold compresses   ■ Cold packs   ■ Ice massage

Prepare cold packs for cryotherapy (cold, moist, or dry treatments) so that they are ready when needed. Always check the skin for signs of whiteness (blanching) or bluishness. If these occur, stop the treatment immediately.

Procedure

Moist Cryotherapy (Cold) Compresses

ALERT: Follow Standard Precautions.

1. Wash hands.
2. Assemble equipment
   a. Cool, wet cloth   c. Dry towel
   b. Plastic cover
3. Apply cool, wet cloth as ordered.
4. Cover wet area with plastic cover.
5. Cover plastic with dry towel.
6. Wash hands.
7. Recheck frequently for
   a. Coolness of cloth
   b. Position
   c. Patient's comfort needs (reapply PRN)
8. Remove as ordered.

9. Dry skin.
10. Dispose of supplies and clean area.
11. Wash hands.
12. Report and document effects of treatment.

Note: Wear gloves if there are broken areas on the skin.

Procedure

Dry Cryotherapy: Ice Bags/Ice Collars

ALERT: Follow Standard Precautions.

1. Wash hands.
2. Assemble equipment.
   a. Ice bag or commercial cold compress
   b. Ice
   c. Cover for ice bag
3. Fill bag with ice. (Run water over cubes to soften sharp edges.)
4. Remove air from bag by pressing sides together.
5. Close end and check for leaks.

Procedure box continued

6. Cover bag with cloth. (Never apply bag directly to skin; it may stick, burn, and tear skin when removed.)
7. Identify patient/client by checking order and name with patient's armband or patient chart.
8. Position ice bag as ordered.
9. Secure bag so that it does not move away from affected area.
10. Provide needed comfort measures for patient.
11. Wash hands.
12. Return frequently to check for
    a. Coolness of ice bag

b. Position of ice bag
c. Color of skin (remove ice if skin is bluish in color and report)
13. Remove ice bag at ordered time.
14. Wash hands.
15. Recheck skin, and report and document effects of treatment.
16. Wash hands.
17. Empty bag, dry, and return to appropriate area for cleaning.

Note: Wear gloves if there are broken areas on the skin.

Hydrotherapy is water therapy. Hydrotherapy is usually given in a whirlpool. The whole body may be treated or just a limb. This treatment is used to

- Apply soothing medication
- Promote relaxation
- Improve circulation and mobility of an injured limb
- Loosen and remove dead skin

This treatment is accomplished in various-sized tubs ranging from small basins to a swimming pool. Your responsibility is to

- Assist the client in disrobing or exposing the area to be treated.
- Ensure that the water temperature is correct (105°F).
- Secure the client to ensure there is no danger of injury.
- Disinfect and clean the equipment.
- Assist the patient when large areas of the body are to be submerged.
- Clean the tub after each treatment.

■ GUARDING TECHNIQUES

Use guarding techniques when moving patients/clients from place to place. These techniques protect the patient while transferring a patient from the bed to a gurney or chair, chair to a chair, chair to a toilet, or commode and back again. You use a variety of techniques to transfer the client.

■ *Pivot technique.* You generally use this technique when moving a patient who can bear weight on at least one foot. It works best when moving from a bed or chair to a chair, toilet, or commode and back again.

■ *Sliding technique.* You use sliding when a client needs to be moved and cannot get up or bear weight on either foot. It works best when moving from bed to gurney, chair, commode, or toilet and back again. Paraplegic and quadriplegic patients may use a flat boardlike device to slide on. This provides security and decreases the chance of separation between chairs and bed and so on.

■ *Lifting technique.* Use this technique when there is ample help and strength to support the client fully while moving him or her from one support to another.

You also use guarding techniques when the patient is ambulating (walking). All patients who can support themselves are encouraged to walk alone or with the assistance of another person. Patients who are uncomfortable usually resist having to move. Your encouragement is needed to keep their body functions as normal as possible. There are a variety of techniques you may use:

■ A guarding belt (walking belt) supports and helps the client feel secure.

■ You may support the patient by placing an arm around the patient's waist and holding one arm firmly.

■ Some patients may need to hold on to you. Just your hand may be enough to steady them in those first few steps after a lengthy stay in bed.

■ Some patients may require two people to assist them. One person on each side of the client should hold each arm and hold the person securely around the waist.

■ Walking next to a rail is helpful. Patients often feel insecure when they are dependent on another person for support. A solid railing provides the extra security they need.

■ EXERCISING

Physical therapy department personnel work with patients to maintain normal functions of all parts of the body. They use range-of-motion exercises to move all joints in the body. This is accomplished through

■ *Active ROM.* The client moves the body part without help.

■ *Passive ROM.* Someone else moves the body part for the patient. (See the procedure "Range of Motion" in Chapter 15.) The physical therapist directs an exercise program that improves strength and mobility. These exercises may use complicated machines or simple items, such as a rubber ball that can be routinely squeezed. Regardless of the technique you use, it is essential that you are secure with the procedure before you attempt to assist a client.

Procedure

Ambulating with a Walking Belt

ALERT: Follow Standard Precautions.

1. Wash hands.
2. Assemble equipment.
   a. Gait belt/walking belt (correct size)
   b. Patient's robe
   c. Patient's footwear
3. Identify patient.
4. Explain what you are going to do.
5. Assist client to sitting position on side of bed.
6. Encourage patient to take a few deep breaths and ask if he or she feels dizzy. (If dizziness is present, let patient sit awhile before walking.)

Procedure box continued

7. Assist patient with robe and slippers.
8. Secure walking belt around patient's waist over clothing.
9. Tighten belt and buckle securely.

Note: Belt is too tight if you cannot put two fingers behind it.

10. Stand in front of patient with broad base of support.
11. Instruct patient to put hands on your shoulder.
12. Ease patient to a standing position and hold hand grip securely at back of belt.

13. Ambulate client as ordered.
14. Observe patient for weakness or discomfort.
15. Return client to room and make comfortable.
16. Document and report patient's tolerance of procedure.
17. Return walking belt to storage area so that it will be available for the next procedure.
18. Wash hands.

■ REHABILITATION EQUIPMENT

Ambulation Devices

Ambulation devices assist patients/clients to walk (see Figure 19–1). Some of the most common devices are described in the next paragraphs.

Canes provide a third base of support for patients who are slightly unstable on their feet. Use a cane when patients are

■ Slightly weaker on one side
■ Easily thrown off balance
■ Insecure walking alone

Special considerations to keep in mind when preparing a cane for use include the following:

■ The patient's height
■ Use of a single-foot cane or multifoot cane
■ Condition of rubber tips
■ Weight and appearance of the cane

Crutches provide support and stability by promoting use of the hands and arms more than the legs. Use them when patients are able to bear weight

■ On one foot or leg
■ Only partially on one leg or on both feet and legs

Special considerations when preparing crutches for use include the following:

■ Adjusting their height for the patient. Keep in mind:

• Axillary pressure—too much pressure causes injury • Hand level

■ The patient's footwear (slippery soles, open toes, etc.)
■ Condition of rubber tips, hand pads, and axillary pads
■ Securing all joints on the crutches

FIGURE 19–1. Ambulation devices: (a) short leg brace; (b) cane; (c) quad cane; (d) wheeled walker; (e, f) crutches.

Walkers provide support and stability. Use them when patients are

■ Relearning to walk
■ On limited weight-bearing
■ Unstable on their feet

Special considerations to keep in mind when preparing walkers for patient use include the following:

■ Adjusting the walker to the patient's height
■ The patient's footwear (open toes, slippery soles, etc.)
■ Securing all joints on walker
■ Condition of rubber tips

Procedure

Walking with a Cane

1. Wash hands.
2. Assemble equipment.
   a. Cane in good repair and with rubber tip
   b. Patient's/client's footwear
   c. Patient's/client's robe
3. Identify patient.
4. Assist client with shoes and robe.
5. Explain what you are going to do.
6. Position client in a standing position (have a co-worker help you if necessary).
7. Check height of cane. Top of cane should be at the patient's hip joint.
8. Check arm position at side of body and hold top of cane. Arm should be bent at a 25° to 30° angle.
9. Have patient hold cane in hand on strongest side of body (unaffected side).
10. Assist client as needed while ambulating. Most physicians order a standard gait procedure.
    a. With cane in hand on strongest side, move cane and weakest foot forward.
    b. Place body weight forward on cane and move strongest foot forward. (Patient will have cane's maximum support when this procedure is used when walking on flat surface, hill, or stairs. Remember: Weak leg and cane move together.)
11. When you have completed ordered ambulation, return patient to the starting place.
12. Provide for patient's comfort.
13. Place cane in proper location. If client is capable and physician permits ambulation without assistance, leave cane in a convenient place for patient.

14. Wash hands.
15. Report and document patient's tolerance of procedure.
    a. Date
    b. Time
    c. Ambulated with cane (e.g., 15 minutes in hall)
    d. How tolerated
    e. Signature and classification

These devices give the patient additional support and aid in balancing while walking or standing. Patients must be able to use their hands and arms to adapt properly to these devices. Some additional devices that aid in ambulation include the following:

Braces provide specific support for weakened muscle joints or immobilize an injured joint. Patients use them when they have

■ Weakened joints or muscles
■ Injuries that need to be stabilized

Procedure

Walking with Crutches

1. Wash hands.
2. Assemble equipment.
   a. Crutches in good repair with rubber tips
   b. Patient's footwear
   c. Patient's robe, if necessary
3. Identify patient.
4. Explain what you are going to do.
5. Help patient with shoes and robe.
6. Check fit of crutches to patient.
   a. Have client stand with crutches in place. (Ask a co-worker to assist if necessary.)
   b. Position foot of crutches about 4 inches to side of patient's foot and slightly forward of foot.
   c. Check distance between underarm and crutch underarm rest. It should be about 2 inches.
   d. Check angle of patient's arm. When hand is on hand rest bar and crutches are in walking position, arms should be at a 30° angle.
7. Remind patient that the hands support most of the body weight, not the underarms (axilla).
8. Assist client to ambulate following gait method ordered. There are a variety of crutch walking gaits. The following will provide guidelines to the most commonly used:
   a. Three-point gait (beginners)
      (1) One leg is weight-bearing.
      (2) Place both crutches forward along with non-weight-bearing foot. Weight will be supported primarily by weight-bearing foot.
      (3) Shift weight to *hands* on crutches and move weight-bearing foot forward.
   b. Four-point gait (beginners) (see figure)
      (1) Both legs are weight-bearing.
      (2) Place one crutch forward.
      (3) Move foot on opposite side of body forward, parallel with forward crutch.
      (4) Place other crutch forward and parallel with first crutch.
      (5) Move other foot forward so that it rests next to first foot.
   c. Two-point gait (advanced) (see figure)
      (1) Both legs are weight-bearing.
      (2) Place one crutch forward and move opposite foot forward with it.

1.   2.   3.   4.
◻ Weak side
Four-point crutch gait

1.   2.
Two-point crutch gait

   (3) Place other crutch forward and parallel with first crutch. Then move opposite foot forward so that it is even with other foot.
   d. Swing-to gait (arm and shoulder strength are needed) (see figure)
      (1) One or both legs are weight-bearing.
      (2) Balance weight on weight-bearing limb.

Procedure box continued

    (3) Place both crutches forward.

    (4) Shift weight to *hands* on crutches.

    (5) Swing both feet forward until parallel with crutches.

Caution: Placing crutches too far forward can result in a fall!

  e. Swing-through gait (advanced: arm and shoulder strength are needed) (see figure)

    (1) One or both legs are weight-bearing.

    (2) Balance weight on weight-bearing limb(s).

    (3) Place both crutches forward.

    (4) Shift weight to *hands* on crutches.

    (5) Swing both feet forward just ahead of crutches.

  9. Return to room.

 10. Ensure that client is comfortable.

 11. Wash hands.

 12. Record the following:

    a. Date

    b. Time

    c. Distance ambulated

    d. How tolerated

    e. Signature and classification

Swing-to gait

Swing-through gait

Special considerations to keep in mind when preparing braces for a patient include the following:

■ They are custom-made for each patient; they are not meant to be shared.

■ They may require padding to protect the skin.

■ There is only one way to apply a brace; be sure that you know the correct way.

A *prosthesis* is an artificial body part or an aid to a part of the body that minimizes a disability. When a body part is missing, the prosthesis gives a natural appearance and provides maximum usability for the person. The prosthesis most commonly dealt with in physical therapy is the artificial arm or leg. Special considerations to keep in mind when preparing a prosthesis for a patient include the following:

Procedure

Walking with a Walker

1. Wash hands.
2. Assemble equipment.
   a. Walker in good condition
   b. Patient's footwear
   c. Patient's robe if necessary
3. Identify client.
4. Tell client what you are going to do.
5. Stand patient up with walker. (Ask a co-worker to help if necessary.)
6. Check to see if walker fits patient properly.
   a. Walker's handgrips should be at top of patient's leg or bend of leg at hip joint.
   b. Arm should be at a 25 to 30° angle.
7. Assist patient to ambulate as ordered. Basic guidelines for walking with a walker are as follows:
   a. Patient begins by standing inside frame of walker.
   b. Patient lifts walker (never slides) and places back legs of walker parallel with toes (never ahead of toes).
   c. Patient shifts weight onto hands and walker (for balance and support).
   d. Patient then walks into walker.
   e. Place yourself just to side and slightly behind client. This position will allow you to observe and be close enough to assist if necessary.
8. When you have completed the ordered ambulation, return patient to his or her starting place.
9. Provide for patient's comfort.
10. Place walker in proper location. If client is capable and physician permits ambulation without assistance, leave walker in a convenient place for patient.
11. Wash hands.
12. Report and document patient's tolerance of procedure.

13. Record the following:
    a. Date
    b. Time
    c. Distance and amount of time ambulated
    d. How tolerated
    e. Signature and classification

■ You must have the right device.
■ The end resting against the patient is padded.
■ All straps must be in good condition.
■ It is clean and the overall appearance is natural.
■ Report tender areas at attachment site.

Transporting Devices

Transport devices include equipment to move patients from one place to another. The most common transporting devices are wheelchairs and gurneys. Gurneys and wheelchairs make it easy to move patients who are unable to walk. You are responsible for a variety of procedures as a physical therapy aide. Be sure that you are knowledgeable and confident about each procedure before you begin work with patients.

Adaptive-Assistive Devices

Adaptive-assistive devices include equipment that helps a person perform daily activities. These devices range from special holders for silverware to devices that help people put on socks or button clothing.

■ JOBS AND PROFESSIONS

- ■ Assistive personnel
- ■ Nurse assistant
- ■ Medical assistant
- ■ Licensed vocational/practical nurse
- ■ Registered nurse
- ■ Physical therapist
- ■ Home health aide

CHAPTER REVIEW *Your link to success*

Thinking Critically:
Check Your Understanding

1. **Communication** Describe what you would say to a patient who was going to have his first hydrotherapy treatment. What special precautions would you take? What would you tell the patient about the possible outcome of his treatment?

2. **Medical Terminology** Use Part One of this text and a medical dictionary to make a list of ten medical terms related to the muscular skeletal systems. Use these terms to write a scenario about a patient with a condition affecting the muscles and/or the skeletal system.

3. **Legal and Ethical** Explain what it means "to know your limitations" as a physical therapy aide working in the physical therapy department.

4. **Patient Education** Describe how and what you would explain to a client about the use of an ambulation device. Explain safety precautions and maintenance of rubber tips and joints on the device. Describe how you would determine the patient's level of understanding.

Portfolio Connection

When you are competent as a physical therapy aide, ask for permission to copy your documentation of treatment for a patient. (Remove all patient identifiers.) Place this copy in your portfolio to document your skills. Place a copy of your on-site trainer's evaluation in your portfolio.

Write a paper describing your doubts and realizations and the barriers that you were able to overcome during your physical therapy experiences. For example, were you concerned about helping care for patients/clients who are experiencing a lot of pain? Describe the ways you plan to use the skills, information, and insights that you gained about people and about this job. This assignment must be in standard report format.

20 CENTRAL SUPPLY/ CENTRAL PROCESSING WORKER

Steps to success

1. Complete Vocabulary Worksheet 1 in the Student Workbook.
2. Read this chapter.
3. Complete Worksheets 2 and 3 as assigned.
4. Practice and demonstrate all procedures.
5. When you are confident that you can meet each objective for this chapter, ask your instructor for the chapter evaluation.
6. Complete "Your Link to Success" at the end of this chapter.

Objectives

When you have completed this chapter, you will be able to do the following:

✓ Complete all objectives in Part One of this book.
✓ Complete vocabulary words in the crossword puzzle.
✓ Identify functions of a central supply/central processing department.
✓ Describe the responsibilities of the central supply/central processing department worker.
✓ Describe the subdepartments of central supply/central processing.
✓ Identify six categories of cleaning agents and their specific functions.
✓ List items of appropriate clothing to be worn in the **decontamination,** preparation, sterilization, and inventory areas.
✓ List three methods of packaging items.

decontamination
Removal of unclean matter and living organisms.

✓ List two types of sterilization and explain two important things to remember about each.

✓ Select items that require special care during sterilization.

✓ Demonstrate proficiency in each procedure pertinent to central supply/central processing.

■ THE CENTRAL SUPPLY DEPARTMENT

Central supply department workers prepare, store, and **distribute** medical supplies throughout a medical facility. This department is responsible for maintaining a ready inventory of supplies and **equipment** for medical services. This department also monitors cleaning and sterilization of areas and equipment in order to maintain infection control within the medical setting.

distribute To deliver.

equipment Instruments, machines, or items used to perform a task.

■ RESPONSIBILITIES OF A CENTRAL SUPPLY WORKER

As a central supply worker, you do the following tasks:

- Answer, screen, record, and direct telephone calls.
- Relay and record messages taken from an intercom.
- Record charges and maintain accurate files.
- Clean **instruments,** containers, and equipment.
- Assemble and wrap procedure trays.
- Operate autoclaves to sterilize items.
- Use antiseptic **solutions** to sterilize items.
- Circulate inventory according to expiration dates.
- Deliver supplies and equipment as needed.
- Maintain accurate inventory of supplies and equipment.

instruments Tools and measuring devices.

solutions Two or more liquids mixed together.

■ STANDARD PRECAUTIONS

When working with equipment contaminated with body substances, always follow Standard Precautions. Review the guidelines in Chapter 12.

■ DECONTAMINATION

There are two main areas in the central supply department that you must be able to recognize. These are clean and dirty areas. They may or may not be marked accordingly. *Clean areas* have items that are unopened or wrapped and dated. *Dirty areas* usually have trash receptacles or unwrapped items that may be clean or soiled. There may also be a hopper (a large toilet-type basin) for washing away contaminated fluids, waste, and so on.

The dirty area is called *decontamination*. All other areas in the department are considered clean areas. Central supply workers wear protective gowns when moving from the decontamination area to a clean area or from clean areas to a dirty area.

The decontamination area receives soiled items that are collected for cleaning and reprocessing. In this area, the workers remove all visible soil on items that are reused. Various types of cleaning agents are used in central supply. Each manufacturer provides directions on how to use each cleaner. Some of the cleaners you use fall under the following categories:

■ *Blood solvents* dissolve dried blood or other proteins on instruments. These solvents must be washed away with a neutral detergent before the cleaning process continues.

■ *Chlorinated detergents* clean heavily soiled items, and they have a bleaching action.

■ *Germicidal detergents* clean large items that cannot be put in a sterilizer. These detergents are allowed to air-dry to maximize the aseptic action.

■ *Neutral detergents* clean most instruments, glass, plastic, and rubber items.

■ *Soap* washes items that can be damaged by stronger detergents (e.g., silicone items, hands, or skin on other parts of the body).

Procedure

Decontamination Area

1. Wear protective equipment.
   a. Head cover
   b. Scrub suit or cover gown
   c. Gloves
   d. Protective eye wear
   e. Mask/shield
   f. Shoe covers (may be required)

   ALERT: Follow Standard Precautions.

2. Determine proper cleaning substance for items to be washed, and dilute according to directions.
3. Unclamp, open, or take apart all items.
4. Soak instruments to loosen dried substances.

5. Scrub instruments under water to decrease the chance of spreading contaminated material through the air.
6. First rinse with tap water and then with distilled or demineralized water to prevent corrosion and mineral deposits on instruments. Wipe large items with a disinfectant and leave to air-dry.
7. Place delicate items into automatic washer baskets and place in washer.
8. Add detergent as directed by manufacturer.
9. Operate automatic washer by following washer directions.
10. Pass items to preparation area.

Procedure

Ultrasonic Cleaning Procedure

1. Wear protective equipment.
   a. Head cover
   b. Scrub suit or cover gown
   c. Protective eye wear
   d. New shoe covers (may be required)

   ALERT: Follow Standard Precautions.

2. Measure detergent and add to water in machine.
3. Follow machine directions for operations.
4. Rinse instruments in tap water.
5. Thoroughly dry each item.
6. Pass items to preparation area.

■ *Washing machine detergent* is more **concentrated** than other detergents but has a low sudsing action.

concentrated Increased strength, strong solution.

NOTE Abrasives are *not* used in central supply, because they make small scratches on instruments that provide a place for pathogens to hide.

Ultrasonic cleaning may be necessary. When it is, it follows the automatic washing step or is in place of the automatic washing step. When hinges or **serrated** areas cannot be cleaned properly by other methods, central supply workers use ultrasonic cleaning. High-frequency sound waves vibrate the detergent solution. This loosens the contaminated material from instruments with hard-to-clean areas.

serrated Sawlike notches.

When the items are clean, they are transferred to the preparation area through a passageway. In a large central supply area, this passage may be a conveyor belt that leads to another room or a sliding window that allows articles to be placed into the clean area. Large items are passed through a doorway or a short hallway. When transferring items from a dirty area to a clean area, remember what you learned in Unit 1, "Nature of Microorganisms," in Chapter 12.

Use good technique so that you do not transfer bacteria from the dirty area to the clean area.

■ PREPARATION AREA

In the preparation area, instruments and supplies are arranged for special procedures on trays or in packages. Items are also checked for damage and for proper working condition.

*P*rocedure

Cleaning Equipment from a Transmission-Based Precaution Patient

1. Wear correct clothing.
   a. Head cover
   b. Cover gown
   c. Mask
   d. Gloves

ALERT: Follow Standard Precautions.

2. Determine proper cleaning substance for items to be washed, and dilute according to directions.
3. Open bag holding items to be cleaned. Remove items from bag.
4. Fold bag and place in trash container.
5. Unclamp, open, or take apart all items.
6. Soak instruments to loosen dried substances.
7. Scrub instruments under water to decrease the chance of spreading contaminated material through the air.
8. First rinse with tap water and then with distilled or demineralized water to prevent corrosion and mineral deposits on instruments. Wipe large items with a disinfectant and leave to air-dry.
9. Place delicate items into automatic washer baskets and place in washer.
10. Place all items into automatic washer.
11. Carefully remove gloves by pulling the cuff over hand, causing glove to be inside out when removed. Dispose of in trash container.
12. Remove cover gown, head cover, and mask, and dispose of according to hospital policy.
13. Add detergent as directed by manufacturer.
14. Operate automatic washer by following washer directions.

The preparation area is a clean area. You are required to wear the following:

■ Scrub suit
■ Head cover
■ Shoe covers (in some departments)

This area may be combined with the sterilization area in small facilities. Each area is separate in larger facilities. Learn the procedures for both areas.

Items being prepared for sterilization are placed on trays or in packages with other items that are used for specific procedures. These are called *procedure trays* or *packs*. When organizing a tray, always check each item for broken areas, and be certain that it works properly.

Packaging Methods

There are different packaging methods. They include the following:

■ Heat-sealed packages that peel open
■ Tape-sealed packages that peel open
■ Packages wrapped in cloth or special paper for sterilization

Procedure

Sterile Wrap, Envelope

1. Select the appropriate size of outer wrap.
   a. Wrapper should be large enough to completely enclose items to be sterilized.
   b. A double thickness is desirable.
   c. Wrapper should not be drawn too tightly, just enough to hold package together.
2. Place items to be wrapped in center of outer wrap. Sides of tray holding items to be sterilized should be aligned with corners of wrapper.

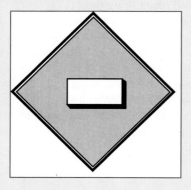

3. Fold corner closest to you past center of pack; holding corner, fold it back, making a flap.

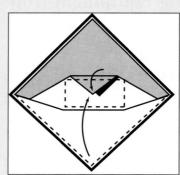

Procedure box continued

4. Fold left corner of wrap just past center and fold corner back, making a flap.

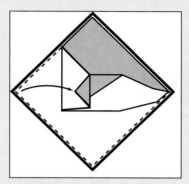

5. Fold right corner of wrap past center (overlap center) and fold back, making a flap.

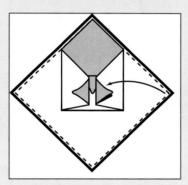

6. Fold corner farthest from you over package.

7. To provide a double thickness, wrap package again following steps 2 through 6.

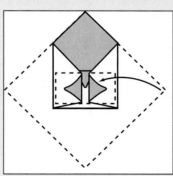

8. Using heat-sensitive tape, secure the edges.

9. Date and label package; follow the procedure "Dating and Labeling Sterile Items."

Procedure

Sterile Square Wrap Fold

1. Select appropriate size of outer wrap.
   a. Wrapper should be large enough to completely enclose the items to be sterilized.
   b. If outer wrap is to be used as a sterile field over a table:
      (1) Wrap should allow at least 6 inches overhang on all four sides of the table.
      (2) A double thickness is desirable.
   c. Wrap should not be drawn too tightly, just enough to hold package together.

2. Place items to be wrapped in center of outer wrap. Corners of tray holding items to be sterilized should be square with corners of wrapper.

3. Fold edge closest to you past center of pack; continue holding edge and fold back to make a 1-inch band.

4. Grasp edge farthest from you and pull over items to be sterilized.

5. Hold the same edge and fold back to make a 1-inch band. (There should be a 2-inch overlap of edges at center of package.)

6. Fold the left edge just past center; holding same edge, fold back to make a band.

7. Fold the right edge just past center; holding same edge, fold back to make a band (overlapping at center).

8. Wrap package again following steps 3 through 7 to provide a double thickness.

Start double wrap

9. Use heat-sensitive tape to secure edges.

10. Date and label package; follow procedure "Dating and Labeling Sterile Items."

Procedure

Linen Preparation

1. Inspection
   a. Spread linen over an illuminated worktable and look for holes, tears, or other defects.
   b. Circle defects with a pencil and send for repair.
   c. Prepare linen without defects for sterilization.
2. Folding
   a. Fold linen according to department procedure.
   b. Sort and stack linen on shelves according to use.
3. Assembly of linen packages
   a. Packages should not exceed 12 by 12 by 20 inches or weigh more than 20 pounds.
   b. Place last item to be used on bottom and first item to be used on top.
   c. Place gauze sponges in the center of the package so that steam can enter each piece of fabric more easily.
4. Wrapping the linen pack
   a. Select an outer wrapper large enough to enclose the items completely.
   b. Wrap the linen as described in the procedure "Sterile Wrap Fold."
      (1) Square fold for large packs
      (2) Envelope fold for small packs
   c. Date and label as described in the procedure "Dating and Labeling Sterile Items."

■ STERILIZATION

In the sterilization area, the clean items are placed in an *autoclave*. The environment in the autoclave kills all microorganisms. The items inside the autoclave are exposed to steam or gas and steam under pressure for a specific period of time. Items that may be damaged from steam, pressure, or gas are placed in a chemical disinfectant. There are some basics that you need to remember when sterilizing. The following serves as a reference guide. (See Chapter 18 for small autoclaves.)

Steam Sterilization

■ The steam and microorganisms must be in contact for a specific amount of time. The time is determined by the temperature of the steam.

■ All items must be completely dry before they are removed from the autoclave. *Remember that pathogens are transported by moisture.*

Gas Sterilization

■ The gas, steam, and microorganisms must be in direct contact for a specific period of time. This time is determined by the concentration of gas and the temperature inside the autoclave.

■ All **ethylene oxide** gas is removed from the sterilized items before they are stored or used.

ethylene oxide Gas that kills living microorganisms.

Sterilizing Plastics, Oils, Powders, and Solutions

■ Plastics require ethylene gas sterilization, as heat deteriorates plastics.

■ Oils and powders require a dry heat sterilization.

■ Solutions require a special steam sterilization method designed just for solutions.

Procedure

Sterilizing with Ethylene Oxide Gas

1. Prepare the gas sterilizer.
   a. Place recording chart in monitor.
   b. Add ink to pens if required.
   c. Check for humidity-sensing element in the chamber.
   d. Preheat sterilizer.
2. Snap master switch "on."
3. Check indicators to ensure that adequate gas supply is available.
4. Depress Sterox selector button.
5. Set timer for length of time required for exposure to gas.

6. Set humidity timer for length of humidification period.
7. Load items into sterilizer.
8. Start the sterilization cycle by depressing the lock door cycle button.
9. Monitor indicators showing when the cycle is complete.
10. Unload sterilizer when cycle is complete.
11. Close door of sterilizer; do not engage holding arm.
12. Aerate sterilized items by following department procedure.

Procedure

Dating and Labeling Sterile Items

1. Date all packages with the day of sterilization.
2. Label packages with name of pack and a listing of items in package.
3. Initial pack as you wrap it.

4. Mark sterilizer number on each package.
5. Rotate sterilized items by date. Packages that are closest to their expiration date are placed forward on the shelf so that they are used first.

Monitoring the Effectiveness of Sterilization

cycle Repeating steps (e.g., a wash cycle).

Each central supply department has procedures for evaluating the effectiveness of the sterilization **cycle.** A permanent record is kept of this monitoring system to ensure infection control. Occasional inspections of the medical facility require inspection of these records. The following gives you an overview of commonly used monitoring devices.

FIGURE 20-1.
Autoclave sterilization indicator tape. Before sterilization (top) the tape is a certain color. After sterilization (bottom) the tape changes color. A chemical change during sterilization causes the tape to change color.

■ *Mechanical monitoring* is accomplished by graphing the pressure/vacuum gauge, temperature gauge, and/or **humidity** gauge readings during the sterilization cycle. These records are then filed by date and time.

■ *Chemical monitoring* is done by using strips of material with a chemical on it that changes color after exposure to enough heat or steam. A tape treated with this chemical secures packages for sterilization. Packages that are sterilized are identified easily by the color change on the tape (see Figure 20–1).

■ *Biological monitoring* is accomplished by placing small containers with live bacteria that are highly resistant in the autoclave during the sterilization cycle. After sterilization, the bacteria are placed in a supportive environment. The bacteria are checked after a specified time. If any bacteria have survived or reproduced, sterilization did not occur.

humidity Wetness, or moisture.

■ INVENTORY AND DISTRIBUTION

The inventory and distribution area maintains an accurate count of supplies and equipment on hand and delivers items as necessary. This is accomplished by replacing discarded items immediately and seeing that broken equipment is repaired in a timely manner. All supplies and sterile equipment are rotated on the shelves to ensure that sterility of items does not expire. Items must be resterilized before use if they are not frequently used and the sterilization time expires.

There are various types of delivery systems in the medical facility. Most medical systems use volunteers to pick up and deliver equipment to departments. Some use the central supply/central processing staff to do these duties. Other facilities use a pneumatic tube system that carries small items from place to place and a dumb-waiter elevator for larger items. Most facilities use freight elevators rather than passenger elevators to deliver very large items. The use of freight elevators keeps medical supplies separate from the general public and lowers the possibility of contamination. It is also better if the visitors are not exposed to equipment.

■ JOBS AND PROFESSIONS

■ Assistive personnel
■ Clinical medical assistant
■ Home health aide
■ Licensed vocational/practical nurse
■ Nurse assistant
■ Registered nurse
■ Surgical assistant

Thinking Critically:
Check Your Understanding

1. **Medical Terminology** Use Part One of this text and a medical dictionary to list ten medical terms describing body fluids and tissues. Use these terms to write a scenario about how the equipment becomes soiled with body fluids and how it looks when it is returned to the decontamination area.

2. **Legal and Ethical** One way to prevent the spread of infection is to use the various sterilization processes found in the central supply/central processing area. Describe these processes and how they are monitored for effective sterilization.

3. **Medical Math** You may handle drainage bottles of different sizes. Determine how many ounces are in containers that measure 250 cc, 2,500 cc, and 1,000 cc.

4. **Case Study** Samual Witt is your co-worker. He likes to work quickly so that he can be done with his work early. You notice that he neglects to wear all of the necessary protective equipment. Sometimes he walks from the decontamination area into the clean area without removing his gown and other protective wear. Describe a way to respond to this observation that would serve to protect Samuel and other co-workers. Explain the possible negative and positive outcomes of your actions.

Portfolio Connection

Once you attain competence as a central supply/central processing worker, ask for permission to photocopy sterilization test strip results. Place copies in your portfolio to demonstrate your understanding of the sterilization process.

Write a paper describing your doubts and realizations and the barriers that you were able to overcome during your central supply/central processing experience. For example, what frightened you, and what moved you beyond your fear? Describe the ways you plan to use the skills, information, and insights that you gained about the people you worked with and about this job. This report must be in standard report format.

ENVIRONMENTAL SERVICES TECHNICIAN/ HOUSEKEEPER

21

Steps to success

1. Read this chapter.
2. Complete Vocabulary Worksheet 1 in the Student Workbook.
3. Practice and demonstrate all procedures.
4. When you are confident that you can meet each objective for this chapter, ask your instructor for the chapter evaluation.
5. Complete the "Your Link to Success" at the end of this chapter.

Objectives

When you have completed this chapter, you will be able to do the following:

✓ Complete all objectives in Part One of this book.
✓ Define new vocabulary words.
✓ Describe the responsibilities of an EVS/housekeeper.
✓ Match department names with their abbreviations.
✓ List seven supplies and types of equipment found on a service cart.
✓ Give two reasons why a service cart is important.
✓ Define *germicidal solution.*
✓ List fourteen guidelines to use in the EVS/housekeeping department.
✓ List five areas to check that are not usually found in your home.
✓ Describe HAI and explain how to prevent it.
✓ List seven general rules to follow when you clean a patient's room.
✓ Explain the cleaning process for preparing a room for a new patient.

✓ List seven specialized departments in the hospital.

✓ Identify the area within a specialized department that requires aseptic cleaning.

✓ Explain why it is important to keep all public areas clean and attractive.

✓ List duties required in the linen area.

✓ Differentiate between general cleaning, cleaning special areas, and cleaning sterile areas.

✓ Demonstrate each procedure pertinent to an EVS/housekeeper.

■ RESPONSIBILITIES OF AN EVS/HOUSEKEEPER

EVS/housekeeper workers are responsible for the cleanliness of the environment. Cleanliness helps prevent the spread of infection and creates a more pleasant environment for patients, employees, and visitors. An EVS/housekeeping employee is an important member of the health care team because he or she provides a therapeutic environment for the delivery of care. The information in this chapter discusses the hospital environment; however, you can transfer these skills to any health care setting, including clinics, medical-professional offices, and private health care agencies.

As a housekeeper, you are required to do the following tasks:

■ Load a service cart with appropriate supplies and materials.

■ Clean assigned areas (for example, room, offices, laboratories):

• Wash floors, furniture, and equipment. • Dust. • Vacuum. • Clean blinds.
• Empty ashtrays. • Empty trash. • Scour sinks, tubs, and mirrors. • Disinfect bedsprings and unit equipment. • Wash walls and ceilings as needed.

■ Replenish soap and towels.

■ Replace cubicle curtains.

■ Replace soiled draperies.

■ Provide daily cleaning of sterile areas.

■ Report malfunctioning equipment.

■ Keep utility and storage rooms orderly.

■ Move furniture, equipment, and supplies.

■ Sweep, mop, wet-wash, and vacuum floors.

■ Polish using a buffing machine.

■ Wash walls, ceilings, and windows.

■ Move furniture.

■ Clean light fixtures.

■ Turn and change mattresses.

■ Hang draperies and blinds.

■ Collect soiled linens and transport them to the laundry.

■ Provide an odor-free environment.

■ ABBREVIATIONS

EVS workers work in many areas of the hospital. They must know the abbreviations that are used for the different departments. They must also be aware of each department's overall responsibilities. As you read the abbreviations for the departments, refer back to Unit 2 of Chapter 2, which discusses the different areas and lists the responsibilities of the workers. Following is a list of many of the departments in the hospital and abbreviations that might be used.

Emergency room	ER
Electrocardiology	EKG/ECG
Environmental services	EVS
Laboratory	LAB
Radiology	X-Ray
Orthopedics	Ortho
Obstetric	OB
Medical-surgical	MED-SURG
Food service	Dietary
Physical therapy	PT
Occupation therapy	OT
Central supply	CS
Neurology	Neuro
Rehabilitation	Rehab
Gynecology	GYN

Other areas are usually not abbreviated:

Respiratory
Pharmacy
Linen room
Billing
Admitting
Medical records
Volunteers
Pulmonary lab
Dialysis
Chapel

■ CARE AND CLEANING OF EQUIPMENT

Use a service cart to keep supplies and equipment where they are easily available as you clean. The carts save many trips to other areas for supplies. They help you be more efficient and save time. Each facility has an equipment list of the things to include on the cart. Not all carts require exactly the same things. Set up your cart according to your assignment. You are also responsible for cleaning your cart at least once a week and as needed. Some standard equipment might include the following:

■ Cleaning brushes
■ Cleaning cloths
■ Dust mop and dustpan

germicidals Solutions that kill most bacteria.

- Toilet bowl brushes
- Cleaners such as **germicidals**
- Deodorizing solutions
- Wet mop
- Paper goods

• Toilet paper • Paper towels and paper towel dispenser key • Tissues • Wastebasket liners

- Gloves (wear gloves according to facility policy)

After you complete your duties for the day, clean your cart and the equipment. Dispose of all trash, and leave the cart ready for the next day's work.

You must keep the equipment clean and in good repair. When equipment is in good repair, your work is much easier. It must also be clean so as to prevent the spread of microorganisms. Review Chapter 12, "Controlling Infection." The patients and other workers *depend on you* to protect them from the spread of disease and infection.

There are some general guidelines that you follow:

Procedure

Stocking the Service Cart

1. Check your service cart to make sure that
   a. Wheels are working.
   b. Storage areas are clean.
   c. Shelves are sturdy.
   d. There are no broken areas.
2. Gather supplies.
   a. Gloves
   b. Mopping bucket
   c. Germicidal solution
   d. Spray bottle with germicidal solution
   e. Paper towel dispenser key
   f. Plastic bags:
      (1) Trash containers (small and large)
      (2) Sanitary napkin containers
      (3) Laundry containers
   g. Mop wringer
   h. Dust mop that has been specially treated
   i. Dustpan
   j. Dust mop with long handle
   k. Cleaning brushes
   l. Cleaning cloths
   m. Toilet bowl cleaner
   n. Toilet paper
   o. Paper towels
   p. Hand soap
   q. Putty knife
   r. Deodorizing solutions
3. Restock your cart at the end of your shift so that it is ready for the next day.
4. Wash hands.

■ Always use Standard Precautions.

■ Read the manufacturer's instructions for operating and maintaining equipment. Follow the instructions.

■ Store equipment properly.

■ Report any defect or problem.

■ Clean, rinse, and wring out a wet mop after use. This helps it last longer and prevents odor and mildew.

■ Never store brooms and brushes on the straw or bristles, because they bend out of shape.

■ Keep cleaning cloths separate from linen to prevent contamination.

■ Empty dust, trash, vacuum bags, and so on, every day.

■ Do not shake dust mops, cleaning cloths, or linen, as this causes the spread of microorganisms.

■ Wipe down all equipment after use, including

• Caution signs • Scraping knives • Ladders • Hoses • Sweepers, vacuums
• Measuring cups • Buckets and pails and their wringers

■ Do not leave solutions in buckets when they are not in use.

■ Do not leave cleaning solutions where a child or confused patient can reach them.

■ Label all containers to prevent mistakes.

■ Do not pull plugs from the socket by the cord.

■ GENERAL CLEANING DUTIES

Everything in the environment must be kept clean, odor free, and safe. Dust and microorganisms are always in the air around us, and it is a daily battle to keep them controlled. It is a very large task to keep everything clean. Areas in a health care facility must be cleaned more frequently than those in the home. The health care environment has many more microorganisms that cause illness and disease. Cleanliness requires following procedure, being aware of all areas around you, and taking pride in keeping everything clean and in tip-top order. Part of your responsibility is to recognize the need to clean an area, change dirty filters, and use detergent, odor-control, and germicidal solutions appropriately. Remember from Part One that a germicide kills bacteria, but a bacteriostatic only slows growth. Odor is controlled by cleanliness, nonaerosol sprays, solutions added to buckets, and small bottles with wicks. The scent must be very light or odorless. You need to be watchful and aware of areas that you might not be as concerned with or need to clean as often in your home. Some of these are as follows:

■ Closets and lockers
■ Cubicle curtains
■ Radiators
■ Heating and cooling ducts
■ Air conditioners
■ Light fixtures
■ Screens
■ Windows
■ Refrigerators
■ Drinking fountains

- Transportable equipment such as wheelchairs, gurneys, and commodes
- Venetian blinds
- Corridors
- Stairways
- Sprinkler heads

Procedure

Cleaning Closets and Lockers

1. Gather equipment.
   a. Bucket
   b. Cleaning solution
   c. Two cleaning cloths
   d. Treated dust mop
   e. Stepstool or ladder
   f. Vacuum
   g. Putty knife
   h. Screwdriver
   i. Spray bottle
   j. Water
   k. Gloves
   l. Deodorizing solution
2. Put on gloves.
3. Prepare cleaning solution.

4. Vacuum and damp-dust inside and outside of closet or locker. (Don't forget the top.)
5. Submerge cloth in cleaning solution.
6. Wring solution out of cloth.
7. Wipe all outside surfaces with cloth. (Wash cloth out frequently to remove dirt; if you don't do this, you will be spreading the dirt around.)
8. Wipe all surfaces with a dry cloth to remove extra solution and water spots.
9. Wipe all inside surfaces with moistened cleaning cloth.
10. Wipe all inside surfaces with a dry cloth.
11. Remove gloves.
12. Wash hands.

Procedure

Cleaning Stairways

1. Gather equipment.
   a. Wet mop
   b. Bucket
   c. Dusting: mop, pan, brush, and cloth
   d. "Caution" sign
   e. Strong cleaning agent
   f. Germicidal solution
   g. Glass cleaner
   h. Hand buffing pad
   i. Gloves
   j. Deodorizing solution
2. Put on gloves.

3. Clean all fixtures around stairway.
   a. Lights
   b. Signs
   c. Windows
   d. Pictures
4. Dust all railings and ledges. (It may be necessary to use extension poles with dusting equipment to reach high places.)
5. Clean all spots on walls and base plates.
6. Dust-mop stairs; start at top using a side-to-side motion. Continue to platform or bottom of stairs, whichever comes first.

Procedure box continued

7. Pick up dust and dirt with a dustpan and brush.
8. Clean area around doors.
   a. Hinges
   b. Knobs
   c. Jambs and ledges
   d. Polish all metal
9. Place "Caution" signs appropriately; rope off half of stairway. (Leave an adequate walkway.)
10. Damp-mop area enclosed by rope.
11. Refinish/wax stairs.

12. Dust-mop again.
13. Move rope and "Caution" sign to other side of stairway and repeat the procedure. (Never remove "Caution" signs before the floor is completely dry.)
14. Recheck area before leaving for missed spots.
15. Clean equipment and return it to its storage area.
16. Remove gloves.
17. Wash hands.

Procedure

Washing Windows

1. Gather equipment.
   a. Vacuum with attachments
   b. Ladder
   c. Double bucket
   d. Cleaning cloth or sponge
   e. Squeegee
   f. Gloves
   g. Lint-free cloth
   h. Paper towel
   i. Window cleaner
   j. Germicidal solution
2. Put on gloves.
3. Remove all objects from window.
   a. Curtains (tie back or take down)
   b. Items on ledge
   c. Blinds (cleaned and pulled up or taken down)
   d. Screens—remove and clean
4. Vacuum ledge, window grooves, and corners.
5. Wash window frame and ledge with germicidal solution.
6. Rinse and dry frame and ledge.
7. Apply window cleaner with spray bottle, brush, or sponge. Be sure to get into corners.
   a. Use a side-to-side movement.

   b. Overlap slightly with each stroke.
8. Rinse if necessary, using the same technique.
9. Remove water with squeegee by doing the following:
   a. Place the rubber edge of the squeegee flat against the window in an upper corner.
   b. Move the squeegee across the window in a sweeping motion to the opposite side.
   c. Wipe rubber edge of squeegee with a cloth.
   d. Repeat this motion across the window until all sections have been wiped.
   e. Wipe bottom edge of window with a cloth.
   f. Wipe all water drops from ledge or floor.
10. Wipe any streaks with a lint-free cloth.
11. Replace all items removed from the window:
   a. Curtains or drapes
   b. Blinds
   c. Decorations, etc.
12. Recheck window for missed spots.
13. Clean equipment and return it to its storage area.
14. Remove gloves.
15. Wash hands.

Procedure

Cleaning Corridors

1. Gather equipment.
   a. Bucket
   b. Disposable gloves
   c. Wet mop
   d. Dusting: mop, pan, and brush
   e. Vacuum
   f. Germicidal solution with deodorizing solution
   g. Stainless steel polish
   h. "Caution" signs
   i. Cleaning cloths
   j. Ladder or stepstool
2. Put on gloves.
3. Clean all fixtures. (Check to see if all fixtures are working properly.)
   a. Lights
   b. Vents
   c. Signs
   d. Drinking fountains
   e. Telephones
   f. Pictures
   g. Window blinds
   h. Mirrors
   i. Drapes or curtains
   j. Ashtrays (if there is an area set aside for smoking)
4. Empty and wash all trash containers in assigned area.
5. Clean windows or glass partitions.
6. Clean marks or spots from walls/wall guards.
7. Clean all ledges.
8. Clean area around door:
   a. Hinges   c. Polish all metal
   b. Knobs   d. Door jambs and ledges
9. Place "Caution" signs appropriately in corridor; rope off half of the corridor. (Always leave adequate walking space.)
10. Dust-mop the floor.
11. Damp-mop or use a floor washing machine.
12. Refinish/wax and buff floors.
13. Dust-mop again.
14. Move rope and "Caution" signs to other side of corridor and repeat procedure. (Never remove "Caution" signs before floor is completely dry.)
15. When finished, check area for missed spots.
16. Clean equipment and return it to its storage area.
17. Remove gloves.
18. Wash hands.

Procedure

Cleaning Drinking Fountains

1. Gather equipment.
   a. Cleaning cloth
   b. Cleaning solution
   c. Metal polish
   d. Gloves
2. Put on gloves.
3. Discard any trash from fountain.
4. Submerge cloth in cleaning solution or use spray bottle with cleaning solution.
5. Wring cloth.
6. Wipe all surfaces on fountain. (Be sure to remove stains or marks of any kind.)
7. Polish all metal parts with a metal polish and soft dry cloth.
8. Wipe up any splashes or spills.
9. Report any fountains that are not working properly.
10. Return all equipment to its storage area.
11. Remove gloves.
12. Wash hands.

■ CLEANING ROOMS THAT ARE OCCUPIED BY PATIENTS

It is difficult to be a patient in a hospital. The patient is in an unfamiliar environment. Patients are sick, and they may have many worries. It is important to make their surroundings as pleasant as possible. It is also very important for you to be pleasant. You must also protect them from further illness or complications caused by a *hospital-acquired infection* (HAI). HAI is a common term used in health care facilities to describe infections that patients acquire in the hospital—they did not have the infection or illness when they were admitted. It is usually caused by a breakdown in asepsis. If you do not clean correctly, the patients' safety is in danger. You have a major responsibility to help prevent HAI. When you clean the patient's room, there are some rules to follow:

■ Follow Standard Precautions.

■ Work quietly, efficiently, and quickly.

■ Be careful around equipment such as IVs, suction machines, and tubing.

■ Do not put one patient's belongings with another patient's things. This causes cross-contamination.

When you clean the room, be sure to do the following:

■ Empty the wastebasket and replace the bedside bag.

■ Pick up any litter that is on the floor.

■ Wipe off the furniture.

■ Clean the phone, call bell, and TV control.

■ Remove spots from around light switches, on walls, and so on.

■ Mop or vacuum the floor.

■ Dust ledges and check light fixtures, vents, and so on.

■ Notice the cubicle curtains. Are there any spots or spills on them? Are they hanging correctly?

■ Clean the bathroom:

• Empty the wastebasket and pick up any litter. • Clean the basin and faucets and polish the mirror. • Clean the shower or tub and the faucets. • Wipe fixtures with an odor-control solution. • Check the shower curtain for mildew or tears. • Wipe down ledges, wall switches, spots on walls, and so on.
• Replace soap, toilet paper, and paper towels. • Clean the toilets and exposed pipes.

■ Replace things just as you found them. Be certain that the telephone, water pitcher, call bell, TV control, tissues, and reading materials are within the patient's reach.

■ Check the overall appearance of the room before you leave, and report any problems or repairs.

■ Notify the nurse if the patient needs anything.

Procedure

Cleaning the Occupied Patient Room

1. Gather equipment.
   a. Cleaning cart with standard supplies
   b. Vacuum
   c. Gloves

ALERT: Follow Standard Precautions.

2. Put on gloves.
3. Dispose of all loose trash and the bedside bag in trash container.
4. Pull plastic over trash in container and tie off. Place in larger trash container to be removed from the area. Repeat process with all trash containers in room.
5. Wipe out the inside of each trash container with cloth dampened in cleaning solution.
6. Place clean plastic liner in all emptied trash containers. Secure top of plastic over edge of container.
7. Use a cloth dampened in germicidal solution to wipe off and dry:
   a. Bedside table
   b. Bed rails
   c. Chairs
   d. Cabinets
   e. Any spots on walls, door jambs, and light switches (*Note:* Don't forget to rinse your cleaning cloth frequently so that you are not spreading dirt.)
8. Place a clean bedside bag at bedside.
9. Clean floors:

Uncarpeted floors—dust mop
   a. Use a treated dry mop.

   b. Start in the corners.
   c. Move mop from left to right.
   d. Work your way toward the door. (Pick up or move light objects and dust under them.)
   e. Dampen wet mop with germicidal solution.
   f. Remop room.

Carpeted floors—vacuum
Note: Start in the corner and work your way toward the door. (Pick up or move light objects and vacuum under them.)

10. Wipe all ledges, vents, sprinkler heads, and lights with cloth dampened in germicidal solution.
11. Wipe all ledges, vents, sprinkler heads, and lights with dry cloth to remove cleaning solution and water spots.
12. Clean bathroom.
    a. Use separate rags and brushes.
    b. Clean toilet according to facility policy.
    c. Clean mirrors.
    d. Polish porcelain.
    e. Wipe tiles and walls.
    f. Clean floor.
    g. Check to be certain that there are soap, toilet paper, and paper towels.
13. Check room for additional needs before leaving.
14. Report any broken items in the room.
15. Return all equipment to its storage area.
16. Remove gloves.
17. Wash hands.

■ CLEANING UNOCCUPIED ROOMS

When patients are admitted to the hospital, their room is their home (see Figure 21–1). Regardless of the reason for their admission, there is cause for some anxiety. The environment is very important for both their feeling of comfort and their protection against infection.

There are specific procedures that must be completed before the room is ready for a new patient.

■ Your supervisor will inspect the room with you and help determine what needs to be done.

■ In some hospitals, the walls and ceilings are washed after each patient is discharged. In other hospitals, this is done according to a rotation schedule. Follow the policy of your facility.

(Text continued on page 542)

FIGURE 21-1. Typical patient unit.

Procedure

Cleaning the Unoccupied Patient Room

ALERT: Follow Standard Precautions.

1. Gather equipment.
   a. Service cart with standard supplies
   b. Vacuum with attachments
   c. Gloves
2. Put on gloves.
3. Evaluate the condition of the room with your supervisor.
4. Clean all furniture thoroughly.
5. Remove furniture from room.
6. Remove curtains and drapes if necessary.
7. In room and bathroom, wash ceiling and walls with germicidal solution, being sure to clean:
   a. Vents
   b. Lights
   c. Sprinkler heads
   d. Television
   e. Doors
   f. Metal protection plates
   g. Curtain rods or tracks
8. Clean windows and window frames.
9. Thoroughly clean floors following the procedure decided upon when the room was evaluated before cleaning.
10. Replace all furniture.
11. Make beds.
12. Replace drapes and curtains if necessary.
13. Inspect room before leaving area.
14. Return all equipment to its storage area.
15. Remove gloves.
16. Wash hands.

Procedure

Dusting

1. Gather equipment.
   a. Dust cloth
   b. Extension for high places
   c. Spray cleaner/wax
   d. Gloves (according to facility policy)
2. Fold dusting cloth in half several times until it is about the size of your hand.

5. Use a spray cleaner/wax or liquid on wood surfaces. Follow manufacturer's directions.
6. Complete all dusting in an area before moving to another area. Conserve your motions by planning.
7. Check the room before leaving for missed areas.

(a)

Fold dusting cloth
(b)

(c)

3. Begin dusting at the highest point near the entrance of a room. Move systematically around the room until you reach the entrance again. (Dust all surfaces in a room.)
4. Use long straight strokes from side to side or up and down.

8. Return all equipment to its storage area.

Use straight strokes

Procedure

Cleaning Furniture

1. Gather equipment.
   a. Cleaning solution
   b. Gloves
   c. Two cloths
   d. Bucket or spray bottle
   e. Vinyl cleaner
   f. Vacuum with appropriate attachments
   g. Furniture polish
2. Put on gloves.
3. Dust furniture.
   a. Wood furniture—use a dry cloth, then furniture polish.
   b. Vinyl and fabric furniture—use a vacuum. Be sure to vacuum in all crevices with a narrow attachment. Use a short bristle brush over surface of fabric.
4. Scrub vinyl with vinyl cleaner.
   a. Spray vinyl cleaner evenly on vinyl.
   b. Let it stand a few minutes (do not allow it to dry).
   c. Scrub very soiled areas with a soft brush.
   d. Wipe vinyl until clean.
5. Rinse vinyl with water-dampened cloth.
6. Wipe vinyl dry with clean dry cloth.
7. Return furniture to its original position.
8. Return all equipment to its storage area.
9. Remove gloves.
10. Wash hands.

Note: Soiled fabric-covered furniture may require professional cleaning or recovering. Some cleaning solutions cause fabric to spot. Ask your supervisor before applying solutions to fabric.

Procedure

Cleaning the Bed

1. Gather equipment.
   a. Bucket
   b. Vacuum with crevice attachment
   c. Cleaning solution
   d. Two cleaning cloths
   e. Cleaning brush
   f. Gloves
2. Put on gloves.
3. Discard all loose trash.
4. Vacuum bed, being sure to clean in all crevices. Use a brush to loosen lint or dust.
5. Remove all tape or stickers from bed. (Use tape remover supplied by your facility.)
6. Dampen a cloth with germicidal solution and wipe:
   a. Pillows
   b. Mattress, both sides
   c. Bedsprings
   d. Side rails
   e. Head- and footboards
   f. Controls
   g. Legs
7. Make a closed bed. (See the procedure "Making a Closed Bed" in Chapter 15.)
8. Remove gloves.
9. Wash hands.

Procedure

Vacuuming Curtains/Drapes

1. Assemble equipment.
   a. Vacuum
   b. Ladder
   c. Gloves
2. Put on gloves.
3. Spread curtains/drapes out, so that more surface area is showing.
4. Place ladder at one end of curtain.
5. Place short bristle brush attachment on vacuum.
6. Vacuum curtains from top to bottom. (Give special care around pleats and valences.)

7. When all surface area of drape has been vacuumed on one side, move to the other side of curtain.
8. Repeat procedure.
9. Return curtains to their original position when cleaning is completed.
10. Return all equipment to its storage area.
11. Remove gloves.
12. Wash hands.

Procedure

Replacing Privacy Curtain and Drapes

1. Gather equipment.
   a. Vacuum
   b. Ladder
   c. Cleaning solution
   d. Two cleaning cloths
   e. Gloves (according to facility policy)
2. Vacuum curtains to remove excess dust. (This will prevent dust and bacteria from being flipped into the air.)
3. Unhook drapes/curtains, being careful not to shake them.

4. Remove hooks from drapes/curtains.
5. Place them in a laundry basket.
6. Wipe curtain track with cleaning solution on a dampened cloth.
7. Wipe track with a dry cloth to remove excess solution and water spots.
8. Place hooks in replacement curtains.
9. Attach hooked curtains/drapes to track.
10. Return equipment to its storage area.
11. Deliver soiled curtains/drapes to the appropriate place for cleaning.

■ Follow the directions for cleaning an occupied room. In addition, you will wash the bed down and make the bed.

■ CLEANING SPECIALIZED AREAS

Specialized areas in the hospital include the following:

- ■ Surgery department
- ■ Labor and delivery
- ■ Nursery
- ■ Catheterization laboratory (cath lab)

- ■ Emergency department
- ■ Central supply
- ■ Medical laboratory

Although some of these are associated with sterile areas, they do not need to be as aseptic as rooms where sterile procedures are done. Always follow facility procedures for cleaning these areas. You follow many of the procedures you have already learned.

■ Remove all trash, litter, and linen. Remember to double-bag in labor and delivery, the emergency room, surgery, and the cath lab.
■ Damp-wipe telephones, furniture, equipment, shelves, ledges, and so on.
■ Clean all sinks, restrooms, utility rooms, and hoppers.
■ Spot-clean where necessary.
■ Clean the floor.
■ Clean isolettes and basinettes.
■ Clean the interiors of autoclaves.

■ CLEANING STERILE AREAS

You have already learned that *sterile* means that there are *no* living microorganisms. The following are sterile areas:

■ Surgery suites
■ Labor and delivery
■ Cath lab

Each area is cleaned daily. You must be very careful when you work around equipment. If you notice anything unusual about the equipment or if you accidentally unplug it or move something, *report it immediately*. Equipment that has been moved or altered in any way can be life threatening. Follow the policy of the facility you work for. However, there are some basic rules for you to learn and follow.

Cleaning After Each Case

Clean sterile areas after each case, and then more thoroughly when the suites are empty and not scheduled for immediate use. Always follow Standard Precautions.

■ All trash and linen that is removed must be bagged according to facility policy.
■ Remove all trash and clean the containers.
■ Clean the linen hampers after you have removed the linen.
■ Damp-wipe all soiled surfaces, including the operating table, back table, and the **Mayo stands.**
■ Spot-check walls and lights.
■ Damp-mop the floor around the operating table.
■ Remake the operating table.
■ You are not expected to clean instruments. This is the responsibility of the operating room personnel.

Mayo stands Adjustable, wheeled, small metal stands that hold equipment and supplies for many procedures.

Additional Daily Cleaning

■ You are expected to clean equipment and furniture:

• All stools • **Kick buckets** and their holders (Figure 21–2) • Operating table • Flat surfaces, counters, cabinets, and so on • **IV poles,** suction units (outside only)

kick buckets Metal buckets on wheels that can be kicked out of the way.

IV poles Poles that raise and lower. IV solutions are hung on these poles.

FIGURE 21–2.
Kick bucket.

■ Spot-clean lights, walls, vents, and so on.
■ Damp-mop floors.
■ Floor-flooding technique may be required.

*P*rocedure

Cleaning Sterile Areas

Note: Daily cleaning using this procedure is necessary in the following areas:

    Surgery

    Labor and delivery

    Catheterization laboratory

1. Gather equipment.
   a. Service cart
   b. Glass cleaner
   c. Gloves

ALERT: Follow Standard Precautions.

2. Put on gloves.
3. Remove all trash from the area.
4. Replace plastic liners in each trash container.
5. Remove soiled linen from hampers.
6. Using a cloth dampened with a germicidal solution, wipe down the linen hamper inside and outside, including wheels.
7. Clean treatment tables.
   a. Remove all parts and clean thoroughly.
   b. Wipe down all visible areas on the table.
   c. Replace mattress pad.
   d. Cover with sheet.
8. Wipe all furniture and equipment in the room, including wheels, etc.
9. Wipe any spots on walls, ledges, doors, etc.
10. Damp-mop floors with clean germicidal solution.
11. Remove gloves.
12. Wash hands.

■ CLEANING PUBLIC AREAS

Patients are cared for in hospitals and health care facilities. There are also visitors, health care workers, and a variety of individuals coming and going. The way the environment looks makes a major impression. A safe, clean, odor-free environment is important because it promotes comfort and a sense of confidence. Patients and families feel encouraged and confident that the staff are caring and competent caregivers.

Every area of the facility is visited by someone each day. It is a major task to keep everything clean and pleasant, especially in facilities that never close.

Your assignment may be in the public areas of the hospital. These areas include the following:

■ Reception area
■ Waiting rooms
■ Offices
■ Nurses' stations
■ Lounges for the staff
■ Public restrooms
■ Stairways, elevators, and corridors
■ Classrooms, meeting rooms, and conference centers

All these areas must be kept clean. Remember that if you do not do a good job, it is obvious to everyone. You have a great responsibility. Take it seriously, and be proud of the appearance of your facility.

■ MAINTAINING THE LINEN AREA

Not all facilities have a separate linen department. Some have all the linens sent out. If your facility has a linen department, you may be assigned to this area. Health care workers in this area have the responsibility to

■ Handle all linen as contaminated; follow Standard Precautions.
■ Maintain the clean linen room and the washer/dryer room.
■ Count linens from the contract laundry, if your facility uses one.
■ Keep the linen carts clean and neat (Figure 21–3).
■ Replenish stock in all clean linen storage areas.
■ Take linens to areas with special requests.
■ Operate the washer and dryer.
■ Sort, inspect, and fold linens.
■ Maintain inventory of linen.
■ Store linen carts out of passageways to prevent congestion.
■ Remove excess lint from area.

FIGURE 21–3.
Linen cart.

Procedure

Cleaning Linen Carts

1. Gather supplies:
   Clean cloths
   Germicidal/detergent solution
   Disposable gloves
   ALERT: Follow Standard Precautions.
2. Put on gloves.
3. Wash all racks and bars of cart with germicidal/detergent solution.
4. Wipe with clean cloth.
5. Spray cover of cart on inside and outside with germicidal/detergent solution.
6. Wipe with dry cloth.
7. Wipe wheels and bumpers with cleaning solution and clean cloth.
8. Inspect covers and carts for condition.
9. Remove gloves.
10. Report items needing repair.
11. Store linen carts out of passageways to prevent congestion.

Procedure

Maintaining Washer/Dryer Room

1. Gather supplies:
   Laundry soap
   Additives according to facility policy
   Disposable gloves
2. Put on gloves.
3. Separate colors and whites.
4. Place in separate piles.
5. Separate linens in piles by weight (all towels together, all sheets together, etc.).
6. Use manufacturer's operating instructions for washer and dryer.
7. Wash and dry linen according to facility policy.
8. Fold laundry according to facility policy.
9. Inspect laundry for tears or stains (handle according to facility policy).
10. Wipe inside and outside of dryer and washer daily with germicidal solution.
11. Remove gloves.
12. Wash hands.

■ JOBS AND PROFESSIONS

- ■ Assistive personnel
- ■ Clinical medical assistant
- ■ Licensed vocational/practical nurse
- ■ Registered nurse

Thinking Critically:
Check Your Understanding

1. **Communication** There is an overhead page for you to come immediately to the labor and delivery area. You just started to wet-mop a hallway. Answer the following questions and justify your responses: (1) Who will you talk to? (2) What will you say? (3) What will you do?

2. **Legal and Ethical** Describe the possible legal results of your leaving a wet floor without signs or a barrier to warn people walking through the area.

3. **Computers** Research and identify ways that computers are used in the environmental services department.

4. **Case Study** Mrs. Summers is a pleasant elderly woman who enjoys talking with you while you are working in her rooms. Today she asks you to do her a favor. She gives you some money to buy her a candy bar from the gift shop. Describe how you will respond to her, and explain your reasoning.

Portfolio Connection

Once you attain competency as an environmental service technician/housekeeper, ask for permission to take pictures of areas you cleaned. Be sure that your photos do not show patients or their guests. Place pictures, along with a description of the area, in your portfolio as evidence of your work. Place a copy of your on-site trainer's evaluation in your portfolio.

Write a paper describing your doubts and realizations and the barriers that you were able to overcome during your environmental services/housekeeping experience. For example, did you have fears about going into the surgery area or the morgue? Describe the ways you plan to use the skills, information, and insights that you gained about the people you worked with and about this job. This assignment must be in standard report format.

22 HEALTH INFORMATION TECHNICIAN

Steps to success

1. Complete Vocabulary Worksheet 1 in the Student Workbook.
2. Read this chapter.
3. Complete Worksheets 2 through 8 as assigned.
4. Practice and demonstrate all procedures.
5. When you are confident that you can meet each objective for this chapter, ask your instructor for the chapter evaluation.
6. Complete "Your Link to Success" at the end of this chapter.

Objectives

When you have completed this chapter, you will be able to do the following:

✓ Complete all objectives from Part One of this book.
✓ Explain why customer service is important.
✓ Differentiate between a positive and negative personal appearance.
✓ Discuss the importance of office appearance.
✓ List nine guidelines when scheduling clients/patients for appointments.
✓ Describe a tickler file.
✓ Discuss two purposes for writing a letter.
✓ Explain how a letter is a legal document.
✓ Discuss the information that is necessary for a medical history form.
✓ List five filing systems.
✓ List two kinds of registration forms.

✓ Explain how to reach the fair dollar amount for determining fees.

✓ Define *professional courtesy*.

✓ Define *insurance assignment*.

✓ Define *managed care*.

✓ Differentiate between an HMO, a PPO, and an EPO.

✓ Define *CPT codes*.

✓ Define *ICD-9 codes*.

✓ Define *HCPCS codes*.

✓ List three types of bookkeeping systems.

✓ List four items to look for when you receive a check from a client/patient.

✓ Define *W-4* and *W-2 forms*.

✓ Match six items that appear on a paycheck.

✓ Explain how to use a petty cash fund.

✓ Recognize the difference between medical and administrative supplies.

✓ Predict what problems might occur if there were no supply ordering procedure.

✓ Identify the questions to ask regarding business equipment.

✓ Demonstrate the following:

  • Looking professional
  • Scheduling appointments
  • Scheduling a new client/patient: first-time visit
  • Scheduling an outpatient diagnostic test
  • Using a pegboard for charges and services
  • Keeping track of petty cash
  • Writing a letter in three styles

■ RESPONSIBILITIES OF A HEALTH INFORMATION TECHNICIAN

Health information technicians facilitate the efficient operation of a provider's (physician, nurse practitioner, physician's assistant) office. They may also work in clinics or other health care facilities and have varied duties in the front office of physician's offices, clinics, and health maintenance organizations (HMOs).

Duties of the health information technician include the following:

■ Answering phones

■ Greeting clients/patients

■ Processing mail

■ Scheduling hospital admissions

■ Scheduling laboratory services

■ Making appointments

■ Preparing insurance forms for Medicare, Medicaid, and workers' compensation

■ Typing medical reports

■ Maintaining client/patient files

■ Handling billing and receipts (in some offices)

■ Preparing payroll for office staff (in some offices)
■ Typing correspondence

■ CUSTOMER SERVICE

Good customer service has different meanings for different businesses. In a department store or bookstore, it means treating the customer politely and having the items the customer needs. What does it mean in a medical office? The definitions are as varied as the number of clients/patients your office sees. In a medical office, good customer service includes the following:

■ Your professional appearance
■ The professional appearance of the office
■ How you answer a phone call
■ The ease in scheduling appointments with the provider
■ The way you make clients/patients feel when they walk into the office
■ How quickly questions are answered
■ How easily billing is done

Be a Professional

The way you are perceived by patients, their family, and other professionals sets the tone for the office. As a health information technician you are responsible for setting a positive tone and image for your employer.

Remember to treat clients/patients the way you expect to be treated when you go to a medical office. Listen to what clients/patients say with their words as well as with their nonverbal communication, and respond paying close attention to your words and nonverbal communication. Review Chapter 5, Unit 1, to reinforce your positive communication skills.

Procedure

Looking Professional

1. Dress according to your facility's dress code.
2. Keep jewelry to a minimum (e.g., watch, stud earrings, and a ring).
3. Wear your name badge every day, in view of clients/patients.
4. Wear clean and polished shoes every day.
5. Keep your hair clean.
6. Wear your hair up and off your collar.
7. Use unscented deodorant.
8. Follow rules of good hygiene.
   a. Brush your teeth at least once a day.
   b. Floss daily.
   c. Use mouthwash or breath mints.
   d. Bathe daily.
9. Keep your nails short and clean. (Use light-colored nail polish, and repair chips.)

Female
10. Keep makeup conservative (e.g., no dark, heavy makeup).
11. Do not use perfume or cologne.
12. Wear full-length hose without runs.

Male
13. Do not use cologne or strong aftershave.
14. Keep beard or mustache neatly trimmed.
15. Shave daily. No stubble!

Procedure

Nonverbal/Body Language

1. Make eye contact with clients/patients as they enter the office.
2. **Maintain** eye contact as you **converse** with clients/patients.
3. Smile.
4. Keep an open **stance.** (Crossed arms or hands indicates an unwillingness or a barrier in communication.)
5. Give your full attention to one client/patient at a time, even when you have multiple tasks (e.g., telephone, other patients).
6. Keep your hands away from your mouth when speaking.

Office Appearance

Office appearance is as important as your appearance. Clients/patients make judgments based on what they see. Clients/patients see the office as a reflection of the quality of care they will receive. Make sure that the office is always clean and orderly. Verify the following:

- Furniture is in its place and in good repair.
- Magazines are neatly arranged in racks or on tables.
- Exam rooms are clean and ready for the next patient. (For example, the table sheet is clean and equipment is clean and ready.)
- Rooms and hallways are well lit.
- Toys are in only one area of the waiting room.
- There is a trash can available for clients/patients.

maintain Keep up.

converse Talk, have a conversation.

stance The way you stand.

Letter Writing

Writing is an important tool of communication between you and your clients/patients. When you write to a client/patient you must communicate clearly, factually, and **concisely.** A letter has many purposes. The two most common are

- To give information
- To ask for information

A letter to a client/patient is a legal record. Always use the following guidelines when preparing a letter:

- Gather all information you need before writing a letter.
- Determine if the letter needs to be formal or informal.
- Understand the purpose of your letter (for example, asking for payment).
- Ask yourself what results you want from the reader of the letter.
- Be specific.
- Use simple wording (for example, *use* instead of *utilize*).
- Be as brief as possible without omitting any important facts.

concisely Brief; to the point.

■ Read the letter carefully.

■ Ask yourself, "Will the reader understand what the writer wants them to do?"

Letter Styles

The most common style is the block-style letter (see Figure 22–1). To write a block-style letter, follow this format:

1. *Date line.*   Six lines from the top of the page
2. *Inside address.*   Three to eight lines from the date
3. **Salutation.**   Two lines from inside address
4. *Message.*   Two lines below salutation
   a. Single space between salutation and first paragraph **b.** Double space between paragraphs
5. *Complimentary closing.*
   a. First letter of first word capitalized (for example, Truly, Sincerely)
   b. Comma after the complimentary close (for example, Sincerely yours,)
6. *Writer's typed name.*   At least five lines from the complimentary closing
7. *Title of writer.*
   a. Typed next to writer's name (for example, Gus Doors, President) or
   b. One line below writer's name:
   Gus Doors
   President
8. If preprinted letterhead is not used, the office name and address follow the writer's title
9. *Identification initials.*   Two lines below title of writer or office name
   a. Initials of writer in capital letters followed by a colon and initials of typist in lowercase letters (for example, GD:mmp)

salutation A greeting (e.g., Dear Sir).

FIGURE 22–1.

THE BLOCK LETTER

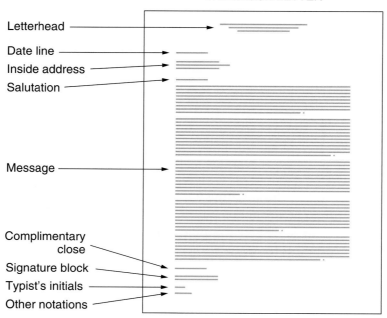

10. *Enclosure notation:* If a letter contains additional paperwork, this notation must be placed one or two lines below the identification initials (for example, Enclosure; if more than one, Enclosure 2, 3, and so on)

There are other styles of letters that your provider may prefer. See Figures 22–2 and 22–3 for other styles.

THE MODIFIED SEMI-BLOCK LETTER   FIGURE 22–2.

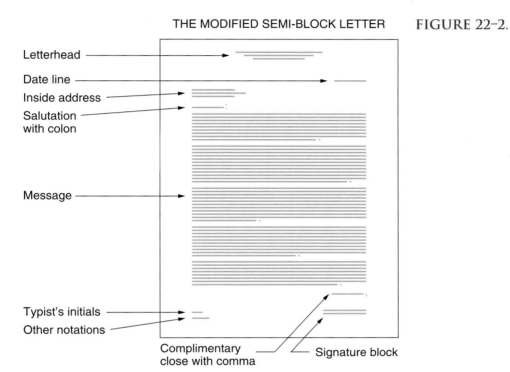

Letterhead

Date line

Inside address

Salutation with colon

Message

Typist's initials

Other notations

Complimentary close with comma   Signature block

THE SIMPLIFIED LETTER   FIGURE 22–3.

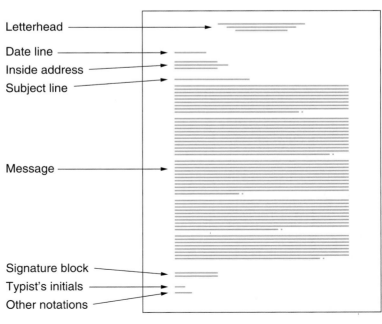

Letterhead

Date line

Inside address

Subject line

Message

Signature block

Typist's initials

Other notations

FIGURE 22–4.

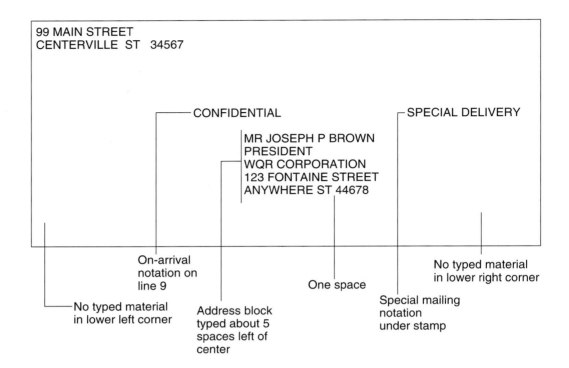

Envelopes

When addressing envelopes, follow the guidelines of the postal service. Remember to put a return address so that the letter can be returned to you if the addressee has moved. Figure 22–4 shows a sample envelope.

■ SCHEDULING

For a smooth-running day it is important to know how to schedule clients/patients for office visits, procedures, and surgeries. Scheduling is done in one of two ways: Appointments are written manually in an appointment book, or a computer system maintains appointment schedules.

Scheduling Office Visits

When scheduling visits, follow these guidelines:

1. A client/patient visit is scheduled every 15 minutes, 30 minutes, or hourly, depending on your provider's specialty (see Figures 22–5 and 22–6).
2. Learn to recognize the clients/patients who require more time with the provider.
3. Always ask the purpose of the appointment (for example, checkup, cold) to allocate enough time for the visit.
4. Ask the client/patient what would be the most convenient time for an appointment.
5. If you are not able to schedule the client/patient at the time and date requested, express regret and ask for a second choice.
6. Ask for a phone number where the client/patient can be reached during the day in case a cancellation is necessary.

FIGURE 22–5.
Standard appointment sheet.

7. Offer to call the client/patient as cancellations occur if the client/patient desires an earlier appointment. Use a tickler file as a reminder. (See page 557.)

8. Always repeat the appointment time and date to the client/patient to avoid confusion.

9. When a client/patient cancels an appointment, note the date, time, and reason for the cancellation in the chart.

10. Give all clients/patients appointment cards when scheduling a follow-up visit. Put the following information on the appointment card:

• Provider's name • Provider's address and phone number • Client's/patient's name • Date and time of next appointment

FIGURE 22–6.
Medical appointment schedule for more than one service at a time.

Procedure

Scheduling Office Visits

1. Assemble materials.
   a. Pen or pencil
   b. Appointment book
   c. Appointment reminder cards for tickler file
   d. Appointment cards
   e. Calendar
   f. Procedure list with approximate time allotments for each procedure
   g. Written instructions for patient/client preparation prior to visit
2. Prepare provider schedules for at least three months.
   a. Mark out vacation or holiday times.
   b. Schedule monthly, weekly, or daily meetings.
   c. Mark schedule to identify hours for client/patient appointments.
3. Follow the correct procedure for the type of appointment system in your office.
4. Write clearly and neatly so that names and procedures are easy to read.
5. Schedule appointments.
   a. By phone:
      (1) Clarify reason for appointment.
      (2) Discuss most convenient time for client/patient (e.g., A.M., P.M.).
      (3) Offer various times.
      (4) Ask for proper spelling of first and last names once a time is chosen.
      (5) Ask for information, such as birthday or Social Security number, if name is common (e.g., Smith, Jones).
      (6) Write client's/patient's telephone number and where he or she can be reached during the day of appointment.
      (7) Allocate **sufficient** time for the visit when scheduling a procedure.
   b. In person:
      (1) Follow steps 1 to 5 of procedure above.
      (2) Give client/patient an appointment card with date and time of appointment.
   c. For appointments more than three months in the future:
      (1) Ask client/patient to address an appointment reminder card.
      (2) Fill in month patient is to return.
      (3) Instruct client/patient that a card will be sent as a reminder to call and make an appointment.
   d. Place appointment reminder card in tickler file so that it is sent at the correct time.

Scheduling Surgeries/Procedures

sufficient Enough.

Learn how your provider wants to schedule surgery and procedures in the hospital or office. Use the following guidelines to help you with this scheduling:

- Determine how long each procedure takes.
- Learn how to schedule clients/patients around these procedures.
- Establish what days and times your provider prefers to do surgeries (for example, Monday, Tuesday, all day, just in the morning).
- Learn the admitting procedure for the hospital where your provider performs surgery.
- Provide the client/patient with the following information:

• Surgery time • Time client/patient needs to arrive at the office or hospital • Registration instructions (admitting forms) if going to the hospital • The hospital's address, telephone, and directions • Written instructions to follow prior to surgery (for example, NPO after midnight)

Procedure

Scheduling a New Client/Patient: First-Time Visit

1. Assemble materials.
   a. Appointment book
   b. Scheduling guidelines
   c. Telephone
   d. Pencil
2. Ask client/patient for the following:
   a. First, last, and middle names
   b. Birth date
   c. Home address
   d. Telephone number
3. Ask client/patient if this is a referral. If yes:
   a. Determine information you need from the referring provider.
   b. Add this information to the medical chart. (Your provider needs to send a consultation report to the referring provider.)
4. Ask what the chief complaint is and when it started.
5. Find the first appointment that allows the appropriate amount of time.
6. Offer a choice of days and times.
7. Enter the following:
   a. Client's/patient's name (NP next to name indicating new patient)
   b. Time and date of appointment
   c. Client's/patient's day telephone number
8. Explain payment procedure (e.g., client/patient must pay for visit, your office will bill).
9. Give directions to the office.
10. Explain parking arrangements.
11. Repeat day, date, and time the appointment is scheduled.

■ Give the client/patient verbal and written instruction, because the person may be nervous or apprehensive and forget what you said.
■ Maintain good lines of communication with the office personnel of all referring providers and assisting providers.

Learning how your office functions allows you to schedule a smooth-running day.

Scheduling Diagnostic Tests

Diagnostic procedures are frequently scheduled to be performed in other facilities. The following is basic information necessary to schedule an appointment:

■ Client's/patient's name
■ Age or date of birth
■ Reason for the diagnostic test

Give the client/patient the appointment information and instructions to prepare for the test. When scheduled for a test like an upper gastrointestinal series [UGI] give written guidelines that explain how to prepare for the test.

Tickler File

A tickler file reminds you of tasks that need to be done at a certain time (for example, by day, week, or month). When you create a tickler file, arrange twelve file dividers in a file. You need one divider for each month and one for each day of the month (1 through 31). When a client/patient needs to be seen at a later date:

Procedure

Scheduling Outpatient Diagnostic Tests

1. Assemble materials.
   a. Written order from provider
   b. Patient's chart
   c. Test preparation instructions for client/patient
   d. Name, address, and phone number of laboratory
   e. Telephone
2. Read provider's order.
3. Ask client/patient when he or she is available.
4. Call test lab.
   a. Order test
   b. Set up time and date
   c. Give name, age, address, and telephone number of client/patient
   d. Ask if there are special instructions for client/patient prior to the test
5. Provide client/patient with the following:
   a. Name, address, and telephone number of laboratory
   b. Date and time
   c. Instructions (in writing) for preparation prior to test
6. Verify instructions with client/patient.
7. Record test time in client's/patient's chart.
8. Put a reminder in the tickler file or on a calendar to check for results.

1. Fill out a reminder card with the client's/patient's name and address.
2. Fill in the blank space with the date of the client'/patient's last visit.
3. Place the card in the file the month prior to the next required visit.
4. Each month, take cards from that month's folder, and mail them to the client/patient.

Check this file routinely. The tickler file tells you what to do and when to do it. The card that is in the file reminds you to notify the client/patient to make an appointment (see Figure 22–7).

FIGURE 22–7.
Appointment reminder card to be placed in a tickler file.

As you requested, Dr. R. C. Smith is reminding you that it has been   since your last visit

Please call (000) 888-0000 to schedule an appointment

R.C. Smith. M.D.
11372 City Drive
Scottsdale, Washington 88888

■ REGISTRATION

New clients/patients must complete two basic forms when registering:

1. Client/patient information forms
2. Medical history forms

Client/Patient Information Forms

The client/patient information form gives the following information:

■ Client's/patient's name, address, and phone number
■ Birth date, sex, marital status, Social Security number
■ Client's/patient's employer name, address, and phone number
■ Insurance company's name, address, and phone number
■ Insured's employer name, address, and phone number
■ If the client/patient is a minor, name of the responsible party

Medical History Forms

The medical history form gives the provider the necessary information to evaluate the client's/patient's physical condition. The client/patient must give you the following information (see Figure 22–8):

■ Previous surgeries
■ Allergies
■ Chronic illness
■ Medications taken
■ General medical history
■ Childhood diseases

Both forms must be completed accurately to serve the needs of both the client/patient and the provider.

■ FILING SYSTEMS

Proper filing helps ensure you can find information when you need it. The filing system serves to

■ Store information and records safely
■ Keep related materials together
■ Retrieve files quickly when needed

The following are the five most common systems:

1. Alphabetical
2. Numerical
3. Color coding
4. Chronological
5. Geographic

GREEN VALLEY MEDICAL GROUP, INC.
MEDICAL HISTORY

NAME _____   DATE OF BIRTH _____

OCCUPATION _____   MARITAL STATUS: S   M   D   W

ALLERGIES:

Are you allergic to:

Penicillin. . . . . Yes _____ No _____

Sulfa . . . . Yes _____ No _____

Aspirin. . . . . Yes _____ No _____

Codeine . . . . Yes _____ No _____

Tetanus Injections . . . . Yes _____ No _____

Iodine . . . . Yes _____ No _____

Foods . . . . Yes _____ No _____

Tape . . . . Yes _____ No _____

Other _____

_____

MEDICATIONS:

List all medications, including over the counter, you are currently taking:

_____

_____

_____

_____

_____

HABITS:

Do you:

Smoke?   Yes _____ No _____ How Much ____

Drink Alcohol? Yes _____ No _____ How Much ____

Drink Beverages That Contain Caffeine?

                Yes _____ No _____ How Much ____

Limit Cholesterol   Yes ____ No ____

Use Other Substances   Yes ____ No ____

                What? _____

EXERCISE:

Do you on a regular basis:

Walk . . . . Yes _____ No _____

Run . . . . Yes _____ No _____

Bike . . . . Yes _____ No _____

Swim . . . . Yes _____ No _____

Aerobic Exercise . . . . Yes _____ No _____

Other . . . . Yes _____ No _____

MENSTRUAL HISTORY (FEMALES):

Date of last **PAP** & results_____

Date of last normal period _____

Date of last mammogram & results _____

Length of cycle (days) _____

Usual duration (days) _____

Number of pregnancies_____

Number of children _____

PRESENT COMPLAINTS:

Do you have:

Headaches . . . . Yes _____ No _____

Fever . . . . Yes _____ No _____

Cough . . . . Yes _____ No _____

Chest Pains. . . . . Yes _____ No _____

Nausea . . . . Yes _____ No _____

Vomiting . . . . Yes _____ No _____

Diarrhea . . . . Yes _____ No _____

Constipation . . . . Yes _____ No _____

Black Stools . . . . Yes _____ No _____

Bloody Stools . . . . Yes _____ No _____

Painful Urination . . . . Yes _____ No _____

Recent Weight Gain or Loss . . . Yes _____ No _____

Other Complaints _____

_____

PAST ILLNESS:

Have you ever had:

High Blood Pressure . . . . Yes _____ No _____

Heart Trouble . . . . Yes _____ No _____

Pneumonia . . . . Yes _____ No _____

Hepatitis . . . . Yes _____ No _____

Cancer . . . . Yes _____ No _____

Diabetes . . . . Yes _____ No _____

Tuberculosis . . . . Yes _____ No _____

Asthma . . . . Yes _____ No _____

Ulcers . . . . Yes _____ No _____

Seizures . . . . Yes _____ No _____

Sexually Transmitted Disease . . Yes _____ No _____

Blood Disorder . . . . Yes _____ No _____

Other _____

_____

OPERATIONS:

Have you had any surgery:

Appendix . . . . Yes _____ No _____

Tonsils . . . . Yes _____ No _____

Gallbladder . . . . Yes _____ No _____

Stomach . . . . Yes _____ No _____

Hemorrhoids . . . . Yes _____ No _____

Female Organs . . . . Yes _____ No _____

Thyroid . . . . Yes _____ No _____

Hernia . . . . Yes _____ No _____

Heart . . . . Yes _____ No _____

Other _____

_____

_____

FIGURE 22–8. Medical history form.

Each filing system involves the same basic procedures:

■ Sorting
■ Coding
■ Indexing
■ Storing or filing

Sorting is the placement of each item according to the particular filing system you are using. Alphabetical sorting requires placing all items with the same letters together. Numerical sorting requires placing all items with the same numbers together. Color sorting requires placing all items with the same colors together. Chronological sorting requires placing all items with the same dates together. Geographical sorting requires placing all items from the same region together.

Coding identifies items that belong to a certain category. For example, surgical files may be assigned a number or letter to identify them as separate from laboratory files.

Indexing organizes items in the order in which they are filed. The American Medical Records Management Association has established rules that provide guidelines for indexing items.

Alphabetical System

The alphabetical system is simple and economical, and it is the most common method for filing records. This system follows the order of the alphabet. If you have not used the alphabet for a long time, take time to review it.

Sorting

To set up an alphabetical filing system, place all charts with the same first letter of the last name together (all A's, all B's, and so on).

■ Samuelsen   ■ Puertas
■ Samuelson   ■ Putnam
■ Masters   ■ Cruz
■ Mendoza   ■ Culver

When there is more than one chart that begins with the same letter, alphabetize by the second, third, fourth letters (or as many as necessary). The boldface letters in the following list determine the files' placement in an alphabetical listing.

■ **Cr**uz   ■ **Pue**rtas
■ **Cu**lver   ■ **Put**nam
■ **Ma**sters   ■ **Samuelse**n
■ **Me**ndoza   ■ **Samuelso**n

Coding

If your files are separated by a code, place all A's with the same code together, all B's with the same code together, and so on. Some systems do not separate coded files. In files that are not separated, the codes identify specific things. For example, an office may have several doctors, and each doctor may be identified by a different color.

All charts can be filed together, or they can be separated, depending on the office procedure.

Indexing

Make three columns on a page and label the columns 1, 2, and 3. When filing by name, place the last name in the column labeled 1, the first name in the column labeled 2, and the middle name or initial in the column labeled 3. For example, if the name is Alec Monroe Goldman, it is indexed as

1	2	3
Goldman	Alec	Monroe

It is important to label charts by this indexing method. This makes placing them in order a simple task.

Charts with initials instead of a first name are placed before spelled-out names. C. Todd Sherman is indexed as

1	2	3
Sherman	C.	Todd

Names that are hyphenated are considered one name, as if the hyphen were not there. For example, Kellie Bell-White is indexed as

1	2	3
Bell-White	Kellie	

Apostrophes are ignored when indexing, so Timothy Gallagher O'Bannon is indexed as

1	2	3
OBannon	Timothy	Gallagher

Last names with prefixes are joined as one name, so Carlos A. De Leon is indexed as

1	2	3
DeLeon	Carlos	A.

Abbreviated names are indexed as if they were spelled out in full. For example, St. Gustov Edward is indexed as Gustov Saint Edward, or

1	2	3
Edward	Gustov	(Saint)

If a title precedes one name or a given name and a middle name, the title is the first indexing number. Father Gerald Rahn, Queen Erin, and Princess Monica are indexed as

1	**2**	**3**
Gerald	Rahn	(Father)
Erin	(Queen)	
Monica	(Princess)	

Titles and degrees before or after a complete name are placed in parentheses after the name for identification. For example, Dr. DeeAnn Marie Sherman or DeeAnn Marie Sherman, M.D., is indexed as

1	**2**	**3**
Sherman	DeeAnn	Marie (Dr.)
Sherman	DeeAnn	Marie (M.D.)

Store or File

Place files in alphabetical order for easy retrieval. Place the names in order by looking for the first letter that is different, indicating the sequence. For example, Gallagher, Kevin DeWayne, is filed before Gallagher, Shaun Patrick Michael, because the K in Kevin comes before the S in Shaun.

Follow the instructions in your Student Workbook to practice sorting, coding, indexing, and filing.

Numerical System

The numerical system is another simple way of maintaining client/patient charts. Use a notebook or computer to record the number assigned to each client/patient. This allows you to find the client/patient name by the assigned number. The assigned number is often referred to as a medical record number or patient/client number.

■ Assigned numbers are placed in numerical order.
■ Assign each new client/patient a number (for example, 001, 002, 003).

Keep a log in a notebook or computer of the client/patient name and number as you assign them. This record must be **accessible** to all staff. For example, assign numbers as follows:

accessible Available to obtain.

File Number	**Client/Patient Name**
001	Mendoza
002	Samuelsen
003	Putnam
004	Puertas
005	Masters
006	Culver
007	Cruz
008	Samuelson

Terminal Digits

terminal Last or ending.

Numbers can indicate many different things. Grouping by **terminal** digits means that you group items according to the last few digits of their assigned number (for example, 432.80, 321.80 or 879.90, 320.90). The terminal digits in these examples are 80 and 90, so all the 80s are filed in order by the first three digits, and all the 90s are filed in the same fashion (for example, 321.80, 432.80 and 320.90, 879.90). Let's pretend that you have items that need to be filed according to their assigned number. First sort these items by grouping all the same number of digits together (for example, all two-digit numbers together, all three-digit numbers together). These are basic rules to follow:

■ When zeros precede numbers, ignore them. Zeros are often added to numbers because computers call for a specific number of digits in a space. For example, the sequence 0001, 0935, 0087 is filed 0001, 0087, 0935. Because you ignore zeros before numbers when filing, you sort 0001 as a one-digit number, 0087 as having two digits, and 0935 as having three digits.

■ Coding is often done by the terminal-digit method. Take the last digits of the assigned numbers and group together all those that are the same. File in ascending order within these groupings. For example, 546.10, 386.30, 957.10, and 752.30 are grouped with all numbers ending with 10 together and all numbers ending with 30 together (546.10, 957.10, 386.30, 752.30).

■ Indexing places items in ascending numerical order within their groups. (For example, 546.10 and 957.10 are in one group, and 386.30 and 752.30 form another group.)

■ Place files according to their numerical order.

Follow the instructions in your Student Workbook for sorting, coding, indexing, and filing numerically.

Color-Coding System

Color coding helps reduce the chance of filing errors. The following are guidelines for using this method.

1. Assign a color sticker to each letter of the alphabet (for example, blue is A, yellow is B, green is C).
2. Determine how many stickers to apply on a client's/patient's chart (depending on chart size). *Example:* If you use three colors on the chart and the client's/patient's name is Mr. Gates, place the stickers in the order that corresponds to the first three letters of the client's/patient's last name (for example, G is yellow, A is blue, and T is purple).
3. Place the color stickers on the side of the chart that faces out when filed.

Chronological System

Chronological filing arranges files in the order of their occurrence, usually by day. This method is most often used in storing research items. Because each day, month, and year can be referred to by number, it is easy to follow the basic numerical system.

1. Sort by placing all items of the same year together.
2. Code each item as in any filing system.
3. Index by placing all files of the same month and year together.
4. File each item by date within the appropriate month and year grouping.

Geographical System

Geographical filing is done according to location. This method is often used for storing records of research studies in specific geographical areas. File alphabetically according to the name of the state, then alphabetically according to the city. File in the following manner:

- Alphabetically according to the state name
- Alphabetically according to the city name
- Alphabetically according to the names of companies

Whichever filing method you use, follow the basic rules for filing under the appropriate system. The following is an example of filing by company name:

Company Name	City	State
A.G. Corporation	Mills	Illinois
Blosson Inc.	Lakewood	California
Gamble Corporation	Reno	Nevada
General Corporation	Redlands	California
K.G. Inc.	Lakes	Utah
K.M.B. Corp.	Mills	Illinois
M.M. General	Lakewood	California
M.W.G. Corporation	Great Lakes	Florida
Water Inc.	Silverton	Illinois

The following items are alphabetized by state and city:

State	City	Company Name
California	Lakewood	Blosson Inc.
California	Lakewood	M.M. General
California	Redlands	General Corp.
Florida	Great Lakes	M.W.G. Corp.
Illinois	Mills	A.G. Corp.
Illinois	Mills	K.M.G. Corp.
Illinois	Silverton	Water Inc.
Nevada	Reno	Gamble Corp.
Utah	Lakes	K.G. Inc.

■ FEES

A fee is a charge for professional services rendered by the provider. The following guidelines help determine how to establish fees:

- All fees must be the same for all clients/patients and insurance companies.
- To arrive at a fair dollar amount, research the following resources:

• Call other providers and/or office staff who have the same type of practice. (For example, if your provider is a family practice provider, talk with another family practice office.) • Ask various insurance companies to provide you with the average dollar amounts they reimburse for services. • Check the state guidelines on charges allowed.

Professional Courtesy

It is a common practice for providers to extend professional courtesy to other providers and some client/patients for services rendered. A provider can decide not to charge a client/patient or other provider for services rendered or charge at a discounted rate. Learn the billing policy in your office so that you can deal appropriately with these types of accounts.

■ BILLING

Each office needs to establish a billing policy. This policy will provide the following information:

■ When to bill a client/patient.

■ When to bill the client's/patient's insurance.

■ When the client/patient pays for services as they are rendered.

■ When to inform the client/patient about your payment policy. (For example, when the client/patient sets up an appointment, tell them: "Mr. Puertas, it's the policy of our office to request payment at the time of service.")

■ Whether you will supply clients/patients with a superbill (Figure 22–9) to send to their insurance company.

■ Whether you will accept assignment. Accepting assignment means that you accept what the client's/patient's insurance allows. *Example:* Your provider charges $55 for an office visit, but the insurance company will only allow a fee of $35 for an office visit. The insurance company then pays you a percentage of the fee allowed (e.g., for example, 80 percent of the allowed fee, or $28). The patient is responsible for the difference between $28 and $35. In this case the provider collects $7 from the client/patient. The provider writes off the remaining $20.

Because there are so many different types of insurance and insurance plans, it is important to have a clear understanding of what companies your provider has contracts with and how those contracts work.

Insurance

You may deal with as many different insurance plans as you do clients/patients. Each insurance company has guidelines and regulations detailing what it considers covered and uncovered benefits. The insurance company also indicates what amount it will pay to the provider of service. It is important that the client/patient insurance information is correct and can be verified. Billing must follow the insurance company's guidelines, or it will not pay. Always request that the client/patient bring his or her insurance card (see Figure 22–10) so that a copy can be kept in the person's chart, insurance forms that are completed and signed, and information that explains policy deductibles.

BRISTOL PARK MEDICAL GROUP, INC.
3160 Redhill Avenue • Costa Mesa, CA 92626

NEW PATIENT
NEW FAMILY **FAMILY PRACTICE**

DATE MO DAY YR	DR	MED REC NO	DOB	LOC	APPT	REASON FOR VISIT		DOCTOR'S USE ONLY
PATIENT NAME					VISIT NO	CO-PAY		
RESPONSIBLE PARTY NAME								

Lab charges are subject to change without notice. You will receive a separate bill from Smith Kline Laboratories

Document Creations (714) 324-3919

MEDICINE 7.50			SMITH KLINE LABORATORY 1.75			INJECTIONS			
LIMITED OV (ROUTINE)	90050	40.00	CHEMZYME	80019	29.75	DPT °C		90701	22.00
INTERMED OV — PELVIC	90060	55.00	CHEMZYME Plus	80019-51	51.00	H.I.B. VACCINE °C		90749	22.00
EXTENDED OV	90070	70.00	W/HDL/LDL			M-M-R		90707	30.00
PERIODIC EXAM	90088	70.00	PRENATAL PANEL	80055	90.50	ORAL POLIO		90712	13.00
COMPREHENSIVE H & P	90080	125.00	W/HbsAg P-5			TETANUS TOX (T-D)		90718	13.00
REDUCED OV	90040	30.00	PAP SMEAR (1 SLIDE)	88150	24.50	T.B. PPD °C		90749	13.00
INIT OV (NEW PATIENT)	90000	50.00	BIOPSY – 1 SPECIMEN	88304	79.75	T.B. TINE		86585	13.00
INIT TREATMENT PROGR	90010	55.00	BIOPSY – MULTI SPECIMENS	88305	86.75	ALLERGY		95150	13.00
UNUSUAL HOURS	99050	35.00	(SPECIFY # OF SPECIMENS)			BICILLIN-CR °C		90749	13.00
HOSPITAL E.R. (INTERM.)	90560	65.00				CORTISONE °C		90749	14.00
						ESTROGEN °C		90749	13.00
						FLU VACCINE		90724	13.00
SURGERY 225.00			SPECIMEN HANDLING	99000	12.00	IV SET-UP °C		99070	28.00
PROCTO-SIGMOIDOSCOPY	45300	90.00	(PAP'S & BIOSPIES ONLY)	—	—	MEASLES MONOVALENT		90705	13.00
FLEXIBLE SIG W/O BIOPSY	45330	190.00	VENIPUNCTURE	90018	7.00				
TENDON INJECTION	20550-58	90.00	BPMG LABORATORY						
INCISION & DRAINAGE	10060-58	90.00	BLOOD-OCCULT (STOOL)	89205	15.00	SUPPLIES			
CRYOCAUTERY — INITIAL	17340-58	79.00	G.C. CULTURE °C	87087	15.00	STERILE TRAY		99070	35.00
CRYOCAUTERY — SUBSQ	17340	45.00	GLUCOSE-METER	82948	12.00	STERILE SETUP		99070	25.00
LAC. SIMPLE (2.5cm)	12001-58	90.00	GRAM STAIN	87205	15.00	SURGERY ROOM CHARGES		99200	50.00
LAC. SIMPLE FACE (2.5cm)	12011-58	157.50	HEMATOCRIT	85014	15.00	ELASTIC BANDAGE		99070	
LAC. SIMPLE (2.5 TO 7.5cm)	12002-58	146.25	KOH ONLY	87220	14.00	CAST MAT'L. (PLASTER)		99070	
ELECTROFUL BODY	17100-58	78.75	KOH/SALINE °C	87999	28.00	CAST MAT'L. (LIGHTCAST)		99070	
ELECTROFUL FACE	17000-58	112.50	MONO-SPOT	86300	15.00	CRUTCHES		99070	40.00
POST-OP CARE	99024	00.00	SALINE ONLY	87210	14.00	EYE TRAY		99070	8.00
			STREP SCREEN	87060	12.00	LAVAGE TRAY		99070	12.00
			URICULT	87087	15.00				
SPECIAL PROCEDURES			URINALYSIS	81000	15.00				
AUDIOGRAM, BASIC	92551-52	36.00	UA DIP ONLY	81002	10.00	BILLING			
EAR LAVAGE	69210-52	10.00	URINE PREG	84703	15.00	COPAY		99095	
ECG — ROUTINE	93000	60.00	WRIGHT'S STAIN	—	—	ADJUSTMENT			
HOLTER MONITOR	93262	325.00	NASAL OR SPUTUM	89190	15.00	COPAY (SPECIAL)		99098	
IPPB	94650	30.00	STOOL	87205	15.00	INFERTILITY (50%)		99092	
MANIPULATION	96600	45.00				FAMILY PLANNING		99091	
SPIROMETRY	94010	45.00	X-RAY 13.00						
			CHEST (2V)	71020	65.00				
NON-COVERED PROCEDURES			CHEST (1V)	71010	50.00				
ALLERGY SERUM	95155	47.00	LUMBOSACRAL SPINE (3V)	72100	65.00	BUSINESS OFFICE USE			
DME/ORTHOTICS	99099		SINUSES COMPLETE (3V)	70220	90.00	DISABILITY FROM:		— —	
DRUG SCREENING	82660	35.00	KNEE (2V)	73560	60.00	DISABILITY TO:		— —	
ELECTIVE PHYSICAL	90750		FOOT (3V)	73630	60.00	ADJUSTMENTS PROF DISCOUNT			
FLU INJECTION	90724	13.00	TOE (3V)	73660	45.00	COURTESY DISCOUNT			
FORM COMPLETION	99080	15.00	WRIST (3V)	73110	65.00	VIP DISCOUNT DO NOT BILL			
			FINGER (3V)	73140	45.00	AUTO ACCIDENT (3RD PARTY)			
			KUB	74000	50.00	PRIME INSURANCE			
						RECALL: YES MONTHS _____			

ICDA-DIAGNOSIS	X	ICDA-DIAGNOSIS	X	ICDA-DIAGNOSIS	X	ICDA-DIAGNOSIS	X	ICDA-DIAGNOSIS	X	ICDA-DIAGNOSIS	X	ICDA-DIAGNOSIS

FIGURE 22–9. Superbill. (Courtesy of Bristol Park Medical Group, Inc.)

Managed Care

Managed care is defined as a cost-effective way of providing service to the clients/patients. The following managed care plans provide this type of benefit for the patient.

FIGURE 22–10.
Insurance card.

You have selected the following Medical Group for you and all your enrolled dependents' care. In order to be covered by your HMO all medical and hospital services must be rendered or authorized by:

GREEN VALLEY MED–SAN FRAN
3160 SUMMIT AVENUE
SAN FRANCISCO, CA 92626

EFFECTIVE
DATE WITH PMG   07-15-96   PMG#   OL2

HMO   ISSUE DATE
                                     08-27-96

GROUP NAME
GREEN VALLEY MEDICAL GROUP

SUBSCRIBER NAME

SUBSCRIBER ID#   GROUP#
                                     52079A

PLAN GI WITH PHARMACY   RERATE AUG
                                     MONTH

Health Maintenance Organization

prepaid Paid ahead of time.

capitation Payment to provide care for a set number of people.

A health maintenance organization (HMO) contracts with a medical group or provider to be the primary care provider for its members. The HMO pays the provider or medical group for its services on a monthly basis. The amount, which is **prepaid,** depends on the number of clients/patients that are enrolled with the medical group or physician. The amount that is paid is called **capitation.** For example, Dr. Smith is a primary care provider who has 10 members of an HMO enrolled with her. The HMO pays Dr. Smith $10 per month per client/patient whether or not the client/patient comes to Dr. Smith. If the client/patient comes to see Dr. Smith once or 10 times in one month, the doctor still receives only one $10 payment per month.

The HMO covers most of the costs for procedures except for a copayment that is the responsibility of the client/patient. If the client/patient needs the care of a specialist (for example, an orthopedist), the primary care provider must direct the client/patient to the appropriate specialist by giving the client/patient a referral authorization.

Preferred Provider Organization

A preferred provider organization (PPO) contracts with a provider or medical group that has agreed to provide care at a reduced rate. The PPO often pays 90 to 100 percent of the cost. The client/patient pays the balance. The client/patient does not have to choose a primary care provider but must see a provider on the contracted list or pay all fees that are higher than the PPO has agreed to pay. There is usually a deductible that the client/patient is responsible for each year.

Exclusive Provider Organization

An exclusive provider organization (EPO) contracts with a medical group or provider to provide services to its members at a reduced cost. The member must see only the providers contracted with the EPO. If the member sees a noncontracted provider, he or she is responsible for all costs.

Always instruct the client/patient to bring the following information to ensure correct billing:

■ Insurance card
■ Insurance forms that are complete and signed
■ All met or paid deductibles

rendered Given or provided.

Remember that if you contract with an insurance plan, you need to follow the company's guidelines when billing for any services **rendered.** Appropriate billing results in correct reimbursement.

Billing Codes

Procedure and diagnostic codes were developed for billing purposes. These codes are accepted universally by programs such as Medicare and Medicaid. There are three types of codes: the Current Procedural Terminology (CPT) system, the Health Common Procedure Coding System (HCPCS), and the International Classification of Diseases 9th Revision Clinical Modification (ICD-9-CM).

Current Procedural Terminology (CPT)

Use the CPT coding system for reporting medical services and procedures performed by providers and other medical professionals. It is a communication method that is nationally accepted by all health insurance programs.

It is important to use the correct CPT code. The code that you use affects the reimbursement your office receives from the insurance plans you do business with. Improper coding can result in loss of payment. Remember that CPT codes

- Are five-digit numeric
- Describe procedures, services, and supplies used
- Are accepted and required by all insurance carriers, with few exceptions
- Are revised annually, and codes are added, changed, or deleted
- Can make a difference in your reimbursement

Health Common Procedure Coding System (HCPCS)

The HCPCS coding system was developed in 1983 by the Health Care Financing Administration (HCFA) to process bills to Medicare for supplies, materials, and injections. Use it when certain procedures and services are not defined in the CPT. Remember that HCPCS codes

- Are five-digit alphanumeric (the first digit is a letter between A and Z)
- Describe supplies, material, and services provided by a medical professional
- Are required when billing Medicare and Medicaid
- Are revised annually, and codes are added, changed, or deleted
- Can make a difference in your reimbursement

International Classification of Diseases 9th Revision Clinical Modification (ICD-9-CM)

Use the ICD-9-CM codes to define the diagnosis. Remember that ICD-9 codes

- Are three- to five-digit numerics (the first three digits represent a **generic** disease; the fourth and fifth digits describe the disease in a more specific manner)
- List the most important diagnosis first if the client/patient has more than one diagnosis

generic Major group (e.g., heart disease or skin disease).

When you are billing, it is **vital** that all the procedural and diagnosis codes coordinate. Insurance companies return any claims that do not have matching procedural and diagnosis codes. For example, suppose that a patient comes in with chest pain, and the procedure that is marked on your superbill or fee ticket is a foot x-ray instead of a chest x-ray. The insurance company will question the claim and return it for clarification.

vital A must, essential.

■ COLLECTIONS

delinquent Late.

Delinquent accounts are a major problem and need careful handling. One person is usually in charge of delinquent accounts. Outside collection agencies may be hired and paid a set fee or percentage for each account they collect. Ask the following questions regarding the collection policy of your facility:

■ When to consider an account delinquent (for example, after 30 or 60 days)

■ When to contact a client/patient regarding the outstanding balance on an account

■ How and when to inform a client/patient that his or her account will be sent to collections

■ What the collection agency's reputation and policies are (some agencies have unusual methods of dealing with clients/patients that may cause problems for your office)

Procedure

Handling Delinquent Accounts

1. Assemble materials.
   a. Delinquent accounts
   b. Office letterhead
   c. Collection letter form
   d. Facility policy for collection of delinquent accounts
2. Sort accounts by number of days delinquent (e.g., 30 days, 60 days, 90 days, and so on).
3. Decide which action to take:

   a. Make phone calls to client/patient as reminders and record response on billing record.
   b. Choose collection letter according to policy.
   c. Prepare collection letter.
   d. Mail collection letter.
   e. Note when letter is sent.
4. Send account information to collection agency according to your facility's policy.

■ BOOKKEEPING

Bookkeeping is the method of recording income for services by the provider. You also use bookkeeping to record expenses, such as office supplies, rent, and telephone, that occur during the daily operations of a business. Your office may select a computerized or manual record-keeping system. As a health information technician you may be responsible for keeping the daily records. To maintain accurate records, you must learn the system your office works with. The following are commonly used methods:

■ Single-entry
■ Double-entry
■ Pegboard

Single-Entry Bookkeeping

This is a simple and inexpensive method of accounting. This system requires the following parts:

■ *General ledger.*   Maintain a logbook with all day sheets.

■ *Day sheets.*   Record all charges for one day for each client/patient.

■ *Accounts receivable ledger.*   Record amount the client/patient pays for service.

■ *Accounts payable ledger.*   Record all fees that you pay for the purchase of equipment, supplies, or services.

Double-Entry Bookkeeping

This system requires recording two entries per financial transaction on a ledger of accounts (see Figure 22–11):

■ *Credit entry.*   An addition or payment

■ *Debit entry.*   A deduction or charge

For example, suppose you need to purchase $400 worth of office supplies with cash. Your ledger reflects a debit to Cash of $400 and a credit to Office Supplies of $400 (see Figure 22–11). This provides an automatic check-and-balance system.

Pegboard (One-Write) Bookkeeping

This method allows you to record information on several kinds of forms at the same time. These forms include the following (see Figure 22–12):

■ *Day sheet.*   A record of all daily financial transactions. One sheet is used per day.

■ *Superbill (statement-receipt).*   A three-part carbon copy form; copies go to the client/patient, insurance company, and office billing.

■ *Ledger cards.*   A financial record of the client's/patient's account. You keep the ledger card where it is easily accessible and separate from the client's/patient's chart.

■ *Clipboard.*   Where the day sheet superbill and ledger card are kept for easy record keeping.

LEDGER OF ACCOUNTS								
	Cash		Equipment		Office Supplies		Medical Supplies	
Date	Credit	Debit	Credit	Debit	Credit	Debit	Credit	Debit

FIGURE 22–11.
Ledger of accounts.

LEDGER OF ACCOUNTS						
	Cash		Equipment		Office Supplies	
Date	Credit	Debit	Credit	Debit	Credit	Debit
10/9/00		−400.⁰⁰			+400.⁰⁰	

FIGURE 22–12.
Day sheet.

PATIENT NAME	PATIENT NUMBER	DEP#	DATE OF SERVICE	SSN FOR OVER 5 YEARS DOB FOR UNDER 5 YEARS	SERVICE CODE	INFORMATION (CRUTCH RETURNS, NAME ON CHECK)	CODE PMT.TYPE	INIT.	DEBIT AMOUNT	CREDIT AMOUNT

GREEN VALLEY MEDICAL GROUP INC.

416776

Costa Mesa (714) 555-3242	Irvine (714) 555-1090	Santa Ana (714) 555-7100	Mission Viejo (714) 555-1600	San Francisco (714) 555-3199	Mountain Valley (714) 555-3130

Payment type codes:
1 = Cash
2 = Credit Card
3 = Insurance check
2 = Check

Service codes:
#901 Co-payment   #998 PMT check
#997 PMT Insurance #999 PMT Cash

GREEN VALLEY MEDICAL GROUP INC.   Facility name _____
                                        Date

PATIENT NAME	PATIENT NUMBER	DEP#	DATE OF SERVICE	SSN FOR OVER 5 YEARS DOB FOR UNDER 5 YEARS	SERVICE CODE	INFORMATION (CRUTCH RETURNS, NAME ON CHECK)	PMT.TYPE CODE	INIT.	DEBIT AMOUNT	CREDIT AMOUNT
Sally Morton	346-72	08	11-22-92	555-55-5555	901		1	DC	15^{00}	15^{00}
1										
2										
3										
4										
5										
6										
7										
8										
9										
10										
11										
12										
13										
14										
15										
16										
17										
18										
19										
20										
21										
22										
23										
24										
25										

Payment type codes:
1 = Cash
2 = Credit Card
3 = Insurance check
4 = Check

Service codes:
#901 Co-payment   #998 PMT check
#997 PMT Insurance #999 PMT Cash

Cash total		
Check total		
Grand total		

X _____
Balanced by

Procedure

Using a Pegboard for Charges and Services

1. Assemble materials.
   a. Pegboard
   b. Calculator
   c. Day sheet
   d. Carbon paper (sheets may be NCR sheets; these do not require carbon paper)
   e. Receipts
   f. Ledger cards
   g. Balance sheet from day before
   h. Pen
2. Set up pegboard.
   a. Put on day sheet.
   b. Put carbon over day sheet.
   c. Put receipts over pegs lined up with first open writing line on day sheet.

Procedure box continued

3. Put in balance from the preceding day.
4. Determine which clients/patients you will see.
5. Pull client/patient ledger cards.
6. Put cards in order of scheduled appointments.
7. Add ledger card to pegboard as clients/patients are seen (one card at a time).
   a. Put card under first receipt.
   b. Line up entry line of ledger with carbon on receipt.
8. Enter information on superbill.
   a. Client's/patient's name
   b. Date
   c. Receipt number
   d. Existing balance from ledger card
9. Remove superbill and clip it to client/patient chart.

After the client/patient sees the provider:

10. Ask client/patient for superbill.
11. Enter fee for service (use fee schedule).
    a. Find receipt on pegboard.
    b. Replace client/patient ledger under receipt.
    c. Put service code and fee on receipt.
12. Record amount paid and new balance.
13. Give completed receipt to client/patient.
14. Repeat steps 7 through 13 for each client/patient.
15. File ledger card at the end of the day or immediately.

At the end of the day:

16. Total all columns on day sheet.

This system allows you to see errors quickly and is easy to learn and maintain.

■ CHECKS (PAYABLE/RECEIVABLE)

If you are responsible for writing checks for bills, the office policy tells you the following:

■ When bills are paid (for example, first or last day of the month)
■ What recording system to use
■ How to write checks clearly to prevent misunderstandings
■ Which accounts are paid in full and which are sent partial payments

If you are responsible for receiving checks from clients/patients, look at the check to verify the following information:

■ The check is made out to the right provider or office name.
■ The written amount is the same as the number amount.
■ The address and telephone numbers on the check are current.
■ The check is signed by the person whose name is on the check.

Confirming this information prevents problems with the bank or client/patient later.

■ PAYROLL

The payroll system is complex. All businesses must follow certain federal and state regulations for payroll. A business may hire an outside agency to prepare its payroll or have an employee complete the payroll. Even if you are not the one responsible for maintaining these records, you must understand the way the payroll system works. Employers must maintain clear records of their payroll system. Every employer must keep the following information for each employee:

Form W-4 (1999)

Purpose. Complete Form W-4 so your employer can withhold the correct Federal income tax from your pay. Because your tax situation may change, you may want to refigure your withholding each year.

Exemption from withholding. If you are exempt, complete only lines 1, 2, 3, 4, and 7, and sign the form to validate it. Your exemption for 1999 expires February 16, 2000.

Note: *You cannot claim exemption from withholding if (1) your income exceeds $700 and includes more than $250 of unearned income (e.g., interest and dividends) and (2) another person can claim you as a dependent on their tax return.*

Basic instructions. If you are not exempt, complete the Personal Allowances Worksheet. The worksheets on page 2 adjust your withholding allowances based on itemized deductions, adjustments to income, or two-earner/two-job situations. Complete all worksheets that apply. They will help you figure the number of withholding allowances you are entitled to claim. **However, you may claim fewer allowances.**

Child tax and higher education credits. For details on adjusting withholding for these and other credits, see **Pub. 919,** Is My Withholding Correct for 1999?

Head of household. Generally, you may claim head of household filing status on your tax return only if you are unmarried and pay more than 50% of the costs of keeping up a home for yourself and your dependent(s) or other qualifying individuals. See line E below.

Nonwage income. If you have a large amount of nonwage income, such as interest or dividends, you should consider making estimated tax payments using Form 1040-ES. Otherwise, you may owe additional tax.

Two earners/two jobs. If you have a working spouse or more than one job, figure the total number of withholding allowances you are entitled to claim on all jobs using worksheets from only one Form W-4. Your withholding will usually be most accurate when all allowances are claimed on the Form W-4 prepared for the highest paying job and zero allowances are claimed for the others.

Check your withholding. After your Form W-4 takes effect, use Pub. 919 to see how the dollar amount you are having withheld compares to your estimated total annual tax. Get Pub. 919 especially if you used the Two-Earner/Two-Job Worksheet and your earnings exceed $150,000 (Single) or $200,000 (Married).

Recent name change? If your name on line 1 differs from that shown on your social security card, call 1-800-772-1213 for a new social security card.

Personal Allowances Worksheet

A Enter "1" for **yourself** if no one else can claim you as a dependent . . . . **A** _____

B Enter "1" if:
- You are single and have only one job; or
- You are married, have only one job, and your spouse does not work; or
- Your wages from a second job or your spouse's wages (or the total of both) are $1,000 or less.

B _____

C Enter "1" for your **spouse.** But, you may choose to enter -0- if you are married and have either a working spouse or more than one job. (This may help you avoid having too little tax withheld.). . . . . **C** _____

D Enter number of **dependents** (other than your spouse or yourself) you will claim on your tax return . . . . **D** _____

E Enter "1" if you will file as **head of household** on your tax return (see conditions under **Head of household** above) . **E** _____

F Enter "1" if you have at least $1,500 of **child or dependent care expenses** for which you plan to claim a credit . . **F** _____

G **Child Tax Credit:**
- If your total income will be between $20,000 and $50,000 ($23,000 and $63,000 if married), enter "1" for each eligible child.
- If your total income will be between $50,000 and $80,000 ($63,000 and $115,000 if married), enter "1" if you have two eligible children, enter "2" if you have three or four eligible children, or enter "3" if you have five or more eligible children . . **G** _____

H Add lines A through G and enter total here. Note: This amount may be different from the number of exemptions you claim on your return. ▶ **H** _____

For accuracy, complete all worksheets that apply.
- If you plan to **itemize or claim adjustments to income** and want to reduce your withholding, see the Deductions and Adjustments Worksheet on page 2.
- If you are **single,** have **more than one job** and your combined earnings from all jobs exceed $32,000, OR if you are **married** and have a **working spouse or more than one job** and the combined earnings from all jobs exceed $55,000, see the Two-Earner/Two-Job Worksheet on page 2 to avoid having too little tax withheld.
- If **neither** of the above situations applies, **stop here** and enter the number from line H on line 5 of Form W-4 below.

- - - - - - - - - - - - - - - **Cut here and give the certificate to your employer. Keep the top part for your records.** - - - - - - - - - -

Form **W-4**	**Employee's Withholding Allowance Certificate**	OMB No. 1545-0010
Department of the Treasury Internal Revenue Service	▶ **For Privacy Act and Paperwork Reduction Act Notice, see page 2.**	1999

1 Type or print your first name and middle initial | Last name | **2** Your social security number

Home address (number and street or rural route) | **3** ☐ Single ☐ Married ☐ Married, but withhold at higher Single rate.
Note: *If married, but legally separated, or spouse is a nonresident alien, check the Single box.*

City or town, state, and ZIP code | **4** If your last name differs from that on your social security card, check here. **You must call 1-800-772-1213 for a new card** . . . ▶ ☐

5 Total number of allowances you are claiming (from line H above or from the worksheets on page 2 if they apply) . **5** _____

6 Additional amount, if any, you want withheld from each paycheck . . . . **6** $ _____

7 I claim exemption from withholding for 1999, and I certify that I meet **BOTH** of the following conditions for exemption:
- Last year I had a right to a refund of **ALL** Federal income tax withheld because I had **NO** tax liability **AND**
- This year I expect a refund of **ALL** Federal income tax withheld because I expect to have **NO** tax liability.

If you meet both conditions, write "EXEMPT" here . . . . ▶ **7** _____

Under penalties of perjury, I certify that I am entitled to the number of withholding allowances claimed on this certificate, or I am entitled to claim exempt status.

Employee's signature
(Form is not valid unless you sign it) ▶ | **Date** ▶

8 Employer's name and address (Employer: Complete 8 and 10 only if sending to the IRS) | **9** Office code (optional) | **10** Employer identification number

Cat. No. 10220Q

FIGURE 22–13. W-4 Form.

1. *W-4 form.* This form gives the number of exemptions the employee claims. It tells the employer how much to withhold from the payroll check for taxes and affects the employee's take-home pay (see Figure 22–13).

2. *Time card.* This is a record of the employee's actual work time (see Figure 22–14). The employee's earnings for the pay period are determined from the person's time card.

3. *Payroll register.* This includes the following information (see Figure 22–15):
   a. Information copied from the time card b. Employee's name c. Number of exemptions (from W-4) d. Hourly rate and hours worked e. **Gross pay** plus overtime f. Taxable earnings for **FICA** g. Unemployment insurance h. Other deductions (for example, savings bonds, insurance) i. **Net pay** j. Check numbers

4. *Employee earnings record.* This record contains the following information (see Figure 22–16):
   a. Employee's name and address b. Social Security number c. Number of exemptions claimed d. Date of birth and marital status e. Rate of pay and hours worked f. Earnings, deductions, and net pay g. Check numbers h. Year-to-date earnings

gross pay Money earned before deductions are removed.

FICA Federal Insurance Contribution Act.

net pay Money earned after deductions are removed.

The amount of employee tax withheld is decided by federal and state regulations. A certain amount of money is withheld from the employee's paycheck to pay federal and state taxes on each paycheck. The following are the taxes withheld (see Figure 22–17):

	Morning In	Noon Out	Noon In	Night Out	Extra In	Extra Out
8						
1 9						
2 10						
3 11						
4 12						
5 13						
6 14						
7 15						

Verified by

\# _____ Loc _____ Dept _____ Super _____

Name _____

Period Ending _____

Scheduled Hours _____ 4–10's _____ Night Shift _____

DO NOT WRITE IN THIS SPACE

Reg Hours _____ Vac Hours _____
OT Hours _____ Sick Hours _____
Dbit Hours _____ SDiff Hours _____
Hol Hours _____ Other Hours _____
Persl _____ Acctg _____

The balance shown above is correct, and receipt is acknowledged.

Signature _____

FIGURE 22–14. Example time card. A time card has 31 days.

NAME	No. Exemp.	Hrly. Rate	Hours Wkd.	EARNINGS			TAXABLE EARNINGS		DEDUCTIONS			Net Pay	Chk. No.
				Reg.	Over-time	Total	FICA	Unemp. Ins.	FICA	FWT	Total		
Bart, Gwen	2	5.60	40	224.00	—	224.00	224.00	224.00	15.01	40.00	55.01	168.99	65
Evans, Sid	1	7.40	42	296.00	22.20	318.20	318.20	318.20	21.32	80.00	101.32	216.88	66
Murray, June	3	10.00	44	400.00	60.00	460.00	460.00	460.00	30.82	69.00	99.82	360.18	67
Sokol, Larry	2	8.00	36	288.00	—	288.00	288.00	288.00	19.16	24.00	43.16	244.84	68
				1208.00	82.20	1290.20	1290.20	1290.20	86.31	213.00	299.31	990.89	

FIGURE 22–15. Payroll register.

FIGURE 22–16. Employee earnings record.

NAME __Bart, Gwen__   SOCIAL SECURITY NO. __046 12 1930__
ADDRESS __14 Pawling Avenue__   DATE OF BIRTH __June 5, 19--__
__Troy, New York 12180__   MARITAL STATUS __Married__
NO. OF EXEMPTIONS __2__   HOURLY RATE __$5.60__

Line No.	Week Ended	Hours Wkd.	EARNINGS			DEDUCTIONS			Net Pay	Check No.	Year-to-Date
			Reg.	Over-time	Total	FICA	FWT	Total			
1	1/7	41	229.60	2.80	232.40	13.60	41.00	54.60	177.80	22	232.40
2	1/14	40	224.00	—	224.00	13.10	40.00	53.10	170.90	65	456.40

BRISTOL PARK MEDICAL GROUP, INC.
3160 REDHILL AVE
COSTA MESA CA   92626   1 - 55

PAYROLL PERIOD FROM	TO	DATE
10-01-99	10-14-99	10-18-99

CONTROL NO.	EMPLOYEE NO.	DEPT.	EMPLOYEE NAME	SOCIAL SECURITY NUMBER	EXEMPTIONS FED.	STATE	OTHER	MAR. STA.

	EARNINGS					TAXES		
TYPE	DESCRIPTION	RATE	UNITS	AMOUNT	TYPE	WITHHELD	YEAR-TO-DATE	
12	REGULAR		40.00	520.00	FIT	71.81	71.81	
21	OVERTIME		.25	4.88	FICA	40.15	40.15	
					SIT	8.94	8.94	
					DI	4.72	4.72	

	DEDUCTIONS					DEDUCTIONS		
NO.	DESCRIPTION	AMOUNT	PERIOD-TO-DATE	NO.	DESCRIPTION	AMOUNT	PERIOD-TO-DATE	

	TOTALS					CHECK NUMBER
Y-T-D GROSS	Y-T-D TAXES	CURRENT GROSS	CURRENT TAXES	DEDUCTIONS	NET CHECK	
524.88	125.62	524.88	125.62		399.26	8018735

FIGURE 22–17. Employee pay stub.

1. Federal income tax (see Table 22–1).

2. Federal Insurance Contribution Act (FICA): This is commonly known as the Social Security tax. The amount of the deduction is **calculated** from the FICA tax tables. The employer must match (also pay) the same amount that is deducted from the employee's gross income.

calculated Figured out.

3. *State income tax.* Like the federal tax, the state tax is withheld from the employee's paycheck for deposit toward the employee's annual taxes. Employers have tax tables to help them determine the amount to withhold.

4. *State disability insurance (SDI).* States establish this fund for persons who are temporarily unable to work. Contributions to this fund are made by the employee.

5. *Unemployment insurance.* The amounts paid and who pays into such funds vary from state to state. This fund is for workers who have lost their jobs.

TABLE 22–1 Example of a Wage Withholding Table

Biweekly Payroll Period—Single Person
for Wages Paid After December 2000

And the wages are—		And the number of withholding allowances claimed is—										
At least	But less than	0	1	2	3	4	5	6	7	8	9	10
		The amount of income tax to be withheld shall be—										
$ 580	$ 600	$ 81	$ 68	$ 54	$ 41	$ 28	$15	$ 1	$ 0	$ 0	$ 0	$ 0
600	620	84	71	57	44	31	18	4	0	0	0	0
620	640	87	74	60	47	34	21	7	0	0	0	0
640	660	90	77	63	50	37	24	10	0	0	0	0
660	680	93	80	66	53	40	27	13	0	0	0	0
680	700	96	83	69	56	43	30	16	3	0	0	0
700	720	99	86	72	59	46	33	19	6	0	0	0
720	740	102	89	75	62	49	36	22	9	0	0	0
740	760	105	92	78	65	52	39	25	12	0	0	0
760	780	108	95	81	68	55	42	28	15	2	0	0
780	800	111	98	84	71	58	45	31	18	5	0	0
800	820	114	101	87	74	61	48	34	21	8	0	0
820	840	117	104	90	77	64	51	37	24	11	0	0
840	860	120	107	93	80	67	54	40	27	14	1	0
860	880	123	110	96	83	70	57	43	30	17	4	0
880	900	128	113	99	86	73	60	46	33	20	7	0
900	920	134	116	102	89	76	63	49	36	23	10	0
920	940	139	119	105	92	79	66	52	39	26	13	0
940	960	145	122	108	95	82	69	55	42	29	16	2
960	980	150	126	111	98	85	72	58	45	32	19	5
980	1,000	156	131	114	101	88	75	61	48	35	22	8
1,000	1,020	162	137	117	104	91	78	64	51	38	25	11
1,020	1,040	167	142	120	107	94	81	67	54	41	28	14
1,040	1,060	173	148	123	110	97	84	70	57	44	31	17
1,060	1,080	178	154	129	113	100	87	73	60	47	34	20

FIGURE 22–18. Example of one type of W-2 form.

A. CONTROL NUMBER B1-049097-0	This information is being furnished to the Internal Revenue Service	OMB NO.	1 Wages, tips, other compensation 32094.40	2 Federal income tax withheld 5559.06
B. EMPLOYER IDENTIFICATION NUMBER 007252			3 Social Security wages 32094.40	4 Social Security tax withheld 1989.85
C. EMPLOYER'S NAME, ADDRESS, AND ZIP CODE GREEN VALLEY MEDICAL GROUP INC 3160 SUMMIT AVE SAN FRANCISCO, CA 92626			5 Medicare wages and tips 32094.40	6 Medicare tax withheld 465.37
D. EMPLOYEE'S SOCIAL SECURITY NUMBER			7 Social Security tips	8 Allocated tips
			9 Advance EIC payment	10 Dependent care benefits
E. EMPLOYEE'S NAME, ADDRESS AND ZIP CODE			11 Nonqualified plans	12 Benefits included in Box 1
			13	14 Other
			15 ☐ Statutory employee ☐ Deceased ☒ Pension plan ☐ Deferred Compensation	
16 State	Employer's state ID number	17 State wages, tips, etc. 32094.40	18 State income tax 1305.46	19 Locality Name CASDI	20 Local wages, tips, etc.	21 Local income tax 412.97

Copy B. To be filed with Employee's FEDERAL tax return
FORM **W-2 Wage and Tax Statement**

Dept. of Treasury - Internal Revenue Service

6. *Other deductions.* Employees can request that other deductions be withheld from their paychecks, such as

a. Health insurance b. Loan repayments c. Credit union payments or deposits d. Christmas club e. Pension funds f. Charitable contributions

The employer must keep an individual record for each employee. The Federal Wages and Hour Law requires the employer to send a wage and tax statement (W-2 form; see Figure 22–18) to the employee no later than January 31 of each year. It contains some of the following information:

- Preceding year's gross earnings
- Federal income tax withholdings
- FICA taxes withheld
- Total FICA wages paid
- Contributions to a retirement plan

If employees terminate employment during the year, a W-2 must be sent to them within 30 days of the last payment of wages.

■ PETTY CASH FUND

Petty cash is an amount of money set aside for the purchase of small items for the office (for example, postage stamps, office supplies). It is important to keep an accurate record of this account. Use the following guidelines for maintaining a petty cash account.

designate To appoint or determine.

disbursement Payment.

auditing Formal checking for correctness.

replenish Refill or build up again.

1. **Designate** an amount to keep in petty cash (for example, $75).
2. Only one person in the office is responsible for handling the petty cash.
3. Design a **disbursement** form (see Figure 22–19) with the following information:

a. Today's date b. Amount given c. Paid to d. Signature of person receiving the cash e. Signature of the person who authorized the expense f. Expense (for example, stamps, copy paper)

4. Attach a receipt to the disbursement form for **auditing** purposes.
5. **Replenish** the fund when necessary by writing a check for the total amount of receipts/disbursement slips. This restores the petty cash account to the starting amount (for example, receipts total $73.25, check written for $73.25 for reimbursement to petty cash fund).

FIGURE 22–19.
Example of one type of disbursement form.

PETTY CASH DISBURSEMENT   No. _22_

Date _1-8-00_ $24.20

Amount

Paid To _Tom Gates_

Expense _Car Fare_

Authorized by _Petty Cash_

Signature

Cash received by _____

Signature

Procedure

Keeping Track of Petty Cash

1. Assemble materials.
   a. Petty cash record form
   b. Disbursement forms
   c. Disbursement journal
   d. Checks as needed
   e. List of petty cash expenditures
2. Decide amount of money to keep for petty cash.
3. Write check to set up fund.
4. Cash check.
5. Write amount of cash in balance column in journal.
6. Write amount to Miscellaneous in disbursement.

7. Use petty cash disbursement form each time a withdrawal is made.
8. Record amount in disbursement journal.
9. Enter new balance.

To replenish petty cash

10. Write check. (Amount spent plus balance must equal beginning balance.)
11. Total the expense column and put charges in correct disbursement column.
12. Record amount added to fund.
13. Record new balance in petty cash fund.

■ SUPPLIES

It is impossible to operate a medical practice without the proper supplies. Keeping supplies stocked is an important responsibility. Following are the two types of supplies and some examples of each type:

■ Medical supplies

• Disposable products (for example, gowns, specimen containers, needles, gloves)
• Medications • Cleaning and disinfectant solutions

■ Administrative supplies

• Expendable items (for example, stationery, pens, registration forms) • Facial tissue, toilet tissue • Paper drinking cups

Your office policy for ordering supplies indicates the following:

■ When to order supplies
■ Names of companies that supplies are purchased from (when placing order, keep in mind the delivery time)
■ What record keeping is done for ordering supplies

■ BUSINESS EQUIPMENT

Your office will have office equipment to help run the medical practice smoothly. Always follow manufacturers' directions when using equipment.

Copier

Identify the following:

■ Where the on/off button is
■ Whether you need to turn the copier off daily or at the end of the week
■ What features the copier has:

• To enlarge and reduce copies • To sort/group copies • To do back-to-back copying • To staple copies • To produce copies in different colors

■ The maximum number of copies that can be made at one time
■ Where the paper tray is
■ How you put the paper in the copier
■ Where the copying paper is kept
■ How a paper jam is cleared
■ Where and how you change ink cartridges
■ The name and phone number of the maintenance/repair company

Facsimile (FAX)

Identify the following:

■ Where the on/off button is
■ All the functions, such as automatic dial, and redial
■ Whether you place the pages to be faxed facing up or down
■ How you dial:

• Whether you need to request an outside line • Listening for a tone before dialing the fax number • Which key is pressed to start the fax operation

■ Where a list of the most frequent numbers faxed is
■ How you put paper in the fax
■ Where the fax paper is kept
■ How you clear a paper jam
■ The name and phone number of the maintenance/repair company

Telephone

Identify the following:

■ How many incoming lines there are
■ What all the features are:

• Transfer • Hold • Speaker • Redial • Phone number memory • Conference calls

■ Whether there are public lines and private lines

Your learning and practicing all the operational guidelines of your office assists in providing good-quality service for your clients/patients. Doing so also makes you an important and valuable part of your office.

Thinking Critically:
Check Your Understanding

1. **Communication** Write a letter to a client whose bill is 10 days past due. Select one of the three letter styles for your letter. Your message must clearly state your request for payment without being intimidating.

2. **Legal and Ethical** Mrs. Smith's husband calls and asks you why his wife has an appointment with the doctor. Write an example of how you would respond to him.

3. **Patient Education** Mr. Morgan is calling to make an appointment with a physician. When you ask what the appointment is for, he does not want to tell you. Write a paper about how you would explain why it is important to know why he needs an appointment. Write the explanation just as you would say it to the patient.

4. **Computers** List the ways computers are used in the health care information department.

5. **Medical Math** Create a spreadsheet to show charges, receipts, and balance due.

6. **Case Study** A patient is upset because he doesn't understand what kind of insurance he has. Write an explanation of the benefit coverage of HMOs and PPOs to help the patient determine what kind of insurance he has. Write the explanation just as you would say it to the patient.

Portfolio Connection

Once you attain competence as a health information technician, ask for permission to copy a letter, a spreadsheet, and other forms and documents that you have completed. (Remove all patient identifiers.) Place these copies in your portfolio as evidence of your skills. Place a copy of your on-site trainer's evaluation in your portfolio.

Write a paper describing your doubts and realizations and the barriers that you were able to overcome during your health information technician experience. For example, were you afraid that you couldn't learn to use the equipment? Describe the ways you plan to use the skills, information, and insights that you gained about the people you worked with and about this job. This assignment must be in standard report format.

23 CLINICAL MEDICAL ASSISTANT

*S*teps to success

1. Complete Vocabulary Worksheet 1 in the Student Workbook.
2. Read this chapter.
3. Complete worksheets 2 through 14 as assigned.
4. Practice and demonstrate all procedures.
5. When you are confident that you can meet each objective for this chapter, ask your instructor for the chapter evaluation.
6. Complete "Your Link to Success" at the end of this chapter.

Objectives

When you have completed this chapter, you will be able to do the following:

✓ Complete all objectives from Part One of this book.
✓ Match vocabulary words with their correct meanings.
✓ Measure and record height and weight of an adult, child, and infant.
✓ Summarize the importance of measuring the circumference of an infant's head.
✓ Explain what a drastic change in growth patterns may indicate.
✓ Explain how to read a visual acuity test and the importance of the results.
✓ Compare and identify examination positions by name.
✓ List four basic examination techniques and explain their purposes.
✓ Compare similarities and differences between a general physical examination and a limited examination to rule out a condition.
✓ Identify symptoms of twelve physical conditions and state the appropriate patient education for each.

✓ Explain two types of pediatric appointments.

✓ List thirteen guidelines to follow when preparing for a surgical procedure.

✓ Reread Chapter 20, "Central Supply/Central Processing Worker":

- Decontamination
- Preparation area
- Sterile wraps
- Sterilization
- Monitoring effectiveness of sterilization

✓ Name five public health issues that require an official report with a public agency.

✓ Match common prescription abbreviations with their meanings.

✓ Match controlled substances with their assigned schedule level.

✓ Name four drug reference books.

✓ Describe methods to ensure safekeeping of medication.

✓ Write a formula for calculating medication dosage.

✓ Match metric measures with their equivalent standard measure.

✓ Name the six "rights" of medication administration.

✓ Recognize the guidelines for preparing and administering medications.

✓ Explain why it is important to observe liquid medication, and describe what to observe.

✓ Match the route of administration with its description.

✓ Explain why injections are given instead of other methods of medication administration.

✓ Describe areas where it is not appropriate to give an injection.

✓ Describe syringe- and needle-handling techniques that prevent accidental needle sticks.

✓ Recognize different types of parenteral medication containers.

✓ Name medications commonly administered by the Z-track method.

✓ Differentiate between intradermal, subcutaneous, intramuscular, and Z-track injections.

✓ Name and explain the purpose of common immunizations.

✓ Demonstrate all procedures in this chapter.

✓ Apply all procedural techniques with confidence.

■ RESPONSIBILITIES OF A MEDICAL ASSISTANT

Medical assistants (MAs) help health care providers examine and treat patients. They perform the tasks that keep a medical office or clinic running smoothly. Some MAs perform both *clinical* and **administrative** tasks. Other MAs are trained in only one of these areas. Some offices require a clinical medical assistant and an administrative medical assistant and do not expect one person to do tasks in both areas.

Clinical duties most commonly include the following:

■ Measuring and recording vital signs

■ Interviewing patients to obtain medical history

■ Explaining medical treatment to patients

■ Preparing patients for examinations

administrative
Pertaining to processing, such as handling of paperwork, that assists in patient care and supports the physician.

■ Assisting the doctor

■ Disposing of contaminated supplies

■ Collecting and preparing specimens for shipment to medical laboratories

■ Practicing aseptic techniques

■ Disinfecting medical instruments

■ Instructing patients in self-care and child care, including medication, diet, and treatments

■ Drawing blood

■ Calling patients and pharmacies as directed by the health care provider

■ Preparing patients for x-ray

■ Performing electrocardiograms (EKGs)

■ Applying dressings and assisting with treatments

■ Cleaning consulting and examination rooms and work areas

■ Performing simple laboratory tests

MAs are an important part of a medical practice. They work in ambulatory care offices as well as those of physicians, chiropractors, optometrists, and podiatrists. The MA position was first recognized in the 1930s, and the position continues to change with advances in medicine. There is a national association that certifies MAs when they meet specific criteria (see Chapter 2).

■ TAKING MEASUREMENTS

To determine a healthy body weight, compare the client's bone size and height. Bone size is identified as small, medium, or large.

Weighing the Patient: Adult and Child over 3 Years of Age

initial First.

Height and weight are recorded during the patient's/client's first visit. Weight is measured in pounds and ounces or in kilograms. The **initial** measurements are a baseline for future visits. Body weight indicates a person's nutritional status. A drastic weight loss or gain can indicate an illness. Patients with edema may need to be weighed daily to help the provider determine the amount of fluid the patient is retaining. Height and weight are also used to determine medication dosage. When weights are closely monitored, always do the following:

■ Use the same scale.

■ Weigh the patient at the same time of day.

■ Determine changes in clothing weight.

Use a scale to measure weight. Measuring accurately is important; always balance the scale at zero before weighing. Two common types of scales are the digital scale, which displays the weight in numbers, and the balance scale.

When weighing a patient/client, guard the person as he or she steps on and off the scale to prevent tripping and falling. Do not allow patients/clients to lean on or hold onto anything while you weigh them, because you cannot get an accurate weight if they do.

Procedure

Measuring Weight on Standing Balance Scale

1. Wash hands.
2. Assemble materials.
   a. Paper/medical record
   b. Pen
3. Balance scale at zero. (Balance-bar pointer must stay steady in center of balance area. If pointer does not center, scale will read weight incorrectly. With the weights on zero, turn balance screw until pointer remains centered.)
4. Ask patient/client to step onto scale.
5. Pointer should rise to top of balance bar.
6. Move large weight on balance bar to estimated patient/client weight. Pointer must continue to rest against top of balance bar.
7. Move small weight to right until pointer hangs free at center of balance bar.
8. Read patient/client weight by:
   a. Reading number next to notch on which biggest weight is resting (e.g., 150).
   b. Add number on upper bar to which smallest weight is pointing (e.g., 21).
   c. Sum of these two numbers is patient's/client's weight (171).
9. Write weight in patient's/client's medical record.

Measuring Height: Adult and Child over 3 years

Height is measured in feet and inches or in centimeters. Most balance scales have a measuring bar to determine height. Compare the size of the bone structure and the height in Table 23–1 to determine a healthy weight range.

Measuring Height, Weight, and Head Circumference: Infants and Toddlers (Under 3 Years of Age)

Infant and toddler growth is rapid and requires frequent monitoring. Infants are usually seen every 2 months to monitor growth and development patterns. Careful measuring and graphing of these patterns can help detect early changes that are important.

Measuring Head Circumference

Measuring head circumference screens infants and toddlers for abnormal head size. Watching head size can alert the provider if a problem such as hydroencephaly is present. Always place the measuring tape over the occipital bone on the back of the head and wrap forward just above the ears to center of forehead.

Measuring Infant and Toddler Height

Infant and toddler heights indicate normal or abnormal growth patterns. Always use the same technique to measure their height and weight. Never estimate height. Use a tape measure or the ruler on the scale or tabletop.

TABLE 23-1   Height and Weight Table for Adults

Men				Women				
		Bone Structure					**Bone Structure**		
Height		**Small**	**Medium**	**Large**	**Height**		**Small**	**Medium**	**Large**
feet & inches	in.				feet & inches	in.			
5'2"	62	128–134	131–141	138–150	4'10"	58	102–111	109–121	118–131
5'3"	63	130–136	133–143	140–153	4'11"	59	103–113	111–123	120–134
5'4"	64	132–138	135–145	142–156	5'0"	60	104–115	113–126	122–137
5'5"	65	134–140	137–148	144–160	5'1"	61	106–118	115–129	125–140
5'6"	66	136–142	139–151	146–164	5'2"	62	108–121	118–132	128–143
5'7"	67	138–146	142–154	149–168	5'3"	63	111–124	121–135	131–147
5'8"	68	140–148	145–157	152–172	5'4"	64	114–127	124–138	134–151
5'9"	69	142–151	148–160	155–176	5'5"	65	117–130	127–141	137–155
5'10"	70	144–154	151–163	158–180	5'6"	66	120–133	130–144	140–159
5'11"	71	146–157	154–166	161–184	5'7"	67	123–136	133–147	143–163
6'0"	72	149–160	157–170	164–188	5'8"	68	126–139	136–150	146–167
6'1"	73	152–164	160–174	168–192	5'9"	69	129–142	139–153	149–170
6'2"	74	155–168	164–178	172–197	5'10"	70	132–146	142–156	152–173
6'3"	75	158–172	167–182	176–202	5'11"	71	135–148	145–159	155–176
6'4"	76	162–176	171–187	181–207	6'0"	72	138–151	148–162	158–179

*P*rocedure

Measuring Height of Adult/Child (over 3 Years of Age)

1. Wash hands.
2. Raise height-measuring rod on back of scale so that tip of height-measuring rod is above patient's/client's head.
3. Instruct patient/client to remove shoes.
4. Ask patient/client to step onto scale and turn around to face away from balance bar.
5. Instruct patient/client to place heels against back of scale and stand straight.
6. Lift measuring rod up so that it points out above patient's/client's head.
7. Lower rod gently until it rests on patient's/client's head.
8. Instruct patient/client to step off scale.
9. Read numbers just above edge of hollow bar of rod at back of scale.
10. Record height on medical record in feet and inches, centimeters, or inches only, according to your provider's policy.

Procedure

Measuring the Head Circumference of an Infant/Toddler (under 3 Years of Age)

1. Wash hands.
2. Obtain measuring tape.
3. Identify the patient.
4. Explain procedure to parent.
5. Place infant in supine position.
6. Position measuring tape over occipital bone and wrap toward forehead. Bring tape just above ears to the center of the forehead.
7. Document measurement.
8. Wash hands.

Procedure

Measuring the Height of an Infant/Toddler

1. Wash hands.
2. Obtain tape measure or measuring bar.
3. Place infant on flat surface.
4. Place zero mark of tape or measuring bar level with top of infant's head.
5. Ask parent or co-worker to hold top of head gently at zero mark.
6. Gently straighten legs.
7. Read measurement that is level with infant's heel.
8. Wash hands.
9. Document measurement.

Procedure

Measuring the Weight of an Infant/Toddler

1. Wash hands.
2. Assemble equipment.
   a. Infant balance scale
   b. Towel
   c. Growth chart
3. Ask parent to remove infant's clothing.
4. Place clean towel on scale cradle to decrease shock of cold metal against infant.
5. Balance the scale at zero with towel in place.
6. Place infant face up on scale. Keep diaper or towel over infant's genital area in case of elimination.

Procedure box continued

7. Place one hand over infant (almost touching) to give a sense of security.
8. Slide weight easily until scale balances.
9. Read scale in pounds and ounces or in kilograms.
10. Return infant to parent.
11. Balance the scale at zero mark.
12. Record weight on growth chart and in patient's chart.
13. If child moves too much to weigh, weigh parent holding infant; subtract parent's weight to get approximate weight of infant or child.

Measuring Weight: Infant/Toddler

Infant and toddler weights are an important measure of growth patterns. Weight in an infant can change very quickly during an illness. Weight loss is an important indicator of dehydration. *Do not* change from weighing with clothes during one visit to weighing without clothes the next visit. Be consistent.

The growth chart in Figure 23–1 is a method of graphing growth patterns. The curved lines flowing across the chart indicate normal growth. Slightly differing levels of growth are normal. A large difference in the expected growth pattern may indicate a problem (for example, glandular imbalance or nutritional deficiency).

Testing Visual Acuity

Vision acuity (clearness) testing helps the provider detect eye disease or injury. Vision acuity tests are usually part of a physical examination. A provider always does a vision acuity test when the patient complains of eye pain, itching, tenderness, or

*P*rocedure

Testing Visual Acuity: Snellen Chart

1. Explain procedure to patient.
2. Position patient 20 feet (6 meters) from Snellen chart.
3. Ask patient to cover left eye and read smallest line of letters that he or she can see.
4. Record the distance patient is from the chart compared to the size of letters patient can see clearly (e.g., 20/20, 20/30, 20/40).
5. Record results with minus number if patient makes an error on a line:

   a. 20/40: with one error = 20/40 − 1
   b. 20/40: with two errors = 20/40 − 2
6. Record results with plus number if patient reads 20/40 line and two symbols in the 20/30 line = 20/40 + 2.
7. Repeat test with right eye covered.
8. Repeat test, allowing patient to use both eyes.
9. Repeat each test with patient wearing glasses (if he or she has prescription lenses).
10. Record results.

FIGURE 23-1. Growth charts for girls and boys from birth to 36 months.

FIGURE 23–2. Snellen eye chart for English readers.

FIGURE 23–3. Snellen eye chart for non-English readers and children. Have young children and non-English-speaking clients use their fingers to indicate directions of the E.

baseline A number, graph, or indication to use as a guideline. A measurement taken at a later time may differ from the baseline, indicating a possible cause for concern.

injury. The provider can identify changes and evaluate the treatment more effectively when there is a **baseline** acuity test.

To read the result of the visual acuity test on a Snellen chart (Figure 23–2), find the fraction to the left of the line the patient is able to read. For example, if the patient reads all the letters in the line marked 20/20 and is unable to read line 20/15, the patient's vision is 20/20. The top number means that the patient is 20 feet from the chart. The bottom number is the distance at which a patient with normal vision can read that row of letters. If line 20/50 is the last line read, the patient's vision is 20/50. This means that the patient is able to read at 20 feet what a person with normal vision sees at 50 feet. The chart in Figure 23–3 is read the same way.

■ STANDARD PRECAUTIONS

When working with patients it is important *always* to follow Standard Precautions to protect yourself when contact with blood or body fluids is possible. Review Chapter 12 and read Tables 23–2 and 23–3.

TABLE 23-2   Standard Precautions with Risk Categorization

Infection-control guidelines exist to protect employees and patients against infectious viruses and bacteria. The Standard Precautions you take depend on the (1) potential for contact with blood, (2) potential for contact with any body fluids, and (3) tasks (procedures) that you perform. This table tells you what to wear when you are doing various tasks. Follow these guidelines to protect yourself and others from infection.

Category	Task Requires:	Protect Yourself By:	Have Available:

I: High risk	Direct contact with blood or other body fluids	Washing hands:
		   If you touch blood/body fluids
		   After removing gloves
		Wearing:
		   Gloves
		   Apron or gown
		   Eye protection
		   Face mask
		Never recapping needles or bending/breaking them
		Placing used needles in a sharps container
		Cleaning off blood/body fluids immediately
		Disposing of waste materials
		Being vaccinated for Hepatitis B	

II: Low risk	When you have close contact with patients but are not likely to come in contact with blood/body fluids	Washing hands	Mask Eye protection Gloves
III: No risk	Your routine work requires no contact with blood/body fluid	Washing hands, as a general rule	

TABLE 23-3   Standard Precautions: Examples of Tasks and Use of Protective Equipment

Task	Gloves	Gown	Mask	Protective Eyewear
Controlling spurting blood	Yes	Yes	Yes	Yes
Controlling minimal bleeding	Yes	No	No	No
Blood drawing	Yes	Yes	Yes	Yes
Oral or nasal suction	Yes	No	Yes	Yes
Handling/cleaning contaminated instruments	Yes	Yes	Yes	Yes
Measuring blood pressure	No	No	No	No

■ ASSISTING WITH EXAMINATIONS

Patients/clients need reassurance during a physical examination. The patient/client may not know what to expect and may feel anxious. To help put him or her at ease, be friendly and efficient.

Equipment

Set up equipment according to the provider's request and check all equipment to be sure it works properly. Equipment varies depending on the body areas to be examined. Learn to anticipate each provider's needs and have equipment and supplies ready before he or she asks for them. Basic equipment includes the following:

■ Blood pressure cuff and sphygmomanometer
■ Stethoscope
■ Opthalmoscope (Figure 23–4)
■ Otoscope (Figure 23–5)

FIGURE 23–4.   Ophthalmoscope.

FIGURE 23–5.   Otoscope.

FIGURE 23–6.   Taylor percussion hammer.

FIGURE 23–7.   Tape measure.

FIGURE 23–8.   Tongue blade.

- Percussion hammer (Figure 23–6)
- Disposable gloves
- Basin/pan
- Tape measure (Figure 23–7)
- Tongue blade (Figure 23–8)

You may need to set up additional equipment. The type of examination determines which equipment the provider will need.

Examination Positions

There are specific positions for each procedure. Putting the patient/client in the correct position makes the examination easier. Always protect the patient's/client's privacy by positioning and draping according to the directions in each procedure.

- *Horizontal recumbent (supine) position.* Use this position for examination, treatment, and surgical procedures of the ventral (anterior) part of the body (for example, for abdominal pain, removal of stitches in chest).

Procedure

Horizontal Recumbent (Supine) Position

1. Wash hands.
2. Explain to client what you are going to do.
3. Assist patient to a position lying flat on his or her back in good alignment, with a small pillow under the head.

4. Drape cover so that he or she is not exposed, leaving all edges of drape loose.

- *Fowler's position.* This position relieves patients who are having trouble breathing (for example, asthma, chest pain). This position allows examination of the anterior and posterior chest (for example, listening to heart and lung sounds).
- *Trendelenburg position.* This position helps restore blood flow to the brain when the body experiences shock. This position also helps promote drainage of congested lungs.
- *Dorsal lithotomy position.* Use this position to examine or perform surgical procedures on the peritoneal and rectal areas (for example, vaginal exam, cystoscopy).
- *Prone position.* Use this position for examination, treatment, or surgical procedures of the dorsal (back) part of the body. (See bottom of p. 595 for other positions.)

Procedure

Fowler's Position

1. Wash hands.
2. Explain to patient what you are going to do.
3. Assist client to a position lying flat on his or her back in good alignment.
4. Keep patient covered so that he or she is not exposed.
5. Knees may bend slightly.
6. Adjust backrest to one of the following positions according to patient's or physician's needs.

7. Drape cover so that patient is not exposed, leaving all edges of drape free.

Procedure

Trendelenburg Position

1. Wash hands.
2. Explain to patient what you are going to do.
3. Assist client to a position lying flat on his or her back in good alignment.
4. Drape cover so that he or she is not exposed, leaving all edges of drape loose.
5. Lower the head of the table until the body is at a 45° angle. Legs may be bent or extended.
6. Reassure patient that he or she will not slide off table.

Procedure

Dorsal Lithotomy Position

1. Wash hands.
2. Explain to client what you are going to do.
3. Assist patient to a position lying flat on his or her back in good alignment.
4. Cover patient so that he or she is not exposed.
5. Gently assist client to bend knees.
6. Separate legs by placing each foot flat on bed about 2 feet apart or in stirrups attached to examination table.
7. Move patient's hips to edge of end of table when stirrups are available.
8. Drape with half-size sheet positioned with one corner toward head and opposite corners between legs. Secure side corner around legs.

Procedure

Prone Position

1. Wash hands.
2. Explain to client what you are going to do.
3. Assist patient to a position lying flat on his or her back.
4. Cover client so that he or she is not exposed.
5. Assist patient to turn onto stomach, keeping him or her covered.

■ *Left lateral position* and *left Sim's position.*   Use this position for minor rectal examinations and treatments.

■ *Knee-chest position.*   Use this position for rectal examinations and surgical procedures. Some examination tables adjust to support the patient's abdomen and chest.

Procedure

Left Lateral Position and Left Sim's Position

1. Wash hands.
2. Explain to client what you are going to do.
3. Assist patient to a position lying flat on his or her back.
4. Cover client so that he or she is not exposed.
5. Assist patient to turn onto left side.
6. Position patient's left arm slightly behind him or her on bed.
7. Gently bend both knees.
8. Place right leg slightly forward of left leg for lateral position.
9. Bend right knee toward chest for Sim's position.

Procedure

Knee-Chest Position

1. Wash hands.
2. Explain to client what you are going to do.
3. Assist patient to a position lying flat on his or her back.
4. Cover patient so that he or she is not exposed.
5. Assist patient to turn onto his or her stomach, keeping client covered.
6. Instruct patient to raise hips upward by kneeling on both knees.
7. Rest patient's head and shoulders on a pillow.
8. Extend arms above head on bed.
9. Drape with a large sheet, allowing edges to hang free.

Examination and Diagnostic Techniques

Examinations require four basic techniques.

1. *Observation/Inspection.* Here the provider looks at the patient/client for normal and abnormal appearance. Skin, eyes, hair, nails, movements, or actions that look unusual may be important in determining an illness (see Figure 23–9a).

2. *Palpation.* In this procedure, the provider feels parts of the body for unusual or abnormal conditions. Feeling and applying pressure also allow the provider to locate tender or painful areas (see Figure 23–9b).

3. *Percussion.* Providers use their fingers to tap over areas of the body. The sounds the provider hears during percussion indicate the fullness, emptiness, and size of internal organs (see Figure 23–9c).

4. *Auscultation.* The provider listens to body sounds through a stethoscope. Sounds of the heart and lungs, bowel sounds, and even the flow of blood through arteries can be heard (see Figure 23–9d).

These four techniques give a provider clues about how the body is working. For example, if a patient complains of a chest cold, the provider listens to the chest with a stethoscope. Gurgling sounds or very little airflow in the lungs tell the provider that the lungs are congested with fluid. A chest x-ray confirms what **auscultation** indicated.

auscultation Listening for sounds within the body.

a

b

c

d

FIGURE 23–9. Methods of physical examinations: (a) inspection; (b) palpation; (c) percussion; (d) auscultation.

When a patient/client complains of pain or other problems, the provider uses the four basic examination techniques. Prepare each patient/client for observation, palpation, percussion, and auscultation. Tell patients/clients what you want them to do. Remember that patients/clients are often nervous. Show patience and understanding.

diagnosis Identification of a disease or condition.

To determine a final **diagnosis** the physician looks for clues from the following sources:

■ Patient/client history

■ Physical examination findings

■ Vital signs

■ Laboratory results

■ Diagnostic test results

■ Symptoms described by the patient

If there is more than one possible diagnosis, the provider needs to rule out each possible condition before determining a final diagnosis. For example, a patient complaining of abdominal pain may need additional tests to

FIGURE 23-10. Patient/client questionnaire. (Courtesy of Bristol Park Medical Group, Inc.)

M E D I C A L
HEALTH QUESTIONNAIRE

NAME _____ AGE _____ DATE _____

HISTORY OF PAST ILLNESS/INJURIES (HAVE YOU HAD?):   MEDICAL RECORD # _____

	YES	NO	UNSURE		YES	NO
MEASLES	□	□	□	HAVE YOU EVER BEEN HOSPITALIZED OR		
MUMPS	□	□	□	BEEN UNDER MEDICAL CARE FOR VERY LONG? □	□	
CHICKEN POX	□	□	□	IF YES, FOR WHAT REASON? _____		
DIABETES	□	□	□			
STROKES	□	□	□	HAVE YOU HAD ANY HEAD INJURIES? □	□	
CANCER	□	□	□	HAVE YOU EVER BEEN KNOCKED UNCONSCIOUS? □	□	
RHEUMATIC FEVER OR HEART DISEASE	□	□	□			
TUBERCULOSIS	□	□	□	**OPERATIONS:**		
SEXUALLY TRANSMITTED DISEASE	□	□	□	HAVE YOU HAD ANY SURGERY? □	□	
CONGENITAL ABNORMALITIES	□	□	□	PLEASE DESCRIBE _____		
OTHER SERIOUS DISEASES	□	□	□			
LIST _____						

FAMILY HISTORY	IF LIVING:		IF DECEASED:		HAS ANY BLOOD RELATIVE EVER HAD?	YES	NO
	AGE	HEALTH	AGE	CAUSE			
FATHER					CANCER		
MOTHER					TUBERCULOSIS		
BROTHER / SISTER					DIABETES		
					HEART TROUBLE		
					HIGH BLOOD PRESSURE		
HUSBAND / WIFE					STROKE		
SON / DAUGHTER					CONVULSIONS		
					SUICIDE OR SEVERE DEPRESSION		
					MENTAL ILLNESS		
					BLEEDING TENDENCY		
					GOUT OR OTHER ARTHRITIS		
					ALCOHOL OR DRUG PROBLEMS		

SOCIAL HISTORY: □ SINGLE   □ MARRIED   □ SEPARATED   □ DIVORCED   □ WIDOWED

	YES	NO		YES	NO
			HAVE PEOPLE EVER ANNOYED		
DO YOU LIVE ALONE?	□	□	YOU BY CRITICIZING YOUR DRINKING? □	□	
DO YOU HAVE DEPENDENTS AT HOME?	□	□	ARE YOU CURRENTLY EMPLOYED?		
DO YOU EXERCISE REGULARLY?	□	□	□ FULL TIME □ PART TIME □ NOT EMPLOYED		
DO YOU SMOKE?	□	□	WHAT IS YOUR JOB? _____		
HOW MUCH? _____			YEARS OF EDUCATION COMPLETED:? _____		
HAVE YOU *EVER* SMOKED?	□	□	HOW MUCH *WORK TIME* HAVE YOU LOST DUE TO YOUR HEALTH?		
HAVE YOU EVER FELT YOU SHOULD CUT DOWN			PAST SIX MONTHS: _____		
			PAST ONE YEAR: _____		
ON YOUR DRINKING?	□	□	PAST FIVE YEARS: _____		

SYSTEMIC REVIEW (DO YOU CURRENTLY HAVE ANY OF THE FOLLOWING?):

GENERAL	YES	NO	HEAD-EYES-NOSE-THROAT (cont'd):	YES	NO
RECENT WEIGHT CHANGE	□	□	SNEEZING OR RUNNY NOSE	□	□
SKIN:	YES	NO	NOSE BLEEDS	□	□
JAUNDICE	□	□	CHRONIC SINUS TROUBLE	□	□
HIVES, ECZEMA OR RASH	□	□	EAR DISEASE	□	□
FREQUENT INFECTION OR BOILS	□	□	IMPAIRED HEARING	□	□
ABNORMAL PIGMENTATION	□	□	ITCHING EYES OR NOSE	□	□
HEAD-EYES-EARS-NOSE-THROAT:	YES	NO	TRANSIENT EPISODES OF UNCONSCIOUSNESS	□	□
EYE DISEASE OR INJURY	□	□	DIZZINESS	□	□
DO YOU WEAR GLASSES/CONTACTS?	□	□	**NECK:**	YES	NO
DOUBLE VISION	□	□	STIFFNESS	□	□
HEADACHES	□	□	THYROID TROUBLE	□	□
GLAUCOMA	□	□	ENLARGED GLANDS	□	□

REC-0100 2/95   (OVER PLEASE)

- Rule out (R/O) appendicitis
- Rule out (R/O) gastroenteritis
- Rule out (R/O) pelvic inflammatory disease (PID)

The provider makes a final diagnosis when tests rule out possible conditions and provide evidence of a specific disease.

General Physical Examination

Regular, routine examinations help identify early signs of illness or conditions that can develop into a disease or illness. The health questionnaire (see Figure 23–10) is a very important part of the routine physical. It provides information about the client's lifestyle. It also gives a history to alert the provider of possible problems. To prepare a patient/client and the exam room, follow the steps in the procedure.

Patient/client teaching is an important part of a medical assistant's responsibilities. Encourage patients to adopt good health habits. Provide written material

FIGURE 23–10.
Patient/client questionnaire *(continued)*.

SYSTEMIC REVIEW: (Cont'd)

RESPIRATORY:	YES	NO
SPITTING UP BLOOD	☐	☐
CHRONIC OR FREQUENT COUGH	☐	☐
ASTHMA/WHEEZING OR DIFFICULTY BREATHING	☐	☐
PLEURISY OR PNEUMONIA	☐	☐

CARDIOVASCULAR:	YES	NO
CHEST PAIN/ANGINA PECTORIS OR HEART ATTACK		
SHORTNESS OF BREATH WALKING OR LYING DOWN	☐	☐
HIGH BLOOD PRESSURE	☐	☐
SWELLING OF HANDS, FEET OR ANKLES	☐	☐
AWAKENING IN THE NIGHT SMOTHERING	☐	☐
HEART MURMUR/PALPITATIONS	☐	☐

GASTROINTESTINAL:	YES	NO
PEPTIC ULCER (STOMACH/DUODENAL)	☐	☐
HEARTBURN/INDIGESTION	☐	☐
VOMITING BLOOD OR FOOD	☐	☐
GALLBLADDER DISEASE	☐	☐
LIVER TROUBLE/HEPATITIS	☐	☐
PAINFUL/BLOODY BOWEL MOVEMENTS	☐	☐
HEMORRHOIDS/PILES OR BLACK STOOLS	☐	☐
CHANGE IN BOWEL HABITS (DIARRHEA, ETC.)	☐	☐
CRAMPING OR PAIN IN THE ABDOMEN	☐	☐
DOES FOOD STICK IN THROAT?	☐	☐

GYNECOLOGICAL: (FEMALE ONLY)
AGE PERIODS STARTED _____
HOW LONG PERIODS LAST _____ DAYS
FREQUENCY OF PERIODS _____ DAYS
NUMBER OF PREGNANCIES _____
NUMBER OF MISCARRIAGES/ABORTIONS _____
DATE OF LAST PAP SMEAR _____ RESULTS_____
DATE OF LAST MAMMOGRAM _____ RESULTS_____

GENITOURINARY:	YES	NO
LOSS OF URINE	☐	☐
FREQUENT URINATION (DAY OR NIGHT)	☐	☐
BURNING OR PAINFUL URINATION	☐	☐
BLOOD IN URINE	☐	☐
KIDNEY TROUBLE (STONES, ETC.)	☐	☐

LOCOMOTOR-MUSCULOSKELETAL:	YES	NO
VARICOSE VEINS	☐	☐
ANY DIFFICULTY IN WALKING	☐	☐
ANY PAIN IN CALVES OR BUTTOCKS ON WALKING, RELIEVED BY REST	☐	☐

NEUROLOGIC:	YES	NO
HAVE YOU HAD FAINTING SPELLS	☐	☐
CONVULSIONS	☐	☐
PARALYSIS	☐	☐

HEMATOLOGIC:	YES	NO
ARE YOU SLOW TO HEAL AFTER CUTS	☐	☐
BLOOD DISEASE	☐	☐
ANEMIA	☐	☐
PHLEBITIS	☐	☐
EXCESSIVE BLEEDING OR ABNORMAL BRUISING	☐	☐

ENDOCRINE:	YES	NO
THYROID DISEASE	☐	☐
HORMONE THERAPY	☐	☐
ANY CHANGE IN HAT OR GLOVE SIZE	☐	☐
ANY CHANGE IN HAIR GROWTH	☐	☐
HAVE YOU BECOME COLDER THAN BEFORE, OR HAS SKIN BECOME DRIER	☐	☐

PSYCHIATRY:	YES	NO
HAVE YOU EVER BEEN ADVISED TO SEEK OR HAVE YOU SOUGHT TREATMENT FOR:		
DEPRESSION	☐	☐
ANXIETY AND/OR PANIC	☐	☐
SEVERE STRESS	☐	☐
ALCOHOL AND/OR DRUG ABUSE	☐	☐

PLEASE LIST ALL KNOWN ALLERGIES (DRUGS, FOOD, ANIMALS, ETC.):

_____   _____
_____   _____
_____   _____

HEALTH RISKS:
I HAVE RECEIVED A HANDOUT COVERING THE FOLLOWING SUBJECTS:
☐ SUBSTANCE USAGE   ☐ PHYSICAL ACTIVITY HABITS   ☐ SAFE SEX PRACTICES
☐ HEALTHY DIETARY HABITS   ☐ STRESS CONTROL   ☐ PERSONAL SAFETY
☐ SELF EXAMINATION (BREAST/TESTICLES)
I UNDERSTAND I CAN ADDRESS ANY CONCERN/QUESTIONS CONCERNING THE ABOVE INFORMATION WITH MY MEDICAL PROVIDER.

SIGNATURE OF PERSON ACQUIRING THIS INFORMATION:_____

SIGNATURE OF PATIENT: _____ DATE _____

QUESTIONNAIRE REVIEWED BY: _____ DATE _____
(MEDICAL PROVIDER)

when the examination is complete. This helps patients/clients understand their role in their care. Following are some examples of patient/client education topics:

- Self-care
- Medication
- Awareness of special condition

Procedure

General Physical Examination

ALERT: Follow Standard Precautions.

1. Wash hands.
2. Take patient/client to scale; measure weight and height; document.
3. Take patient/client to examination room. If patient is new, review patient questionnaire and clarify unclear information. (Some providers prefer that the MA complete the patient questionnaire.) See example of patient questionnaire in Figure 23–10.
4. Interview patient and document the following:
   a. Date and time
   b. Principal complaint or purpose of visit. Document verbatim the patient's description of the injury.

Note: If injury occurred at work or may be work related, special authorization is required prior to treatment.

   c. Age
   d. Any known allergies
   e. Current medications
   f. Medications recently stopped
   g. Date of last rectal exam
   h. Female's date of last
      (1) Normal menstrual period
      (2) Mammogram
      (3) Pap smear
5. Measure body temperature and blood pressure; document.
6. Count pulse and respiratory rate; document.
7. Note any visible symptoms.
8. Instruct patient/client to have a seat while waiting for physician.
9. Notify or signal provider that patient is ready for conference.
10. Prepare patient for examination when provider indicates.

11. Instruct patient/client to
    a. Remove all clothes. (Offer to assist patients.)
    b. Put gown on with opening in back. (Some providers prefer opening in front when doing breast examination.)
    c. Have a seat while waiting for physician.
12. Check room and have the following equipment and supplies ready:
    a. Opthalmoscope
    b. Otoscope with ear shields
    c. Percussion hammer
    d. Disposable gloves
    e. Basin/pan
    f. Tape measure
    g. Tongue blade
    h. Lubricant
    i. Anal scope
    j. Vaginal speculum for women
13. After the examination:
    a. Give medication or treatment if ordered.
    b. Instruct patient to dress. (Offer to help patients.)
    c. Remove instruments and tray to cleaning area.
14. Wash hands.
15. When patient/client is dressed:
    a. Complete patient teaching as necessary.
    b. Direct client according to provider's order (for example, to laboratory for lab work, to radiology department for x-ray, to receptionist to make next appointment and payment arrangements).
16. Document treatments, procedures, and medication given.
17. Clean examination room for next patient/client.
18. Wash hands.

- Self-examination
- Breast exam
- Blood pressure
- Lifestyle changes that promote good health
- Dietary habits
- Balancing work, family, and private time
- Exercise
- Smoking cessation

A patient may complain of symptoms that require an examination other than his or her general physical examination visits. The following information guides you in preparing for the most common types of examinations.

Procedure

Limited Examination

ALERT: Follow Standard Precautions.

1. Wash hands.
2. Take patient/client to scale; weigh and document.
3. Take patient/client to examination room and instruct him or her to have a seat.
4. Interview the patient/client and document the following:
   a. Date and time
   b. Principal complaint
   c. Age
   d. Allergies
   e. Current medication
5. Measure body temperature; document.
6. Count pulse and respiration; document.
7. Measure blood pressure; document.

Eye, Ear, Nose, and Throat Examinations

Eye, ear, nose, and throat examinations are known as EENT examinations. This type of examination may be routine or may be done when a patient complains of the following:

- Decreased hearing
- Congested nose
- Sore throat
- Red and irritated eyes
- Runny nose
- Earache
- Head and facial pain

The physician examines the eyes, ears, nose, and throat and may also examine the chest if these symptoms occur.

The eye may need a light eye patch to prevent further damage from trauma. After surgery, instillation of a local anesthetic may be needed for therapeutic use. A pressure eye patch is used for corneal abrasions, to control postoperative edema and hemorrhage from trauma.

During an EENT examination, the provider may decide to culture drainage in the throat. The culture helps identify the specific bacteria causing an ear or throat infection. Use good technique when obtaining a specimen for culture. If a specimen is contaminated, the test results will be incorrect. Review "Obtaining a Specimen for Culture" in Chapter 18. See Table 23–4 for common EENT conditions, possible treatments, and patient teaching. The following procedures may be necessary to treat or diagnose various eye, ear, nose, and throat conditions.

Procedure

Eye Irrigation (Continuous)

ALERT: Follow Standard Precautions.

1. Wash hands.
2. Explain what you are going to do.
3. Assemble equipment.
   a. Sterile towel
   b. Sterile basin
   c. IV tubing
   d. IV pole
   e. 1,000 cc IV normal saline
   f. Cotton balls
   g. Litmus/pH paper for chemical burn
   h. Topical anesthetic
   i. Plastic trash bag
   j. Disposable gloves
4. Perform a visual acuity test unless severity of situation or physician's order contraindicates.
5. Wash hands thoroughly.
6. Place client in supine position.
7. Put on gloves.
8. Turn client's head to side affected to prevent solution flowing over nose and into other eye.
9. Place towel under patient's head and/or place basin beneath eye.
10. Use litmus paper to determine if irritant is acid or alkaline.
11. Spike 1,000 cc IV bag with IV tubing (chemical burn: use at least 1,000 cc of normal saline to dilute and wash out harsh chemical).
12. Close clamp.
13. Invert IV bag on IV pole.

Instill topical anesthetic to eye according to policy and/or physician orders.

14. Separate patient's eyelid with thumb and index finger on nondominant hand.
15. Open clamp on IV tubing and begin irrigation.
16. Hold tubing at 45° angle.
17. Ask patient to rotate eye clockwise.
18. Direct stream at inner canthus so that the normal saline solution flows across the cornea to the outer canthus.
19. Stop the flow of solution periodically and ask patient to close eye. (This will move secretions from upper to lower conjunctival sac.)
20. Dry eyelid with cotton balls.
21. Wipe from inner to outer canthus.
22. Use new cotton ball for each wipe.
23. Remove gloves.
24. Wash hands thoroughly.
25. Perform visual acuity test on physician's direction.
26. Document the following on client's chart:
    a. Date
    b. Time
    c. Duration of irrigation
    d. Type of solution
    e. Amount of solution
    f. Visual acuity test before and after irrigation
    g. Patient's tolerance of procedure
    h. All instructions given patient
    i. Signature and classification

TABLE 23–4   Common EENT Conditions, Possible Treatments, and Patient Education

Condition	Possible Treatments	Patient Education
Cataracts	Surgery	1. Encourage patient. 2. Provide patients and family with written information as to pre- and postoperative expectations.
Conjunctivitus	Medication Eye irrigation (wash) Warm compresses Allergy testing	1. Teach ways to prevent reinfection and cross infection. 2. Teach need for good lighting. 3. Teach to rest eyes periodically. 4. Teach application of medication.
Glaucoma	Medication Surgery Close observation	1. Instruct patient not to lift heavy objects. 2. Teach stress-reduction techniques. 3. Teach importance of taking prescribed medication.
Sty	Warm compress Incision and drainage Medication	1. Teach application of warm compress. 2. Instruct to reduce reading or straining of eye. 3. Instruct to keep out of direct sunlight. 4. Instruct not to rub eyes. 5. Teach ways to keep eye clean.
Otitis	Medication Heat Removal of fluid from behind the membrane Surgery (myringotomy)	1. Teach recognition of symptoms. 2. Teach use of vaporizers and decongestants.
Otosclerosis	Surgery (stapedectomy)	1. Encourage patient. 2. Provide written postoperative care instructions.
Deviated nasal septum	Surgery	1. Encourage patient. 2. Provide written postoperative care instructions.
Nasal polyps	Surgery	1. Encourage patient. 2. Provide written postoperative care instructions.
Laryngitis	Vaporized cool mist medication Reduction of irritants	1. Teach use of vaporizer. 2. Teach medication administration. 3. Teach need for environment free of smoke or irritants.

Procedure

Fluorescein Staining of the Eye

ALERT: Follow Standard Precautions.

1. Wash hands.
2. Assemble equipment and supplies.
   a. Normal saline solution
   b. Fluorescein strip
   c. Tissues
   d. Cobalt blue light
   e. Cotton balls
   f. Disposable gloves
3. Explain procedure to patient/client.
4. Place patient flat on examination table or in a semi-Fowler's position.
5. Tilt patient's head toward affected side.
6. Provide patient with tissue.
7. Put on gloves.
8. Remove fluorescein strip from sterile package.
9. Moisten tip of fluorescein strip with drop of sterile solution.

Procedure box continued

10. Hold strip in one hand. *Do not contaminate tip.*
11. Gently evert patient's lower eyelid with other hand.
12. Touch lower conjunctival sac gently with tip of fluorescein strip.
13. Instruct patient to blink eyes gently. This will spread dye over corneal and conjunctival surfaces.
14. Assist physician with examination.
    a. Hand cobalt blue light to physician.
    b. Irrigate eye after examination to prevent chemical conjunctivitis from fluorescein.
    c. Dry eye with cotton ball.
    d. Apply eye patch if ordered by physician.

15. Remove gloves.
16. Wash hands and document the following on client's chart:
    a. Date
    b. Time
    c. Vital signs
    d. Affected eye
    e. Irrigation solution used
    f. Amount of irrigation
    g. All instructions given patient
    h. Patient's condition on discharge
    i. Medications given
    j. Signature and classification

*P*rocedure

Light Eye Patch Application

ALERT: Follow Standard Precautions.
1. Wash hands.
2. Assemble supplies.
    a. Gauze, 4 × 4
    b. Tape
    c. Plastic or metal eye shield
    d. Gauze eye patch
    e. Disposable gloves
3. Explain what you are going to do.
4. Place client flat or in semi-Fowler's position on exam table.
5. Wash hands thoroughly.
6. Put on gloves.
7. Instruct patient to close eye.
8. Gently apply gauze eye patch over patient's closed eye.
9. Secure gauze patch with two pieces of tape.

10. Apply a metal or plastic shield over eye patch per physician order.
11. Remove gloves, wash hands.
12. Instruct patient that monocular (one eye) vision alters
    a. Depth perception
    b. Field of vision
13. Tell patient:
    a. Not to drive
    b. Not to operate machinery
14. Document the following on patient's chart:
    a. Date
    b. Time
    c. Type of patch applied
    d. All instructions given patient
    e. Patient's condition on discharge
    f. Signature and classification

Procedure

Pressure Eye Patch Application

ALERT: Follow Standard Precautions.

1. Wash hands.
2. Assemble supplies.
   a. Gauze, 4 × 4
   b. Tape
   c. Plastic or metal eye shield
   d. Gauze eye patch
   e. Disposable gloves
3. Explain to client what you are going to do.
4. Place patient flat or in semi-Fowler's position on examination table.
5. Wash hands.
6. Put on gloves.
7. Instruct patient to close eye.
8. Gently apply two or three gauze eye patches over patient's closed eye.
9. Secure gauze patch with two pieces of tape.
10. Apply a head dressing to secure patch for burn patients or patients allergic to tape.
11. Ask patient to try to open his or her eye after patch application.
12. Reapply patch if patient *is* able to open affected eye.
13. Apply a metal or plastic shield over eye patch per physician order.
14. Remove gloves, wash hands.
15. Instruct patient that monocular vision alters
    a. Depth perception
    b. Field of vision
16. Tell patient:
    a. Not to drive
    b. Not to operate machinery
17. Document the following on patient's chart:
    a. Date
    b. Time
    c. Type of patch applied
    d. All instructions given patient
    e. Patient's condition on discharge
    f. Signature and classification

Procedure

Audiometric (Hearing) Examination

1. Wash hands.
2. Assemble and prepare equipment.
   a. Acoustically shielded booth
   b. Earphones and cushions (clean before using)
   c. Audiometric report form
   d. Otoscope
   e. Manual audiometer
3. Take client to examination room.
4. Check both ears with otoscope to ensure clearness of ear canals. (Eardrum should be visible.)
5. Seat patient in acoustically shielded booth so that he or she cannot see manipulation of dials of audiometer.
6. Begin test with better ear, if patient can hear better with one ear than the other.
7. Instruct client prior to putting on earphones:
   a. He or she will hear a series of tones of various sound levels.
   b. First one ear will be tested and then the other.
   c. He or she is to raise a finger each time he or she hears a tone.

Procedure box continued

    d. Client should keep his or her finger up for as long as he or she hears tone, *no matter how faint it is.*

    e. Instruct patient to lower finger *only* when he or she no longer hears sound.

    f. Instruct patient to push button on response terminal (in place of raising finger) if booth is used.

8. Place earphones over patient's ears. Make sure that each earphone is centered over ear canal and that cushions fit snugly.

9. Place blue earphone over left ear.

10. Place red earphone over right ear.

11. Do not allow patient to handle earphones.

12. Close door to audiometric test booth.

13. Present one or two tones of different frequencies at easily heard levels so that patient becomes familiar with procedure.

14. Set frequency dial at 500 Hz, hearing dial at 30 dB.

15. Decrease dB level by 10 until patient responds by lowering his or her finger or depressing response terminal. For example,

500 Hz	30 dB
	20 dB
	10 dB
	0 dB
	−10 dB
	−20 dB

16. When there is no response from patient, increase dB level by 5 until patient responds by raising his or her finger or depressing response terminal. For example,

500 Hz	0 dB
	5 dB
	10 dB
	15 dB
	20 dB
	25 dB
	30 dB
	35 dB
	40 dB

17. *Interrupt tone, present at same level to confirm that patient has heard sound.*

Follow preceding instructions for dB. Increase Hz value to

    1000
    2000
    3000
    4000
    6000
    8000

18. Do *not* set up rhythm in turning tone off and on. Patients may respond based on rhythm anticipation and not on "true" hearing levels.

19. Do *not* prolong test unnecessarily. If responses become inconsistent beyond reasonable expectation, terminate test and repeat at later date.

20. Document results on graph (blue ink for left ear and red ink for right ear), fill in all areas, sign and date side 2 of the audiometric form.

Procedure

Ear Irrigation

ALERT: Follow Standard Precautions.

1. Wash hands.
2. Assemble equipment and supplies.
   a. Irrigation syringe
   b. Basin
   c. Waterproof drape
   d. Towels (two)
   e. Container for solution
   f. Irrigating solution
   g. Cotton-tip applicators
   h. Otoscope
   i. Debrox (if ordered)
   j. Disposable gloves
3. Take allergy history. (If known or possible allergies to irrigation solution exist, notify physician.)
4. Check with patient/client for the following:
   a. History of eardrum perforation
   b. Complications from previous ear irrigations
5. Explain procedure to patient.
6. Position patient in one of two ways:
   a. Sitting with head tilted slightly forward and toward affected side
   b. Lying on examination table with head tilted toward affected side
7. Check auditory canal with otoscope.
8. Wash hands thoroughly.
9. Put on gloves.
10. Instill ear wax softener according to physician's order.
11. Prepare solution as specified by physician.
12. Place emesis basin close to patient's head, under ear.
13. Ask patient to hold basin.
14. Test irrigating solution. (Temperature of solution should be between 95° and 105° F.)
15. Gently pull outer ear to straighten ear canal.
16. Draw solution into syringe.
17. Insert tip of irrigating syringe at opening of auditory canal.
18. *Do not occlude (block) opening.*
19. Point tip of syringe upward and toward posterior end of ear canal.
20. Gently instill solution against canal wall.
21. Observe return flow for debris.
22. Observe patient for
    a. Pain
    b. Dizziness

Note: Discontinue procedure immediately if symptoms occur.

23. Continue irrigation until return flow is clear, or 500 cc of solution is used.
24. Inspect ear canal with otoscope for cleanliness.
25. Remove basin.
26. Dry ear and neck with towel.
27. Turn patient on affected side to facilitate drainage of residual debris.
28. Measure and record amount of solution returned.
29. Remove gloves, wash hands.
30. Document the following on client's chart:
    a. Date
    b. Time
    c. Which ear irrigated
    d. Volume of solution
    e. Temperature of solution
    f. Appearance of canal before and after irrigation
    g. Appearance of return flow
    h. Patient's tolerance of procedure
    i. Instructions given patient
    j. Condition on discharge
    k. Signature and classification

Respiratory Tract Examination

Respiratory tract examinations include the ears, nose, throat, and chest. Prepare the room with an otoscope, nasal speculum, tongue blade, penlight, and stethoscope. The upper respiratory system is usually examined when the patient experiences the following symptoms:

■ Fever
■ Chest pain
■ Cough
■ Discharge from nose or ears
■ Difficult breathing
■ Headache
■ Tiredness
■ Nasal congestion
■ Watery eyes

See Table 23–5 for common respiratory conditions, possible treatments, and patient teaching.

Cardiovascular Examinations

Cardiovascular examinations focus on the heart and blood vessels of the body. The provider checks the cardiovascular system during a routine physical. He or she also examines this system when a patient complains of the following:

TABLE 23–5 Common Respiratory Conditions, Possible Treatments, and Patient Education

Condition	Possible Treatments	Patient Education
Rhinitis	Medication to relieve symptoms	1. Instruct patient to gently blow nose. 2. Inform patient of complication of closing nostrils when blowing nose (sinus drainage is forced into eustacian tube). 3. Instruct patient to call physician if nasal drainage is yellow or greenish, or puslike (purulent).
Pharyngitis (sore throat)	Medication to relieve symptoms and to kill bacteria if present	1. Perform throat culture if bacteria is suspected cause.
Tonsilitis	Medication Possible surgery	1. Provide pre- and postoperative instruction. 2. Provide instructions for medications.
Laryngitis	Inhalation of steam or medicated cool mist Antibiotics Warm gargle	1. Explain need for steam and/or cool medicated mist. 2. Instruct patient to rest voice.
Bronchitis	Medication	1. Instruct patients who smoke to stop. 2. Explain that bronchi in lungs are irritated.
Pneumonia	Inhalation of steam or medicated cool mist Hospitalization may be necessary Bedrest Medication to relieve symptoms Antibiotics if bacterial pneumonia	1. Obtain sputum for culture and sensitivity. 2. Explain need for sputum specimen. 3. Instruct patient to cough into tissue.
Emphysema	Medication Postural drainage Breathing treatments	1. Stress importance of balanced diet and reduced dairy product intake. 2. Recommend exercise program. 3. Encourage patient to stop smoking.

- Headaches
- Nervousness
- Dizziness
- Chest pain or a squeezing feeling in the chest
- Pain in neck, jaw, and arms
- Fatigue (feeling very tired)
- Shortness of breath
- Enlarged (distended) neck veins
- Rapid heartbeat (palpitations)
- Cold extremities
- Numbness in the extremities
- Hot, reddened area on legs
- Varicose veins

The provider may order an electrocardiogram (EKG/ECG) to measure the heart's activity. Follow the procedure "EKG/ECG" in Chapter 17. The provider orders an echocardiogram if he or she suspects heart structure damage or disease. The echocardiogram allows the provider to see the inner structure and motion of the heart. The echocardiogram is usually performed in radiology.

The provider may also order tests of the patient's/client's blood. The following blood tests tell the most about the cardiac (heart) muscle:

- Lactic dehydrogenase (LDH)
- Creative phosphokinase (CPK)

When the EKG/ECG indicates changes and the LDH/CPK are abnormal, the provider assumes heart muscle damage is present. If you are certified and are required to draw blood, refer to Chapter 18 and follow the procedure "Drawing Blood with a Vacutainer" or "Using a Needle and Syringe to Draw Blood." Process the blood sample according to laboratory guidelines. Remember: Always follow Standard Precautions when drawing blood. See Table 23–6 for common cardiovascular conditions, possible treatments, and patient teaching.

Digestive System Examination

The digestive system examination focuses on the mouth, teeth, tongue, pharynx, esophagus, stomach, and the small and large intestine. The pancreas, liver, and gallbladder are the accessory organs that help digest food. When examining the digestive system, the provider also examines the accessory organs. The provider examines this system during a routine physical or when a patient/client complains of the following:

- Heartburn (burning sensation around and below the location of the heart)
- Abdominal pain
- Abdominal cramps
- Fever
- Vomiting
- Nausea
- Bloating
- Frequent loose stools (diarrhea)

TABLE 23–6   Common Cardiovascular Conditions, Possible Treatments, and Patient Education

Condition	Possible Treatments	Patient Education
Coronary artery disease (narrowing of arteries of the heart)	Medication Surgery Diet	1. Explain importance of low-salt, low-fat diet; weight control; prescribed exercise program. 2. Reduce stress factors. 3. Stress importance of taking prescribed medication. 4. Provide written information on condition.
Myocardial infarction (heart attack, MI)	Medication Rehabilitation	1. Encourage patient to follow prescribed diet, medication program, and exercise. 2. Provide written instructions and information about condition.
Congestive heart failure (CHF) (tissue of heart and lungs are edematous)	Medication Rest Diet Antiembolism stocking	1. Encourage patient to follow prescribed diet and medication program. 2. Provide written instructions and information about condition.
Hypertension (blood pressure above 140/90)	Medication Diet therapy Exercise program	1. Warn patient not to stop medication without seeing physician. 2. Stress importance of diet and exercise. 3. Explain why blood pressure increases with weight gain and poor dietary habits.
Varicose veins (veins that allow blood to pool and not return to the heart)	Ace bandages Warm soaks Surgery	1. Explain importance of changing position frequently (sitting, standing). 2. Explain application of elastic wrap or elastic stockings and their purpose. 3. Stress importance of elevating legs. 4. Stress importance of loose clothing so that circulation is not impaired.
Thrombophlebitis	Medication Surgery Warm compresses	1. Instruct in application of warm compresses. 2. Instruct in elevation of legs. 3. Teach to watch for danger signs.
Cerebral vascular accident (CVA/stroke)	Hospitalization Physical therapy Occupational therapy Speech therapy Medication	1. Encourage patient to reach highest potential. 2. Teach awareness of adaptive devices and assist in selection.

■ Constipation
■ Hernias
■ Blood in the stool
■ Pain or burning with bowel movement

To prepare a patient/client and room for the digestive system examination, follow the procedure "Limited Examination." The initial examination may indicate the need for further examinations and tests. The results of a hematocrit and hemoglobin test tell the provider if there is a significant blood loss. Refer to Chapter 18 and follow the procedures "Microhematocrit" and "Using a Hemoglobinometer."

Endoscopy procedures allow the provider to see the inside of the digestive system. The provider uses an endoscope for this examination. The inside of an endoscope is lined with special mirrors and a light. These scopes are fragile and require special care. There are several types of endoscopes. The following procedures are used to view different areas of the digestive system with endoscopes:

■ *Gastroscopy.* Views the pharynx, esophagus, stomach using an endoscope inserted through the mouth.
■ *Colonoscopy.* Views the inside of colon and intestines using an endoscope inserted through the rectum.
■ *Sigmoidoscopy.* Views the lower colon using a sigmoidoscope inserted through the rectum

The following are common x-ray procedures to help diagnose digestive system disorders:

■ *Upper gastrointestinal series (UGI).* Allows fluoroscope viewing of the esophagus, stomach, duodenum, and small intestine. The patient swallows barium, a **radiopaque** liquid. The barium shows the shape and size of the inside of each organ it moves through. If a growth or ulcer is present, the UGI allows the radiologist to see it.
■ *Lower gastrointestinal series (LGI)–barium enema (BE).* Views the entire large intestine. Barium is administered as an enema. The radiopaque barium shows tumors, **polyps,** ulcers, **diverticulitis,** changes in **mucosa,** and other changes.
■ *Sonograms.* XDisplays on a monitor the movement and shapes of organs inside the body. High-frequency sound waves from the ultrasound equipment reflect these movements and shapes. The radiologist can determine if growths are present or if normal movement or function is absent.

Each radiology procedure requires special patient preparation before the test. Instruct patients in writing and verbally to ensure that they understand. When directing patients, always follow the radiology department guidelines for each test. See Table 23–7 for digestive system conditions, possible treatments, and patient teaching.

radiopaque Shows as a white material when a fluoroscope x-ray is taken.

polyps Small tumor-like growths.

diverticulitis Inflammation of the small sacs in the wall of the colon.

mucosa Thin lining on the inside of the intestines.

Urinary System Examination

The urinary system examination focuses on the kidneys, ureters, urinary bladder, and urethra. In the male the prostate, as deferens, testes, scrotum, and penis are also examined. This system is examined once a year during a general physical and when a patient complains of the following:

■ Frequent urination with a feeling of urgency, burning sensation, small amounts of urine
■ Pain in kidney area
■ Blood in the urine
■ Swelling (edema) around eyes and in the feet

Most patients complaining of urinary system disorders require a urinalysis. To collect a routine urine specimen or a clean-catch specimen, follow the procedures in Chapter 18. Remember to use Standard Precautions when handling body fluids. The provider may require blood chemistries to see if waste products are being filtered out of the blood. If you are certified and are required to draw blood chemistries, follow the procedure "Drawing Blood with a Vacutainer" or "Using a Needle and Syringe to Draw Blood" in Chapter 18. Remember to observe Standard

TABLE 23–7   Common Digestive System Conditions, Possible Treatments, and Patient Education

Condition	Possible Treatments	Patient Education
Gastroesophageal reflux (burping gastric juices into esophagus)	Antacids Frequent small meals Surgery	1. Instruct patient to sit up during and after eating. 2. Teach to elevate head when sleeping.
Hiatal hernia	Medication Alteration of diet and eating patterns Surgery	1. Teach diet modifications. 2. Teach need for frequent small meals. 3. Teach weight control. 4. Teach to elevate head when sleeping.
Peptic ulcer	Medication Stress reduction Stopping smoking Alteration of diet	1. Teach diet modification. 2. Instruct patient to watch for bloody or tarry stools.
Appendicitis	Surgery	1. Provide pre- and postoperative instruction.
Colitis	Medication Diet therapy Psychotherapy to relieve anxiety Surgery	1. Encourage patient to follow diet. 2. Teach importance of reducing stress. 3. Provide pre- and postoperative instruction.
Abdominal hernia	Surgery	1. Instruct in signs of strangulated hernia. 2. Provide pre- and postoperative instruction. 3. Provide written material about condition.
Hemorrhoids	Diet therapy Surgery	1. Instruct in diet restrictions. 2. Provide written material about condition.

Precautions when handling blood. See Table 23–8 for urinary system conditions, possible treatments, and patient teaching.

Male Reproductive System Examination

The male reproductive system examination focuses on the penis, scrotum, urethra, prostate, epididymis, vas deferens, and testes. This system is examined once a year and when a male patient complains of the following:

TABLE 23–8   Common Urinary System Conditions, Possible Treatments, and Patient Education

Condition	Possible Treatments	Patient Education
Cystitis	Medication Increase in water intake	1. Instruct in importance of drinking enough water to dilute bacteria (unless physician restricts fluids). 2. Instruct women always to wipe themselves from front of perineum to back.
Pyelonephritis	Medication Increase of fluids	1. Encourage large intake of water.
Nephrolithiasis	Diet therapy Medication Increase in fluid intake Heat application Surgery	1. Instruct patient to strain all urine and inspect for stones. 2. Provide list of low-calcium foods. 3. Provide pre- and postoperative instruction.

TABLE 23–9　Male and Female Reproductive System Conditions, Possible Treatments, and Patient Education

Condition	Possible Treatments	Patient Education
Epididymitis	Bedrest Ice application Medication Increase in fluid intake	1. Provide instruction in ice application. 2. Provide written material explaining condition. 3. Encourage increased fluid intake.
Prostatitis	Medication Increase of fluids	1. Provide written material about the condition and surgical considerations.
Gonorrhea	Medication	1. Instruct patient to reveal condition to all sex partners and arrange for medical care. 2. Instruct patient to abstain from sexual activity. 3. Provide written material about condition that promotes responsible sexual habits.
Syphilis	Medication	1. Instruct patient to reveal condition to all sex partners and arrange for medical care. 2. Instruct patient to abstain from sexual activity. 3. Provide written material about condition that promotes responsible sexual habits.
Chlamydia	Medication	1. Instruct patient to reveal condition to all sex partners and arrange for medical care. 2. Instruct patient to abstain from sexual activity. 3. Provide written material about condition that promotes responsible sexual habits.
Genital warts	Medication Surgery	1. Provide written material about condition that promotes responsible sexual habits.
AIDS	Medication to relieve symptoms Incurable	1. Provide emotional support and information about local support groups. 2. Provide written material about condition that promotes responsible sexual habits. 3. Instruct in Standard Precautions to prevent infection of others.

- Frequent and urgent urination
- Pain or swelling in the scrotum
- Painful or difficult urination
- Discoloration of the scrotum
- Enlargement of the scrotum
- Urethral discharge
- Genital sores, rash, blistering, or warts

Prepare the patient for a limited examination. Provide gloves, lubricant, and a small light for the doctor. The provider may order a culture, routine urinalysis, or a clean-catch specimen. See Table 23–9 for reproductive system conditions, possible treatments, and patient teaching.

Female Reproductive System Examination

The female reproductive system examination focuses on the perineum, vagina, uterus, cervix, clitoris, ovaries, fallopian tubes, and breasts. The female reproductive system is examined once a year and when the patient complains of the following:

- Vaginal itching or discharge
- Swollen, painful breasts
- Lump or mass felt in breast
- Pelvic pain
- Abnormal uterine bleeding

  • Heavy bleeding • Scant menstrual flow • Spotting between periods

- Absence of regular menstrual flow
- Inability to become pregnant

cervix Neck (e.g., the cervix of the uterus is the neck of the uterus).

Women should have a pelvic (vaginal) examination and Papanicoulaou test (Pap test) yearly. General practitioners, internists, gynecologists, and obstetricians routinely perform pelvic exams and Pap tests to identify tissue abnormalities. A Pap smear can help identify unusual cells (for example, cancer cells) on the **cervix.**

The Pap smear requires gentle scraping of the cervix during the pelvic exam. Tissue scraped from the cervix is smeared on a slide. Later the slide is examined under a microscope. Tissue cells and fluids help detect early signs of cancer. Pap smear results are reported using the Bethesda System (see Table 23–10).

Equipment for a pelvic examination and Pap smear is shown in Figure 23–11. Prepare the patient and room for a pelvic examination according to the procedure on page 615.

TABLE 23-10   Bethesda System/Cytology Reporting

Cytology Report	Patient Information and Instructions
A. Negative for malignancy, within normal limits (WNL)	1. Notify patient by telephone or letter. 2. Instruct patient to return for repeat Pap smear as the physician directs.
B. Squamous cell changes associated with inflammation; atypical squamous cells of undetermined significance; atypical squamous cells associated with human papillomavirus (HPV) infection; low-grade squamous intraepithelial lesion	1. Notify patient by telephone or letter. 2. Treatment is individualized, depending on history, and may include the following: a. Medication b. Repeat Pap smear in 1–3 months 3. Provide patient information.
C. Atypical squamous cells associated with human papillomavirus (HPV) infection; low- to high-grade squamous intraepithelial lesion; mild to moderate dysplasia/CIN-1 CIN-2	1. Notify patient by telephone. 2. If unable to reach patient after two calls, send a registered or certified letter. 3. Treatment is individualized, depending on history, and may include the following: a. Medication b. Repeat Pap smear c. Immediate colposcopy d. Referral to gynecologist 4. Educate patient to reduce anxiety and promote understanding; stress importance of follow-up.
D. Lesions associated with human papillomavirus (HPV) infection; high-grade squamous intraepithelial lesion; severe dysplasia/CIN-3; carcinoma-in-situ (CIS); malignant lesions	1. Notify patient by telephone. 2. If unable to reach by telephone after one call, send a registered or certified letter. 3. Treatment on order of physician: a. Immediate colposcopy b. Referral to gynecologist if not already seen

Cotton applicators   Wooden tongue blade   Microscope slides   Pap smear fixative

Glove   Lubricant   Uterine dressing forceps   Vaginal speculum

FIGURE 23–11. Equipment for a pelvic examination and Pap smear.

Procedure

Pelvic Examination and Papanicolaou (Pap) Test

1. Wash hands.
2. Take patient/client to scale; weigh and document.
3. Take patient to examination room.
4. Interview patient/client and document the following:
   a. Date
   b. Time
   c. Principal complaint/reason for visit
   d. Age
   e. Allergies
   f. Current medication
   g. Last normal menstrual period
   h. Date of last Pap smear
5. Instruct patient to
   a. Void (empty bladder).
   b. Disrobe from waist down.
   c. Put drape over knees.
6. Assemble equipment and supplies.
   a. Exam gloves

   b. Physician's gown
   c. Eye protection
   d. Vaginal speculum
   e. Light source
   f. Lubricant
   g. Cotton-tip applicators
   h. Cervical scraper
   i. Glass slides
   j. Fixative solution
   k. Slide container
   l. Lab requisition

ALERT: Follow Standard Precautions.

7. Explain procedure to patient to promote cooperation and lessen anxiety.
8. Assist patient into dorsal recumbent position with buttocks extended slightly beyond end of table, feet in stirrups (see the procedure "Dorsal Lithotomy Position").
9. Tell provider when patient is ready.
10. Put on exam gloves.

Procedure box continued

11. Hold slides for proper placement of specimens. Prepare slides when exam is completed:
    a. Spray with fixative.
    b. Write patient's/client's name on frosted end of slide.
12. Remove gloves, wash hands.
13. Complete lab requisition with all necessary information.
14. Assist patient/client to sitting position after examination.

15. Instruct patient/client that she will be notified about test results.
16. Send slide and requisition to lab.
17. Document the following:
    a. Pap test, sent to lab
    b. Patient notified that test results will be sent to her
18. Clean room for next patient.

Breast Exam

When the provider is going to perform a breast exam, it is necessary to instruct the patient/client to remove all clothes above the waist and place the examination gown on with the opening in the front. Take a minute to instruct the patient/client in the simple breast self-examination. Reinforce the fact that just a few minutes each month can save her life. Tell the patient/client to follow the steps in Figure 23–12 once a month about a week after the menstrual cycle ends. Patients/clients who have experienced menopause should perform the check the first day of each month.

See Table 23–11 for female reproductive system conditions, possible treatments, and patient teaching. Figure 23–13 provides guidelines for early detection of cancer in women without symptoms.

TABLE 23–11   Conditions of the Female Reproductive System, Possible Treatments, and Patient Education

Condition	Possible Treatments	Patient Education
Vaginitis	Medication Vaginal irrigation	1. Instruct patient in use of vaginal creams, suppositories, or irrigation. 2. Encourage patient to wear cotton underwear.
Pelvic inflammatory disease (PID)	Medication Heat application Vaginal irrigation Surgery	1. Instruct about general hygiene. 2. Provide written material and explanation of condition, and promote responsible sexual habits.
Mastitis	Medication Hot and cold applications	1. Provide information on diet modification (e.g., decrease caffeine and chocolate intake). 2. Instruct patient in use of hot and cold compresses.
Endometriosis	Medication Surgery	1. Instruct patient in use of medication. 2. Provide written information about condition. 3. Provide pre- and postoperative instruction.
Premenstrual syndrome (PMS)	Medication	1. Instruct in diet modification (salt restriction; avoidance of alcohol and caffeine). 2. Instruct to reduce stress.
Breast cancer	Medication Surgery Radiation Radiation Implants	1. Provide written information on condition. 2. Provide pre- and postoperative instruction. 3. Inform about local support groups.

■ BREAST SELF-EXAMINATION: A NEW APPROACH

All women over 20 should practice monthly breast self-examination (BSE). Regular and complete BSE can help you find changes in your breasts that occur between clinical breast examinations (by a health professional) and mammograms.

Women should examine their breasts when they are least tender, usually seven days after the start of the menstrual period. Women who have entered menopause, are pregnant or breast-feeding, or who have silicone implants should continue to examine their breasts once a month. Breast-feeding mothers should examine their breasts when all milk has been expressed.

If a woman discovers a lump or detects any changes, she should seek medical attention. Nine out of ten women will not develop breast cancer, and most breast changes are not cancerous.

Remember the seven P's for a complete BSE:

1. Positions
2. Perimeter
3. Palpation
4. Pressure
5. Pattern
6. Practice with Feedback
7. Plan of Action

1. Positions

Visual Inspection: Standing

In each position, look for changes in contour and shape of the breasts, color and texture of the skin and nipple, and evidence of discharge from the nipples.

Palpation: Side-Lying and Flat

Use your left hand to palpate the right breast, while holding your right arm at a right angle to the rib cage, with the elbow bent. Repeat the procedure on the other side. The side-lying position allows a woman, especially one with

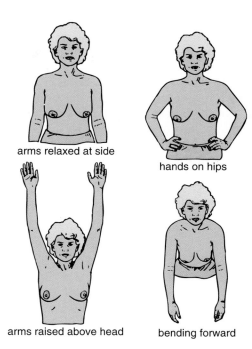

arms relaxed at side / hands on hips / arms raised above head / bending forward

large breasts, to most effectively examine the outer half of the breast. A woman with small breasts may need only the flat position.

Side-Lying Position

Lie on the opposite side of the breast to be examined. Rotate the shoulder (on the same side as the breast to be examined) back to the flat surface.

Flat Position

Lie flat on your back with a pillow or folded towel under the shoulder of the breast to be examined.

FIGURE 23–12. How to examine your breast. (Courtesy of the American Cancer Society, California Division, Inc.)

2. Perimeter

The examination area is bounded by a line which extends down from the middle of the armpit to just beneath the breast, continues across along the underside of the breast to the middle of the breast bone, then moves up to and along the collarbone and back to the middle of the armpit. Most breast cancers occur in the outer area of the breast (shaded area below).

3. Palpation with Pads of the Fingers

Use the pads of three or four fingers to examine every inch of your breast tissue. Move your fingers in circles about the size of a dime.

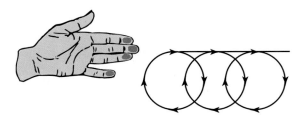

Do not lift your fingers from your breast between palpations. You can use powder or lotion to help your fingers glide from one spot to the next.

4. Pressure

Use varying levels of pressure for each palpation, from light to deep, to examine the full thickness of your breast tissue. Using pressure will not injure the breast.

light
medium
deep

5. Pattern of Search

Use one of the following search patterns to examine all of your breast tissue. Palpate carefully beneath the nipple. Any incision should also be carefully examined from end to end. Women who have had any breast surgery should still examine the entire area and the incision.

Vertical Strip

Start in the armpit, proceed downward to the lower boundary. Move a finger's width toward the middle and continue palpating upward until you reach the collarbone. Repeat this until you have covered all breast tissue. Make at least six strips before the nipple and four strips after the nipple. You may need between 10 and 16 strips.

start in armpit

Wedge

Imagine your breast divided like the spokes of a wheel. Examine each separate segment, moving from the outside boundary toward the nipple. Slide fingers back to the boundary, move over a finger's width and repeat this procedure until you have covered all breast tissue. You may need between 10 and 16 segments.

American Cancer Society Guidelines for Breast Cancer Detection

Breast Self-Examination: Age 20 and over: Monthly
Clinical Breast Examination: Age 20–39: every 3 years — Age 40 and over: yearly

FIGURE 23–12. How to examine your breast *(continued)*.

Circle

Imagine your breast as the face of a clock. Start at 12 o'clock and palpate along the boundary of each circle until you return to your starting point. Then move down a finger's width and continue palpating in ever smaller circles until you reach the nipple. Depending on the size of your breast, you may need 8 to 10 circles.

Nipple Discharge

Squeeze your nipples to check for discharge. Many women have a normal discharge.

Axillary Examination

Examine the breast tissue that extends into your armpit while your arm is relaxed at your side.

6. Practice with Feedback

It is important that you perform BSE while your instructor watches to be sure you are doing it correctly. Practice your skills under supervision until you feel comfortable and confident.

7. Plan of Action

Every woman should have a personal breast health plan of action:

■ Discuss the American Cancer Society breast cancer detection guidelines with your health care professional.

■ Schedule your clinical breast examination and mammogram as appropriate.

■ Do monthly BSE. Ask your health professional for feedback on your BSE skills.

■ Report any changes to your health care professional.

American Cancer Society Guidelines for Breast Cancer Detection

Mammography: Age 40–49: every 1–2 years
                Age 50 and over: yearly

FIGURE 23–12. How to examine your breast *(continued)*.

FIGURE 23–13. Cancer-related checkups. (Courtesy of the American Cancer Society, California Division, Inc.)

GUIDELINES
For the early detection of cancer in people without symptoms
TALK WITH YOUR DOCTOR
Ask how these guidelines relate to you.

AGE 20–40	AGE 40 AND OVER

CANCER-RELATED CHECKUP EVERY 3 YEARS

Should include the procedures listed below plus health counseling (such as tips on quitting tobacco use) and examinations for cancers of the thyroid, testes, prostate, mouth, ovaries, skin, and lymph nodes.

Some people are at higher risk for certain cancers and may need to have tests more frequently.

BREAST
- Exam by doctor every 3 years
- Self-exam every month
- One baseline breast x-ray between ages 35 and 39.
    > Higher Risk for Breast Cancer: Personal or family history of breast cancer, never had children, first child after 30

UTERUS
- Pelvic exam every 3 years

Cervix
- All women who are or have been sexually active, or have reached 18 years, have an annual Pap test and pelvic examination. After three or more consecutive satisfactory normal annual examinations, the Pap test may be performed less frequently at the discretion of her physician.
    > Higher Risk for Cervical Cancer: Early age at first intercourse, multiple sex partners

---

Remember, these guidelines are not rules and only apply to people without symptoms. If you have any of the Seven Warning Signals, see your doctor or go to your clinic without delay.

CANCER-RELATED CHECKUP EVERY 3 YEARS

Should include the procedures listed below plus health counseling (such as tips on quitting tobacco use) and examinations for cancers of the thyroid, testes, prostate, mouth, ovaries, skin, and lymph nodes.

Some people are at higher risk for certain cancers and may need to have tests more frequently.

BREAST
- Exam by doctor every year
- Self-exam every month
- Breast x-ray every year after 50; between ages 40 and 49, one every 1–2 years as recommended.
    > Higher Risk for Breast Cancer: Personal or family history of breast cancer, never had children, first child after 30

UTERUS
- Pelvic exam every 3 years

Cervix
- All women who are or have been sexually active, or have reached 18 years, have an annual Pap test and pelvic examination. After three or more consecutive satisfactory normal annual examinations, the Pap test may be performed less frequently at the discretion of her physician.
    > Higher Risk for Cervical Cancer: Early age at first intercourse, multiple sex partners

Endometrium
- Endometrium tissue sample at menopause if at risk
    > Higher Risk for Endometrial Cancer: Infertility, obesity, failure of ovulation, abnormal uterine bleeding, estrogen therapy

COLON & RECTUM
- Digital rectal exam every year
- Stool slide test every year after 50
- Procto exam—*after two initial negative tests 1 year apart*—every 3 to 5 years after 50
    > Higher Risk for Colorectal Cancer: Personal or family history of colon or rectal cancer, personal or family history of polyps in the colon or rectum, ulcerative colitis

TABLE 23–12   Conditions Affecting Bones, Possible Treatments, and Patient Education

Condition	Possible Treatments	Patient Education
Arthritis	Medication Heat Rest, sometimes Therapy Surgery	1. Provide written information on activities of daily living, medication, exercise, diet, and treatments. 2. Promote a lifestyle that encourages patient's highest physical potential.
Fracture	Medication Bedrest Heat or cold applications	1. Teach cast care. 2. Teach safe movement while wearing a cast. 3. Teach signs of circulation changes. 4. Teach importance of good nutrition.
Scoliosis	Brace Exercise Surgery	1. Teach importance of routine exercise. 2. Encourage the wearing of brace if ordered.
Herniated vertebral disk	Bedrest Traction Therapy Medication Surgery	1. Instruct in use of traction. 2. Provide pre- and postmenstrual instructions.
Bursitis	Medication Removal of joint fluid Sling Heat Therapy	1. Instruct in application of sling. 2. Instruct in application of heat packs. 3. Provide written instructions on how to prevent bursitis.
Gout	Medication Rest Increased fluid for weight reduction in obese	1. Provide information on medication. 2. Provide instruction in proper diet and provide handout.

Orthopedic Examination

Orthopedic examinations may require examination of any bony area of the body. All bones of the body are covered with skin and other tissue. X-rays allow the provider to see bones. When injury to a bone occurs, the muscle, tendons, and soft tissue around the injury also require treatment. See Chapter 19 regarding physical therapy for various treatments. See Table 23–12 for conditions affecting bones, possible treatments, and patient education.

■ PEDIATRICS

Pediatrics pertains to providing care for children. A pediatrician is a medical doctor specializing in the care of children and infants. Family practice providers also provide medical services for children and infants as well as their parents. There are two types of pediatric appointments:

1. Well-child appointment
2. Sick-child appointment

The well child is checked routinely to evaluate growth and development patterns. Early identification of abnormal development allows quick, effective treatment. Children also receive immunizations at regular intervals. Immunizations prevent many life-threatening diseases.

Education of parents is important with each well check. Giving parents child development information can make your job easier. Parents who are informed about normal development and growth patterns are more relaxed and require less direction. Routine well-child appointments are usually scheduled at the following ages:

- 1 month
- 2 months
- 4 months
- 6 months
- 9 months
- 12 months
- 15 months
- 18 months
- 24 months, and yearly thereafter

The sick child shows signs of infection or disease. Often, sick children wait in a separate waiting room away from well children. This separation helps prevent the spread of infection and disease.

When possible, take the time to show children instruments and other items and to explain how they are used in their care. Children's knowledge and sense of safety make your job more interesting and rewarding.

Childproof your examination and waiting rooms so that they are safe. Never leave a small child alone on an examination table. When weighing infants or giving care, *always* keep one hand on the child to secure its position. When infants or children need treatment that requires them to be absolutely still, restraining procedures are needed. Proper restraint is important to protect the infant/child and ensure accuracy of the procedure.

The parent of a sick child is usually distressed. Take time to explain what you are doing and why you are doing it. Provide the parent with handouts about care and answer questions. Refer a question to the provider if it is out of your scope of training. Your active listening and patience will help calm the parent.

Review Chapter 9 to better understand normal development and birth defects. Review Figure 23–1 for an example of growth charts.

■ MINOR SURGICAL PROCEDURES

Surgeries that do not require a general anesthetic or complicated equipment are often considered minor. The following are common minor surgical procedures:

- Suturing lacerations—sewing cuts or separated tissue
- Incision and drainage (I & D) procedures—opening an abscess (infected area) or cyst (pocket of fluid) and allowing it to drain
- Removal of foreign bodies from subcutaneous tissue
- Removal of warts, moles, and skin tags
- Biopsy—taking small pieces of tissue for microscopic examination
- Cauterization—burning of small areas of tissue to remove tissue or stop bleeding

FIGURE 23-14.
Types of suture
material.

Guidelines to Follow When Preparing for Surgical Procedures in the Office

1. Reinforce all instructions given patient by physician/surgeon.
2. Explain all procedures simply, clearly, and calmly.
3. Obtain witnessed informed operative consent for all surgical procedures.
4. Patients having surgical procedures that require IV push, preoperative medication, and local anesthesia must have someone to drive them home following the procedure.
5. Assess the patient's stress level. Note symptoms, address them appropriately, and document them.
6. Assess vital signs every 15 minutes during surgery.
7. Follow Standard Precautions.
8. Complete surgical skin preparation following the physician's order.
9. Have emergency equipment available.
10. Maintain sterile technique during procedures.
11. Apply sterile dressings according to the physician's order.
12. Monitor patients for ½ hour following procedure or until stable for discharge.
13. Discharge all patients from surgery by wheelchair or according to facility policy.

Familiarize yourself with the most common surgical instruments. Give special attention to details. You are responsible for quick, easy identification of instruments when assisting a physician (see pictures of surgical instruments in your Student Workbook).

Suture material and needles are a part of most surgical trays. Familiarize yourself with needle types (see Figure 23–14) and various suture materials (cotton, silk, nylon, catgut, and wire are a few). The size or gauge of sutures is labeled in 0s. A suture label reading 0 contains a thick suture material; a package label that reads 00,000 (5-0) contains a thin suture material. Most suture materials are measured in 0s ranging from 0 to 0,000,000,000 (10-0). Suture packages indicate the type and size of suture needle in the package, if no needle is included, the picture of the needle is absent.

Prepare a patient and surgical room as follows:

Procedure

Surgical Setup

1. Wash hands.
2. Assemble equipment and supplies.
   a. Mayo stand or surgical table
   b. Sterile items:
      Fenestrated drape
      Nonfenestrated drape
      Medicine glass for anesthesia
      Sponges, 4 × 4
      5-cc syringe or control syringe
      Needles: 18 gauge–1 inch, 25 gauge–½ or 1½ inch (or size physician prefers)
      Cautery (physician preference—electric or battery)
      Suture material (physician preference)
      Instruments
      Gloves
      Gowns (physician preference)
      Specimen containers
   c. Mask
   d. Cap
   e. Goggles and/or face shield
   f. Lab requisitions
   g. Anesthetic (physician preference)
3. Take patient/client to surgical area.
4. Explain the procedure and check to see if informed consent is signed.
5. Reassure patient.
6. Instruct patient to remove clothing and put exam gown on.
7. Wash hands.
8. Open a sterile drape or towel and place on Mayo stand, or place largest package on a flat surface and open. The outer wrap will serve as a barrier between table and sterile items. This creates a sterile field to work on.

Note: Be sure Mayo stand is dry. A wet drape allows microorganisms to enter sterile field.

9. Position package so that first edge unfolded will be pulled away from you. (By opening away from you with first motion, you will not have to reach across area again.)
   a. Remove tape.
   b. Loosen corner tucked in at taped edge.
   c. Open by pulling away from you and placing open edges straight across from you (see Figure a).

d. Slowly pull corners at right and left of package, opening sides. This exposes inside of package (see Figure b).

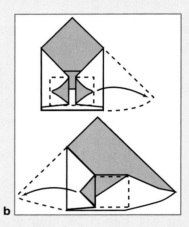

e. Carefully pull back on corner pointing toward you (see Figure c).

10. Open all supplies and equipment and drop onto sterile field.
11. Cover sterile field with a sterile drape.
12. Position patient at physician's request.
13. Assist as physician requests.
14. Document procedure.

Note: If you need to handle sterile items, follow next procedure for putting on sterile gloves and removing gloves.

Procedure

Putting on Sterile Gloves and Removing Gloves

1. Wash hands.
2. Pick up wrapped gloves.
3. Check to be certain that they are sterile.
   a. Package intact
   b. Seal of sterility
4. Place on clean, flat surface.
5. Open wrapper by handling only the outside. (Figures a and b).
6. Use your left hand to pick up the right-handed glove at folded cuff edge, touching only the inside of glove (Figure c).
7. Put glove on right hand (Figure d).
8. Use gloved right hand to pick up left-handed glove (Figures e–f).
   a. Place finger of gloved right hand under cuff of left-handed glove.
   b. Lift glove up and away from wrapper to pull onto left hand.
   c. Continue pulling left glove under wrist. (Be certain that gloved right thumb does not touch skin or clothing.)
9. Place fingers under cuff of right glove and pull cuff up over right wrist with gloved left hand.
10. Adjust fingers of gloves as necessary.

If either glove tears, remove and discard. Begin with new gloves!

11. Turn gloves inside out as you remove them; dispose of with hazardous materials.

b

c

a

Procedure box continued

d

e

f

Following surgery it is important to clean up and process equipment and used supplies. Always remember to follow Standard Precautions and dispose of hazardous materials according to facility procedures.

Procedure

Taking Down a Surgical Setup

1. Assemble supplies.
   a. Exam gloves
   b. Sharps container
   c. Double red bags in red container
   d. Double red bags
   e. Laundry hamper
   f. Basins
   g. Gown and mask
   h. Detergent
   i. Bacteriocidal
   j. Nonpermeable gloves
   k. Face shield/eye goggle and nose/mouth shield
   l. Non-permeable gown

   ALERT: Follow Standard Precautions.

2. Wash hands thoroughly.
3. Put on nonpermeable disposable gloves, gown, and face shield.

4. Check Mayo stand to ensure that specimen has been placed in properly labeled specimen container.
5. Place container on counter with lab requisition.
6. Using a Kelly clamp or long-handle forceps, remove all items from tray. Place
   a. Syringes and needles in sharps container
   b. Suture needles in sharps container
   c. Scalpel blade and handle in sharps container
   d. Cautery blade (if it is disposable) in sharps container
   e. Used sponges in biohazardous waste
   f. All instruments in basins with cleaning/disinfecting solutions
   g. All paper material (drapes, towels, etc.) in biohazardous waste
   h. Bloody linens (cloth towels and/or drapes), if used, in double red bag in laundry hamper

Procedure box continued

7. Remove and discard exam gloves in biohazardous waste.
8. Wash hands thoroughly.
9. Put on disposable gloves.
10. Spray surgical table and Mayo stand with germicide.
11. Discard disposable suction tip (if used) in biohazardous waste.
12. Empty suction bottle (if used) in hopper or toilet.
13. Thoroughly rinse suction tubing and bottle with clear water.
14. Soak suction bottle and tubing (if used) in cleaning agent for 10 minutes, then rinse with water.
15. Discard gloves in biohazardous waste.
16. Put on nonpermeable gloves.
17. Soak suction bottle and tubing (if used) in bacteriocidal for 10 minutes.
18. Rinse suction bottle and tubing (if used) with water.
19. Wash instruments according to facility procedure.
20. Remove gloves.
21. Wash hands thoroughly.
22. Take specimen to lab with completed requisition.

Note: Carefully follow facility policies and procedure when working with hazardous material.

*P*rocedure

Changing a Sterile Dressing

1. Wash hands.
2. Assemble supplies.
   a. Pair of nonsterile examination gloves
   b. Pair of sterile examination gloves
   c. Sterile dressing material
   d. Tape
   e. Biohazardous waste container

ALERT: Follow Standard Precautions.

3. Explain procedure to patient.
4. Position patient/client.
5. Put on nonsterile gloves.
6. Remove soiled dressing and examination gloves.
7. Discard in biohazardous waste container.
8. Wash hands.
9. Set up sterile tray.
   a. Place sterile drape on Mayo stand.
   b. Open and place all sterile dressing supplies on sterile field.
   c. Pour wound-cleaning solution or antiseptic into sterile container.

10. Put on sterile gloves.
11. Medicate wound as directed by physician.
12. Apply a double layer of gauze to wound or incision.

Note: If moderate to heavy drainage is expected, reinforce dressing. If drainage seeps through to outer layer, wound will be contaminated.

13. Remove gloves and place in biohazardous waste container.
14. Wash hands.
15. Secure dressing with tape.
16. Document the following:
   a. Date
   b. Time
   c. Type of dressing applied
   d. Appearance of wound
   e. Your name and classification

PUBLIC HEALTH REPORTING

Some conditions require filing an official report. These reports concern public health issues.

1. Communicable, reportable diseases are identified by the local health agency.
2. Animal bites and scratches are usually reportable to the local public health agency or animal control authority.
3. Real or suspected child abuse is reported to local authorities according to your facility's policy. Child abuse is defined as abuse to a person under the age of 18. The following are examples of abuse:

   a. A physical injury that is inflicted on a child by other than accidental means b. Sexual assault of a child c. Sexual **exploitation** of a child d. Willful cruelty or unjustifiable punishment of a child e. **Corporal** punishment or injury f. **Neglect** g. Abuse in out-of-home care

4. Real or suspected elder abuse or abuse of a dependent adult is reported to local authorities according to your facility's policy.
5. Disorders characterized by a lapse of consciousness are usually reported to the department of motor vehicles or a local health agency.

Reporting conditions such as those listed above protect others from disease or injury. Each state's requirements differ. Learn what reports your state or county requires to protect public health.

exploitation To use another person for profit or enjoyment.

corporal Bodily. For example, corporal punishment involves hitting or harming the body.

neglect To ignore or not provide for.

PHARMACOLOGY AND MEDICATION ADMINISTRATION

Working with medication and administering medication are serious responsibilities. As a medical assistant you are responsible for the following:

- Administering medication
- Being aware of side effects
- Interpreting prescriptions
- Reinforcing the provider's instructions
- Recognizing adverse effects of medications
- Reporting accurate observations
- Using references to obtain directions

Common Prescription Abbreviations

Special abbreviations and symbols are used when working with medication. To understand and communicate about medication use the following abbreviations:

cap(s)	capsule(s)
dil	dilute
dr	dram
D/W	dextrose in water
fl or fld	fluid
gal	gallon
gt or gtt	drop

IM	intramuscular
IU	international units
IV	intravenous
kg	kilogram
L	liter
liq	liquid
m or min	minum
mcg	microgram
mEq	milliequivalent
mg	milligram
ml	milliliter
NS	normal saline
OD	right eye
oint	ointment
OS	left eye
OU	both eyes
oz	ounce
pt	pint or patient
pulv	powder
sc or subc or subq	subcutaneous
tinc or tr or tinct	tincture

Legal Issues

There are federal guidelines regulating the manufacture, distribution, dispensing, and sale of medication. Federal regulations are monitored by the Drug Enforcement Agency (DEA) of the Department of Justice. Federal legislation controls the distribution of drugs. State regulations are monitored by the State Department of Health and Human Services.

The medical assistant assists the provider by

- Monitoring expiration dates of the physician's DEA registration.
- Keeping records and inventory that are legally acceptable.
- Controlling access to all drugs, controlled substances, and prescription pads.
- Destroying medication when expired. Disposal of controlled substances must be witnessed.

Drugs that can cause addiction and abuse are divided into five groups, called schedules. Each schedule names the drugs and explains their ability to become addicting and/or abused (see Table 23–13).

Prescriptions

Prescription drugs are medications that require monitoring by a licensed physician. The Federal Drug Administration determines which drugs must be prescribed by a physician. Prescriptions are instructions to a pharmacist to supply the patient with

TABLE 23-13	Schedule of Controlled Substances
Schedule I	Addiction and abuse are likely. Not accepted for medical use in the United States. Limited to approved research. *Examples:* heroin, LSD, and mescaline.
Schedule II	Drugs are easily addicting and abuse is likely. Accepted for medical use in the United States. *Examples:* amobarbital, amphetamines, cocaine, codeine, meperidine, methadone, methamphetamine, morphine, opium, and secobarbital.
Schedule III	Addiction and abuse are possible. Accepted for medical use in the United States. *Examples:* APC with codeine, butabarbital, methyprylon, nalorphine, and paregoric.
Schedule IV	Addiction and abuse are possible but less likely. Accepted for medical use in the United States. *Examples:* Chloral hydrate, diazepam, meprobamate, paraldehyde, and phenobarbital.
Schedule V	Addiction and abuse are limited or not likely. Accepted for medical use in the United States. *Example:* Low-strength codeine mixed with nonnarcotic drugs, including those listed in Schedule III.

medication in a specified amount. The prescription also provides directions for taking medication. The prescription is a legal document. There are six parts to complete in a prescription:

1. Patient information and superscription

• Date • Client's name • Client's address • Age, if child • Rx, meaning "recipe" or "take thou"

2. Inscription

• Name of medication • Amount of medication

3. Subscription

• Directions to pharmacist

4. Sig or signa

• Directions to patient

5. Physician's signature and address, registry number, and controlled substances approval number (BNDD)

6. Number of times, if any, the prescription can be refilled

Medication/drugs are described in three ways:

1. A brand name is assigned to a drug by the manufacturer. The brand name is commonly used in advertising a medication.

2. A generic name often describes the chemical makeup or classification of a drug. Generic names are adopted by the U.S. Adopted Name Council (USAN); Pharmacopia (USP), *a database catalogue;* or the United States National Formulary (NF), *the dictionary of drug names.*

3. The chemical name reflects the chemicals in the drug and its structure.

The cost of generic medication is usually less than that of brand-name medication. Patients save money if the doctor prescribes the generic form or tells the patient that a generic medication is acceptable.

Drug Reference Books

There are so many medications available that it is difficult to remember all the important information. To determine the best medication for a patient, doctors often refer to reference books. The following paragraphs briefly describe the most frequently used reference books.

The *United States Pharmacopia* (USP)–*National Formulary* (NF) is published every five years. The publication lists only official drugs, and it identifies drug standards. The NF chapter explains the ingredients of each drug. Drug information includes the following:

■ Description of drug
■ Standards for purity
■ Strength and composition
■ Storage
■ Use
■ Dosage

American Medical Association Drug Evaluations is a periodically revised book of officially established and recognized drug names and standards.

The *Physician's Desk Reference* (PDR) is not an official drug reference book but is the most commonly used. It is published annually; periodic (twice yearly) supplements provide information on newest medications. The PDR contains the following information:

■ Partial list of drug manufacturers, including their addresses
■ Emergency telephone number
■ Brand-name drugs (Section 2, pink pages)
■ Drugs listed by category or classification (Section 3, blue pages)
■ Drugs listed by generic and chemical names (Section 4, yellow pages)
■ Locations of poison control centers (following Section 4) (Section 5)
■ Pictures of drugs with their manufacturers
■ Each drug's composition, uses and action, administration, dosage, precautions, contraindications, and side effects, and its common, generic, and chemical names (Section 6, the largest section of white pages)
■ List of manufacturers of diagnostic drugs and the uses of those drugs (Section 7, green pages)

American Hospital Formulary Services (AHFS) provides periodic supplements that maintain current information. This publication gives unbiased drug information. Drugs are listed by generic names according to their therapeutic or pharmacological class.

It is important for MAs to understand how to use reference books. MAs are responsible for giving medication correctly. Drug reference books provide guidelines for responsible administration of prescribed medication. The *Physician's Desk Reference* is the most available reference.

Using the Physician's Desk Reference (PDR)

The PDR can be used in a variety of ways. To demonstrate this we will use the example of a patient who hands you an oval-shaped pill with Wallace 200 stamped on it. You can take that pill to the PDR and compare it with the pictures in Section 5. An exact comparison indicates that Wallace is the manufacturer and 200 is the dose. To become more familiar with the PDR, follow the steps in this procedure.

Procedure

Using the *Physician's Desk Reference* (PDR)

1. Identify the name of the manufacturer by going to Section 5, compare the tablet with pictures to identify the medication.
   a. Wallace is the manufacturer.
   b. Turn to the page where Wallace pills are displayed.
   c. Match the pill with pictures of pills displayed.
   d. A yellow oval pill marked "Wallace 200" matches "Soma Compound with Codeine 200 mg" in the display.
2. Turn to Section 2, the pink pages. Find "Soma Compound with Codeine 200 mg." Two page numbers are listed.
   a. The first page number refers to Section 5, the picture of the medication.
   b. The second page number refers to Section 6 and provides product information.
3. Turn to the page number indicated in Section 6 to find specific drug information.
   a. Description of drug

   b. Clinical pharmacology
   c. Indications and usage (describes the reasons for using the drug)
   d. Contraindications (reasons not to give this drug)
   e. Warnings
   f. Precautions
   g. Dosage and administration
   h. How supplied
   i. Storage recommendations
4. Go to Section 1 for more information about a drug. Find the manufacturer:
   a. Wallace Laboratories is listed with the W's in the alphabetical list.
   b. Write requests for information using the address supplied.
   c. Call for assistance using the professional services telephone number or night and weekend emergency number if available.

Storage and Handling of Drugs

Medication requires special handling. To ensure the safekeeping of medications, always:

■ Keep medications in a locked area away from other supplies.
■ Keep medications in original containers.
■ Refrigerate medications that require storage at lower than room temperatures.
■ Rotate medications so that the oldest are used before expiration dates.
■ Destroy expired medications. (Follow office policy when destroying medication.)
■ Keep medications requiring darkness out of the light (in a dark cupboard or container).
■ Be aware of medications that react with other materials (for example, some medications react with plastic so must be stored in glass).

To organize the storage of drugs, use a simple, logical system. One example of a system is alphabetic arrangement by classification—for example, all **antibiotics** together, **contraceptives** together, **diuretics** together. Within each classification, separate oral, **parenteral, topical,** and other medications. Federal law requires that you place all controlled substances (see Table 23–13) in a locked cabinet safely separated from other medications. Any controlled substances that are lost or stolen must be reported by the physician to the Drug Enforcement Agency.

Drug Dosage

Giving the right medication dosage is an important part of administering medication. Many medications are prepackaged and ready to give. Some medications require dosage calculation. A simple **formula** for calculating dosage is

$$\frac{\text{dosage you want}}{\text{dosage you have}} = \text{dosage you give}$$

Example: The physician orders 200 mg (milligrams) of a medication. You have 100-mg tablets of the medication.

$$\frac{\text{dosage you want}}{\text{dosage you have}} = \frac{200 \text{ mg}}{100\text{-mg tablets}} = \text{you give two tablets}$$

Divide 200 mg by 100 mg:

$$100\overline{)200} \atop \underline{200}$$

The patient needs to take two tablets to receive 200 mg of the ordered medicine.

The medication that the doctor orders must be measured in the same terms as the medication you have on hand. For example, if the physician orders a medication in milligrams and you have doses measured in grams, you must convert milligrams to grams. To convert measures, see Table 23–14 or use the following easy steps:

■ To convert grams to grains or grains to grams, you must learn that 1 g = 15 gr.
■ To convert grams to grains, multiply the number of grams × 15. *Example:* 30 g × 15 = 450 gr
■ To convert grains to grams, divide the number of grains by 15. *Example:* 450 gr ÷ 15 = 30 g
■ To convert grams to milligrams, move the decimal three places to the right. *Example:* 1 g = 1,000 mg (1 g = 1,000. mg)
■ To convert milligrams to grams, move the decimal three places to the left. *Example:* 1,000 mg = 1 g (1,000. mg = 1.000 g)

Review Chapter 7, Unit 2. This review will help you remember common medical weights and measures. Use the formula in Chapter 7 to review and practice changing or converting the following:

■ Ounces (oz) to cubic centimeters (cc) or milliliters
■ Milliliters (mL) to ounces (oz)

antibiotics Substances that slow growth of or destroy microorganisms.

contraceptives Items that serve to prevent pregnancy.

diuretics Drugs that increase urine output.

parenteral Not in the digestive system (e.g., injections are parenterally administered).

topical Surface of the body.

formula Accepted rule (e.g., a math formula and a baby formula are both guidelines or rules).

TABLE 23–14 Metric Dosage and Apothecary Equivalents

Liquid Measure		Weight	
Metric	Approximate Apothecary Equivalents	Metric	Approximate Apothecary Equivalents
1000 mL	1 quart = 1 L	30 g	1 ounce
750 mL	1½ pints	15 g	4 drams
500 mL	1 pint	10 g	2½ drams
250 mL	8 fluidounces	7.5 g	2 drams
200 mL	7 fluidounces	6 g	90 grains
100 mL	3½ fluidounces	5 g	75 grains
50 mL	1¾ fluidounces	3 g	45 grains
30 mL	1 fluidounce	2 g	30 grains (½ dram)
15 mL	4 fluidrams	1.5 g	22 grains
10 mL	2½ fluidrams	1 g	15 grains
8 mL	2 fluidrams	0.75 g	12 grains
5 mL	1¼ fluidrams	0.6 g	10 grains
4 mL	1 fluidram	0.5 g	7½ grains
3 mL	45 minims	0.4 g	6 grains
2 mL	30 minims	0.3 g	5 grains
1 mL	15 minims	0.25 g	4 grains
0.75 mL	12 minims	0.2 g	3 grains
0.6 mL	10 minims	0.15 g	2½ grains
0.5 mL	8 minims	0.12 g	2 grains
0.3 mL	5 minims	0.1 g	1½ grains
0.25 mL	4 minims	75 mg	1¼ grains
0.2 mL	3 minims	60 mg	1 grain
0.1 mL	1½ minims	50 mg	¾ grain
0.06 mL	1 minim	40 mg	⅔ grain
0.05 mL	¾ minim	30 mg	½ grain
0.03 mL	½ minim	25 mg	⅜ grain
		20 mg	⅓ grain
		15 mg	¼ grain
		12 mg	⅕ grain
		10 mg	⅙ grain
		8 mg	⅛ grain
		6 mg	1/10 grain
		5 mg	1/12 grain
		4 mg	1/15 grain
		3 mg	1/20 grain
		2 mg	1/30 grain
		1.5 mg	1/40 grain
		1.2 mg	1/50 grain
		1 mg	1/60 grain
		0.8 mg	1/80 grain
		0.6 mg	1/100 grain
		0.5 mg	1/120 grain
		0.4 mg	1/150 grain
		0.3 mg	1/200 grain
		0.25 mg	1/250 grain
		0.2 mg	1/300 grain
		0.15 mg	1/400 grain
		0.12 mg	1/500 grain
		0.1 mg	1/600 grain

TABLE 23-14   *(continued)*

Some measurements and equivalents* for pouring medicines (to be memorized):

4 mL (4–5 mL)	=	1 teaspoon	or	1 dram	or	60 drops (gtt)	
1 mL	=	¼ teaspoon	or	¼ dram	or	15–16 drops (gtt)	
2 mL	=	½ teaspoon	or	½ dram	or	30–32 drops (gtt)	
15 mL	=	3 teaspoons	or	4 drams	or	½ ounce (oz)	
30 mL	=	6 teaspoons	or	8 drams	or	1 ounce (oz)	
1 tablespoon	=	3 teaspoons	or	15 mL	or	½ ounce (oz)	
2 tablespoons	=	6 teaspoons	or	30 mL	or	1 ounce (oz)	
6 fluidounces	=	1 teacupful	or	150–180 mL			
8 fluidounces	=	1 glassful	or	240–250 mL			
2 pints	=	1 quart	or	1,000 mL			
4 quarts	=	1 gallon	or	4,000 mL			

*These equivalents are approximate only. In practice, the cubic centimeter and the milliliter are equal. Actually, the cubic centimeter is less than the milliliter by 0.000028 cc.

■ Pounds (lb) to kilograms (kg)
■ Kilograms (kg) to pounds (lb)

Administering Medications

To prevent mistakes and injury to the patient, always follow carefully the six "rights" of medication administration:

1. Right drug
2. Right dose
3. Right route of administration
4. Right time
5. Right patient
6. Right documentation

Guidelines for Preparing and Administering Medications

1. Wash hands.
2. Follow only written medication orders.
3. Do not allow yourself to be distracted while preparing medication.
4. Always read the medication label three times:
   a. When taking it from the shelf (do not use medication that is not clearly labeled) **b.** Before measuring the ordered amount **c.** When returning the container to the shelf or discarding it
5. Know the drug you are giving. Look it up in one of the reference books to confirm the expected action, dosage, and route of administration.
6. Calculate the ordered dosage if necessary. Verify calculations with a co-worker.
7. Measure medications.
   a. Measure solid medications such as pills, tablets, or capsules by dropping the medication from the package into a medicine cup. **b.** Observe liquid medications for
   • Color change • Cloudiness • Sedimentation
   Note: If these conditions exist, discard the medication.

c. Always have a second nurse verify order, dose, and measured medication in syringe when giving

- Insulin • Heparin

d. Gently shake emulsions and suspensions to mix ingredients completely. Shaking distributes all of the ingredients equally. This allows you to give accurate amounts of all ingredients. e. When pouring liquids, place the label of the bottle in the palm of your hand to keep liquid from dripping on label. f. Pour the liquid into a medicine cup; hold at eye level to achieve an accurate measure. g. Clean the neck of the medication bottle before capping. h. Never mix two or more medications unless ordered (check compatibility).

ALERT: Follow Standard Precautions.

8. Apply topical medications to the skin, mucous membrane (including vaginal creams and suppositories), or the cornea of the eye. Always follow the specific directions on the medication. Use aseptic technique to prevent contamination of medication.

9. Never leave medication unattended. Prepare medication and administer immediately. Watch the patient swallow oral medication.

10. Never administer medication prepared by another person.

11. Always verify the patient's name and the order on the chart to ensure that the right medication is given to the right patient.

12. Check patient allergies before administering medication. Look at allergies listed on patient's chart and ask patient if he or she is allergic to the medication.

Note: Medication can be given in a rectal suppository if the client/patient cannot take by mouth. Use the following procedure when a suppository is ordered.

Procedure

Administering a Rectal Suppository

1. Wash hands.
2. Assemble supplies.
   a. Gloves
   b. Suppository
   c. Lubricant

ALERT: Follow Standard Precautions.

3. Verify medication with physician's order.
4. Identify patient/client.
5. Confirm known medication allergies with patient.
6. Position patient in left Sim's position (see the procedure).
7. Put on examination gloves.
8. Remove suppository from wrapper.
9. Lubricate tip of suppository.
10. Separate buttocks with gloved hand.
11. Instruct patient to take a deep breath.
12. Insert suppository, tapered end first, into rectum.

13. Use forefinger to advance suppository along rectal wall toward the umbilicus for approximately 3 inches.
14. Hold patient's buttocks together for several seconds or until urge to defecate subsides.
15. Encourage patient to retain suppository for at least 20 minutes.
16. Clean excess lubricant from anus.
17. Remove gloves and discard in biohazardous waste.
18. Document the following:
    a. Time
    b. Date
    c. Route
    d. Medication
    e. Dose
    f. Expiration date
    g. Lot number
    h. Signature and classification

TABLE 23–15   Medication Administration Procedures

Administration Route	Type of Medication	Administration Procedure
Buccal	Tablets	Tablet placed between the gums and cheek of the mouth; absorbed as tablet dissolves
Inhalation	Medicated aerosols, mists, sprays, streams	Liquid medication inhaled through nebulizer, respirator, or inhalation device
Irrigation	Solution	Solution washed through a body cavity or over a membrane
Installation	Solution	Medication dropped into area requiring treatment, such as ear or eye
Injunction or topical	Liniments, lotions, ointments, powders, solutions, sprays, tinctures	Medication applied to skin (use gloves to apply)
Oral	Capsules, pills, solutions, spansules, tablets	Medication taken by mouth and swallowed
Parenteral	Sterile solution	Medicated solution injected into body tissue and absorbed
Rectal	Suppositories, solutions	Medicated solution or suppository inserted into rectum
Sublingual	Tablets	Tablet placed under the tongue to dissolve
Vaginal	Creams, foams, liquids, ointments, solutions, suppositories	Medication applied, inserted, or irrigated (douche)

13. Observe the patient for unusual reactions. It is good practice to keep the patient for 15 to 20 minutes after:
   a. A first-time dose of antibiotic **b.** A large dose of antibiotic **c.** An insulin injection **d.** Administration of allergy serums
14. Discard unused or refused medications. *Never return medication to original containers.*
15. Notify the physician immediately if medication is refused.
16. Record the following on the correct chart:
   a. Date **b.** Time **c.** Drug **d.** Amount given **e.** Route of administration **f.** Lot number of medication **g.** Manufacturer's name **h.** Expiration date

See Table 23–15 for a description of how medications are given.

Medication Administration by Injection

Injections, shots, and hypodermics are parenteral methods of giving medication. The word *hypodermic* means "under the skin." Hypodermic injections put medication under the skin. The medication and needle size determine the depth of the injection. Medications are given by injection to

■ Achieve a fast response
■ Ensure that the correct amount is administered
■ Provide medication when it cannot be given another way

FIGURE 23-15. A hypodermic needle.

- Provide anesthesia to a specific part of the body
- Place medication in a specific area, such as a joint

Do not give injections in body areas that are

- Burned
- Cyanotic (bluish color)
- Close to large blood vessels, bones, or nerves
- Swollen
- Bruised, injured, or scarred
- Unusual in skin texture or color, or enlarged (for example, moles or warts)

Syringes

Syringes are measuring devices that allow you to force medication through a needle at the tip of the syringe. See Figure 23-15 to identify the parts of a syringe. Syringe sizes vary from very small to 60 mL. The most commonly used syringe is 3 cc/mL.

Tuberculin Syringe

Special syringes are used for administration of small doses. A tuberculin syringe measures up to 1 cc/mL (see Figure 23-16). Note the very fine calibrations on the syringe. These special syringes allow you to measure as small as 0.1 cc. Use this type of syringe for allergy testing and tuberculin skin testing.

Insulin Syringe

An insulin syringe measures insulin in unit measures (see Figure 23-17). Syringe size is determined by the patient's required dosage. The most commonly used are U50 or U100 syringes.

FIGURE 23-16.
Tuberculin syringe.

FIGURE 23-17.
Insulin syringes measure in units.

Needles

Needles that attach to syringes for injection come in different lengths and diameters of needle opening **(lumen).** Length of needles for medication administration ranges from ½ to 2 inches. You determine needle length according to where you want the medication in the tissue. For example:

lumen Opening (e.g., opening in a tube or needle).

■ An intradermal injection requires a short, ½- to ⅝-inch needle for medication that goes just under the skin.
■ An intramuscular injection requires a needle that is long enough to reach the muscle, usually 1½ to 2 inches.
■ A subcutaneous injection requires a ⅝- to 1-inch needle to reach subcutaneous tissue.

Needle diameter, also called needle gauge, describes the size of the opening in the needle. Needle gauges range between 14 and 27. As the number of the gauge increases, the diameter of the needle opening *(lumen)* decreases. For example, a 25-gauge needle has a small opening (lumen). A 16-gauge needle has a large opening (lumen).

Preventing Needle Sticks

Needle sticks injure the skin and introduce infectious agents into the body. Accidental needle sticks that occur after an injection is given can be serious. An accidental needle stick can transfer a disease from one person to another. Transfer of Hepatitis B and AIDS is of greatest concern. (See Tables 23–2 and 23–3 for Standard Precaution task categorization, page 591.) To prevent accidental needle sticks:

1. *Never* recap a needle after giving an injection.
2. *Never* lay a syringe down after giving an injection.
3. Immediately place the syringe in a puncture-resistant, leakproof container (a sharps container) (see Figure 23–18).
4. Empty sharps containers when they are three-fourths full.
5. Close lid tightly on a sharps container when moving it.

Preparing Parenteral Medication

Medication comes in many different types of containers. The following are the most common:

■ *Prefilled unit-dose disposable syringes or cartridges* (see Figure 23–19).
■ *Ampule.* Small glass container with a narrow neck, allowing for **aspiration** of medication.

aspiration Withdrawal of a fluid.

■ *Vial.* Closed glass container with rubber stopper. Vials are simple unit-dose or multidose containers. Some vials contain powdered medicine and require mixing

FIGURE 23–18.
Sharps containers.

AVOID INFECTION

THE FOLLOWING PROCEDURES ARE RECOMMENDED:

1. DON'T RECAP NEEDLES. AVOID needlesticks.

2. Immediately DISPOSE OF SYRINGE (with needle intact) into puncture-resistant, leak-proof container with one-way entry. Per: Calif. Administration Code Title 22 and Attachment A–2

3. DON'T OVERFILL. Look into see-through entry for syringe level.

4. CLOSE LID WHEN FULL. Snap top lid on securely, "Tupperware Fashion."

5. CARRY AT ARM'S LENGTH. USE SAFETY HANDLE. Avoid physical contact with contaminated containers.

reconstituting
Adding water to a powdered drug.

diluent Liquid added to powder that dissolves the powder.

(**reconstituting**) with a **diluent.** A thin metal flap covers the rubber stopper. Take precautions to prevent cutting your finger when lifting this metal flap.

Various Methods of Giving Injections

There are five common methods for giving injections. Each method allows the medication to be absorbed in a different way. The following paragraphs and procedures describe four of these methods. (Medical assistants are not legally approved to use the fifth method, intravenous injection.)

FIGURE 23–19.
Unit-dose cartridge.

Procedure

Opening an Ampule and Aspirating Medication

1. Wash hands.
2. Assemble supplies.
   a. Alcohol wipe
   b. Medication ampule
   c. Ampule file
   d. Gauze, 2 × 2
3. Check medication label against physician's order when taking ampule from shelf.
4. Tap stem of ampule lightly to empty medication into ampule.
5. Cleanse neck of ampule with alcohol wipe.
6. Place gauze at neck.
7. Hold ampule between fingers at top and bottom.

8. Snap the top off of ampule with quick movement so that glass fragments catch in gauze.
9. File across narrowest part of neck when difficult to break.
10. Discard top of ampule in sharps container.
11. Check medication label against physician's order.
12. Aspirate medication:
    a. Insert tip of needle into ampule below fluid level.
    b. Draw plunger back to pull appropriate amount of medication into syringe.

Procedure box continued

13. Remove needle from ampule, being careful not to touch edge of container.
14. Check medication label and dosage against physician's order and discard ampule in sharps container.

15. Turn syringe so that needle is pointing up, tap syringe to move air bubble to tip of syringe, then push air through needle if air bubbles are present.
16. Cover needle according to facility policy.

Procedure

Aspirating Medication or Diluent from a Vial

1. Wash hands.
2. Assemble supplies.
    a. Medication vial
    b. Syringe
    c. Alcohol wipe
3. Select the appropriate syringe and needle (attach needle to syringe if necessary).
4. Check medication label against physician's order when taking medication vial from shelf.
5. Remove metal flap from vial and clean top of rubber stopper with alcohol wipe.
6. Carefully remove cap from needle.
7. Draw the same amount of air into syringe as that of medication to be given. (*Example:* Physi-

cian's order calls for 1 cc of medication; draw 1 cc of air into syringe.)
8. Check medication label against physician's order before drawing up medication.
9. Puncture rubber stopper on vial top with needle.
10. Push air into medication vial to equalize pressure when medication is aspirated.
11. Aspirate (withdraw) medication into syringe.
12. Remove needle from vial and cover.
13. Check medication label and dosage against physician's order.
14. Return vial to shelf or discard in sharps container.

Procedure

Reconstituting Powder Drugs

1. Wash hands.
2. Assemble supplies.
    a. Syringe   c. Sterile diluent
    b. Alcohol wipes   d. Medication
3. Check medication label against physician's order when taking vial from shelf.
4. Read reconstitution/dilution instructions on medication vial.
5. Take sterile diluent fluid from shelf and check against medication label.
6. Aspirate diluent (see aspiration procedure).
7. Check medication label against physician's order.

8. Remove metal flap from vial.
9. Clean rubber stopper with alcohol.
10. Select syringe and needle.
11. Remove cap from needle.
12. Puncture rubber stopper of medication vial.
13. Push appropriate amount of diluent into medication vial.
14. Remove needle from vial and dispose of in sharps container.
15. Gently roll medication vial between hands to mix medication powder and diluent.

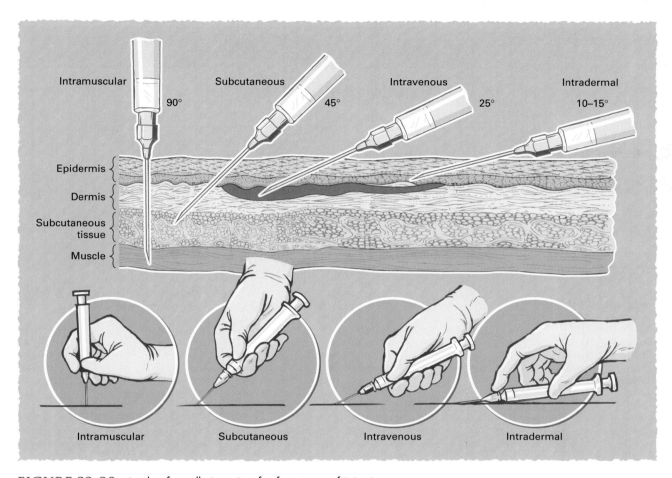

FIGURE 23–20. Angle of needle insertion for four types of injection.

Intradermal (ID) injections are given just under the surface of the skin (Figure 23–20).

■ *Purpose.*   To administer allergy tests and tuberculin skin test
■ *Amount.*   Usually between 0.1 and 0.3 mL
■ *Sites.*   Anterior forearm, distal to the anticubital space

Subcutaneous ("sub Q") injections are given in the subcutaneous tissue layer.

■ *Purpose.*   To achieve quick absorption of medication into the bloodstream
■ *Amount.*   No more than 2 mL
■ *Sites.*   Upper outer arm, abdomen, anterior thigh, or scapular portion of the back

Intramuscular (IM) injections are given in muscle tissue.

■ *Purpose.*   Maximum gradual absorption of medication into the bloodstream.
■ *Amount.*   2 to 5 mL. Doses of 4 to 5 mL should be divided in half and administered in two injections.
■ *Sites.*   Deltoid, dorsal gluteal, vastus lateralis of the thigh, or ventral gluteal.

*P*rocedure

Intradermal Injection

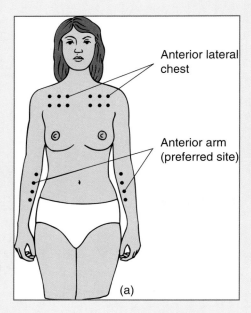

Anterior lateral chest

Anterior arm (preferred site)

(a)

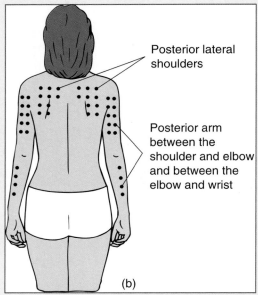

Posterior lateral shoulders

Posterior arm between the shoulder and elbow and between the elbow and wrist

(b)

1. Wash hands.
2. Assemble supplies and medication.
   a. Tuberculin syringe
   b. Needle, 25- or 26-gauge, ⅜- or ⅝-inch long
   c. Substance for injection
   d. Alcohol wipe
   e. Gloves
3. Verify medication label against physician's order. Put gloves on.
4. Cleanse vial stopper. Draw up medication in a tuberculin syringe.
5. Ask patient/client to identify himself or herself.
6. Confirm any known medication allergies. (If known or possible allergies to medication exist, do not administer medication. Report to physician.)

ALERT: Follow Standard Precautions.

7. Locate injection site: Measure two to three fingers' width distal (toward the wrist) to the antecubital space.

Note: If skin at preferred site is burned, irritated, scarred, or highly pigmented, use the following:
   a. ***Anterior lateral area of chest***
   b. ***Posterior lateral shoulder***
   c. ***Posterior lateral arm between shoulder and elbows or elbow and wrist***

8. Put on gloves.
9. Cleanse site with alcohol in a circular motion from center, moving outward.

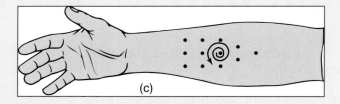

(c)

10. Allow skin to dry completely.
11. Holding patient's forearm in one hand, stretch skin taut.
12. Rotate syringe until bevel of needle is facing up.
13. Position syringe so that the needle is almost flat against patient's skin.
14. Insert needle through epidermis so that point of needle is still visible through skin.
15. Advance needle approximately ⅛ inch below skin's surface.
16. Inject medication slowly until a wheal (raised area) appears.
17. Remove needle and discard in sharps container.

Never massage the area.

18. Apply small bandage if necessary.

Procedure box continued

19. Remove gloves and dispose of according to facility policy.
20. Wash hands.
21. Document administration in patient's chart.
    a. Time
    b. Date
    c. Route
    d. Site
    e. Medication
    f. Dose
    g. Expiration date
    h. Lot number
    i. Signature and classification

Procedure

Subcutaneous Injection

1. Wash hands.
2. Assemble supplies and medication.
   a. Syringe
   b. Needle: 25 gauge, ⅝-inch long
   c. Alcohol wipe
   d. Medication
   e. Disposable gloves
3. Verify medication label against physician's order.
4. Put gloves on.
5. Cleanse top of medication vial.
6. Draw up medication into appropriate syringe.
7. Ask patient/client to identify himself or herself.
8. Confirm any known medication allergies. (If known or possible allergies to medication exist, do not administer medication. Report to physician.)

ALERT: Follow Standard Precautions.

9. Identify injection site. The preferred sub-Q site to inject insulin is the abdomen.

(a)   (b)

10. Cleanse injection site with an alcohol wipe starting at center of site and moving outward with circular motion.
11. Allow skin to dry.
12. Grasp skin firmly between thumb and forefinger to elevate subcutaneous tissue.

13. Smoothly and quickly thrust needle into tissue at 45° angle **except** when giving insulin or heparin; then insert needle at 90° angle.

14. After needle is inserted:
    a. Release grasp on skin.
    b. Pull back on plunger to check for blood. (If blood is aspirated, remove needle, discard needle and syringe, and repeat procedure.)
    c. Slowly inject medication into tissue if no blood is aspirated.
15. Remove needle from tissue quickly and smoothly.
16. Apply pressure over injection site and massage area unless contraindicated due to type of medication given.
17. Dispose of syringe in sharps container.
18. Remove gloves and dispose of according to facility policy.
19. Wash hands.
20. Document administration in patient's chart.
    a. Time
    b. Date
    c. Route
    d. Site
    e. Medication
    f. Dose
    g. Expiration date
    h. Lot number
    i. Signature and classification

Procedure

IM Injection (Adults)

1. Wash hands.
2. Assemble supplies and medication.
   a. Syringe
   b. Needle: 22 gauge, 1½-inch
   c. Alcohol wipes
   d. Medication
   e. Disposable gloves
3. Verify medication label against physician's order.
4. Put gloves on.
5. Cleanse stopper on vial.
6. Draw up medication into appropriate syringe.
7. Ask patient/client to identify himself or herself.
8. Confirm any known medication allergies. (If known or possible allergies to the medication exist, do not administer medication. Report to physician.)
9. Choose an appropriate site.

ALERT: Follow Standard Precautions.

10. Cleanse injection site with alcohol wipe starting at the center of site and moving outward with circular motion.
11. Allow skin to dry.
12. Give injection.
    a. Grasp skin firmly.
    b. Hold syringe firmly perpendicular to skin.
    c. Thrust needle into muscle with one quick, smooth motion.

   d. Hold syringe with one hand.
   e. Pull back on plunger with other hand, to aspirate. (If blood appears, remove needle, discard needle and syringe, and repeat procedure.)
   f. Inject the medication slowly, allowing time (10 seconds) for distension of space in muscle to accommodate fluid if no blood appears.
13. Withdraw needle smoothly and quickly.
14. Immediately apply direct pressure to site using alcohol wipe.
15. Massage site unless contraindicated.
16. Discard syringe in sharps container.
17. Remove gloves and dispose of according to facility policy.
18. Document administration in patient's chart.
    a. Date
    b. Time
    c. Route
    d. Site
    e. Medication
    f. Dose
    g. Expiration date
    h. Lot number
    i. Signature and classification

Procedure

IM Injection (Infants and Children)

1. Wash hands.
2. Assemble supplies and medication.
   a. Syringe
   b. Alcohol wipes
   c. Needle: 25 gauge, ½- to ⅝-inch
   d. Medication
   e. Disposable gloves

3. Follow steps 3–5 in the procedure "IM Injection (Adults)."

Note: It is recommended that 1 mL be the maximum volume administered in a single site to small children and infants. The muscles of small infants may not tolerate more than 0.5 mL.

6. Ask child's parent to identify child and confirm known allergies.

Procedure box continued

ALERT: Follow Standard Precautions.

7. Select injection site.

    a. Preferred site of IM injection for *infants and toddlers to the age of 3* is lateral thigh (vastus lateralis), using upper outer quadrant. Pinch lateral thigh to raise muscle during injection.

(a)

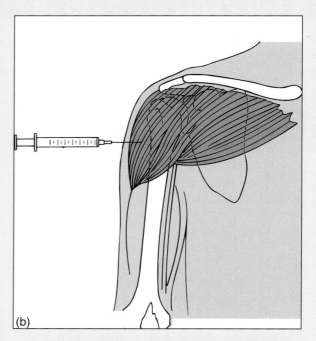

(b)

    b. Preferred sites of injection for children over age of 3 are same as for adults. *The dorso-gluteal area should not be used until the child has been walking for at least one year.*

8. Ask a second person (nurse or MA) to help restrain patient.

9. Follow steps 9–18 in "IM Injection (Adults)."

(c)

The Z-tract technique is another method of giving an intramuscular injection. Z-tract is recommended when

■ Medication is irritating to subcutaneous tissue.
■ Medication discolors or stains the tissue.
■ Complete absorption of medication in the muscle is important.

The following medications are given by the Z-tract method:

■ Immunoglobulin	■ Gamma globulin	■ Imferon
■ Antibiotics	■ Estrogen	■ Testosterone
■ Vistaril	■ Procaine	■ Narcotics

In the Z-tract technique, the medication is given in the upper outer quadrant of the gluteal muscle of the hips. Pull the tissue laterally away from the injection site. While holding the tissue, give the injection. Remove the needle. Then release the tissue. See the figure in the procedure "IM Z-Track Injections" for a clear view of how the medication is deposited in the muscle.

Procedure

IM Z-Track Injection

Follow steps 1–4 of the procedure "IM Injection (Adults)."

 5. Draw up medication in appropriate syringe and add 0.3 mL of air to syringe.

 6. Tap air bubble to end of syringe so that it is beside tip of plunger.

 7. Change needle used to draw up medication.

 8. Attach sterile 22-gauge 2-inch needle to syringe.

 9. Follow steps 6–8 in the procedure "IM Injection (Adults)."

ALERT: Follow Standard Precautions.

 10. Cleanse injection site with alcohol starting at center of site and working outward with circular motion.

 11. Allow skin to dry.

 12. Pull skin laterally away from injection site.

 13. Remove needle cap.

 14. Insert needle at 90° angle in one swift motion.

 15. Pull back on tip of plunger to aspirate. (If blood is aspirated, remove needle, discard needle and syringe, and repeat procedure.)

 16. Inject medication slowly, followed by 0.3 mL of air.

 17. Wait 10 seconds after completing injection before removing needle.

 18. Remove needle and allow retracted skin to move back into position. *Do not massage site of injection.*

Z track tissue displacement

 19. Document administration in patient's chart.

    a. Date

    b. Time

    c. Medication

    d. Lot number

    e. Expiration date

    f. Route-Z track

    g. Location

    h. Signature and classification

■ IMMUNITY AND IMMUNIZATIONS

Immunity is the body's resistance to disease and infection. The body develops immunity in the following ways.

toxins Poisons.

■ The body has a natural resistance to specific viruses, bacteria, or their **toxins.** Natural immunity is present at birth and lasts a lifetime.

■ The body produces antibodies. Antibodies attack foreign substances called antigens, or their toxins. *Example:* When the measles virus enters the body, the patient experiences measles. Antibodies are formed to attack and destroy the virus. If the measles virus enters the body again, the antibodies that destroyed the measles virus before quickly destroy the virus. The patient does not get the measles again. This is called a natural **acquired** immunity.

acquired Refers to a condition, disease, or characteristic that began after birth.

■ The body receives a **vaccine** of a dead or weakened organism. The body then produces antibodies that destroy the organism. This is called immunization by vaccination.

vaccine Dead or weakened organisms that stimulate the body to make antibodies.

■ The body receives an **antitoxin** that provides an immediate resistance to toxins formed from an invading organism.

antitoxin Substance that provides immunity to a toxin.

Immunization by Vaccination

Immunization by vaccination is commonly used to prevent the following illnesses:

■ Whooping cough
■ Diptheria
■ Measles: rubella (3 days, causes birth defects) and rubeola (7 to 14 days)
■ Tetanus
■ Smallpox
■ Hepatitis
■ Haemophilus influenzae
■ Polio

inoculation Instill, to put into the body.

ALERT If live virus is indicated on vial, always wear eye protection to prevent self-**inoculation** if a splash from syringe-and-needle separation should occur.

The ability to control these diseases has saved many lives. It is important for everyone to be immunized. As a medical assistant, encourage patients to be immunized and to have their children complete each immunization series (see Table 23–16). *Important:* Do not immunize ill patients or those who experienced a fever in the previous 24 hours. When giving flu or rubella vaccine, ask patients if they are sensitive to egg protein or feathers. If they are, do not give flu or rubella vaccine. Federal regulations require patients to read specific information and to sign an informed consent *before administration* of DTP, OPV, or MMR.

The following lists briefly describe the diseases for which immunization is routinely provided.

Pertussis or Whooping Cough

■ Highly contagious

listlessness A state of being without energy.

■ Most prevalent in infants and children under 4 years of age
■ Gradual in onset, with sneezing, cough, slight fever, and **listlessness**

TABLE 23-16 Recommended Schedule for Active Immunization of Normal Infants and Children

Vaccines	Ages to Administer	Protects Against	Comments
Diptheria and tetanus toxoids, pertussis (DTP)	2 months, 4 months, 6 months, 18 months, 5 years	Diptheria, tetanus, whooping cough	Can be given earlier than 2 months. Diptheria and tetanus toxoids should be repeated every 10 years.
Oral polio vaccine (OPV)	2 months, 4 months, 18 months, 4 to 6 years	Poliomyelitis	Allow 6 weeks to 2 months between doses; if risk is high for getting polio, an additional dose may be given at 6 months.
Haemophilus influenza b vaccine hibtiter	2 months, 4 months, 6 months, 15 months	Haemophilus influenza b	
Measles (rubeola), mumps, rubella (MMR)	12 months, 5 years	Measles (rubeola), mumps, German measles (rubella)	

■ Characterized after 10 to 14 days by a cough that sounds like a whoop (that is, a series of short, quick coughs)
■ Treated with antibiotics to help reduce other infections (secondary to pertussis)

Diptheria

■ Contagious
■ Serious because it produces a false membrane in the throat that makes it difficult to eat, drink, and breathe
■ Damaging to the heart and central nervous system
■ Often fatal if untreated

Tetanus

■ An infection of the central nervous system
■ Introduced into the body through any opening in the skin or through the umbilical cord of the newborn
■ **Characterized** by headaches, fever, and muscle spasms of the jaw (lockjaw) and throat; eventually all body muscles spasm
■ Often fatal

Poliomyelitis

■ Caused by one of three polio viruses
■ Introduced into the body through the mouth
■ Characterized by fever, **malaise,** headache, nausea, vomiting, slight abdominal pain (these symptoms may disappear and recur with pain and **paralysis**)
■ Uncommon today, but occurred in **epidemic** proportions before vaccine was discovered

characterized Distinguished by; refers to a trait or quality.

malaise Weakness or discomfort.

paralysis Loss of sensation and muscle function.

epidemic Disease that spreads rapidly among people.

Haemophilus Influenza B

■ The main cause of inflammatory diseases in young children
■ Very serious, causing diseases from **meningitis** to **septic arthritis**
■ Difficult to treat; causes death if treatment is not successful

Measles (Rubeola)

■ Contagious
■ Caused by virus that affects the skin and respiratory system
■ A serious **preventable** childhood infectious disease
■ Occasionally complicated by **pneumonia** and/or **encephalitis**
■ Preventable by a preparation of human antibodies called **gamma globulin,** which may be given to prevent or modify measles after exposure in individuals who have not received measles vaccine

Mumps

■ An infectious disease caused by a virus
■ Noticeable when the glands under the ear swell, followed a day or two later by fever, diarrhea, and malaise
■ Responsible for swelling and inflammation of the **testicles** or ovaries, in rare cases causing **sterility**
■ Occasionally complicated by meningitis

German Measles (Rubella)

■ Contagious
■ Caused by a virus
■ Characterized by slight fever and swollen glands under the ear, down the neck, and around the back of the neck
■ Known to cause damage to a baby developing in the uterus. (A pregnant woman should be notified immediately if she is exposed to a person with rubella, as she needs to see a physician as quickly as possible.)

meningitis Inflammation of the membrane covering the brain.

septic arthritis Bacterial inflammation of the joint caused by bloodborne bacteria carried from another place in the body.

preventable Able to be kept from happening.

pneumonia Inflammation of the lungs.

encephalitis Inflammation of the brain.

gamma globulin Substance that acts as an antibody to increase immunity.

testicles Site of production of the male sex cell.

sterility Absence of living organism or inability to produce offspring.

Thinking Critically: Check Your Understanding

1. **Communication** Write a paper explaining why it is important to report certain health issues. Your paper must include at least five reportable conditions and two different agencies to which these conditions are reported.

2. **Cultural Competency** Research different cultures and identify those that require the husband to be present when the wife is examined by a medical provider.

3. **Patient Education** Mrs. Jones is being scheduled for a mammogram. Write a paper that explains the procedure and describes how you can reassure her that it is not a difficult procedure.

4. **Computers** Describe ways computers are used in the clinical setting of a medical office.

5. **Medical Math** Describe the equivalencies of millimeters and inches, centimeters and ounces, and pounds and kilograms. Convert 36 inches into millimeters, 4 ounces into centimeters, and 120 pounds into kilograms. Determine the dose to give when 10 grains of a medication are ordered and you have 300-mg tablets available.

6. **Case Study** You are educating a new mother on the importance of immunizing her child. During your explanation she interrupts you and says she has a friend with a child who is mentally impaired. The friend blames early immunizations for her child's impairment. Explain how you will respond to the mother and what you will do.

Portfolio Connection

Once you attain competence as a clinical medical assistant, ask for permission to copy an example of patient charting that you have completed. (Remove all patient identifiers.) Place these copies in your portfolio as evidence of your skills. Place a copy of your on-site trainer's evaluation in your portfolio.

Write a paper describing your doubts and realizations and the barriers that you were able to overcome during your clinical medical assistant experience. For example, were you afraid that you couldn't learn to use the equipment? Describe the ways you plan to use the skills, information, and insights that you gained about the people you worked with and about this job. This assignment must be in standard report format.

24 DENTAL ASSISTANT

CO-AUTHORED BY VIVIAN MUENSTERMAN

*S*teps to success

1. Complete Vocabulary Worksheet 1 in the Student Workbook.
2. Read this chapter.
3. Complete Worksheets 2 through 10 as assigned.
4. Practice and demonstrate all procedures.
5. When you are confident that you can meet each objective for this chapter, ask your instructor for the chapter evaluation.
6. Complete "Your Link to Success" at the end of this chapter.

Objectives

When you have completed this chapter, you will be able to do the following:

✓ Complete all objectives in Part One of this book.
✓ Match vocabulary words with their correct meanings.
✓ Describe the responsibilities of a dental assistant.
✓ List eight recognized dental specialties.
✓ Differentiate between posterior and anterior teeth and their functions.
✓ Identify the following:
  • Deciduous and permanent teeth by name on a diagram
  • Surfaces of a tooth
  • Charting symbols and abbreviations
  • Dental office equipment by name
  • Specific OSHA infection control guidelines for the dental office

- Common dental instruments
- Basic dental tray setups

✓ Apply charting symbols and abbreviations to indicate conditions of teeth on a dental chart.

✓ Label the following:
  - Parts of the oral cavity on a diagram
  - Teeth on a diagram using the universal method
  - Anatomical structures of a tooth on a diagram

✓ Explain the following:
  - How to position a patient for a dental procedure
  - The importance of observing patients before, during, and after procedures

✓ Describe the following:
  - Admitting and seating a patient for a dental procedure
  - The dental assistant's position related to the patient and the dentist during a procedure
  - Oral evacuation, rinsing, and drying techniques
  - Steps for cleaning the treatment room following procedures and between patients

✓ Teach the following:
  - How to use disclosing tablets/solution
  - The Bass toothbrushing technique
  - Dental flossing techniques

✓ Demonstrate the following:
  - Basic instrument transfer techniques
  - Preparation and transfer of an anesthetic syringe
  - Procedure for completion of treatment and dismissing a patient
  - How to make a study model
  - Assisting techniques during basic restorative procedures

✓ Prepare impression materials.

✓ Mount a full-mouth and bite-wing x-ray series.

✓ Apply all procedural techniques with confidence.

■ RESPONSIBILITIES OF A DENTAL ASSISTANT

Dental assistants are valued members of the dental health care team. Their primary duty is chairside assisting during oral care procedures. Their basic duty is to maintain **visibility** in the mouth. They also provide instruments and materials as the dentist needs them to complete the dental treatment. Constant observance and consideration of the patient's/client's comfort level and health status are important in the role of a dental assistant. The responsibilities of a dental assistant include the following:

visibility Ability to see.

■ Working directly with the dentist in the treatment room

■ Preparing and cleaning dental treatment rooms following infection control guidelines

■ Preparing necessary equipment and instrumentation for dental procedures

■ Processing and mounting dental x-rays

■ Caring for and maintaining dental equipment

- Teaching patients oral hygiene methods
- Taking and pouring study models (may be an expanded role in your state)
- Possibly performing some front office duties
- Exposing x-rays (radiographs) (requires completion of a state-approved radiology course or examination)

■ DENTAL SPECIALTIES

ADA American Dental Association.

The dental profession has eight recognized specialties. A dental assistant requires specialized training to work in these areas. Specialized training may occur through on-the-job training in the dental office, through study courses given by the dental societies, or at a school certified by the **ADA.** Dental assistants need to know what the specialties are when their dentist refers patients to the specialist. The following are the eight specialties:

periapical Around the apex (e.g., of the tooth).

- *Endodontist.*   Diagnoses and treats diseases of the dental pulp and **periapical** tissues
- *Oral pathologist.*   Studies causes, processes, and effects of diseases of the mouth
- *Oral surgeon.*   Performs oral surgery
- *Orthodontist.*   Treats and prevents irregularities of the teeth and dental arches
- *Pedodontist.*   Cares for teeth and oral conditions of children
- *Periodontist.*   Treats and prevents disease of the bone and soft tissues surrounding the teeth
- *Prosthodontist.*   Replaces missing teeth or oral tissues by artificial means, such as crowns, bridges, dentures, and implants
- *Public health dentistry.*   Concerned with the dental health of the population

General dentists may have training in some specialized areas; however, they may choose to refer to a specialist when they feel it is better for the patient.

■ INTRODUCTION TO DENTISTRY

The oral cavity and the teeth are very important in the total health of the body. The mouth is related directly to eating, physical health, and a sense of well-being. A healthy mouth allows the digestive system to function properly. The mouth allows communication through speaking. When we think our teeth do not look nice, we may hide our mouth with our hand while talking. This makes it hard for others to understand what we are saying. The physical appearance of teeth plays a major role in personal relationships. If we feel unattractive, we may withdraw from social events. Unpleasant breath odor causes others to avoid getting close. Physical appearance of the mouth also effects mental attitudes about ourselves. Poor self-image causes us to lose our self-confidence. As a dental assistant, you are an important member of the dental team. The care that you give the patient helps keep them healthy physically and mentally.

accessory Helping.

masticate Chew.

primary First.

deciduous Falling out (e.g., primary teeth fall out to make room for permanent teeth).

■ ODONTOLOGY

Odontology is the study of teeth. Teeth are **accessory** organs that help **masticate** food. There are two sets of teeth. They are the **primary** or **deciduous** (baby) teeth and the permanent teeth. When a baby is born it has 44 tooth buds. The tooth buds begin to **erupt** when the baby is about 6 months old. Deciduous teeth are the 20 baby teeth (primary teeth). Each tooth has a specific function in processing food and acting as a guide for a permanent tooth.

When the child is between 5 and 12 years old, the deciduous teeth begin to fall out and the permanent teeth erupt through the gingiva/gums. Permanent teeth are the 32 adult teeth. The child who has some deciduous teeth and some permanent teeth has mixed **dentition.**

erupt Push through.

dentition Natural teeth in the dental arch.

■ INTRODUCTION TO THE TEETH AND ORAL CAVITY

Teeth are identified by name, number, and the function they perform in the digestion of food. The following information teaches you how to identify teeth, where the teeth are located, and the anatomy of a tooth.

Face and Oral Cavity

When dentists examine patients they look at the face first. Dentists ask themselves:

- ■ Is the bone structure normal and balanced?
- ■ Do the skin and lips (labia) look healthy?

Next, the dentist does an oral examination (see Figure 24–1). This examination tells the dentist things about the patient's health and habits (for example, whether

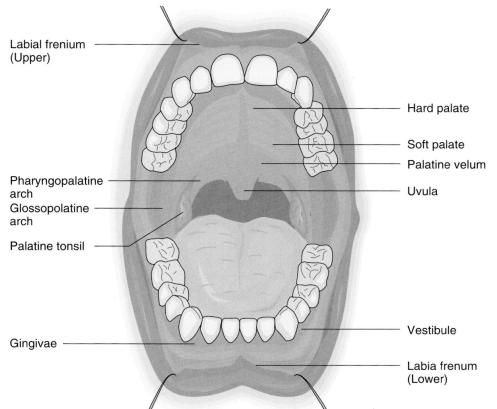

FIGURE 24–1.
Mouth and oral cavity.

Labial frenium (Upper)

Pharyngopalatine arch

Glossopolatine arch

Palatine tonsil

Gingivae

Hard palate

Soft palate

Palatine velum

Uvula

Vestibule

Labia frenum (Lower)

restorative To return to as close to normal conditions as possible.

he or she practices good oral care). Often, a nondental disease shows up in the oral cavity first and is identified during the examination. The complete oral examination is one of the most important procedures that a dentist performs. As a dental assistant, you help the dentist during this examination and during **restorative** care. To assist the dentist, you need to know the following:

■ Simple anatomy of the face and oral cavity
■ Tooth numbers, parts, surfaces, and structures

Maxillary and Mandibular Arches

Refer to Figure 24–2, an illustration of the skull.

■ *Maxilla.*   The arched bone in the face where the roots of the upper teeth fit into the sockets (alveolus)
■ *Mandible.*   The arched lower bone (jawbone), where the roots of the lower teeth fit into the alveolus
■ *Median line or midline.*   Divides the teeth into left and right sides

Placement and Function of Teeth

The following are the anterior teeth (see Figure 24–3):

■ *Incisors.*   Located in the very front of the mouth. Their thin cutting edge cuts food by biting pieces. They include the central and lateral incisors.
■ *Cuspids/canines.*   Located next to the lateral incisors. Their sharp points/cusps tear food that is too tough for the incisors to cut. Cuspids have the longest roots of all teeth.

The following are the posterior teeth (see Figure 24–3):

FIGURE 24–2.
Skull.

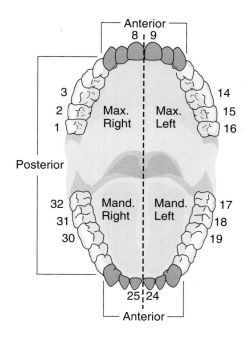

FIGURE 24-3.
Location of posterior and anterior teeth.

■ *Premolars.* Located next to the cuspids/canines. They are also called *bicuspids* because the have two **cusps** for tearing and grinding.

■ *Molars.* Located next to the bicuspids. These are the largest teeth in the mouth. They have broad grinding surfaces that grind down large chunks of food.

cusps Pointed or rounded raised areas on the surface of the tooth.

Identification of Teeth by Name and Location

There are 32 permanent teeth in the dentition (Figure 24–4). The following are the maxillary teeth:

> 2 central incisors in the center next to the midline.
> 2 lateral incisors next to the central incisors.
> 2 cuspids under the **ala** next to the lateral incisors.
> 2 first premolar/bicuspids next to the cuspids.
> 2 second premolar/bicuspids next to the first bicuspids.
> 2 first molars next to the second bicuspid.
> 2 second molars next to the first molar.
> 2 third molars or "wisdom teeth" in the back of the mouth. Not everyone has these molars. Some molars remain under the gingiva/gums line or in the alveolar bone and are often removed if the mouth does not have room for them.

ala Outer side of the nostril.

The mandibular teeth:

> 2 central incisors in the center next to the midline.
> 2 lateral incisors next to the central incisors.
> 2 cuspids under the corner of the nose next to the lateral incisors.
> 2 first premolar/bicuspids next to the cuspids.
> 2 second premolar/bicuspids next to the first bicuspids.
> 2 first molars next to the second bicuspid.

FIGURE 24–4.
Universal method of identifying permanent teeth.

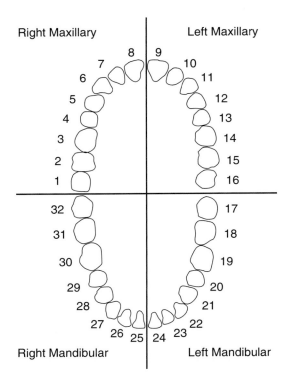

2 second molars next to the first molar.

2 third molars or "wisdom teeth" in the back of the mouth. Not everyone has these molars. Some molars remain under the gingiva/gums line and are often removed if the mouth does not have room for them.

There are 20 deciduous teeth in the dentition (Figure 24–5).

2 central incisors in the center next to midline
2 lateral incisors next to the central incisors

FIGURE 24–5.
Universal method of identifying deciduous teeth.

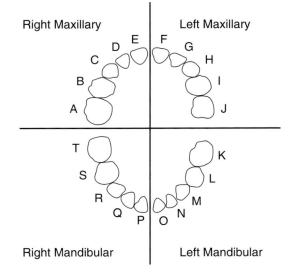

2 cuspids just under the ala wing of the nose
0 THERE ARE NO BICUSPIDS IN THE DECIDUOUS DENTITION
2 primary first molars
2 primary second molars

The mandibular arch:

2 central incisors in the center next to midline
2 lateral incisors next to the central incisors
2 cuspids just under the ala wing of the nose
0 THERE ARE NO BICUSPIDS IN THE DECIDUOUS DENTITION
2 primary first molars
2 primary second molars

Identification of Teeth by Letter and Number

One method of identifying teeth is the *universal method*. In this method, deciduous/primary teeth are identified by letter, and permanent teeth are identified by number.

When identifying deciduous teeth, begin lettering with the right second molar in the maxillary arch (see Figure 24–5). It is labeled A. Continue lettering from upper right to upper left, then lower left to lower right. The last molar on the right mandibular arch is labeled T.

When identifying permanent teeth, begin numbering with the right third molar in the maxillary arch (see Figure 24–4). It is numbered 1. Continue numbering from upper right to upper left, then lower left to lower right. The last third molar on the mandibular arch is numbered 32. A tooth that has not erupted or is missing is still counted.

■ ANATOMY OF THE TOOTH

The dental assistant works directly with the dentist. It is important to communicate with the dentist during **intraoral** procedures. You must know the anatomy of the tooth to communicate effectively with the dentist.

intraoral Within the oral cavity.

Sections of the Tooth

A tooth is divided into three main sections (see Figure 24–6):

■ *Crown.* Covered with enamel. The enamel is the white part of the tooth that we can see in our mouth.
■ *Cervix.* Neck of the tooth. It begins where the enamel stops and the **cementum** begins. Dentists call this the CEJ (cemento-enamel junction)
■ *Root.* Covered with cementum, lies below the gingiva/gums. It holds the tooth in the bony sockets of the jaw. A tooth may have more than one root, depending on where it is in the mouth.

cementum Hard, thin covering or shell covering root of tooth.

• Mandibular molars have two roots. • Maxillary molars have three roots.

FIGURE 24–6.
Sections of a tooth.

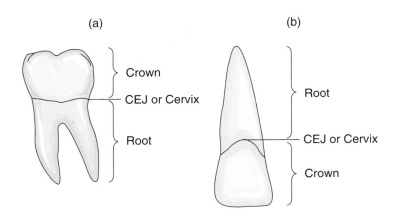

Parts of the Tooth

Each tooth has several parts (see Figure 24–7):

decay Breaking down; rot.

■ *Enamel.*   The hardest tissue in the body. It covers the crown section of the tooth. Enamel is a protective sheet made of calcium and phosphorus that protects the dentin of the tooth.

■ *Dentin.*   Harder than bone but softer than enamel. Dentin makes up the bulk of a tooth. It does not have nerves but it senses pain caused by **decay,** temperature, and chemical changes. Dentin may grow a second layer or wall of defense to try to keep decay from entering the pulp or nerve of the tooth.

■ *Cementum.*   The hard, thin covering or shell that covers the root.

■ *Periodontal ligaments/periodontal membranes.*   Small fibers that are anchored in the cementum and attached to the bone socket. They act as a shock absorber for the tooth and help the tooth withstand **functional stress.**

functional stress Stress to tooth caused by its normal function (e.g., force of pressure when biting something hard).

■ *Pulp.*   The soft tissue inside the hard wall of enamel and dentin. It has veins, arteries, and nerve tissue that nourish the tooth and sense pain.

■ *Apex.*   The very tip of each root. The blood vessels and nerves of the tooth enter through the **apical foramen** in the apex of the tooth.

apical foramen Opening in the apex.

Tissues Around the Teeth

The structures that surround the teeth are also important. They are as follows:

■ *Alveolar processes (bone).*   Form the sockets that hold and support teeth in their position.

■ *Gingiva/gums.*   Cover the alveolar bone, protecting the tooth and deeper tissues from injury or infection.

sulcus Depression, groove, area where gingival tip meets tooth enamel.

■ *Gingival sulcus.*   The open space between gingiva/gums and a tooth. This is the area where dental floss is applied to remove bacteria and food particles.

Surfaces of the Teeth

Dentists use terms that specify surfaces (sides of the tooth) to record information about the condition of each tooth. To chart conditions of the teeth, the dental assistant must know the crown surfaces. Each tooth has a crown and root. Each tooth also has four sides and a biting or chewing surface (see Figure 24–8).

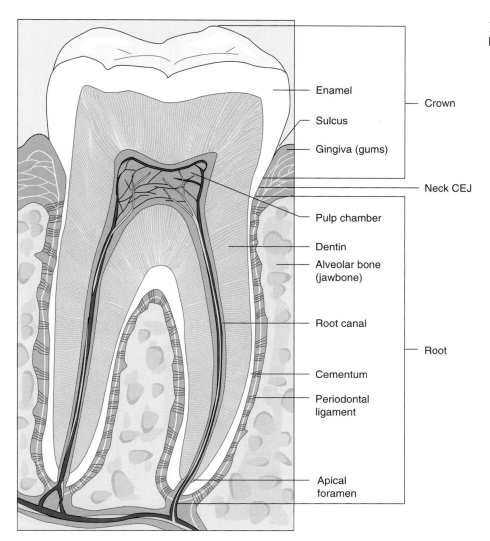

FIGURE 24-7.
Parts of the tooth.

- Enamel
- Sulcus
- Gingiva (gums)
- Crown
- Neck CEJ
- Pulp chamber
- Dentin
- Alveolar bone (jawbone)
- Root canal
- Root
- Cementum
- Periodontal ligament
- Apical foramen

■ *Anterior teeth.*   Central and lateral incisors and the cuspids
■ *Posterior teeth.*   Bicuspids and molars

The surfaces of the anterior teeth (see Figure 24–8) are called

■ *Labial.*   Surface that touches the lips
■ *Lingual.*   Surface facing toward the tongue
■ *Incisal.*   Edge of the tooth that we bite with
■ *Distal.*   Surface away from midline, toward the back
■ *Mesial.*   Surface toward the midline

The surfaces of the posterior teeth (see Figure 24–8) are called

■ *Buccal.*   Surface that touches the cheeks
■ *Lingual.*   Surface facing toward the tongue
■ *Occlusal.*   Large chewing surface where food is ground
■ *Distal.*   Surface away from midline
■ *Mesial.*   Surface toward the midline

FIGURE 24–8.
Surfaces of the anterior and posterior teeth.

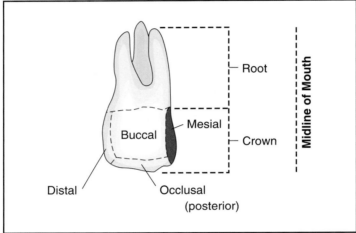

proximal Nearest or next to.

All teeth have mesial and distal sides that touch each other. The mesial side of one tooth touches the distal side of the tooth next to it. These sides are **proximal** to each other and are called proximal surfaces.

■ CHARTING CONDITIONS OF THE TEETH

legal record Record that can be used in a law suit (e.g., the patient chart).

Charting is an important responsibility. The chart is a **legal record.** Your charting must be neat, complete in detail, and correct. When charting the condition of a tooth, use abbreviations, symbols, and specialized forms. Dental offices may use different forms, but the basic guidelines are the same.

Dental Chart

Every patient has a dental chart. The dentist uses this chart for each visit. It provides a record for each dental visit (see Figure 24–9). The dental chart usually has three parts.

   1. Personal information about the patient/client:

   • Name, address, phone number • Insurance coverage, billing address • Medical precautions such as allergies to medication, bleeding, etc.

FIGURE 24-9.
Dental chart. (Courtesy of SYCOM)

(a)

EXAMINATION RECORD

Last name   First name   Spouse's first name   Home phone   Patient number

Address   Physician's name and phone number   Date of examination

City   State   Zip   Copy of diagnosis to be sent   Birth date   Age

| 1 | 2 | 3 | 4 | 5 | 6 | 7 | 8 | 9 | 10 | 11 | 12 | 13 | 14 | 15 | 16 |

| X-rays |
| Date |
| Diagnostic models |
| Date |
| Photograph |
| Clinical exam |
| Vitality test |
| Test results |

| 32 | 31 | 30 | 29 | 28 | 27 | 26 | 25 | 24 | 23 | 22 | 21 | 20 | 19 | 18 | 17 |

| a | b | c | d | e | f | g | h | i | j |

| t | s | r | q | p | o | n | m | l | k |

Summary:

Health Alerts

MEDICAL HISTORY — SUMMARY

General health

Existing illness

Medicine/Drugs

Allergies _____ Blood pressure S_____/D_____/

DENTAL HISTORY — SUMMARY

Attitude

Home care

CLINICAL DATA

General condition of teeth

Plaque _____ Stains _____ Abrasions _____

Condition of present restorations

Overhangs _____ Contact points _____

Inflammation of gingival tissue: Slight _____ Moderate _____ Severe _____

Color _____ Recession _____ Pockets _____

Condition of the floor of mouth

Palate: Hard _____ Soft _____ Cheeks _____

Lips _____ Frenum _____ Tongue _____

Ridges _____ Presence of exudate _____

Areas of food retention _____ Saliva _____

Calculus: Slight _____ Moderate _____ Excessive _____

Oral cancer exam _____ TMJ _____ Neck _____

Occlusion _____ Results of X-ray: Bone _____

Root tips _____ Impactions _____

Supernumerary _____ Abscesses _____

Item 1019V   05/94

(b)

Name _____   Fees

Tooth	Services necessary			
1				
2				
3				
4				
5				
6				
7				
8				
9				
10				
11				
12				
13				
14				
15				
16				
17				
18				
19				
20				
21				
22				
23				
24				
25				
26				
27				
28				
29				
30				
31				
32				
33				
34				
35				
36				
37				
38				
39				
40				

2. Diagram of the teeth on which to chart/document

3. Other information:

• Patient medical conditions affecting treatment • Radiographic history • Treatment given • Services performed • Estimated fee • Amount charges/paid

Charting Abbreviations

The following abbreviations apply to crown surfaces (see Figure 24–10):

M	mesial
La/F	labial facial
I	incisal
B, Bu/F	buccal/facial
D	distal
Lin, Li, L	lingual
O, Occ	occlusal
F	facial

FIGURE 24–10.
Abbreviations for the surfaces of the teeth.

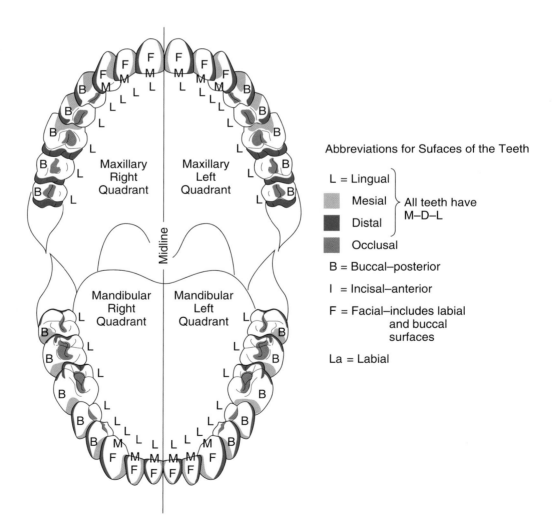

Abbreviations for Sufaces of the Teeth

L = Lingual
Mesial   } All teeth have
Distal   } M–D–L
Occlusal

B = Buccal–posterior

I = Incisal–anterior

F = Facial–includes labial and buccal surfaces

La = Labial

Abbreviations are also used for other dental terms. The following are suggested terms. Use the terms that your dentist prefers.

Abs	abscess
Adj	adjustment
Amal	amalgam
Anes	anesthetic
BWX	bite-wing x-rays
CA	corrective appliance
C & B	crown and bridge
cb	cement base
CMX	complete mouth x-rays
Com	composite
Cr	crown
Dent	denture
Diag	diagnosis
DR	denture repair
DS	denture service
Est	estimate
Exam,Ex	examination
Ext	extraction
FGCr	full gold crown
Fix Br	fixed bridge
FL	full lower
FM	full mouth
FT	fluoride treatment
FU	full upper
GI	gold inlay
GO	gold onlay
GR	gold restoration
GT	gingiva/gums treatment
Imp	impression
Lido	lidocaine
occ adj	occlusal adjustment
OS	oral surgery
PA	preparatory appointment
PFM	porcelain fused to metal
PL	partial lower
POH	personal oral hygiene instruction

POT	postoperative treatment
Prep	preparation
Prophy	prophylaxis
PU	partial upper
Radiogr	radiographs
RCT	root canal therapy
Rem	removable
RR	resin restoration
SM	study models
SR	silver restoration
ST	sedative treatment
Temp	temporary
X-ray/X	x-rays
Xylo	xylocaine

Types of Diagrams on Dental Charts

A dental chart has an anatomical or geometric diagram of the teeth.

■ The *anatomical diagram* (Figure 24–11) may show the crowns of the teeth, the crowns of the teeth and the root, or the crowns of the teeth and a small part of the root.

■ The *geometric diagram* (Figure 24–12) is another type of diagram the dentist may use for charting. The teeth are identified by number and show all sides and the crown in a geometric drawing.

Charting Symbols

Basic symbols identify conditions of the teeth and procedures. There are many different ways to chart these conditions, required procedures, and completion of the necessary care. Examples of charting symbols are shown in Figure 24–13.

Match the following conditions with the appropriate tooth number on the anatomical diagram in Figure 24–14 and the geometric diagram in Figure 24–15. This will help you understand how to use charting symbols.

Tooth Number	Condition
2	Full gold crown bridge abutment (anchor tooth)
3	Pontic-fake tooth of bridge
4	Veneer with gold bridge abutment (anchor tooth)
8	Mesial decay
9	Mesial fracture
11	Distal decay
13	Full porcelain crown

Anatomical Diagram of Permanent Teeth

Anatomical Diagram of Deciduous Teeth

FIGURE 24–11.
Anatomical diagrams of the permanent and deciduous teeth.

FIGURE 24–12.
Geometric diagram of the teeth.

FIGURE 24–13.
a Examples of charting symbols.

ANATOMICAL DIAGRAMS	GEOMETRICAL DIAGRAMS	ANATOMICAL DIAGRAMS	GEOMETRICAL DIAGRAMS
Missing Tooth	Missing Tooth	To Be Extracted	To Be Extracted
Unerupted or Impacted	Unerupted or Impacted	Upward/Downward Drifting	Upward/Downward Drifting
Mesial Distal Drifting Tooth	Mesial Distal Drifting Tooth	Buccal Lingual 3/4 Crown	Buccal Lingual 3/4 Crown

16	Needs to be extracted
17	Impacted toward mesial
18	Buccal decay
19	Occlusal decay
20	Mod restoration already done filled in
24	Root canal
25	Periapical abscess (around the root)
29	Two occlusal pit decays
30	MO (mesiocclusal) decay
31	DO (distocclusal) decay
32	Missing

A common procedure is to use red and blue color codes on the chart. *Red* indicates that treatment is necessary. Use the following guidelines to chart conditions needing treatment.

ANATOMICAL DIAGRAMS	GEOMETRICAL DIAGRAMS	ANATOMICAL DIAGRAMS	GEOMETRICAL DIAGRAMS
Full Crown	Full Crown	Porcelain Crown Fused to Metal	Porcelain Crown Fused to Metal
3/4 Crown Full Crown Fixed Bridge	Unerupted or Impacted	Fracture	Fracture
Abscess	Abscess	Root Canal	Root Canal

FIGURE 24–13.
b Examples of charting symbols.

■ Outline fractures and dental **caries** in red.

■ Use red for **impaction, abscesses,** overhanging margins, extractions, and periodontal pockets.

■ Outline in red an old restoration that needs replacing and fill in with solid blue.

Blue indicates that the treatment is completed or that there is a condition that does not require treatment but must be watched carefully.

■ Use blue to outline and shade amalgam restorations that are in good condition.

■ Outline and draw diagonal lines in blue for gold restorations.

■ Use blue to indicate missing teeth and root canals.

■ Outline tooth-colored restorations in blue (e.g., restorations that match the teeth).

Indicate a cavity (carie/decay) that covers more than one surface by writing, "Tooth #1 has an MO," which means a mesioocclusal cavity.

Learn the procedure that your dentist prefers.

caries Decay.

impaction Any tooth that does not erupt when it should (e.g., tooth blocked by bone and/or tissue, keeping it under the surface of the gum).

abscesses Pockets of pus in a limited area.

FIGURE 24–13.
c Examples of charting symbols.

ANATOMICAL DIAGRAMS	GEOMETRICAL DIAGRAMS	ANATOMICAL DIAGRAMS	GEOMETRICAL DIAGRAMS
4mm 4mm	4 4		
Periodontal Pocket	Periodontal Pocket	Periodontal Abscess	Periodontal Abscess
Occ MOD Amalgam Restoration	Occ MOD Amalgam Restoration	D(III) MO(II) MI(IV) Composite Restoration	D(III) MO(II) MI(IV) Composite Restoration
Overhanging margin	Overhanging		

LINGUAL

FULL MOUTH DIAGRAM USING SYMBOLS
TO INDICATE MISSING TEETH

FIGURE 24–14. Examples of charting an anatomical diagram.

FIGURE 24–15. Examples of charting a geometric diagram.

■ DENTAL EQUIPMENT

A dental treatment (operatory) room is designed and organized to ensure that the dentist and assistant perform procedures in a safe and time-efficient manner. Treatment room equipment includes the following:

■ Dental chair
■ Dental unit
■ Operational light
■ Mobile carts or cabinets
■ Operatory stools
■ X-ray machine and view box

The type of equipment varies depending on the office. As a dental assistant, you are responsible for learning how to use the various types of equipment. Dental equipment is costly and requires special care. It is important that you follow the manufacturers' cleaning and operating instructions.

Dental Chair

Parts of a dental chair are as follows (see Figure 24–16):

- The body of the chair includes the backrest, seat, and leg support.
- The armrest is usually movable.
- The headrest supports the patient's head and is movable.
- The control panel is on the side or back of the chair. Foot pedals are attached to base of chair or rest on the floor. These are used to move the chair into either a sitting or reclining (supine) position.
- The swivel lever is at the base of the chair, which allows the chair to rotate.

Dental Unit

A dental unit is attached to the dental chair or to a separate movable cart (Figure 21–16). The basic parts of a dental unit are as follows:

FIGURE 24–16. (Photos courtesy of A-dec, Inc.) a. Dental unit; b. Chair; c. Air/water syringe; d. Mobile dental unit (note foot-controlled rheostat).

FIGURE 24–16. *(continued).* e. Assistant's cart; f. and g. Operative stools.

- ■ Master switch/control for
- • Water and air • Handpiece
- ■ Dental handpiece with burs or drills:
- • High speed • Slow speed
- ■ Foot control **(rheostat),** which provides power to the handpiece.
- ■ Air/water syringe to rinse and dry teeth.
- ■ Oral **evacuation** system to **aspirate** saliva and drainage from the mouth. This system has two hoses attached to
- • A suction tip • A small saliva ejector
- ■ Cuspidor, the bowl that patients spit into (modern offices use suction in place of a cuspidor).

rheostat Control for flow of electric current.

evacuation Removal.

aspirate Remove substances.

Operational Light

The operational light is attached to the chair or the ceiling. It has handles to move the light. The light must focus on the site where the dentist is working.

Dental Mobile Carts or Cabinets

The dental cart/cabinet provides storage for a small number of sterile instruments, treatment trays, dental materials, and supplies. Large amounts of supplies are stored in areas away from the patient treatment room.

Operatory Stools

Operatory stools vary in design. There may be a footrest ring near the base on some stools, but all include the following:

- ■ Padded seat
- ■ Five casters at the base to prevent tipping

■ Height-adjustment lever to position:

• Dental assistant 4 to 6 inches above the dentist • Dentist stabilized below the assistant, with thighs parallel to floor when feet are flat on the floor

■ Adjustable back support

Radiology Machine

A radiology machine uses radiation to take x-rays. All radiology machines must operate according to state regulations to ensure safety. State regulations tell how to prevent **overexposure** to radiation and provide safety guidelines for machine operations. These regulations require the following:

overexposure Too much contact with radiation.

■ Registration of each radiology machine
■ **Periodic** inspection of equipment to ensure safe operation
■ A licensed person to operate a radiology machine

periodic Occurring at regular intervals.

■ INFECTION CONTROL

Infection control guidelines exist to protect employees and patients against infectious viruses and bacteria. The Standard Precautions you follow depend on

■ The potential for contact with blood
■ The potential for contact with any body fluids
■ The tasks that you perform

OSHA directs health care workers and their employers to follow specific guidelines to protect against infection (review Unit 1 of Chapter 12). As a dental assistant, you wear gloves, mask, and protective eyewear when assisting with or performing procedures. You are also required to wear a long-sleeve lab coat or top to protect against being scratched by an instrument. Table 24–1 helps you understand Standard Precautions and protective wear guidelines.

Infection control measures are necessary to prevent infecting other patients, yourself, and co-workers. Cleaning the treatment area is one way to control infection. Read the following Chapter 20 topics:

■ Decontamination
■ Preparation area

TABLE 24–1 Standard Precautions: Examples of Tasks and Use of Protective Equipment

Task	Gloves	Gown	Mask	Eye Wear
Controlling spurting blood	Yes	Yes	Yes	Yes
Controlling minimal bleeding	Yes	No	No	No
Oral or nasal suction	Yes	No	Yes	Yes
Handling/cleaning contaminated instruments	Yes	Yes	Yes	Yes

Procedure

Cleaning the Treatment Room Between Patients/Clients

1. Wash hands.
2. Assemble equipment.
   a. Latex gloves or utility gloves
   b. Disinfectant solution
   c. Disposable towel
   d. Protective wear (see Table 24–1)
   ALERT: Follow Standard Precautions.

3. Put on protective wear.
4. Discard all disposable items.
5. Place soiled instruments in disinfectant container, and cover.
6. Spray/wipe disinfectant solution on all surfaces. Follow directions on disinfectant for the drying procedure.

Procedure

Preparing the Treatment Area for a Patient/Client

1. Wash hands.
2. Assemble equipment.
   a. Procedure tray/instruments
   b. Plastic **barriers**
   c. Patient's chart
   d. Most recent x-rays
   e. Headrest cover
   f. Patient drape
   g. Alligator clips
   h. Two pairs of latex gloves
   i. Mask/safety shields or glasses
   ALERT: Follow Standard Precautions.
3. Open procedure tray or place instruments on treatment tray in the order of use, and cover.
4. Place all barriers on chair and handpieces.

5. Position patient chair in lowest position.
6. Raise armrest on patient-access side of chair.
7. Place chart for easy access by the dentist.
8. Display most recent x-rays on view box.
9. Place patient drape and alligator clips for easy access.
10. Use plastic barriers to cover:
    a. Handpiece and hoses
    b. Air/water syringes, tips, and hoses
    c. Suction hose and plastic tip
    d. Operative light handles
    e. X-ray tube head
11. Place latex gloves, mask, and protective glasses for easy access to dentist and dental assistant.

■ Sterile wraps
■ Monitoring effectiveness of sterilization

This information tells you how to clean, wrap, and sterilize instruments.

The treatment area must be clean and free of any items from the preceding patient. Prepare the room for the next client by doing the following procedure.

Clients may be nervous about seeing the dentist. The way you greet the patient and bring him or her to the treatment area helps set the atmosphere for that appointment. Once the treatment area is prepared for the patient, follow the steps below to admit and seat the patient.

barriers Items that prevent infectious material from contacting surface.

■ BASIC SETUP FOR DENTAL PROCEDURES

Always have the patient's chart, x-rays, and recently taken study models available when you set up the area. Be sure that you have pencils in all the colors that you may need.

The basic setup tray contains the following:

1. *Mouth mirror.*   To reflect light to see the surfaces of the teeth; to inspect teeth, tongue, gingiva, and oral cavity; and for retraction (hold cheek back)
2. *Explorer.*   To feel teeth for decay or other problems
3. *Cotton forceps.*   To pick up gauze/cotton to dry areas of mouth/teeth
4. *Periodontal probe.*   To check and measure sulcus area
5. *Gauze squares.* $4 \times 4s/2 \times 2s$ to dry and hold slippery tissues
6. *Suction tip/saliva ejector.*   To keep mouth dry and structures visible
7. *Air/water syringe tip.*   To rinse and dry
8. *Dental floss.*   To check contacts between teeth

Procedure

Admitting and Seating a Patient/Client

1. Greet patient by name. Verify that chart and patient's name match.
2. Say, "We are ready for you now, Mr./Mrs. _____, I'll show you to the examination room." (Keep the discussion pleasant; follow the dentist's instructions when answering questions. If you are unsure of an answer, instruct the patient to ask the dentist; for example, "Dr. _____ can answer that question when he comes in" or "Please ask Dr. _____ when he comes in.")
3. Show patient where to place personal items. (It's best to indicate a place for personal items within the patient's view.)
4. Seat patient and lower armrest.
5. Place patient drape over chest and secure with alligator clips.
6. Review and document patient's health history and current dental concerns.
7. Measure vital signs if required by dentist.

8. Provide patient with protective eyewear if necessary.
9. Wash hands.
10. Put on protective wear.
11. Notify dentist that patient is ready.
12. Adjust chair at time of examination/treatment. The patient's toes should be at the same level as his or her nose.

■ BASIC CHAIRSIDE ASSISTING SKILLS DURING DENTAL TREATMENT

There are specific guidelines that the dental assistant follows whenever he or she is assisting the dentist at chairside. These guidelines are as follows:

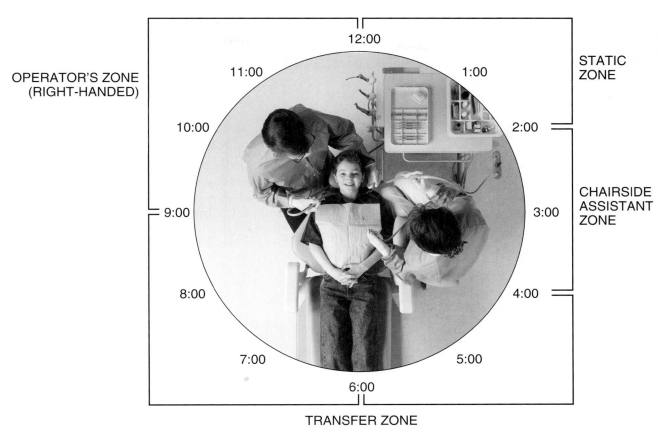

FIGURE 24–17. Clock positions/working zones. (Photo courtesy of A-dec, Inc.)

- Position light 36 inches away from mouth.
- Adjust the light to ensure that the area being worked on is always visible during treatment.
- Use the suction tip and air/water syringe as needed to ensure visibility.
- Pass instruments and materials as needed.

Instrument Transfer

Remember to pass instruments over the patient's chest and below the patient's chin. The positions of the dentist, dental assistant, and patient are compared to the positions of a clock. The patient's head is always at 12 o'clock. The right-handed dentist is usually at 9 to 11 o'clock. The dental assistant works between 2 and 3 o'clock. Familiarize yourself with the "clock" positions (see Figure 24–17).

■ ORAL EXAMINATION

During the oral examination, the dentist examines the face, joints, muscles, glands, tissue, and oral cavity with his or her fingers. This method of examination is called **palpation.** Next the dentist uses a mirror and explorer to check the teeth and gingiva/gums. The dentist examines each tooth, and the dental assistant uses symbols to draw needed services on the tooth chart. After a thorough examination, the dentist explains the findings and the recommended procedures.

palpation Examine by feeling for unusual or abnormal conditions.

Procedure

Assisting During the Oral Examination

1. Seat and drape patient/client.
2. Wash hands.
3. Assemble equipment.
   a. Patient chart
   b. Pencils in colors you may need
   c. X-rays
   d. Current study models
   e. Sterile package with basic setup instruments
   f. Gauze
   g. Protective wear
4. Open sterile package and place on sterile field.
5. Put on protective wear.
6. Pass mouth mirror and explorer to dentist at same time. Use both hands to place mirror in dentist's left hand and explorer into right hand. (This is reversed if dentist is left-handed.)

Pain Control

Controlling pain is an important part of patient care. There are different types of pain control.

■ An analgesic helps relieve pain or causes it to disappear. In dentistry the analgesia is often given in a gas and inhaled through a face mask. The advantages are that

• The patient feels relaxed and awake. • The medication is short acting and easy to control.

sedate Calm.

Other forms of analgesia are pills or injections that help **sedate** the patient. These are usually longer acting than gases. *Never leave a patient/client alone when he or she is sedated.*

injectable Medication given by needle.

■ Local anesthetics take away feeling in a specific area. Local anesthetics are topical and **injectable.** The dentist often uses both.

saturating Soak.

• Topical anesthetics such as lidocaine (Xylocaine) ointment are rubbed over the gingiva/gums and absorbed into the tissue. The surface tissue loses feeling. This lessens the discomfort of the injection. • Injectable anesthetic such as lidocaine (Xylocaine) is placed in the gingiva/gums tissue, either blocking a nerve or **saturating** the tissue around nerves.

The dentist decides which type of anesthetic to give the patient. When he or she orders an injectable anesthetic, the dental assistant prepares and passes the syringe to the dentist. The dental assistant selects the needle length depending on the site of injection. The dentist orders anesthesia for

■ *Maxillary infiltration,* which requires a separate injection for each tooth. The anesthesia is injected near the nerve endings. It requires a 1-inch needle (see Figure 24–18a).

■ *Mandibular nerve block,* which blocks the main nerve, causing several teeth to be free of pain. It requires a 1⅝-inch needle (see Figure 24–18b).

Anesthetic medication is available in narrow glass tubes called carpule/cartridges. The carpule/cartridge is placed into an aspirating syringe. Follow the steps in the procedure "Loading and Unloading a Carpule/Cartridge in an Aspirating Syringe."

FIGURE 24–18. Injection sites for anesthesia.

(A) Maxillary infiltration   (B) Mandibular nerve block

Procedure

Loading and Unloading a Carpule/Cartridge in an Aspirating Syringe

1. Wash hands.
2. Assemble equipment. (Keep syringe and medication out of patient's view to prevent anxiety.)
   a. Lidocaine carpule
   b. Aspirating syringe
   c. Sterile needle
   d. Alcohol wipe
   e. Protective wear
3. Inspect the carpule for
   a. Large bubbles (more than 2 mm), which are usually caused by freezing. **Do not use.**
   b. Bulging/protruding plunger, which means either
      (1) The cartridge was left in a chemical disinfectant solution too long. **Do not use.**
      (2) The cartridge was frozen. **Do not use.**
   c. Cracks and chips, which can cause a cartridge to break during injection. **Do not use.**
   d. Expiration date. **Do not use after the last day of the month the medication expires.**
4. Put on protective wear.
5. Disinfect cap end of cartridge with 70 percent ethyl alcohol.
6. Pull piston/plunger all the way back on syringe.
7. Place plunger end of the cartridge into syringe at base of piston.
8. Move body of cartridge into syringe and gently secure in place by applying slight pressure to the plunger (harpoon).
9. Attach needle to syringe.
10. Loosen needle cover. **Do not remove it.**
11. Pass syringe to dentist. (See the procedure "Passing and Receiving the Syringe."

To remove cartridge after the injection:

12. Draw cartridge back from needle and remove from syringe.
13. Remove needle according to office procedure and place in sharps container.
14. Disinfect syringe and sterilize.

dominant hand
Hand used for writing, eating, working.

Passing the Syringe

Always pass syringe to the dentist below the patient's chin or behind the patient's head to help reduce his or her anxiety.

Procedure

Passing and Receiving the Syringe

ALERT: Follow Standard Precautions.

1. Hold syringe in your **dominant hand.**
2. Apply topical anesthetic to applicator, and hand it to dentist with your other hand.
3. Lay thumb ring/cradle of syringe at the dentist's thumb, making sure his or her fingers are in position to grasp the syringe before you release it.
4. Remove needle cap as you slide your hand away from syringe. Place cap on tray in position to slip used needle in place easily after injection.
5. Place your hand near patient's hands to prevent sudden movements from hitting syringe (especially important for new patients).
6. Observe patient before, during, and after injection for signs of fainting or allergic reaction.
7. Receive syringe by holding barrel, taking care to prevent needle sticks.
8. Recap needle by holding syringe with both hands and scooping cap into position on needle.
9. Carefully secure cap and remove needle.
10. Place needle in sharps container.
11. Loosen cartridge and place in sharps container.

Procedure

Instrument Exchange

ALERT: Follow Standard Precautions.

1. Use thumb and forefinger of your left hand to pick up instruments from tray.
2. Stick little finger out.
3. Turn instrument and your hand **parallel** to instrument dentist is already holding.
4. Approach slowly.
5. Curl little finger around and pick up unwanted instrument. Squeeze instrument into your wrist.
6. Place new instrument into position between dentist's thumb and forefinger.
7. Turn used instrument with thumb and return it to tray in order of use.

parallel Same direction and at a distance, so that two points do not touch.

rotary Move in a circular fashion.

■ ORAL EVACUATION/RINSING/DRYING TECHNIQUES

When a tooth restoration such as removing decay and filling the tooth is necessary, the dentist uses instruments called handpieces. Handpieces, which hold small drills (burs) to cut and shape the tooth, operate at very high speeds. A small cutting device called a **rotary** cutting instrument (or bur) is placed in the end of the handpiece. Water comes out of the handpiece to cool the tooth because cutting (drilling) on the tooth creates heat that is painful.

The dental assistant picks up water and tooth debris with the high-volume evacuation tip. This tip is called an HVE, vacuum tip, suction, or aspirator (see Figure 24–19).

The plastic tip (usually disposable) is placed into the handle at the end of the suction hose. There are two ways to grasp the suction tip (see Figures 24–20 and 24–21):

1. Thumb-to-nose grasp
2. Pen grasp

CAUTION Be gentle when using the suction tip in the patient's mouth to prevent injury to fragile tissue. Keep a good grasp to ensure constant control of the suction.

Proper placement and use of the suction tip save operating time and reduce by 80 percent the debris that flies out of the mouth during procedures (Figure 24–22).

The dental assistant usually sits on the left side of the patient and holds the suction tip in his or her right hand. Reverse this if working with a left-handed dentist.

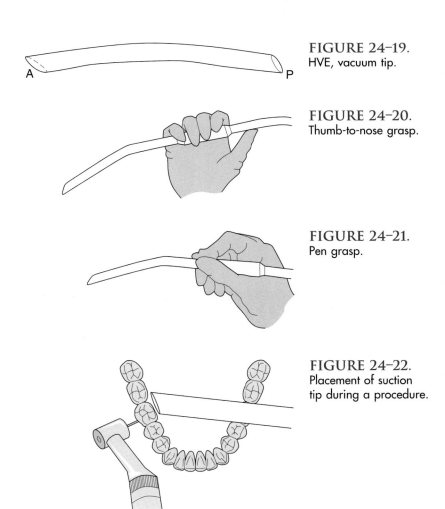

FIGURE 24–19.
HVE, vacuum tip.

FIGURE 24–20.
Thumb-to-nose grasp.

FIGURE 24–21.
Pen grasp.

FIGURE 24–22.
Placement of suction tip during a procedure.

Procedure

High-Velocity Evacuation

1. Wash hands.
2. Assemble equipment.
   a. Long-sleeved lab coat
   b. Gloves
   c. Eye protection
   d. Mask
   e. Suction tip

ALERT: Follow Standard Precautions.

3. Put on protective wear.
4. Grasp HVE (suction tip) according to area of mouth to suction.
5. Position tip before dentist places handpiece and mirror into position.
6. Place beveled edge parallel to buccal or lingual side of tooth being treated.
7. Keep tip close to treated tooth to pull debris and water over tooth into tip.

Procedure

Air-Water Spray or Triplex Syringe

1. Wash hands.
2. Assemble equipment.
   a. Gloves
   b. Gown/lab coat
   c. Eye protection
   d. Mask
   e. Air/water syringe and tip
   f. Plastic protective covers for hoses

ALERT: Follow Standard Precautions.

3. Put on protective wear.

4. Test syringe by pressing
   a. "A" to spray a stream of air
   b. "W" to spray a stream of water
   c. "A" and "B" to combine water and air in a spray
5. Place air/water tip near opening of oral cavity and aim at surfaces to be rinsed. Position suction tip close to water spray.
6. Immediately dry area with air, allowing dentist to continue treatment. (Avoid spraying directly into a surgical wound and use short burst of air.)

Procedure

Completion of Treatment and Patient/Client Dismissal

1. Fold client drape to collect debris as you remove alligator clip and drape.
2. Return patient to sitting position. (Place hand on patient's shoulder and caution him or her not to stand up too fast, allowing time to balance.)
3. Lower chair to a safe height.

4. Check area to see that patient collects all belongings.
5. Escort patient to reception desk.
6. Chart completion of procedures.
7. Wash hands.
8. Perform the procedure "Cleaning the Treatment Room Between Patients/Clients."

■ STUDY MODELS

Study models or casts of teeth, gingiva/gums, and soft tissues provide the structure necessary to make dentures, partial dentures, bridgework, and other corrective/prosthetic devices. An impression of these structures is made before making a model. The impression creates a mold to pour plaster/stone material into. The study model is made when the plaster/stone dries and is removed from the impression/mold. There are four steps to follow:

1. Make an **alginate** impression of the mandibular/lower teeth first, then of the maxillary/upper teeth. The maxillary impression procedure may cause gagging, so it is best to take it second.
2. Make a wax bite impression. A wax bite shows the relationship of the occlusal (touching) surfaces of the maxillary and mandibular teeth.
3. Mix the plaster.
4. Pour into impression mold, and trim.

To make a study model, take each step in the following procedures.

alginate Material for making impressions.

nondominant hand Hand that is not used for writing or other tasks.

seating Putting firmly in place to prevent moving.

Procedure

Preparing to Take Alginate Impressions

1. Wash hands.
2. Assemble equipment.
   a. Gloves
   b. Protective eyewear
   c. Mask
   d. Gown
   e. Basic setup (see "Basic Setup for Dental Procedures")
   f. Alginate powder
   g. Rubber bowl
   h. Measuring scoop (with alginate powder)
   i. Water measure (with alginate powder)
   j. Water at room temperature
   k. Spatula (shaped like a beaver's tail)
   l. Impression trays
   m. Round pencil-like strips of beading wax
   n. Plastic drape
   o. Clock/watch

   ALERT: Follow Standard Precautions.

3. Seat and drape client. Leave seat in upright position while taking impressions, to minimize gagging.
4. Ask patient if he or she has ever had an impression taken.

5. Explain what you are going to do, including what the patient will feel/experience.
6. Put on protective wear.
7. Remove any removable items (bridge, loose crown, dentures, etc.) from patient's mouth, rinse, and place on paper towel.
8. Rinse patient's mouth with water syringe.
9. Fit impression trays (upper and lower) by placing a tray size you think will fit in patient's mouth. (The correct size will not stretch lips.) The teeth must be in center of tray, not touching tray sides.
10. Rinse and dry selected trays.
11. Apply beading wax around edge of each tray to form impression edge and prevent pressure on gingiva/gums tissue (vestibule).
12. Place prepared trays on covered treatment tray ready for use.

Mixing–Loading Trays

13. Verify whether alginate is fast set or regular set. Fast or regular set determines length of time alginate takes to mix and become firm in patient's mouth.
14. Follow mixing directions on alginate container.
    a. Place measured room-temperature water into rubber bowl.

Procedure box continued

b. Place measured alginate powder into bowl.

c. Mix water and powder until powder is completely wet.

d. Hold bowl sideways in your **nondominant hand.** Holding spatula in your dominant hand, mix by rubbing mixture against sides of bowl in a figure-eight motion until creamy smooth.

15. Load mandibular tray with a spatula, as you would frost a cake. Be sure to fill tray without leaving air bubbles.

16. Wipe and smooth surface of alginate mixture with wet gloved finger before placing tray in patient's mouth.

17. Stand in front of patient.

18. Instruct patient to open mouth just enough to allow tray to be placed in mouth.

19. Insert tray into mouth one side at a time.

20. Line up tray handle with patient's midline (nose).

21. Press back of tray over molars.

22. Press onto front teeth, while easing lip away from impression material.

23. Instruct client to lift tongue; at same time press down, **seating** impression material around teeth and gingiva/gums.

24. Hold tray in position until alginate is firm enough to stay in shape or to set. (Alginate directions will give the approximate time period.)

25. Feel alginate to see if it holds its shape, before removing tray.

26. Run your gloved index and middle fingers along labial edge of tray to release seal around teeth when alginate is set.

27. Lift front of tray first, then lift back.

28. Turn tray sideways and remove from mouth one side at a time.

29. Rinse and suction patient's mouth.

30. Gently rinse impression with water and spray with disinfectant.

31. Display impression for dentist to inspect.

32. Place in plastic bag for a minimum of 10 minutes before pouring plaster/stone to make model.

33. Load maxillary tray as described in steps 13 and 14.

34. Provide patient with tissue to blot moisture if necessary.

35. Instruct patient to breathe through his or her nose and slightly lean forward once tray is in place.

36. Stand behind patient.

37. Instruct patient to open mouth just enough to accept tray.

38. Insert tray one side at a time and position over teeth.

39. Center tray by placing handle in line with patient's nose.

40. Press impression material over back teeth first.

41. Press over front teeth while easing lip away from impression material.

42. Press tray in place, seating impression material over gingiva/gums line.

43. Allow client to lean slightly forward and to breathe through the nose.

44. Hold tray in place until alginate is set (see step 24).

45. Follow steps 26 to 32 to complete procedure.

46. Remove protective wear.

47. Wash hands.

Procedure

Registering a Wax Bite

1. Wash hands.
2. Assemble equipment.
   a. Bowl of warm water
   b. Wax bite wafer (thin, U-shaped)
   c. Lab knife
   d. Protective wear
3. Explain what you are going to do.
4. Put on protective wear.
5. Trim back edges of wax to fit patient's mouth if necessary.
6. Place wax in warm water to soften.
7. Grasp wax so that U shape can be placed in mouth to align with U shape of teeth.
8. Instruct patient to open mouth.
9. Place wax in position over lower teeth.
10. Instruct client to bite down on wax hard enough to make an impression but not enough to bite through wax. Ask the patient to hold the bite.
11. Spray air onto wax to gently cool.
12. Ask patient to open mouth when cool.
13. Gently remove wax, being careful not to bend or tear impression.
14. Gently rinse wax and spray with disinfectant.
15. Mark patient's initials in upper right corner of wax impression.
16. Place wax impression with alginate impressions.
17. Remove protective wear and wash hands.

Procedure

Preparing and Pouring Plaster/Stone into Impressions to Make Casts

1. Wash hands.
2. Assemble equipment.
   a. Modeling plaster/stone
   b. Scale or measuring device for plaster
   c. 100-mL graduated cylinder
   d. Rubber bowls/flexiboles
   e. Plaster spatula
   f. Vibrator
   g. Impressions
   h. Wax paper/glass slab/tile square
   i. Scale
3. Place 45 to 50 mL of water into bowl.
4. Measure 100 g of plaster.
5. Mix plaster powder into water by pouring a slow, steady stream of powder and stirring carefully.
6. Mix until material looks like sour cream.
7. Hold mixing bowl on vibrator for approximately 2 minutes, allowing bubbles to rise to surface.
8. Remove bowl from vibrator and mix ingredients with spatula again.
9. Secure impression in your hand by holding tray handle.
10. Rest impression tray on vibrator.
11. Secure impression tray to keep from falling.
12. Scoop plaster/stone mixture with spatula.
13. Pour small portions of plaster/stone from spatula into one end of impression.
14. Watch plaster/stone vibrate into each tooth form.
15. Turn impression tray as you gradually fill each tooth form with plaster/stone.
16. Remove impression tray from vibrator when all tooth forms are filled with plaster/stone.
17. Pour plaster to fill remainder of impression tray.
18. Use spatula to smooth and fill total impression tray.

Procedure box continued

19. Form a ½-inch-thick round patty on a glass slab or tile. The patty must be the size of the impression tray.

(Patty of stone)

Tray

Base

20. Turn impression tray filled with plaster/stone onto patty. Keep tray level with countertop.

21. Inspect to ensure that plaster/stone impression and base are joined together. **Make sure that edge of impression tray is not covered with plaster.**

22. Flatten inside area of tray where the tongue normally is when placing mandibular impression on base.

23. Allow at least 29 to 60 minutes for plaster/stone to set/harden.

24. Hold plaster/stone model and impression tray under running water.

25. Gently slide plaster/stone model out of impression tray.

26. Dispose of impression material.

27. Clean trays if they are reusable.

Procedure

Trimming Study Models

1. Wash hands.
2. Assemble equipment.
   a. Protective eyewear
   b. Laboratory knife
   c. Model trimmer
   d. Bowl of water
3. Soak models in water at least 5 minutes. (Wet models are easier to trim and do not break as easily.)
4. Put on protective eyewear.
5. Turn on model-trimmer water.
6. Allow time for water to moisten grinding wheel.

Safety precaution: Hold model securely with steady pressure against grinding wheel. Always keep fingers away from wheel.

7. Place base of model against grinding wheel to smooth and level surface. The base must be at least ½-inch thick and parallel to biting surface of teeth.

8. Place heel of mandibular model against wheel and trim to approximately ¼ inch behind third molar.

9. Hold heel at a 90-degree angle (perpendicular) to the base.

10. Measure maxillary model against mandibular model and trim to match.

11. Trim side of
    a. Maxillary model at a 63-degree angle to heel.
    b. Mandibular model at a 55-degree angle to heel.
    c. Keep edge of models between ¼ and ⅜ inch of bicuspids.

Procedure box continued

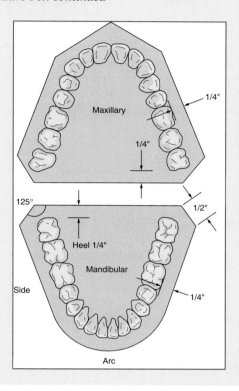

12. Trim heel points to ½ inch to a 125-degree angle to heel.
13. Mark by making a small cut on the
    a. Maxillary model on each side of cuspid and central incisors, to form a point.
    b. Mandibular model to form an arc at cuspids.
14. Clean trimmer according to manufacturer's instructions.
15. Clean area and return equipment to its storage area.
16. Wash hands.

Procedure

Cavity Preparation

ALERT: Follow Standard Precautions.

1. Wash hands.
2. Assemble equipment.
   a. Gloves
   b. Gown
   c. Protective eyewear
   d. Mask
   e. Anesthetic solution
   f. Aspirating syringe
   g. Lidocaine ointment
   h. Cotton rolls
   i. Basic procedure tray
   j. Restoration instruments
   k. Suction tips
   l. Air/water tips
   m. Handpieces and burs
3. Prepare anesthetic syringe.
4. Put on protective wear.
5. Position yourself, suction, and water/air devices for easy access.
6. Perform suction, rinsing, and drying procedures as needed during restorative process. This is referred to as "keeping the operating field clear."

Note: When you learn to prepare materials to line and fill the cavity, you may begin performing these duties.

■ ASSISTING DURING BASIC RESTORATIVE PROCEDURES

Restoring a tooth to a healthy state is a frequently performed procedure in a dental office. The dental assistant is very important in this procedure. Be certain to learn your dentist's preferences. It is important to become familiar with the materials that your dentist uses in these procedures. Always read all product directions carefully when preparing to assist with restorative procedures. Be prepared to provide the dentist with all materials and equipment needed during a procedure. (See procedure on p. 689.)

■ ORAL HYGIENE

Human teeth are meant to last a lifetime. Remember that enamel is the hardest tissue in the body. Why, then, do we lose teeth? The bacteria that live in everyone's mouth cause disease. There are two main reasons why we lose teeth:

■ Disease of the gingiva/gums, periodontal tissues, and/or the alveolar process (bony socket)
■ Holes in the enamel and/or dentin (cavities)

Proper toothbrushing and flossing plus good nutrition can help prevent disease and destruction (review Chapter 10).

Dental assistants explain and demonstrate proper toothbrushing and flossing techniques to their patients. The instruction must be clear and meet each patient's needs (for example, working around a bridge). Correct flossing and brushing helps

plaque Soft deposit of bacteria and bacterial products on teeth.

■ Remove **plaque**
■ Prevent bad breath (halitosis)
■ Prevent periodontal infection
■ Prevent bleeding gingiva/gums

■ TEACHING ORAL HYGIENE

Your dentist may ask you to use disclosing tablets or solution to show the client that there is plaque in the mouth. The disclosing tablets are usually red and stain the plaque to help the patient see the areas where plaque has formed. Patients can see that even when they think plaque is removed, it may not be. This is a very good way to help patients understand that correct brushing and flossing is important.

There are several types of brushing techniques. Use the technique your dentist prefers. The Bass technique is a common one.

Common abbreviations for charting patient education:

■ *OHI.*   Oral hygiene, complete cleansing of oral cavity
■ *TBI.*   Toothbrushing instruction
■ *DFT.*   Dental floss instruction

interproximal surfaces Sides between teeth.

Flossing removes the plaque from the **interproximal surfaces** (between teeth). It removes plaque and food. Flossing cleans areas where brushing cannot reach. Correct flossing is very important because tooth decay often begins on the interproximal surfaces.

Procedure

Disclosing Tablet/Solution

1. Wash hands.
2. Put on gloves.
3. Assemble equipment.
   a. Disclosing tablets or solution
   b. Toothbrush recommended by dentist
   c. Mirror
   d. Cup
   e. Towels
   f. Protective wear if required
4. Explain why brushing/flossing is important.
   a. To prevent disease
   b. To prevent halitosis
   c. To prevent bleeding gingiva/gums
   d. For total body health

5. Follow directions for preparing disclosing tablets/solution.
6. Ask patient to swish solution around in mouth and spit solution into container.
7. Have patient rinse mouth.
8. Have patient look at teeth in mirror.
9. Explain that red areas are plaque.
10. Explain that this plaque must be removed to keep the mouth healthy. The best way to remove it is by toothbrushing and flossing. All surfaces of the teeth must be brushed carefully.

Procedure

Bass Toothbrushing Technique

1. Wash hands.
2. Assemble equipment.
   a. Tooth model (if using a model for teaching)
   b. Protective wear (if brushing patient's teeth or if there is contact with saliva)
   c. Toothbrush
3. Explain importance of toothbrushing.
4. Demonstrate correct brushing using model or on patient.
Note: Put on gloves if demonstrating on patient.
   a. Place soft brush on upper right molars (maxillary).
   b. Position brush at 45-degree angle to teeth.
   c. Gently move bristles into gingival sulcus.
   d. Move brush in short strokes at least 10 to 20 times, keeping brush in place (wiggle-jiggle motion).

   e. Move brush to next two or three teeth and repeat until all buccal/labial surfaces are brushed.
Note: Place brush in vertical or horizontal position for anterior teeth.
   f. Repeat technique beginning at upper right molars until all maxillary teeth are brushed.
   g. Use short, vibrating motion to scrub occlusal surfaces.
   h. Repeat this procedure for lower teeth (mandibular).
5. Ask client if he or she has any questions.
6. Remove and clean equipment.
7. Remove protective wear.
8. Wash hands.
9. Chart TBI (toothbrushing instruction).

Procedure

Dental Flossing

1. Wash hands.
2. Assemble equipment.
   a. Tooth model (if using a model for teaching)
   b. Gloves (if flossing patient's teeth or if there is contact with saliva)
   c. Dental floss (waxed or unwaxed according to policy)
3. Explain importance of flossing.
4. Demonstrate correct flossing technique using model or patient.

Note: Put on protective wear if demonstrating on patient.

   a. Cut floss 18 inches (measure from finger to elbow).
   b. Wrap floss around middle or index finger of both hands, leaving 1 to 2 inches between fingers.
   c. Stretch floss between fingers and gently guide floss in between teeth. *Do not snap floss;* it can damage gingiva/gums.
   d. Pass floss through **contacts** (where teeth touch) and wrap it around tooth in a C shape.
   e. Move floss up and down several times on sides of each tooth.

Note: Make sure that floss goes beneath gingiva/gums into the sulcus.

   f. Unroll new floss from one hand and wrap used floss around middle finger of other hand.
   g. Repeat for each tooth until all teeth in maxilla and mandible are completed.
5. Explain that there may be some bleeding of the gingiva/gums the first few times the patient does this procedure.
6. Ask patient if he or she has any questions.
7. Remove protective wear.
8. Remove and clean equipment.
9. Wash hands.
10. Chart DFI (dental flossing instruction).

---

contacts Place where surface of teeth touch.

resorption Loss of substance or bone.

■ DENTAL RADIOGRAPHS

Dental assistants must have special training before they can take radiographs of the mouth. (Call your state dental board or association for information.) As an entry-level dental assistant, you may mount dental radiographs after they are developed. To mount radiographs correctly, you need some basic information.

Dental radiographs are photographs of the teeth. The radiographs allow the dentist to see between the teeth, the pulp of each tooth, and the bone (for example, caries, metallic restorations, poorly fitted crowns, root end infection, **resorption** of alveolar bone). Radiographs allow the dentist to identify problems and make repairs before the problems cause further damage.

Radiography Terminology

■ *Radiopaque* structures do not allow radiation to pass through. Enamel, metallic restorations, and dentin are radiopaque. They are very white on the film.

■ *Radiolucent* structures allow rays to penetrate through them. Pulp and caries are radiolucent. They are dark areas on the film.

■ *Periapical* films (PA) show two or three teeth and their surrounding bone structure (see Figure 24–23).

■ *Bite wings* (BWX) show the crowns of the maxillary and mandibular teeth. These are often called the cavity detector films (see Figure 24–24).

■ *Occlusal* (OCC) is a large film that shows the whole arch from the occlusal view (see Figure 24–25).

■ *Panographic* (PANX) is a long film taken from outside the mouth (extra oral) by a special machine. It shows all structures and teeth (see Figure 24–26).

The radiographs serve as a guide that helps determine the treatment plan. After the radiograph is taken, it must be developed and mounted. Mounting film may be one of your duties.

(a) Anterior

(b) Posterior

FIGURE 24–23.
Periapical views.

(a)   (b)

FIGURE 24–24.
Bite wings.

FIGURE 24–25.
Occlusal view.

FIGURE 24–26.
Panoramic survey.

Types of Mounts

Mounts come in different sizes. They may have 1, 2, 4, 7, 14, 16, 18, 20, and 28 windows. Bite-wing mounts have 2 or 4 windows. Common periapical mounts have 16 or 18 windows. When mounting films, you must remember the following:

- Periapical films show the crown and roots.
- Maxillary molars have three roots.
- Maxillary cuspids are the longest teeth in the mouth.
- Maxillary lateral incisors are larger than mandibular lateral incisors.
- Maxillary central incisors are larger than mandibular central incisors.
- Mandibular molars have two roots.
- Mandibular lateral incisors are wider than mandibular central incisors.
- The center of the mount is the median line.
- If the distal portion is on the right margin, it is the left-hand side of the dental arch.
- If the distal portion is on the left margin, it is the right-hand side of the dental arch.
- Dental film has a raised dot on a corner of the film.
- Place all films with the dot facing upward, which is a convex view.

convex Raised.

- **Convex** is a facial surface view.
- Concave is a lingual surface view.
- A full-mouth series usually includes 14 periapical films plus two or four bite wings.

Procedure

Mounting Dental Films

1. Wash hands.
2. Assemble equipment.
   a. Developed x-rays
   b. X-ray mounts
   c. View box
3. Turn on view box.
4. Lay out x-rays. (Make certain that raised dot is facing upward.)
5. Arrange film on view box before placing into mount.
6. Mount the two or four bite-wing films.

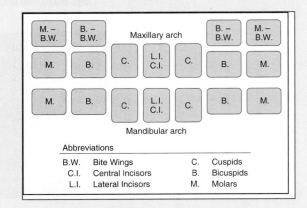

Procedure box continued

Note: Bicuspid views are closest to the center of the mount.

7. Mount two central (CI) and lateral (LI) incisor films. Place mandibular films with roots downward and maxillary films with roots upward.

8. Mount the four cuspid (C) films. The two longest cuspids are maxillary teeth.

9. Mount the four bicuspid (BC) films.

10. Mount the four molars (M) films. The molars with three roots are the maxillary molars.

11. Review the anatomical charts to check mount for accuracy.

12. Turn off view box.

13. Clean and replace equipment.

14. Wash hands.

15. Record the following on patient chart and dental x-ray mount:

   a. Patient's name

   b. Date x-rays were taken

   c. Name of person who took x-rays

   d. Dentist's name and address

Thinking Critically: Check Your Understanding

1. **Communication** You have learned that patients may be nervous when they arrive for their dental appointment. Explain ways that you can help patients relax and feel less nervous when they arrive. Describe how to set up the environment and greet your patients so that they will feel less nervous.

2. **Medical Terminology** An eight-year-old boy fell off of his bike and knocked his top two front teeth out. Using appropriate terminology and identifiers, write a description for a dental record of the dentition on this boy.

3. **Legal and Ethical** Review earlier chapters about legal and ethical issues to help you respond to the following dilemma. A vendor who provides paper products to dental offices tells you that his products are better than his competitors, and he is really pressuring you to use his products. When you explain that you are happy with your current products, he offers you two free cases of each product he supplies if you will only sign a twelve-month contract. He also hands you a $75.00 gift certificate to an elite clothing store. What legal and ethical concerns should be addressed in this situation?

4. **Patient Education** Describe what you would tell a patient about taking an alginate impression, including why it is necessary and how long it will take. Include instructions about how the patient will be positioned in the chair, how the patient should place his or her tongue, and how the patient should breathe.

5. **Computers** Describe ways computers are used in dental care.

6. **Case Study** You are preparing the instruments and aspirating syringe for a patient who is scheduled to have two teeth, numbers 5 and 31, extracted. Using medical terminology, describe the size of the needles you will prepare for each anesthesia injection and where you will place the topical anesthesia.

Portfolio Connection

Once you attain competence as a dental assistant, ask for permission to copy an example of your charting. (Remove all patient identifiers.) Place this copy in your portfolio as evidence of your skills. Place a copy of your on-site trainer's evaluation in your portfolio.

Write a paper describing your doubts and realizations and the barriers that you were able to overcome during the dental assistant experience. For example, were you afraid that you couldn't learn to use the equipment? Describe the ways you plan to use the skills, information, and insights that you gained about people and about this job. This assignment must be in standard report format.

GLOSSARY

A

abbreviations Words that have been shortened.

abdominal thrust Forceful thrust on the abdomen, between the sternum and the navel, in an upward motion toward the head.

abnormalities Things that are not usual, that differ from the standard (e.g., congenital heart disease means that the heart is different from a normal heart).

abrasive Compound used to rub away or scrape away another substance.

abreast Side by side.

abscesses Pockets of pus in a limited area.

absorption Passage of a substance through a body surface into body fluids and tissues (e.g., nutrients from digested food pass through the wall of the small intestine into the blood).

accessible Available to obtain.

accessory Helping.

accurate Exact, correct, or precise.

acids Substances that cause the urine to have an acid pH.

acquired Refers to a condition, disease, or characteristic that began after birth.

ADA American Dental Association.

adapt To change, to become suitable, to adjust.

adaptation Changing to work better.

adequate Enough, sufficient.

administrative Pertaining to processing, such as handling of paperwork, that assists in patient care and supports the physician.

admit To let someone in, take in.

adolescent Pertaining to the period of life between childhood and maturity.

aerobic Requiring oxygen.

agglutination Clumping together (e.g., red blood cells clump together).

aggressiveness Tendency to start fights and quarrels or to attack without reason.

airborne Particles that float in the air.

ala Outer side of the nostril.

alginate Material for making impressions.

alignment Keeping a resident in proper position.

alimentary canal Long muscular tube beginning at the mouth and ending at the anus.

alveolar-capillary Pertaining to air sacs in the lungs.

ambulation Walking.

amniotic fluid Liquid that surrounds the fetus during pregnancy.

amplify To increase or elevate a sound (e.g., the ossicles of the ear amplify sound waves).

amputation Removal of a body part.

anaerobic Able to grow and function without oxygen.

anesthesia Loss of feeling or sensation.

annoyance Irritation (e.g., to feel irritated with a co-worker or patient).

anorexia nervosa Loss of appetite with serious weight loss; considered a mental disorder.

antagonist Something that works against.

anterior Located in the front; opposite of posterior (e.g., the abdominal wall is anterior to the back).

antibiotics Substances that slow growth of or destroy microorganisms.

antibodies Substances made by the body to produce immunity to an antigen.

antigen Foreign matter that causes the body to produce antibodies.

antiseptic Substance that slows or stops the growth of microorganisms.

antitoxin Substance that provides immunity to a toxin.

anus Outlet from which the body expels solid waste.

anxiety Upset or distress felt over a real or imagined problem.

apex Pointed end of something (e.g., the pointed end of the heart is called the apex of the heart).

apical foramen Opening in the apex.

apparatus Equipment needed to perform a task (e.g., blood pressure apparatus includes a blood pressure cuff and a stethoscope).

appendicular Pertaining to any body part added to the axis (e.g., arms and legs are attached to the axis of the body).

appropriate Suitable, correct.

arteriosclerosis Condition of hardening of the arteries.

artifacts Unwanted marks on an electrocardiogram.

asepsis Sterile condition, free from all germs.

aseptic technique Methods used to make the environment, the worker, and the patient as germ-free as possible.

aspirate Remove substances.

aspiration Withdrawal of a fluid.

assure To guarantee; to promise positively.

asymptomatic Without visible symptoms.

atherosclerosis Condition of hardening of the arteries due to fat deposits that narrow the space blood flows through.

auditing Formal checking for correctness.

augmented Increased (e.g., augmented voltage leads show an increase in graph size).

auscultation Listening for sounds within the body.

autoclaves Sterilizers that use steam under pressure to kill all forms of bacteria on fomites (objects that pathogens live on and can transfer infection).

automated Method of lab testing that uses equipment to perform a series of steps, as compared to a manual method.

autopsy Medical procedure after death to determine the cause of death.

axial Pertaining to the central structures of the body (e.g., vertebrae, skull, ribs, and sternum).

axillary Referring to the armpit.

axis A center point that can be rotated around.

B

barriers Items that prevent infectious material from contacting surface.

baseline A number, graph, or indication to use as a guideline. A measurement taken at a later time may differ from the baseline, indicating a possible cause for concern.

biases Tendencies; prejudices.

biconcave Having a depressed surface on both sides.

bingeing Eating excessively.

biocular Having two eyepieces.

biohazard Substance that has potential to transmit disease.

birth defects Defects present at birth.

blood pressure Highest and lowest pressure against the walls of blood vessels.

boundaries Legal limits (e.g., you may know how to perform a task, but you may not do it because you are limited by your license, certification, registration, or rules and regulations).

bounding Leaping, strong, or forceful (e.g., a very strong pulse is a bounding pulse).

brittle Fragile, easy to break.

C

calcify To harden by forming calcium deposits.

calculate Figure out.

calculated Figured out.

calibration Standard measure (e.g., each line on a thermometer or a ruler is a calibration).

calories Units of measurement of the fuel value of food.

capitation Payment to provide care for a set number of people.

carbon dioxide A gas, heavier than air; a waste product from the body.

cardiopulmonary Having to do with the heart and lungs.

caries Decay.

cartilage Tough connective tissue; forms pads at end of bones, is found in the nasal septum and external ear, and forms the major portion of the embryonic skeleton.

catheters Tubes inserted into body opening or cavity.

cell Smallest structural unit in the body that is capable of independent functioning.

cell membrane Thin, soft layer of tissue that surrounds the cell and holds it together.

Celsius Measure of heat; in medicine, a Celsius thermometer is sometimes used to measure body heat. Also called centigrade.

cementum Hard, thin covering or shell covering root of tooth.

cerebrospinal fluid Liquid that flows through and around brain tissue.

cerebrovascular accidents (CVA) Complete or partial loss of blood flow to brain tissue caused by blood vessel spasms, intracranial bleeding, and/or obstruction of the blood vessels in the brain.

cervix Neck (e.g., the cervix of the uterus is the neck of the uterus).

characterized Distinguished by; refers to a trait or quality.

chronic Continuing over many years or for a long time (e.g., chronic illness).

chyme Creamy semifluid mixture of food and digestive juices.

cilia Hairlike projections that move rhythmically.

circulation Continuous one-way movement of blood through the heart and blood vessels to all parts of the body.

clammy Moist, cold skin.

classify To put like items together.

clumped Stuck together.

colitis Inflammation of the colon.

coma Deep sleep; unconscious state for a long period of time.

communicable Capable of passing directly or indirectly from one person or thing to another.

communication Act of exchanging information.

competent Capable or able to perform a skill or task.

complex Having two or more related parts.

comply To follow directions, do what you are asked to do.

components Parts or elements of a whole, an ingredient.

composed Formed by putting many parts together.

compromising Giving up something important.

concave Curved inward, depressed; dented.

concentrated Increased strength, strong solution.

conception Occurs when the male sperm fertilizes the female ovum and a new organism begins to develop.

concisely In a brief manner; to express in a few words.

confidential Private, personal, restricted, secret.

connective tissue Tissue specialized to bind together and support other tissues.

consecutive Following one after the other.

conserve Save (e.g., when you shorten a word to save space).

consistency Thickness.

constipation Infrequent or difficult emptying of the bowel.

contacts Place where surface of teeth touch.

contaminated Soiled, unclean, not suitable for use.

contingency Event that may occur but is not intended or likely to happen.

continuum Progression from start (birth) to finish (death).

contraceptives Items that serve to prevent pregnancy.

contract To shorten, to draw together; muscles shorten when you flex a body part.

contraction Drawing up.

contusion Condition in which the skin is bruised, swollen, and painful, but is not broken.

convents An establishment of nuns.

converse Talk, have a conversation.

convex Raised.

convey To say, tell, or express.

coordination State of harmonized action, such as eye and hand coordination.

coping Handling difficult situations.

corporal Bodily. For example, corporal punishment involves hitting or harming the body.

courteous Polite; considerate toward others.

crouch To stoop, using the large muscles of the legs to help maintain balance.

cusps Pointed or rounded raised areas on the surface of the tooth.

custodial Marked by watching and protecting rather than seeking to cure.

cycle Repeating steps (e.g., a wash cycle).

cylinder Long, narrow, circular container.

cystitis Inflammation of the urinary bladder.

cytoplasm All of the substance of a cell other than the nucleus.

D

debilitating Causing weakness or impairment.

decade Period of 10 years.

decay Breaking down; rot.

deciduous Falling out (e.g., primary teeth fall out to make room for permanent teeth).

decimal A number containing a decimal point.

decompose To decay; to break down.

decontamination Removal of unclean matter and living organisms.

defamatory Statement that causes injury to another's reputation.

defecation The pushing of solid material from the bowel.

deficiency Shortage (e.g., a deficient diet causes the body to function poorly because it is missing an important element).

deficient Lacking something (e.g., a deficient diet causes the body to function poorly because it is missing an important element).

definitive Clear, without question, exacting (e.g., when giving emergency care, each treatment should be done in a definitive manner).

dehydration Severe loss of fluid from tissue and cells.

delegates Gives another person responsibility for doing specific tasks.

delinquent Late.

dentition Natural teeth in the dental arch.

dentures False teeth.

designate To appoint or determine.

deteriorates Breaks down.

dexterity Skill in using one's hands.

diabetes mellitus Condition that develops when the body cannot change sugar into energy; there is an insufficient amount of insulin, leading to an increased amount of sugar in the blood.

diagnosis Identification of a disease or condition.

diagnostic Pertaining to the determination of the nature of a disease or injury by examining (e.g., using x-ray and laboratory tests).

dialysis Process of removing waste from body fluids.

diarrhea Passage of watery stool at frequent intervals.

diastolic pressure Lowest pressure against the blood vessels of the body. It is measured between contractions.

digestion Process of breaking down food mechanically and chemically.

diluent Liquid added to powder that dissolves the powder.

disbursement Payment.

discretion Caution about what one says and does.

disinfection Process of freeing from microorganisms by physical or chemical means.

dismantles Takes apart.

disorientation State of being confused about time, place, and identity of persons and objects.

disoriented Being confused about time, place, and identity of persons and objects.

disposition Act of disposing of (e.g., a person desires that his or her monies be given to an organization after his or her death).

dissection Act or process of dividing, taking apart.

distal Farthest from the point of attachment.

distribute To deliver.

diuretics Drugs that increase urine output.

diverticulitis Inflammation of the small sacs in the wall of the colon.

document Written record.

do not resuscitate Do not perform cardiopulmonary resuscitation (CPR).

dressings Gauze pads that are used to cover a wound.

droplet A small drop of fluid.

duct Narrow, round tube that carries secretions from a gland.

dysfunction Impaired or abnormal functioning.

E

edema Swelling; abnormal or excessive collection of fluid in the tissues. Usually, the swelling is in the hands, ankles, legs, or abdomen.

efficiency Ability to accomplish a job with the least possible difficulty.

EKG/ECG Graphic record of the electrical currents produced by the heart.

elastic Easily stretched.

electrocardiograph Instrument that records electric currents produced by the heart.

elimination Process of getting rid of.

embryo Living human being during the first eight weeks of development in the uterus.

embryonic Pertaining to the embryo.

emesis Vomit.

encephalitis Inflammation of the brain.

endometrium Interlining of the uterus.

endowments Gifts of property or money given to a group or organization.

enemas Solution introduced into the rectum.

enterotoxin Poisonous substance that is produced in, or originates in, the contents of the intestine.

environment Surroundings we live in. Environmental disease can occur in any area around us (e.g., hospital, restaurants, public places, home, school).

environmental sanitation Methods used to keep the environment clean and to promote health.

enzyme Substance that causes a change to occur in other substances.

epidemic Disease that spreads rapidly among people.

epidermis Outer layer of skin.

epigastric Pertaining to the area over the pit of the stomach.

epilepsy Chronic disease of the nervous system.

episodes Events in a series.

epithelial Pertaining to covering of the internal and external organs of the body.

equilibrium State of balance.

equipment Instruments, machines, or items used to perform a task.

era Period of time.

ergonomic Related to the study of the work environment.

erupt Push through.

essential Necessary (e.g., certain food elements are necessary for the body's functions).

estrogen Female hormone.

ethics Social values, conduct, description of what is right and wrong.

ethylene oxide Gas that kills living microorganisms.

evacuated Emptied out.

evacuation Removal.

excreted Thrown off or eliminated as waste material.

excretion Process of eliminating waste material.

exorcise To force out evil spirits.

expiration/exhalation Process of forcing air out of the body during respiration.

exploitation To use another person for profit or enjoyment.

exposed Left unprotected.

extemporaneous Completed with little preparation.

extract Identify and take out or emphasize.

extremities Arms, legs, hands, and feet.

F

facilities Places designed or built to serve a special function (e.g., hospital, clinic, doctor's office).

Fahrenheit Measure of heat; in medicine a Fahrenheit thermometer is often used to measure body heat.

familiar Known.

faulty Defective or imperfect.

feces Solid waste that is evacuated from the body through the anus.

feedback Information received as a result of something done or said.

fetus Infant developing in the uterus after the first three months until birth.

FICA Federal Insurance Contribution Act.

fixation Repair or fix.

flexibility Ability to bend easily.

flexible Able to bend easily.

flushed Showing reddening of the skin.

formula Accepted rule (e.g., a math formula and a baby formula are both guidelines or rules).

foster To develop; to promote; to stimulate.

fracture Broken bone.

frayed Worn away or tattered (e.g., electrical cords may be worn, causing wires to be exposed).

friction Disagreement because of a difference of opinion.

frustration Deep, chronic sense of insecurity.

functional stress Stress to tooth caused by its normal function (e.g., force of pressure when biting something hard).

functions Action or work of tissues, organs, or body parts (e.g., the heart's function is to pump blood).

G

gamma globulin Substance that acts as an antibody to increase immunity.

ganglia Mass of nerve tissue composed of nerve cell bodies. Ganglia lie outside the brain and spinal cord.

gastrointestinal Pertaining to the stomach and intestine.

gauge Standard scale for measurement.

generalized Affecting all of the body.

generic Major group (e.g., heart disease or skin disease).

geriatric Pertaining to old age.

germicidals Solutions that kill most bacteria.

gestures Motions of a part of the body to express feelings or emotions (e.g., nodding the head yes or no).

gravity Natural force or pull toward the earth. In the body, the center of gravity is usually the center of the body.

Greenwich time Standard time, a 12-hour clock.

gross pay Money earned before deductions are removed.

H

hazardous Dangerous.

heart block Interference with the conduction of the electrical impulses of the heart that is either partial or complete.

HEDIS Health Plan Employer Data and Information System; an organization that provides quality care guidelines.

Heimlich maneuver Forceful upward thrust on the abdomen, between the sternum and the navel.

hematoma Collection of blood beneath the skin.

hemoglobin Complex chemical in the blood; carries oxygen and carbon dioxide.

hemorrhage Large amount of bleeding.

heparinized Containing heparin, an anticoagulant.

hereditary Passed from parent to child.

heredity Characteristics passed from parent to child.

holistic Pertaining to the whole; considering all factors.

homeostasis Constant balance within the body. This balance is maintained by the heartbeat, blood-making mechanisms, electrolytes, and hormone secretions.

hormones Protein substances secreted by an endocrine gland directly into the blood.

horseplay Rowdy behavior; acting inappropriately in a work environment.

host The organism from which a microorganism takes nourishment. The microorganism gives nothing in return and causes disease or illness.

hostility Unfriendliness; ill will toward another.

humidity Wetness, or moisture.

hydrotherapy Treatment that uses water therapy for disease or injury.

hypertension High blood pressure.

hypotension Low blood pressure.

I

idolizing Loving to excess.

ileitis Inflammation of the ileum (the lower three-fifths of the small intestine).

immunizations Substances given to make disease organisms harmless to the patient; may be given orally or by injection (e.g., tetanus, polio).

impaction Any tooth that does not erupt when it should (e.g., tooth blocked by bone and/or tissue, keeping it under the surface of the gum). Also, being tightly wedged into a part (e.g., fecal material wedged into the bowel that requires mechanical means to remove).

impaired Weakened; deteriorated; not functioning in the usual manner.

impatience Unwillingness to tolerate.

impending About to happen.

implement To accomplish; make it work.

impulses Measures of electrical activity to the heart tissue recorded on a graph.

incontinent Unable to control the bowel or bladder.

inferior Lower (e.g., one product is inferior in quality to another product).

infirmity Unsound or unhealthy state of being.

inflated To swell or fill up with air.

infuses Flows into the body by gravity (e.g., IV drips through a tube into the body).

ingestion By mouth.

initial First.

injectable Medication given by needle.

inoculation Instill, to put into the body.

inspiration/inhalation Process of breathing in air during respiration.

instruments Tools and measuring devices.

insulin Hormone secreted by the pancreas; essential for maintaining the correct blood sugar level.

insulin shock Condition caused by too much insulin.

interact To work together; to have an impact on each other.

interdisciplinary Involving two or more disciplines.

interproximal surfaces Sides between teeth.

interstitial Space between tissues.

interstitial fluid Liquid that fills the space between most of the cells of the body.

intoxication State of poisoning or becoming poisoned.

intracranial Inside the skull.

intraoral Within the oral cavity.

intravenously Directly into a vein.

invasive Entering the body.

involuntary Not under control (e.g., muscle twitching).

irregularities Different than normal.

irreversible Cannot be changed; condition will remain the same.

isolated Limited in contact with others.

IV poles Poles that raise and lower. IV solutions are hung on these poles.

K

kick buckets Metal buckets on wheels that can be kicked out of the way.

L

labeling Describing a person with a word that limits them (e.g., lazy, stupid).

laceration Wound or a tear of the skin.

lacrimal Pertaining to tears.

lactation Body's process of producing milk to feed newborns.

lateral Relating to the sides or side of.

laxative Liquid or pill that causes evacuation of the bowel.

legal record Record that can be used in a law suit (e.g., the patient chart).

legible Capable of being read easily.

licensing Giving an agency or person permission to carry on certain activities and telling what they may not do as well as what they are authorized to do.

limb Arm, leg.

lipid Fat.

listlessness A state of being without energy.

localized Affecting one area of the body.

lumen Opening (e.g., opening in a tube or needle).

lymphocytes Type of white cell.

M

magnify Enlarge.

maintain Keep up.

malaise Weakness or discomfort.

malfunctioning Not working as it is supposed to.

malignant Cancerous.

mandates Commands, orders.

manual Book with guidelines.

masticate Chew.

maternal Relating to the mother or from the mother.

matures Becomes fully developed.

Mayo stands Adjustable, wheeled, small metal stands that hold equipment and supplies for many procedures.

mechanism Process or a series of steps that achieve a result.

meningitis Inflammation of the membrane covering the brain.

menstruation Cyclic deterioration of the endometrium.

metabolic Pertaining to the total of all the physical and chemical changes that take place in living organisms and cells.

metabolism The body's process of using food to make energy and use nutrients.

microns Units equaling one millionth of a meter.

microorganisms Organisms so small that they can only be seen through a microscope.

microscopic Too small to be seen by the eye but large enough to be seen through a microscope.

millimeters Measure of length.

minerals Inorganic elements that occur in nature; essential to every cell.

minute Exceptionally small.

misrepresentations Untruths; lies.

monasteries Homes for men following religious standards.

monocular Having one eyepiece.

monocytes Large single-nucleus white cell.

mucosa Thin lining on the inside of the intestines.

N

neglect To ignore or not provide for.

nephron Functional part of the kidney that filters liquid waste.

net pay Money earned after deductions are removed.

neurological Pertaining to the nervous system.

neuron Nerve; includes the cell and the long fiber coming from the cell.

nondominant hand Hand that is not used for writing or other tasks.

noninvasive Not involving penetration of the skin.

nonpathogenic Not causing disease.

nosocomial Infection acquired while in a health care setting, such as a hospital.

nucleus The part of a cell that is vital for its growth, metabolism, reproduction, and transmitted characteristics.

nutrients Food.

O

obesity Extreme fatness; abnormal amount of fat on the body.

obligation Moral responsibility (e.g., to give the best possible patient/client care, to be on time for work).

observant Quick to see and understand.

observation Act of watching.

obsolete Out of date.

obstruction Blockage or clogging.

occult Hidden, unseen.

omission Neglect of duty.

opportunistic infections Infections that occur when the immune system is weakened. Common organisms that the body normally resists cause infection.

oral Referring to the mouth.

osseous Bonelike.

ossicles Three small bones in the middle ear: incus, stapes, and malleus.

outpatients Patients/clients who do not require hospitalization but are under a physician's care.

overexposure Too much contact with radiation.

ovum Female reproductive cell that when fertilized by the male develops into a new organism.

oxidation The mixing together of oxygen and another element.

oxygen Element in the atmosphere that is essential for maintaining life.

oxygenated Contain oxygen.

P

palpation Examine by feeling for unusual or abnormal conditions.

parallel Same direction and a distance, so that two points do not touch.

paralysis Loss of sensation and muscle function.

parasites Organisms obtaining nourishment from other organisms they are living in or on.

parasitic Pertaining to an organism that lives in or on another organism, taking nourishment from it.

parenteral Not in the digestive system (e.g., injections are parenterally administered).

pathogenic Disease causing.

Patient's/Client's Bill of Rights Document written by the American Hospital Association outlining expected patient/client rights while in a hospital.

penetrates Enters or passes through (e.g., a fractured bone passes through the skin).

periapical Around the apex (e.g., of the tooth).

pericardial fluid Liquid that surrounds the heart.

perineal Region between the vulva and anus in a female, or between the scrotum and anus in a male.

periodic Occurring at regular intervals.

peripheral Situated away from a central structure.

peristalsis Progressive, wavelike motion that occurs involuntarily in hollow tubes of the body.

peritoneal cavity Area of the body containing the liver, stomach, intestines, kidneys, urinary bladder, and reproductive organs.

peritoneal fluid Liquid in the peritoneal cavity.

personnel People who work in an establishment; a personnel office is where a worker goes to apply for a job.

phagocytes Cell that surrounds, eats, and digests microorganisms and cellular waste.

philosophy Theory; a general principle used for a specific purpose.

physiological Pertaining to normal body functions.

pigmented Colored; relating to various parts of the body (e.g., iris of the eye, lips, moles, freckles).

plaque Soft deposit of bacteria and bacterial products on teeth.

plasma Liquid part of the blood, consisting of water, nutrients, wastes, hormones, antibodies, and enzymes. Watery, colorless fluid containing leukocytes, erythrocytes, and platelets.

pleural fluid Liquid that surrounds the lungs.

pneumonia Inflammation of the lungs.

pollutants Things that contaminate the air (e.g., smoke, smog).

polycythemia Condition of having too much blood.

polyps Small tumorlike growths.

porous Filled with tiny holes.

posterior Behind, to the rear, toward the back (e.g., the heel is posterior to the toes).

postmortem After death.

postural supports Soft restraints used to protect resident.

potential Possible.

pouch Small bag or sac.

predators Organisms or beings that destroy.

prejudge To decide or make a decision before having the facts.

prejudices Judgments or opinions formed before the facts are known.

prepaid Paid ahead of time.

prestige Influence obtained through success, wealth, or some other source.

preventable Able to be kept from happening.

primarily For the most part; chiefly.

primary First.

priorities Those things that are most important.

prioritize To put in order of importance.

procedures Methods used to accomplish a desired result.

progressive Moving forward, following steps toward an end product.

prohibit To not allow.

project To show or reflect.

prone Lying on the stomach.

prosthetics Artificial parts made for the body (e.g., teeth, feet, legs, arms, hands, eyes, breasts).

proteins Complex compound found in plant and animal tissues, essential for heat, energy, and growth.

protrusion Pushing through.

provider Physician, physician assistant, nurse practitioner.

proximal Nearest or next to.

prudent Careful or cautious.

psychiatric Pertaining to the mind.

psychological Pertaining to the mind.

psychotherapy Method of treatment using mental applications, such as hypnotherapy.

purging Causing oneself to vomit.

Q

quackery Practice of pretending to cure diseases.

R

radiopaque Shows as a white material when a fluoroscope x-ray is taken.

range of motion (ROM) Moving all joints of the body, can be active or passive.

rapport Harmony; a close relationship with another.

reagents Chemical substances that react to the presence of other substances in the blood and urine.

receptors Nerves that respond to stimuli.

recipient One who receives.

recognition Acknowledgment as being worthy of approval.

reconstituting Adding water to a powdered drug.

rectal Referring to the far end of the large intestine just above the anus.

refer To send to.

reflexes Result when a nerve is stimulated and an involuntary action occurs (e.g., touch a hot stove, and the muscles react involuntarily to move the fingers away).

regulate To control or adjust.

rehabilitation Process that helps people who have been disabled by sickness or injury to recover as many of their original abilities for activities of daily living as possible.

reimburse To pay back for something given or spent.

relevant Pertaining to, or having to do with, the patient/client.

rendered Given or provided.

replenish Refill or build up again.

reproduction Process that takes place in animals to create offspring.

resident Able to protect itself.

residual Left over.

resistance Ability of the body to protect itself from disease.

resorption Loss of a substance or bone.

responsibility One's answerability to an employer in areas such as dependability and honesty.

restorative To return to as close to normal conditions as possible.

restrict To keep within limits; to confine.

resultant Resulting from an action.

retention Keeping elements within the body that are normally eliminated (e.g., waste products such as urine and feces).

rheostat Control for flow of electric current.

rickettsiae Parasitic microorganisms that live on another living organism and cause disease.

rotary Move in a circular fashion.

S

sacral region The area where the sacrum is located; forms the tail end of the spinal column.

salutation A greeting (e.g., Dear Sir).

saprophytes Organisms that live on dead organic matter.

saturated Soaked; filled to capacity.

saturating Soak.

scattering Spreading in many directions, dispersing.

seating Putting firmly in place to prevent moving.

sebaceous Pertaining to fatty secretions.

secretion Producing and expelling a special substance (e.g., sebaceous glands secrete oil; salivary glands secrete saliva).

sedate Calm.

seizure Involuntary muscle contraction and relaxation.

self-esteem Belief in oneself.

semen Fluid from the testes, seminal vesicles, prostate gland, and bulbourethral glands. Contains water, mucin, proteins, salts, and sperm.

sensory Pertaining to the ability to hear, see, feel, smell, and taste.

septic arthritis Bacterial inflammation of the joint caused by bloodborne bacteria carried from another place in the body.

serrated Sawlike notches.

sex cells Cells that allow reproduction to occur.

shocks Convulsion of muscles and extreme stimulation of nerves when an electric current passes through the body.

sloughed Discarded; separated from (e.g., to shed dead cells, as from the outer skin).

soluble Able to break down or dissolve in liquid.

solutions Two or more liquids mixed together.

specialties Fields of study or professional work (e.g., pediatrics, orthopedics, obstetrics).

specifications Exact way something should be done.

spermatozoa Male sex cells.

sphincter Circular muscle that allows the opening and closing of a body part (e.g., anus, pylorus).

sphygmomanometer Measuring device used to measure the pressure against the arteries of the body.

spirochetes Slender, coil-shaped organisms.

splints Firm object used to support an unstable body part.

spontaneous Occurring naturally without apparent cause.

spurts To force out in a burst; to squirt.

stability Ability to maintain a balance, both mentally and physically.

stamina Body's strength or energy.

stance The way you stand.

Standard Precautions Guidelines designed to reduce the risk of transmission of microorganisms from recognized and unrecognized sources of infection in the hospital.

sterility Absence of living organism or inability to produce offspring.

sterilized Made free from all living microorganisms.

stethoscope Instrument used to hear sound in the body (e.g., heartbeat, lung sounds, bowel sounds).

stimuli Elements in the external or internal environment that are strong enough to set up a nervous impulse.

stoma Opening, e.g., opening in abdomen in an ostomy.

structure Form in which the body is made.

subcutaneous Beneath the skin.

sufficient Enough.

sulcus Depression, groove, area where gingival tip meets tooth enamel.

superstitious Trusting in magic or chance.

supine Lying on the back.

suppository Bullet shaped mass inserted into rectum to stimulate bowel movement.

surgical Repairing or removing a body part by cutting.

susceptible Capable of being affected or infected (e.g., body can be attacked by microorganisms and become ill).

swathe Bandage.

syncope Fainting.

syndrome A number of symptoms occurring together.

systolic pressure Highest pressure against blood vessels. Represented by first heart sound or beat heard when taking a blood pressure.

T

terminal Last or ending.

terminology Specialized terms used in any occupation.

testicles Site of production of the male sex cell.

testosterone Male hormone.

therapeutic Pertaining to the treatment of disease or injury (e.g., physical therapy, radiology, diet, nursing).

therapies Methods of treatment of disease or injury (e.g., physical therapy, radiology, diet, nursing).

tissues Group of cells of the same type that act together to perform a specific function.

tomography X-ray technique that produces film of detailed cross sections of tissue.

tone Firmness or tightness.

topical Surface of the body.

toxins Poisonous substances.

TPR Stands for "temperature, pulse, respiration."

traditional Customary beliefs passed from generation to generation.

translate To make understandable.

transmitting Causing to go from one person to another person.

trauma Damage to the body caused by an injury, wound, or shock; mental trauma occurs from emotional shock.

trend General direction or movement.

tuberculosis Disease caused by Tubercle bacilli; may cause death if untreated.

24-hour time/military time Method of telling time by counting each hour consecutively for 24 hours (i.e., . . . 11, 12, 13, . . .).

U

ulcerations Open areas, or sores.

uniformity A state of being all the same; does not vary.

unoxygenated Lacking oxygen.

urethritis Inflammation of the urethra.

V

vaccine Dead or weakened organisms that stimulate the body to make antibodies.

value Importance, worth.

venipuncture Puncture of a vein.

vessels Tubes that carry fluid in the body.

viable Capable of living.

villi Tiny projections.

visibility Ability to see.

vital A must, essential.

vitality Ability of an organism to go on living.

vitamins Group of substances necessary for normal functioning and maintenance of health.

voluntary Under the control of the person (e.g., you voluntarily raise your arm; it does not rise automatically).

W

waste products Elements that are unfit for the body's use and are eliminated from the body.

Z

zygote Any cell formed by the coming together of two reproductive (sex) cells.

Index